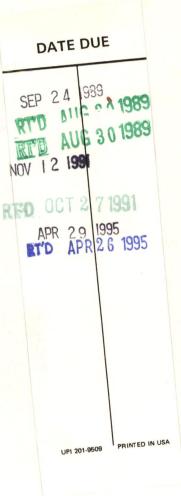

PRINCIPLES AND METHODS OF
ADAPTED PHYSICAL EDUCATION
AND RECREATION

PRINCIPLES AND METHODS OF

ADAPTED PHYSICAL EDUCATION AND RECREATION

WALTER C. CROWE, Ed.D.

Professor of Physical Education,
California State University at Long Beach,
Long Beach, California

DAVID AUXTER, Ed.D.

Professor of Developmental Physical Education,
Slippery Rock State College,
Slippery Rock, Pennsylvania

JEAN PYFER, P.E.D.

Professor of Physical Education,
University of Kansas,
Lawrence, Kansas

FOURTH EDITION

with **543** illustrations

The C. V. Mosby Company

ST. LOUIS • TORONTO • LONDON   1981

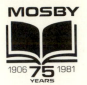

MOSBY

1906 **75** 1981
YEARS

A TRADITION OF PUBLISHING EXCELLENCE

Cover photo by James Bryant

FOURTH EDITION

The C. V. Mosby Company
11830 Westline Industrial Drive, St. Louis, Missouri 63141

Library of Congress Cataloging in Publication Data

Crowe, Walter C.
 Principles and methods of adapted physical education and recreation.

 Third ed. by D. D. Arnheim, D. Auxter, and W. C. Crowe.
 Includes bibliographies and index.
 1. Physical education for handicapped children—Collected works. 2. Physical education for handicapped persons—Collected works. 3. Handicapped children—Recreation—Collected works. 4. Handicapped—Recreation—Collected works. 5. Individualized instruction—Collected works. I. Auxter, David. II. Pyfer, Jean. III. Arnheim, Daniel D. Principles and methods of adapted physical education and recreation. IV. Title.
GV445.C74 1981   371.9′044   81-1004
ISBN 0-8016-0327-7   AACR2

C/VH/VH 9 8 7 6 5 4 3 2 1   02/C/228

To
our families

Preface

The fourth edition has been extensively revised to reflect changes required by Public Law 94-142, which defines the process by which education of the handicapped shall be conducted. This far-reaching legislation requires that school districts include in their programs Individual Education Programs and due process guarantees for handicapped persons. It is implied in this law that every teacher education agency should provide prospective teachers with experience in formulating individualized performance objectives based on assessment and in planning suitable programs that will enable handicapped persons to accomplish measurable objectives and goals. The number of individuals requiring special services for various disabling conditions is expanding at an ever-increasing rate. There is today a pressing need for programs and specialists that will aid handicapped individuals in developing their full potentials. Physical education and recreation can play an integral role in this development.

In the early 1970's the Bureau of Education of the Handicapped, part of the United States Office of Education, listed physical education and recreation as national educational priorities for the handicapped. This emphasis at the federal level has stimulated innovation in physical education programming for the handicapped. Educators are becoming more aware that each child can learn and develop at his or her own rate. Since each handicapped child is intrinsically different from other children, programming for individual handicapped persons based on their development and learning, in accord with their needs, should be emphasized.

This edition has retained descriptions of specific handicapping conditions and has included new sections on principles of normalization and the Individual Education Program. The book alerts the reader to educational processes that tend to view children as children, irrespective of their handicaps. Therefore, chapters have been updated to provide information for delivery of services for severely handicapped individuals. Materials contained within the text that are particularly applicable to the motor development of the severely handicapped are reflex maturation, conversion of perceptual prerequisites to instructional objectives, application of learning principles to instruction, and extensive normative data on preschool motor behaviors. Furthermore, chapters on handicapping conditions, relaxation, therapeutic exercise, musculoskeletal disorders, facilities, and equipment have undergone thorough revision. More than 60 new illustrations and numerous examples have been added to the book to clarify concepts presented.

This book is designed for the elementary and secondary school physical educator and the recreation specialist in adapted physical education. More specifically, it is intended as a text for colleges offering courses in adapted and corrective physical education and therapeutic recreation. The physical educator, recreational therapist, corrective therapist, school administrator, physician, school nurse, and physical therapist should all find the contents of this book pertinent to their particular fields.

Every effort has been made to show the reader both an academic and a practical approach to the field of adapted physical education. In all possible areas, theoretical material has been reinforced with information that is useful, practical, and feasible and that applies directly to the teaching situation. The basic organization of this text is designed to describe the comprehensive aspects involved in the implementation of adapted physical education programs. There are four major divisions: The Scope, Key Teaching and Therapy Skills, Programming for Specific Problems, and Organization and Administration.

Part One provides the reader with an understanding of the diverse and complex nature of the handicapped individual. In this section, we have focused attention on the principles of normalization, the psychological implications of disability, the pertinent aspects of growth and development, and the perceptual implications for both nonhandicapped and handicapped persons. A chapter on the Individual Education Program directly relates these materials to meeting the individual needs of the handicapped person in our society.

Part Two is designed to provide an in-depth discussion of therapeutic exercise, tension reduction, low vitality and physical fitness, and adapted sports and games as they relate to all types of handicapped persons. Furthermore, prerequisite abilities that relate to motor skills and contribute to efficient task analysis are identified. These prerequisites of perceptual, physical, and motor tasks are essential to the development of programmed instruction for the Individual Education Program. Both individual and group approaches are presented to aid students and teachers in preparing to readily apply these techniques and materials to their respective learning and teaching situations.

Part Three supplies the reader with specific information about the most prevalent types of disabilities found in the elementary school, high school, and college groups and discusses the implications of these disabilities for the physical education program. Every attempt has been made to give timely and intensive coverage of these conditions and to discuss procedures for assessment and program planning.

Part Four includes information about the organization and administration of a district or school program, illustrates means of organizing adapted physical education classes for instruction in a variety of situations, and provides extensive coverage of facilities and equipment used in the adapted physical education and therapeutic recreation program.

Many hours and much hard work have gone into the creation of this edition. As is true of most productions of this type and magnitude, many individuals have assisted us. Therefore appreciation is accorded to those persons who have given their suggestions and comments on the first three editions, for their ideas have been incorporated into this edition. We wish to thank Dr. Dawn Chaney, Bennett College, Greensboro, N.C., for reviewing the manuscript and for providing many helpful comments. For their excellent photographic contributions, special thanks are extended to Dr. Julian Stein, Director of Programs for the Handicapped, AAHPERD; Dr. Tom Songster, Sports Director of Special Olympics; Carolyn Williams, Slippery Rock State College Swimming Program for the Handicapped; and the Special Education Early Childhood Intervention Program of the University of Kansas, Lawrence.

Dr. Jean Pyfer, Professor of Physical Education at the University of Kansas, is a contributing author to this edition. Dr. Pyfer has been an active professional in adapted physical education for many years. She has held several positions of leadership in the profession and has a wealth of background in direct services to handicapped persons. She is the recipient of several personnel preparation grants from the U.S. Office of Education, Bureau of Education for the Handicapped. Her services are sought for consultation and in-service training of implementation procedures of P.L. 94-142. Her professional work has cut across most disciplines that serve handicapped persons. Dr. Pyfer has been active in research in the area of perceptual-motor dysfunction for the more than 10 years and has received such awards as the Outstanding Educator in America Award for Educational Leadership by the Optometric Association. She has over fifty articles and invited presentations to her credit. Indeed, Dr. Pyfer is one of the outstanding professionals in the field of adapted physical education, and she has made invaluable contributions to this fourth edition.

Walter C. Crowe
David Auxter

Contents

PRINCIPLES AND METHODS OF

ADAPTED PHYSICAL EDUCATION
AND RECREATION

PART ONE

The scope

Part One is prepared for the reader as an introduction to the diverse and complex nature of disability and, more specifically, to the role of physical education for the handicapped. We have focused the reader's attention on how the handicapped child is cared for in our society, on the psychosocial implications of the handicapped child's disability, and on pertinent aspects of growth and development that affect typical and atypical individuals. In keeping with recent federal legislation and a trend of increased importance in several states, information is included on implementation of the Individual Education Program.

1

Serving the disabled individual

I introduce . . . a bill . . . to insure equal opportunities for the handicapped by prohibiting needless discrimination. . . . The time has come when we can no longer tolerate the invisibility of the handicapped in America. . . . I am calling for public attention to . . . facilities which are functionally inadequate and designed simply to isolate these persons from society. . . . These people have the right to live, to work to the best of their ability—to know the dignity which every human being is entitled. But too often we keep children who we regard as ''different'' or a ''disturbing influence'' out of our community activities altogether. These are people who can and must be helped to help themselves. That this is their constitutional right is clearly affirmed in a number of recent court decisions.[8] Senator Hubert Humphrey, chief sponsor of the Rehabilitation Act of 1973.

Physical educators are working in an era in which assumptions about the nature of handicapped persons are changing. Changing assumptions and changing facts about the handicapped give rise to new legal policies for conducting physical education for the handicapped. Judgments from the courts that have been converted into federal statutes give rise to new responsibilities to physical education and recreation personnel who conduct programs for handicapped individuals.

In enacting Section 504 of the Rehabilitation Act of 1973 (P.L. 93-112),[25] Congress has in effect codified the constitutional right to equal protection (Fourteenth Amendment) of the United States Constitution. As Broderick noted, Section 504 was originally introduced in 1971-1972 as a bill to include the handicapped in the Civil Rights Act of 1964.[13]

Section 504 was directed at the broad aspects of discriminatory practices. To fully implement Section 504 subsequent corollary legislation—the Education of All Handicapped Children Act of 1975 (P.L. 94-142)—was enacted.[27] In this legislation physical education was the only educational curriculum specifically referenced. Thus, physical educators have unique opportunities and responsibilities for serving handicapped children.

It is the purpose of this chapter to clarify the expectations of educational practices of adapted physical educators as compared to public policy formulated in the courts and incorporated in legislative statutes at federal and state levels.

The problem that physical education teachers of the handicapped must resolve is how to conduct instruction that conforms to the practices that have been laid down by federal statutes. Thus, in a transitional phase that involves changing instructional patterns in teaching, it is not uncommon for confusion to exist as to how to conduct physical education programs for the handicapped. A question that may exist for some time is what constitutes legal and ethical practice. To partially answer this critical question we have attempted to determine the meaning of Section 504 and of P.L. 94-142.

This is a time of great transition in the professional fields that deliver assistance to the mentally, physically, and emotionally inconvenienced. In our affluent society, no longer must the less fortunate person be relegated to living outside the mainstream of life.

HISTORICAL IMPLICATIONS
Early history

In the highly developed countries of the world, the present level of concern for the well-being of the individual has evolved gradually over a period of many thousands of years. One of the characteristics of the typical early primitive cultures was their preoccupation with survival. Historians speculate that members of many early primitive societies who were unable to contribute to their own care were either put to death, allowed to succumb to a hostile environment, or forced to suffer a low social status. In some societies, persons displaying

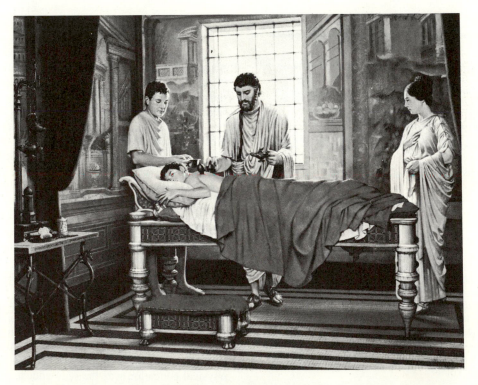

Fig. 1-1. Galen treating an ill child by cupping. (Courtesy Parke, Davis, & Co., Detroit.)

obvious behavioral deviations were considered—from a religious point of view—evil or, conversely, touched with divine powers.

These early inhabitants learned to fear the unknown and unexplained. Out of this anxious anticipation of danger or pain, they developed highly organized superstitions and religious expressions of the good and evil they saw in nature. The deviant individual, as the result, represented the unexplained and was often thought to be fraught with evil spirits.

Early sophisticated civilizations, such as China, Babylonia, and Egypt, depict in their writings the fear and superstition commonly associated with the atypical person. Even with the advent of modern science, the severely impaired or disabled were often regarded with disdain and suspicion, an attitude that is held by many persons in today's society.

The body perfection of the ancient Greeks and the rugged self-denial of the Spartans offered little, if any, place for the deformed or less endowed. Many deviant adults and children were made fools,

jesters, and entertainers by the aristocrats of that period. Greek medicine, with the aid of Hippocrates (460-370 B.C.), made some inroads into changing man's reliance on supernaturalism by introjecting the logic of scientific reasoning. However, the chain of fear and superstition was not broken for long. After Greece's fall to the Roman Empire, its culture and scientific spirit degenerated. Even the brilliance of such persons as Claudius Galen (130-200 A.D.), a noted Greek physician, surgeon, and writer, could not impede the downward spiral (Fig. 1-1).

The medieval period brought with it self-denial for reasons of piety. As a result, the maimed, infirm, and mentally disturbed were often allowed to perish from a lack of care or become the recipients of cruel and inhuman treatment. Fear continued to cloud man's thoughts and found expression in the guise of religious doctrine. Any person different in behavior or appearance was thought to be a witch or possessed by the devil. Not until the late Renaissance period were man's primitive attitudes

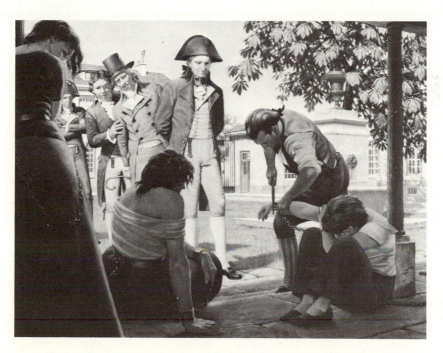

Fig. 1-2. Pinel unchains the insane. (Courtesy Parke, Davis, & Co., Detroit.)

about the handicapped to be chipped away by scientific reason.

Humanitarianism and humanism

The Middle Ages gave way to the more positive period of the Renaissance, in which human dynamism again fulminated. Great social and cultural upheavals took place. The seed of social consciousness had been planted. A genuine concern for the individual developed, giving the individual dignity. With a desire for social reform came a multitude of movements to improve man's life. Reforms dealing with peace, prison conditions, poverty, temperance, and insanity were organized and many social and moral problems were attacked in the first decade of the nineteenth century (Fig. 1-2). However, the main impetus for aiding the disabled did not occur until early in the twentieth century and as late as the early 1960's for the mentally retarded and the emotionally disturbed. The contributions of such figures as President Franklin D. Roosevelt, supporting the fight against crippling diseases such as poliomyelitis, and the Kennedy family, working to help the mentally retarded, can hardly be overlooked when discussing this country's humanitarian concerns.

Humanism is concerned with the individual's knowledge, understanding, and full, unconditional acceptance of the self, without which there cannot be acceptance by others.

Influences of war

Surges of social change often just precede or follow in the wake of great national upheaval. Such was the case with the United States just before and just after the Civil War. The national climate during the period that preceded the Civil War was gradually changing from the coldness of Puritanism to a greater warmth and a beginning acceptance of man's imperfection. A social awareness at this time indicated an interest in making the world a better place for all to live. However, social welfare institutions could not keep pace with the enigma created by the industrial revolution and the human exploitation that accompanied it. Not until public legislation, which occurred later, would many of these problems be resolved.

By the twentieth century, the public's interest in the physically handicapped had heightened to the extent that legislative action was taken to alleviate some of the financial burden on individuals. The stimuli for action were the great number of permanently injured industrial workers, the influenza pandemic, the crippling infantile paralysis of 1916, and the multitude of maimed World War I veterans who returned from fighting overseas.

World War I is marked as a period that greatly advanced medical and surgical techniques designed to help ameliorate many physically disabling conditions. In addition, individuals were restored to usefulness by vocational and workshop programs. The interim between World War I and World War II was a time in which state and federal legislation was enacted to promote vocational rehabilitation for both the civilian and the military disabled. The Smith-Sears Act of 1918 and the National Civilian Vocational Rehabilitation Act of 1920 were the forerunners of the Social Security Act of 1935 and the Vocational Rehabilitation Act of 1943, which provided the handicapped both physical and vocational rehabilitation.

With World War II came thousands of ill and incapacitated service personnel. Means were employed to restore them to function as useful and productive members of society. Physical medicine became a new medical speciality. Many of the heretofore hospital services became autonomous ancillary medical fields. The paramedical specialties of physical therapy, occupational therapy, and corrective therapy considerably decreased the recovery time of many patients.

The present and future

How many handicapped persons currently reside in the United States? Until the 1970 census, this was a difficult question to answer. Reports indicate that there are over 11 million persons between the ages of 16 and 64 years who are not in institutions and are disabled and unable to work for 6 months or longer. In other words, 1 out of 11 Americans or 9% of its working force of 121 million were disabled by some chronically disabling condition. In general, the 1970 census revealed that those individuals who were handicapped and not in the mainstream of life earned less income had less education, were employed less often, and represented more poverty than their working counterparts.[1,20] In contrast to the proportion of handicapped persons of working age, there are estimated to be over 7.5 million handicapped children in America, representing 12% of the school-aged population.

Many disabling conditions are becoming extinct, whereas others are coming to the forefront. Poliomyelitis is almost a disease of the past and the destructive effects of German measles are being controlled, but as society imposes new and different demands on humans other conditions emerge and become important. In recent years, more public and professional attention is being paid to mentally retarded, learning disabled, and multiply handicapped persons.

The court decisions and subsequent legislation of the early 1970's provide guidelines for mainstreaming handicapped children. Mainstreaming enables handicapped children to receive their education with their peers in regular classes. Such placement in an educational setting enables handicapped children to prepare for more normalized living.

Gilhool and Stutman point out that to determine the meaning of a legislative statute the starting point is "the plain language of the statute itself."[11] In addition, one must look to the historical context of the statute, previous related legislation, the overall legislative scheme, the evil the statute was designed to remedy, the spirit of the legislation, and its legislative history.

LEGISLATION
History

A quarter of a century ago, in the case of *Brown vs. the Board of Education*,[7] the Supreme Court expressed a theme that has recurred in P.L. 94-142, that of integration as a constitutional presumption of equal protection as applied to the segregation of children. The case addressed segregation by race. Subsequent court decisions addressed segregation on the basis of handicapping conditions. In the Brown case, which is not unrelated to the segregation of children because of handicap, the same parallel can be made for placement in the least restrictive environment.

In 1954, the Supreme Court, established the principle that all children must be guaranteed equal educational opportunity. The court presented the following statement:

[Education] is required in the performance of our most basic responsibilities. . . . It is the very foundation of good citizenship. Today it is a principal in preparing him for later . . . training, and in helping him adjust normally to his environment. In these days, it is doubtful that any child may reasonably be expected to succeed in life if he is denied the opportunity of an education. Such an opportunity, where the state has undertaken to provide it, is a right which must be made available *to all on equal terms*.[7] (Italics added.)

In drafting P.L. 94-142 a similar relationship was observed between the effects of segregation by handicapping conditions and the effects of segregation by race. Therefore, Congress articulated a familiar theme from the Brown case, namely, that segregation is inherently unequal because it does not provide the segregated children with culturally relevant social learning experiences. In plain language, the Congress has required states to employ "procedures to assure that to the maximum extent appropriate handicapped children . . . are educated with children who are not handicapped. . . ."[27]

Integration of the handicapped

Although it is well recognized from a legal point of view that handicapped children are to be educated with nonhandicapped children (mainstreaming), there is confusion as to whether this is a trend that will continue. The educational measures that were promoted by the U.S. Office of Education in the 1960's and 1970's encouraged innovative ways to accommodate individual differences. These programs enriched educational programming for culturally disadvantaged, minority, and handicapped children. A wide array of different programs and strategies were introduced, which lead educators to believe that innovations were far from permanent.

Testimony from social scientists in the Brown case indicated that segregation of children deprived both groups of culturally relevant social learning experiences. Using this theme, Senator Stafford, the ranking minority member of the subcommittee for the handicapped, again expressed the educational values of integrating handicapped children

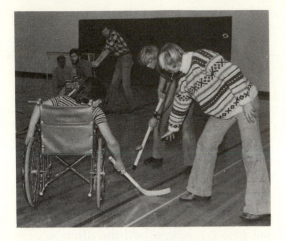

Fig. 1-3. Handicapped and nonhandicapped persons participating in a game of floor hockey. (Courtesy of Julian Stein, American Alliance for Health, Physical Education, Recreation, and Dance, and Courage Center, Minneapolis, Minn.)

with their nonhandicapped peers. Senator Stafford made the following points:

For far too long handicapped children have been denied access to the regular school system because of an inability to climb the steps to the schoolhouse door, and not for any other reason. This has led to segregated classes for those children with physical handicaps. This is an isolation that is in many cases unnecessary. It is an isolation for the handicapped child and for the "normal" child as well. The sooner we are able to bring the two together, the more likely that the attitudes of each toward one another will change for the better.

I firmly believe that if we are to teach all of our children to love and understand each other, we must give them every opportunity to see what "different" children are like.

If we allow and, indeed, encourage handicapped children and nonhandicapped children to be educated together as early as possible, their attitudes toward each other in later life will not be such obstacles to overcome. A child who goes to school every day with another child who is confined to a wheelchair will understand far better in later life the limitations and abilities of such an individual when he or she is asked to work with, or is in a position to hire, such an individual.[24a]

The subject of integration of handicapped children is a critical portion of P.L. 94-142 because integration prepares handicapped children and non-

handicapped children for life in a world that includes handicapped people. It is not consistent with the Congress's intentions to maintain segregated, handicapped-only special education centers or schooling in such institutions.

Consider the following statement of Gilhool and Stutman: "Under the statutes any degree of segregation can be maintained only if it is necessary to the appropriate education of a child. There is no cognizable reason under the statutes—that is, no learning reason and no disability reason—for handicapped-only centers, certainly not on the scale they now exist."[11] There are few if any legitimate teaching strategies that require the complete isolation of a child from interaction with other children, and the few such strategies that do exist apply to a very limited number of children for very short periods.

Brown et al.[6] address the learning reasons for schooling severely handicapped children with nonhandicapped children. For the most part, these reasons are similar to those of Congress for enacting the integration concept. Brown et al. maintain the following position:

Long-term, heterogeneous interactions between severely handicapped and nonhandicapped students facilitate the development of the skills, attitudes, and values that will prepare both groups to be sharing, participating, contributing members of complex, postschool communities. Stated another way, separate education is not equal education.

Segregated service delivery models have at least the following disadvantages:
1. Exposure to nonhandicapped student models is absent or minimal;
2. Severely handicapped students tend to learn "handicapped" skills, attitudes, and values;
3. Teachers tend to strive for the resolution of handicapping problems at the expense of developing functional community referenced skills;
4. Most comparisons between students are made in relation to degrees of handicap rather than to criteria of nonhandicapped performance;
5. Lack of exposure to severely handicapped students limits the probability that the skills, attitudes, and values of nonhandicapped students will become more constructive, tolerant, and appropriate.

Certainly, it is possible that interaction may not take place even if severely handicapped students are in the physical presence of nonhandicapped students. However, unless severely handicapped and nonhandicapped students occupy the same physical space, interaction is impossible. . . . In the future, severely handicapped students, upon the completion of formal schooling, will live in public, minimally segregated, heterogeneous communities, where they will constantly interact with nonhandicapped citizens. Thus, the educational experience should be representative and help prepare both severely handicapped students and nonhandicapped students to function adaptively in integrated communities.[6]

Discrepancy between what exists and what should be

Although it is explicitly stated in the legislative statutes that handicapped children should be placed in the least restrictive environment, Brown et al. point out that "While there may appear to be a continuum of service delivery options available, the predominant models currently in use are self-contained schools on the grounds of residential facilities, and self-contained private and public schools."[6]

The Congress has required that inequitable practices be changed, and the courts have made it clear that the integration of handicapped children into the schools and handicapped adults into the mainstream of society must be effected. The case of *Hairston vs. Drosick,* presented to a West Virginia federal district court, illustrated the application of Section 504's integration principle to education.[12] In this case the parents of a spina bifida child who was offered homebound instruction, a special education class, or a regular class if her mother would come to the school two or three times per day to attend to the child sued for admission to the regular class without conditions. Their claim was based upon Section 504. The court conducted an extensive investigation and concluded the following:

There are a great number of other spina bifida children throughout the State of West Virginia who are attending public schools in the regular classroom situation, the great majority of which have more severe disabilities than the plaintiff child Trina Hairston including children having body braces, shunts, Cunningham clips and ostomies, and requiring the use of walkers and confinement to wheelchairs. The needless exclusion of these children and other children who are able to function adequately from the regular classroom situation would be a great disservice to these children. . . . A major goal of the educational process is the socialization process that takes place in the regular classroom, with the result-

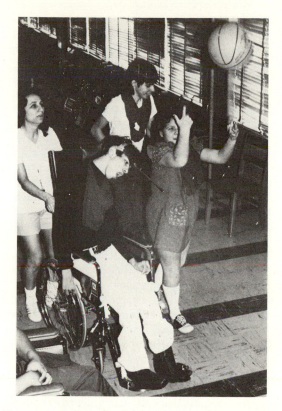

Fig. 1-4. Severely handicapped persons can take their physical education in the public schools. (Courtesy of Julian Stein, American Alliance for Health, Physical Education, Recreation, and Dance, and Omaha Public Schools, Omaha, Neb.)

ing capability to interact in a social way with one's peers. It is therefore imperative that every child receive an education with his or her peers insofar as it is at all possible. This conclusion is further enforced by the critical importance of education in this society.[12]

Normalization

The discussion to this point has dealt with legislation for the integration of handicapped persons in the mainstream of school and society. There has been little discussion of the qualitative human relationships that are to exist between handicapped and nonhandicapped persons. Indeed, there are many who might believe that all that is needed to provide optimal educational benefit to all children is exposure to one another. The outcome of such placement assumes positive values for both groups as a result of the transfer of values and characteristics. The acceptance of handicapped children into society after years of social stereotyping and stigmatization, which deny these citizens value and respect, presents critical problems for effectively implementing federal mandates in handicapped physical education. We believe that one must deal with the complex concept of *normalization*[28]—a different concept but one not unrelated to that of mainstreaming. It is desirable that normalization principles be accepted by society at large and particularly by professionals who deliver services to the handicapped. Thus, subsequent discussion will focus on the principles of normalization as they relate to handicapped persons.

A component of the stereotyping and prejudice that historically attends disabled persons is the view that disabled people cannot function productively. In P.L. 94-142, Congress determined that ''developments in the training of teachers and in diagnostic and instructional procedures and methods have advanced to the point that, given appropriate funding, state and local agencies can and will provide effective special education to meet the needs of handicapped children.''[27] It is clear that Congress found that all handicapped children, however severely handicapped, can learn to some degree to function in society.

The concept adopted by the Congress requires that the handicapped be provided with educational methods and procedures that prevent stigmatization, with opportunities to take full advantage of their cultures, with access to the same privileges and institutions that foster valued roles and lives, and with the highest technical competence, equipment, and processes to attain as normal lives as possible. In short, the Congress has adopted the principles of normalization.

Ideology must be recognized as an important determining factor for developing normalized status for the handicapped. Other factors with which the present-day physical education teacher must cope are the discrepancy between the requirements of federal mandates and expectancies of parents and society at large and the current technical capabilities of personnel to implement individualized programs for handicapped children in the least restrictive environment in the most normalized fashion.

Despite the clear intention of the legislature pertaining to integration, there are at least two crucial problems in providing entitled benefits to handicapped citizens that are in accord with the principles of normalization. First, the instructional technology available has not been incorporated into physical education programming for the handicapped. Second, the physical education teacher may not have had appropriate training to utilize new instructional processes and techniques and, depending on his or her attitudes toward handicapped children, may have little motivation to acquire the training.

Perception of deviance and social consequence

It is clear that Congress used the principles of normalization to formulate public policy through legislation for the handicapped. The attitudes of personnel who are to implement this policy can have great impact for handicapped children, for such policy has implications for the skill development, educational progress, personal growth, self-image, public image, and social acceptance of the handicapped.

In the past, many handicapped persons have been considered social deviants. Wolfensberger indicates that a person may be regarded as deviant if some characteristic or attribute is judged different by others who consider the characteristic or attribute of importance and who value this difference negatively.[28] An overt and negatively valued characteristic that is associated with a deviance is called *stigma*. For instance, members of ethnic minorities, persons with cosmetic disfigurements, dwarfs, and children with handicapping conditions have been considered deviant.

Deviance is a social perception. It is not characteristic of a person but rather of an observer's values as they pertain to social norms.[28] When a person is perceived as deviant or is stereotyped, as is the case with many handicapped children, he or she is prescribed to a role that carries great expectancies by the nonhandicapped. Furthermore, most of these social perceptions clearly reflect prejudices that have little relationship to reality. As Wolfensberger indicates, the lack of objective verification is not a crucial element in the shaping of a social judgment or social policy.

Legislation supports the principles of normalization

It is our position that educational programming for the handicapped should not be growth inhibiting but should be developmental in nature, integrative rather than segregative, and normalizing rather than stigmatizing.

During the 1970's the courts raised the issue that handicapped persons placed in mental health and mental retardation residential facilities have a *right to treatment*.[13,29] It was the position of the courts that the reason for placement of an individual in a residential institution was either for habilitation or treatment purposes. However, the courts brought to light the fact that the conditions of some of the handicapped persons worsened as a result of institutionalization.

The same evidence was uncovered in cases concerning severely handicapped children and their right to education. For instance, in the case of *Fialkowski vs. Pittenger*[10] the child in question had acquired the skill of walking prior to training and the skill regressed while the child was in the educational program. This is of significance to the physical education teacher, because walking falls under the purview of physical education as defined in P.L. 94-142. Regression of physical skill, an area in which physical educators are involved, is more observable than regression of cognition. The court decreed that handicapped persons had a right not to be subjected to deterioration as a result of treatment, habilitation, and educational programming. Of course, the logical question raised by these litigations is "why is it that the intended outcomes of these programs were not achieved?"

Benefits for handicapped children

Section 504 indicates that handicapped children shall not be denied benefit from programs. It is also abundantly clear that benefits from physical education programs are measured in terms of the development of the child in motor skills and the physical and motor prerequisites. As the courts reviewed the programs that were provided for handicapped persons, it became obvious that many persons who conducted the programs believed they were of benefit to the children. However, in many instances it was found that there were few data to indicate that such development occurred. Purported benefits that could not be objectively measured were called *imagined benefits*. Those that could be objectively documented were called *actual benefits*. The question that was asked of the care providers (adapted physical education teachers included) was "are there real benefits for handicapped children in education?" Actual benefits must assist the development of skills that help the handicapped to cope with community living arrangements, that provide the prerequisites for vocation, and that enable participation in recreational activity, which will enhance their personal and social vantage. These questions will be addressed in Chapter 4.

Out of the concern of parents and small groups for the welfare of individuals grew many major organizations devoted to obtaining funds, establishing programs, and carrying on treatment and research activities. A sampling of some of these organizations follows:

1. Alexander Graham Bell Association for the Deaf, Inc.
   1537 30th St., NW
   Washington, D.C. 20007
2. American Academy for Cerebral Palsy
   University Hospital School
   Iowa City, Iowa 52240
3. American Alliance for Health, Physical Education, Recreation, and Dance
   1900 Association Dr.
   Reston, Va. 22043
4. American Association on Mental Deficiency
   5201 Connecticut Ave., NW
   Washington, D.C. 20016
5. American Cancer Society, Inc.
   219 East 42nd St.
   New York, N.Y. 10017
6. American Diabetes Association
   18 East 48th St.
   New York, N.Y. 10017
7. American Foundation for the Blind
   15 West 16th St.
   New York, N.Y. 10011
8. American Legion
   National Child Welfare Division
   P.O. Box 1055
   Indianapolis, Ind. 42206
9. American Medical Association
   535 North Dearborn St.
   Chicago, Ill. 60610
10. American Occupational Therapy Association, Inc.

6000 Executive Blvd.
Rockville, Md. 20854

11. American Physical Therapy Association
1156 15th St., NW
Washington, D.C. 20005

12. American Psychiatric Association
1700 18th St., NW
Washington, D.C. 20009

13. American Public Health Association, Inc.
1015 18th St., NW
Washington, D.C. 20036

14. Arthritis Foundation
1212 Avenue of the Americas
New York, N.Y. 10036

15. Association for the Aid of Crippled Children
345 East 46th St.
New York, N.Y. 10017

16. The Council for Exceptional Children
1920 Association Dr.
Reston, Va. 22091

17. Epilepsy Foundation of America
111 West 57th St.
New York, N.Y. 10019

18. Goodwill Industries of America, Inc.
9200 Wisconsin Ave.
Washington, D.C. 20014

19. ICD Rehabilitation and Research Center
340 East 24th St.
New York, N.Y. 10010

20. International Council for Exceptional
Children
1201 16th St., NW
Washington, D.C. 20006

21. Joseph P. Kennedy, Jr., Foundation
719 13th St., NW
Washington, D.C. 20005

22. Muscular Dystrophy Association of America, Inc.
1790 Broadway
New York, N.Y. 10019

23. National Association for Mental Health
10 Columbus Circle, Suite 1300
New York, N.Y. 10019

24. National Association of the Deaf
1575 Redwood Ave.
Akron, Ohio 44301

25. National Association for Retarded Citizens
2709 Avenue E
Arlington, Tex. 76010

26. National Cystic Fibrosis Research Foundation
521 5th Ave.
New York, N.Y. 10017

27. National Easter Seal Society for Crippled
Children and Adults
2023 West Ogden Ave.
Chicago, Ill. 60612

28. National Education Association
1201 16th St., NW
Washington, D.C. 20036

29. National Epilepsy League
203 North Wabash Ave.
Chicago, Ill. 60601

30. National Foundation for Asthmatic Children
5601 West Trials End Rd.
P.O. Box 5114
Tuscon, Ariz. 85703

31. National Foundation for Neuromuscular
Diseases
250 West 57th St.
New York, N.Y. 10019

32. National Foundation—March of Dimes
1275 Momaroneck Ave.
White Plains, N.Y. 10695

33. National Hemophilia Foundation
25 West 39th St.
New York, N.Y. 10018

34. National Kidney Disease Foundation
342 Madison Ave.
New York, N.Y. 10010

35. National Multiple Sclerosis Society
257 Park Ave., South
New York, N.Y. 10010

36. National Paraplegia Foundation
333 North Michigan Ave.
Chicago, Ill. 60601

37. National Rehabilitation Association
1522 K Street, NW
Washington, D.C. 20005

38. National Therapeutic Recreation Society
1700 Pennsylvania Ave., NW
Washington, D.C. 20006

39. National Tuberculosis Association
1790 Broadway
New York, N.Y. 10019

40. United Cerebral Palsy Association, Inc.
66 East 34th St.
New York, N.Y. 10016

41. United States Office of Education,
Department of Education
7th and D Sts., SW
Washington, D.C. 20202

CLINICAL SERVICES

Professional care of the handicapped is broadly based, encompassing the talents and dedication of many disciplines. All clinical services ideally join together, having as their common goal the development of the physical, mental, social, cultural, and vocational potential of each disabled person they serve.

A number of disciplines are described herein to acquaint the reader with those hospital and institutional services concerned with the handicapped. These services may be presented under three categories, namely, direct medical services, psychological services, and rehabilitative and habilitative services.

Direct medical services

In most clinical settings there is direct medical service to the patient, including physicians' and nurses' care and support. Laboratory and x-ray services are important adjuncts to the effective delivery of direct medical care to the patient.

All medical specialties lend their particular talents to the disabled; for example, a child with cerebral palsy might require the diagnostic or surgical ability of a neurologist, a muscle transplant by an orthopedic surgeon, and medical rehabilitation by the physiatrist. A child with behavioral problems would be seen by the psychiatrist or psychologist, whereas a case complicated by growth factors would require consultation with a pediatrician.

Today's physicians, whatever their specializations, are beginning to see the value of taking the patient's care beyond the immediate pathological condition. In the rehabilitation or habilitation setting physicians are concerned that their patients may live as fully as possible within the scope of specific handicaps and abilities. As members of intradisciplinary groups physicians are usually charged with the responsibility of leadership and with final authority as to the care of the patient.

Psychological services

Almost always associated with any clinical setting concerned with the handicapped are the psychological services that deal with the client's emotional problems. The professional fields that usually come under this heading are psychiatry, psychology, clinical social work, and vocational counseling.

The psychiatrist is a physician who specializes in the study and treatment of mental illnesses. The psychiatrist focuses on the psychopathology that makes the individual unable to function effectively in society.

The psychologist, in contrast to the psychiatrist, is not a physician, but specializes in both normal and abnormal human behavior. Disciplines under the heading of psychology include clinical, educational, and counseling psychology. The clinical psychologist places the greatest emphasis on psychopathology, which stems from the disordered personality. In comparison, the educational and counseling psychologists place their emphasis on the normal personality. The educational psychologist is concerned with learning problems and maladaptation to the school setting, whereas the counseling psychologist deals primarily with normal personalities that exhibit problems.

As a specialist working with the handicapped, the psychologist must understand the many psychological problems that confront the patient and his or her family. A major handicap forces the individual to make many extreme personality adjustments. Faulty adjustments to these problems may result in psychopathological conditions requiring professional help. The rehabilitation psychologist serves to aid the patient by offering counseling on personal and occupational levels, making personality and vocational evaluations, and making referral to the psychiatrist in case of severe maladjustments.

The clinical social worker must have an understanding of the broad spectrum of intraprofessional specialties and how they affect each patient. The primary concern is with the personal effects of a disability, such as economics and the interpersonal relationship of family and friends. Often almost insurmountable problems involving social and environmental pressures are resolved by the professional and empathetic handling of the patient by the clinical social worker.

Vocational counseling in the total rehabilitation setting is one of the newest professions. The counselor is a specialist who has a broad knowledge of handicapping conditions, the rehabilitative process, and the needs of the disabled. Persons with physical, mental, or emotional handicaps are encouraged to achieve optimum development of their capacities and abilities for employment. The fact must be emphasized that in our society occupational independence is directly related to socioeconomic status and personal feelings of worth.

Rehabilitative and habilitative services

The term *rehabilitation* can generally be defined as the process of returning a disabled person to an effective level of physical, mental, and emotional

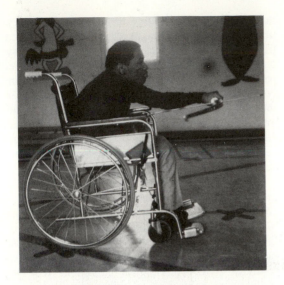

Fig. 1-5. Physical education for the handicapped involves lifetime sport skills. (Courtesy of Julian Stein, American Alliance for Health, Physical Education, Recreation, and Dance, and Coldwater State School and Hospital, Coldwater, Mich.)

health. On the other hand, the term *habilitation* refers to the process of assisting the disabled individual to live as effectively as the impairment will allow. There are many disciplines in the clinical setting (some of which have already been discussed) that are concerned with the optimum functioning of the handicapped. Under this heading is an array of services for the disabled, depending on the type and scope of the clinical facility. Some of the more common professional practices are music therapy, orthotics and prosthetics, and the large number of therapies that concentrate on the movement of the patient.

Music therapy

Because of its value as a recreational, creative, and therapeutic medium, music is becoming an increasingly important part of the treatment programs in many hospitals and mental institutions. Music is known to produce varying degrees of physiological, psychological, and emotional responses in the human organism. Therefore its employment can serve as an important therapeutic adjunct to the total rehabilitation program. The music therapist can also encourage socialization of the patient through singing, dancing, and playing instruments.

Orthotics and prosthetics

When discussing the various kinds of professional assistance that are provided the physically impaired it would be remiss to omit orthotics and prosthetics. Each has developed into a highly defined technology that aids the crippled patient in becoming more self-sufficient within the limitations of the particular disability. *Orthotics* offers the patient a number of possible benefits, namely, the prevention and correction of structural deformities, aid in supporting the body, and an adjunct to the control of involuntary movements. It provides a variety of self-help devices and splints made for the patient's own requirements. *Prosthetics*, on the other hand, is the specialty of making and fitting artificial limbs and is becoming increasingly precise and sophisticated as new procedures and materials become available.[22]

Movement therapies

Of special interest to the physical educator are the many therapies found in institutions and hospitals that are based on movement behavior.

Physical therapy. Massage and heat have been used since the dawn of humankind for the amelioration of various illnesses. Physical therapy today is the process of treating physical impairments by the use of various physical modalities as prescribed by a qualified physician. The physical therapist utilizes a number of treatment devices to bring about a healing or rehabilitative response from the patient, namely, deep heat (diathermy, ultrasound), superficial heat (infrared heat, hydromassage, etc.), cryotherapy (cold therapy), electrical muscle stimulation, massage, mobilization techniques, manual muscle testing, and specific exercises for affected muscles and joints. The physical therapist may also instruct the patient in the use of braces, wheelchairs, crutches, and prosthetic appliances and in activities of daily living.

Occupational therapy. Occupational therapy is a medically prescribed program that provides the patient with interesting activity that will develop varying degrees of physical strength, endurance, and, above all, hand dexterity. Through this medium functional skills are learned that aid the pa-

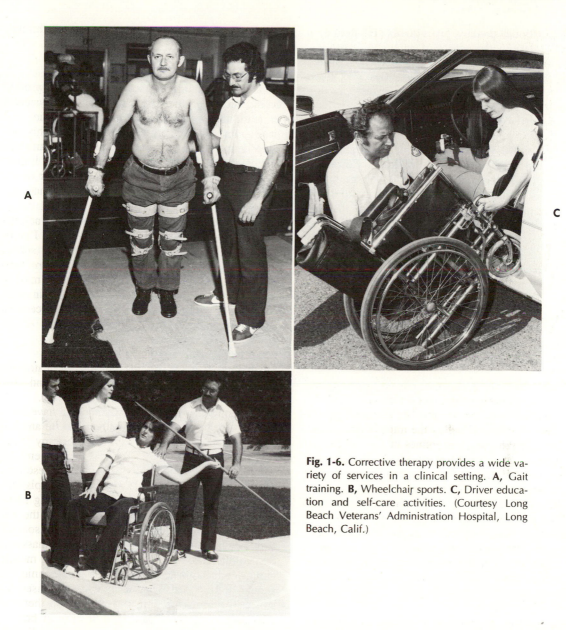

Fig. 1-6. Corrective therapy provides a wide variety of services in a clinical setting. **A,** Gait training. **B,** Wheelchair sports. **C,** Driver education and self-care activities. (Courtesy Long Beach Veterans' Administration Hospital, Long Beach, Calif.)

tient's psychological outlook as well as help him or her to become self-sufficient and perhaps occupationally independent. In many institutions the occupational therapists train the patient in the use of special upper extremity self-help splints.

Recreational therapy. Therapeutic recreation, as defined by the National Therapeutic Recreation Society, is "a special service within the broad area of recreation services. It is a process which utilizes recreation services for purposive intervention in some physical, emotional, and/or social behavior to bring about a desired change in that behavior and to promote the growth and development of the individual."[21]

Recreational therapy gives to the rehabilitation armamentarium the aspect of enjoyable activities. The therapist, through gross motor movements, uses the patient's physical capacities and those abilities that may give an impetus to restoring important physical or mental functions.

Corrective therapy. The profession of corrective therapy emerged as a result of the needs created by World War II and the reconditioning programs instituted by Dr. Howard Rusk. Corrective therapy is defined as the application of the principles, tools, techniques, and psychology of medically oriented physical education to assist the physician in the accomplishment of prescribed objectives.

Corrective therapy is contrasted to adapted physical education primarily in its delivery of services. Adapted physical education functions as an integral part of the various educational levels, including elementary, secondary, college, and university, whereas corrective therapy takes place within hospitals, clinics, and centers dedicated to physical, mental, and emotional restoration and/or habilitation.

The primary procedures employed by the corrective therapist are the following:

1. Offering conditioning and reconditioning exercises for the development of specific and/or general physical requirements
2. Supplying socialization and resocialization activities for the handicapped, employing psychiatric objectives
3. Teaching fundamentals of transfer activities in daily living and the utilization of all types of orthotic and prosthetic devices, including manually controlled motor vehicles
4. Instructing the individual in postural alignment and bodily movement through neuromuscular reeducation
5. Instructing the individual in developmental movement activities, employing basic motor-learning principles
6. Teaching adapted sports, games, and other activities

Coordination of services

There has been considerable emphasis on the belief that programs for the handicapped should be of an interdisciplinary nature. However, according to Stone,[25] problems have existed in the delivery of services within the system. Professionals within the system have taken on the roles, functions, and goals of each other. This has happened because of inadequate planning or coordination and without consideration of the effectiveness of the various professionals in their new roles. As a result we have homogenized professionals who no longer have defined expertise and programs that are less than desirable. Although Stone was not addressing physical education specifically, his view may well relate to the coordination of physical education and the related services (therapies). Role confusion can lead to duplication of services in some programs and voids in others, which result in a lack of comprehensive programming for handicapped children.

Congress has attempted to resolve this problem and has been specific in assigning roles to the professions. According to P.L. 94-142, physical educators provide *direct services*. The activities of other professionals such as recreation therapists, physical therapists, dance therapists, and occupational therapists are referred to as *related services*. Related services are for the purpose of "assisting handicapped children to benefit from special education,"[27] in this case special physical education. Thus, Congress has set forth specific roles and functions to be performed by direct and related services.

The concept of related services

Before a related service such as physical therapy, occupational therapy, or recreational therapy can be implemented in the curriculum it must be determined that the limitations of the child are such that special education—or special physical education in this case—cannot effectively deal with the child's educational problem. A related service should be provided when a child cannot make the expected progress in skill development in physical education. For instances, if it is decided that a handicapped child does not have the prerequisite strength of a specific muscle group to acquire a sport skill and that the physical educator cannot rectify the problem, a physical therapist may be called upon to provide a related service. The function of the physical therapist becomes one of providing programming to the specific muscle group to establish prerequisite strength so that the child

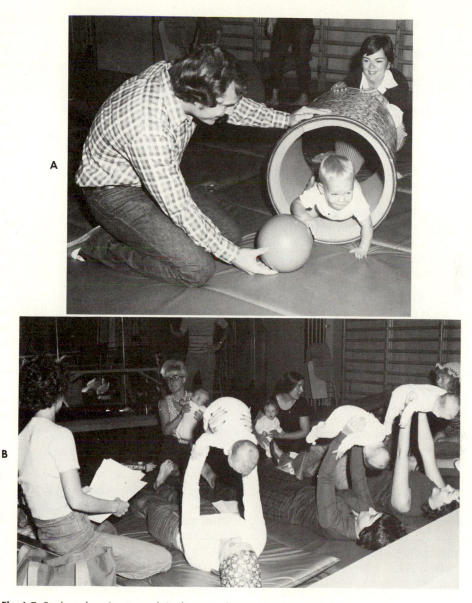

Fig. 1-7. Students learning to work in the area of motor therapy. **A,** Helping a child gain an awareness of spatial relationships. **B,** Infant stimulation through movement. (**B,** Courtesy California State University, Audio-Visual Center, Long Beach, Calif.)

may acquire the skills to be taught by the physical educator. The physical therapist's plan should include measurement of developmental progress in terms of the strength of the specific muscle group. In addition to the measurement of progress the physical therapist and those who plan for the related service should indicate the dates of initiation of services, the dates of termination of services, and the duration of the training. However, the development of the skill to be taught in the physical education class is the responsibility of the physical educator. The development of the physical prerequisites (of a pathological nature) to the skill is the responsibility of the related service provider. Such a procedure streamlines services with greater emphasis on the education of the child and upgrades the quality of instruction.

THE CHALLENGE

The challenge for physical educators and those who deliver related services for the handicapped is formidable, because at present there is, we believe, only a modest number of technically competent, trained personnel who can provide programs of physical education for the handicapped that conform with the recent federal legislation. The solution is to develop trained personnel who possess the necessary technical skills and capabilities.

JOINT RESPONSIBILITY OF THE PARENTS AND THE SCHOOLS

As a result of previous legislation, education for the handicapped is the joint responsibility of the school and parents. In the past, teachers could direct the instruction of handicapped children as they saw fit. Indeed, once the classroom door was closed the teacher controlled what was taught and how class was conducted. The role of the parents was to reinforce the desired educational goals proposed by the school.

The autonomy of the school to control the destiny of handicapped children has changed. The parents, school, and child (when possible) share in the responsibility of the educational development of the child. Representatives of the school and the child's parents (or a representative for the family) meet at least annually to plan an educational program for the child. Such a procedure of cooperative planning between the school and the parents has its roots in constitutional doctrine and has been incorporated into federal statutes for the conduction of educational programs for the handicapped. It is likely that the emphasis placed on the parent's responsibility for the education of the handicapped child will continue to increase.

The United States Supreme Court articulated more than 50 years ago in the case of *Meyers vs. Nebraska* the themes of integration, parental influence, and an individual appreciation and pursuit of competence for all people.[19] Justice McReynolds made the following statement:

The American people have always regarded education and acquisition of knowledge as matters of supreme importance which should be diligently promoted. . . . Corresponding to the right of control, it is the natural *duty of the parent to give his children education suitable to their station in life,* and nearly all states enforce this obligation by compulsory laws.

The right of parents to engage [a teacher] to instruct their children . . . is within the liberty of the Amendment. The *legislature has attempted* [unconstitutionally] *to interfere . . . with the opportunities of pupils to acquire knowledge, and with the power of parents to control the education of their own.*[19] (Italics added.)

Thus, constitutional precedent was established for parent participation in planning the Individual Education Program.

The parent has the option to participate with the school in planning and implementing the educational program by (1) consulting with the school in the Individual Education Program planning conference; (2) monitoring the child's educational progress by comparing behavior in the home with data reported by the school; (3) implementing the Individual Education Program in the home; and (4) using due process to resolve discrepancies in views on placement, educational content, and appropriate delivery of the content.

INCIDENCE OF HANDICAPPING CONDITIONS

The United States census of 1970 estimated that 30% of the population is under 21 years of age and that there are over 46 million persons between 5 and 17 years of age.

The National Health Survey determined that children under 15 years of age have approximately three bouts with acute illness annually. Respiratory conditions constituted about 55% of the reported conditions. Injuries from accidents also constitute a serious problem affecting one child in three.[4,14,23] It has been estimated that almost one child in five, or 18% of the population under 17 years of age, has one or more chronic disorders. During one 2-year period over 11 million children had one or more chronic conditions. Of those conditions reported, the most prevalent, which were hay fever, asthma, other allergies (accounting for

32.8%), sinusitis, bronchitis, and other respiratory diseases (accounting for 15.1%), made up almost half of the chronic conditions of children under the age of 17.[14,23] Paralysis, orthopedic disorders, hearing defects, speech defects, and heart disease also represented a considerable number of those conditions reported.

An ever increasing number of children with congenital malformations are surviving to a greater age each year. The conditions having the highest incidence are heart disorders, congenital dislocation of the hip, cleft palate and lip, spina bifida occulta, and meningocele.[14]

The number of individuals with multiple disabilities is also increasing. The reasons are many, but the primary ones seem to be the higher rate of survival among infants born prematurely and advanced techniques of medical science that are keeping children with one or more disabilities alive.

It has been determined from national public and private agencies and from state and local directors of special education programs that over 12% of the school-aged population, which ranges from 6 to 19 years of age, is handicapped to the extent of needing special education assistance.

The hypothetical incidence of handicapping conditions in the United States is approximately 12%, although estimates for the total handicapped population range from 6.5% to 13.7%. Under P.L. 94-142 states are required to make a count of unserved handicapped children. Thus, there are reasonably accurate data on the number of handicapped children served. A discrepancy between the percentage of children served and the hypothetical 12% would indicate the percentage of children who are unserved in a given state.[16] The assumed prevalence rates of handicapping conditions for the major categories are as follows:

1. Speech impaired   3.5%
2. Learning disabled   3.0%
3. Mentally retarded   2.3%
4. Emotionally disturbed   2.0%
5. Other conditions   1.2%
   a. Crippled and other health impaired   0.500%
   b. Deaf   0.075%
   c. Hard of hearing   0.5%
   d. Visually handicapped 0.1%
   e. Deaf and blind and other multihandicapped   0.060%

Kennedy and Danielson report the number of unserved children by handicapping conditions in 1977-1978 of the 15 states ranked by the net unserved children. The data also indicate that there is considerable variation among states of the number of handicapped children who are unserved.[16] Such information enables a state to focus on finding those children who need special education.

DEFINITIONS OF HANDICAPPING CONDITIONS

Prior to the enactment of P.L. 94-142 there were several definitions of handicapping conditions. There were operational definitions for local school districts and state departments of education and there were professional definitions. At present, however, the federal regulations have definitions of handicapping conditions that possess general application. These definitions appear below:[27]

(1) "Deaf" means a hearing impairment which is so severe that the child is impaired in processing linguistic information through hearing, with or without amplification, which adversely affects educational performance.

(2) "Deaf-blind" means concomitant hearing and visual impairments, the combination of which causes such severe communication and other developmental and educational problems that they cannot be accommodated in special education programs solely for deaf or blind children.

(3) "Hard of hearing" means a hearing impairment, whether permanent or fluctuating, which adversely affects a child's educational performance but which is not included under the definition of "deaf" in this section.

(4) "Mentally retarded" means significantly subaverage general intellectual functioning existing concurrently with deficits in adaptive behavior and manifested during the developmental period, which adversely affects a child's educational performance.

(5) "Multihandicapped" means concomitant impairments (such as mentally retarded-blind, mentally retarded-orthopedically impaired, etc.), the combination of which causes such severe educational problems that they cannot be accommodated in special education programs solely for one of the impairments. The term does not include deaf-blind children.

(6) "Orthopedically impaired" means a severe orthopedic impairment which adversely affects a child's educational performance. The term includes impairments caused by congenital anomaly (e.g., clubfoot, absence

of some member, etc.), impairments caused by disease (e.g., poliomyelitis, bone tuberculosis, etc.), and impairments from other causes (e.g., cerebral palsy, amputations, and fractures or burns which cause contractures).

(7) ''Other health impaired'' means limited strength, vitality, or alertness due to chronic or acute health problems such as a heart condition, tuberculosis, rheumatic fever, nephritis, asthma, sickle cell anemia, hemophilia, epilepsy, lead poisoning, leukemia, or diabetes, which adversely affects a child's educational performance.

(8) ''Seriously emotionally disturbed'' is defined as follows:

(i) The term means a condition exhibiting one or more of the following characteristics over a long period of time and to a marked degree, which adversely affects educational performance:

(A) An inability to learn which cannot be explained by intellectual, sensory, or health factors;

(B) An inability to build or maintain satisfactory interpersonal relationships with peers and teachers;

(C) Inappropriate types of behavior or feelings under normal circumstances;

(D) A general pervasive mood of unhappiness or depression; or

(E) A tendency to develop physical symptons or fears associated with personal or school problems.

(ii) The term includes children who are schizophrenic or autistic. The term does not include children who are socially maladjusted, unless it is determined that they are seriously emotionally disturbed.

(9) ''Specific learning disability'' means a disorder in one or more of the basic psychological processes involved in understanding or in using language, spoken or written, which may manifest itself in an imperfect ability to listen, think, speak, read, write, spell, or to do mathematical calculations. The term includes such conditions as perceptual handicaps, brain injury, minimal brain dysfunction, dyslexia, and developmental aphasia. The term does not include children who have learning problems which are primarily the result of visual, hearing, or motor handicaps, or mental retardation, or of environmental, cultural, or economic disadvantage.

(10) ''Speech impaired'' means a communication disorder, such as stuttering, impaired articulation, a language impairment, or a voice impairment, which adversely affects a child's educational performance.

(11) ''Visually handicapped'' means a visual impairment which, even with correction, adversely affects a child's educational performance. The term includes both partially seeing and blind children.

The scope of special education for the exceptional child is broad. Programs of instruction can be offered in a number of places, depending on the needs of the child. Special education is available in hospitals and special residential and day schools as well as in home instruction and special classes for the handicapped within the regular schools. However, the majority of handicapped students are attending regular schools.

The concern of all persons is that every handicapped individual should have the opportunity to reach full potential through the Individual Education Program.

Implications

Physical education is the only specifically mentioned curriculum area in P.L. 94-142. Therefore, the physical education curriculum has been specifically defined in the regulations as follows: ''The term means the *development* of: (a) physical and motor fitness; (b) fundamental motor skills and patterns; and (c) skills in aquatics, dance, and individual and group games and sports (including intramurals and lifetime sports)''[27] (italics added). Thus, the parameters of the physical education curriculum are well defined. A full preplacement evaluation that determines specific areas of physical education needs should test the pertinent areas of development.[27] Thus, what is needed in the preplacement evaluation of handicapped children are educational data on the full spectrum of the physical education curriculum. A discussion of evaluation will be included in Chapters 2, 3, 4, and 5.

The necessity of data collection on the educational performance is again emphasized when the definition of handicapped conditions is studied for specific populations. A common theme in many of the definitions of handicapping conditions expresses disapproval of programs that adversely affect a child's educational performance. As will be discussed in Chapters 2 and 4, a sound data base that compares the discrepancy between normative levels of physical educational performance and actual levels of performance must be studied to make such judgments.

Furthermore, the last passage of the physical education regulations of P.L. 94-142 clearly states that all of the other definitions previously associated with physical activity for the handicapped were to be incorporated into the definition of physical education.

It is abundantly clear that physical education for the handicapped takes on the characteristics of traditional physical education for normal children. However, the critical word that specifically delineates the nature of activity is *development*. The concept of development of the individual in the mentioned curricular areas is consistent with the goals of the Individual Education Program (Chapter 4).

ADAPTED AND THERAPEUTIC PHYSICAL EDUCATION

Physical activity as a remedial modality has been recognized since recorded history. Early man became aware that movement of the body through massage, passive manipulation, and active exercise had an ameliorating effect on various physical and mental disorders. However, it was not until more recent times that concise systems of *medical gymnastics* were devised as a means to correct certain physical anomalies. One well-known system was that created by Per Henrik Ling of the Royal Institute of Gymnastics, Stockholm, in 1814. The Ling system, as it became known, consisted of specific formalized movements performed with the intent of developing or restoring the participant's health through proper body mechanics and posture. This system was brought to America in 1884 by Nissen and Posse. Requiring an exactness of movement, it soon won favor among American educators whose principal goals followed the European tradition of discipline and health through exercise. Harvard University became the first school in America to conduct a remedial physical education program. The school's program was designed by Dr. Dudley Sargent to help the students gain health through correct postural alignment and to prevent bodily deterioration from an increasingly sedentary life.

After World War I, physical education changed gradually from formality to play and sports activities. Even though many schools accepted the play concept, they still provided a special physical education class for students unable to take part in regular activities. At first, the primary concern of this special physical education class was to improve posture, but gradually the scope expanded to include a variety of handicapping conditions.

Special physical education programs were gradually expanded to incorporate sports, games, and rhythms adapted to the needs of the handicapped child. Through the efforts of such pioneers as George Stafford,[24] numerous physical education and recreational activities were found to benefit the total development of the exceptional person.

In 1947, the Committee on Adapted Physical Education of the American Association of Health, Physical Education, and Recreation defined *adapted physical education* as ". . . a diversified program of developmental activities, games, sports, rhythms, suited to the interest, capacities, and limitations of students with disabilities who may not safely or successfully engage in unrestricted participation in the vigorous activities of the general [physical] education program."[1a] It is generally agreed that adapted physical education classes should be provided for the severely disabled within each school. Also, classes should be provided for the subfit and for persons with moderate disabilities, postural deviations, or obesity, all of whom cannot be adequately cared for in the regular physical education program. However, wherever possible, provisions within the regular physical education class should be made for the handicapped. The developmental concept in which activities are individualized should be employed in all physical education programs, not only in programs for the handicapped. A high-quality regular physical education program utilizes the developmental concept by offering individualized instruction and opportunities for developing physical fitness, skill in sports activities, good body mechanics, and fundamental motor patterns and skills for all the students in the program.

WHERE ARE WE GOING?

Adapted physical education has burgeoned in the past 10 years. An ever growing number of schools, hospitals, and institutions is utilizing the services of the adapted physical educator.

This current increase of interest in adapted physical education has been a result mainly of three factors: increased private and public funding, a broader scope of programming, and integration of disciplines. More money than ever before is being spent in research and program development in the area of special physical education. Universities and colleges are researching teaching methods and approaches in dealing with the exceptional child. School districts are innovating and putting into practice experimental plans for physically educating the handicapped child.

The scope of programming has broadened decidedly in the past 10 years. In the past most adapted physical education took place at the elementary and secondary school levels, whereas now it is conducted with the very young child, on every school level, and with citizens in retirement centers. Program coverage has expanded to involve almost all exceptional persons who can respond to physical education activities.

More and more frequently the physical educator is coming together with the classroom teacher to talk about common problems. This type of cooperation is particularly effective in the cases of the adapted physical educator and the special education classroom teacher. More than ever before, physical education is respected for the many positive effects it has on the exceptional child. No longer can disciplines dealing with aspects of the exceptional child work independently. The current trend is one of an interdisciplinary approach to the problems of children, with each expert joining his or her talents with those of others in the child's best interests.

Physical educators interested in the challenge of individuals with problems will find adapted physical education one of the most personally rewarding of all the many facets of physical education. Its future is bright.

REFERENCES

1. Abeson, A., editor: A continuing summary of pending and completed litigation regarding the education of handicapped children, Arlington, Va., 1973, The Council for Exceptional Children, State-Federal Information Clearinghouse for Exceptional Children.
1a. American Medical Association: Physicians and schools, Report of a conference on the cooperation of the physician in the school health and physical education program, Chicago, 1947, Bureau of Health Education.
2. Arnheim, D. D., and Sinclair, W. A.: The clumsy child: a program of motor therapy, ed. 2, St. Louis, 1979, The C. V. Mosby Co.
3. Ayres, A. J.: Sensory integration and learning disorders, Los Angeles, 1973, Western Psychological Services.
4. Better education for handicapped children, Annual report fiscal year 1969, Washington, D.C., 1970, U.S. Department of Health, Education, and Welfare.
5. Berstein, P. L.: Theory and methods in dance movement therapy, Dubuque, Iowa, 1971, Kendall/Hunt Publishing Co.
6. Brown, L., et al.: Toward the realization of the least restrictive educational environments for severely handicapped students, The American Association for the Education of the Severely/Profoundly Handicapped, 2(4):13-17, December 1977.
7. Brown vs. the Board of Education, 347 U.S., 483, 1954.
8. Congressional Record 118:525, January 20, 1972.
9. Denhoff, E.: Cerebral palsy: the preschool years, Springfield, Ill., 1967, Charles C Thomas, Publisher.
10. Fialkowski vs. Pittenger, In the United States District Court for the Eastern District of Pennsylvania, Civil Action 74-2262, 1976.
11. Gilhool, T., and Stutman, N.: Integration of severely handicapped students: toward criteria for implementing and enforcing the integration imperative of P.L. 94-142 and Section 504, Philadelphia, 1977, Public Interest Law Center of Philadelphia.
12. Hairston vs. Drosick, 423 F. Suppl. 180 (S.D. W. Va., 1976).
13. Halderman vs. Pennhurst, In the United States District Court for the Eastern District of Pennsylvania, Civil Action 74-1345, 1977.
14. Health of children of school age, Washington, D.C., 1966, U. S. Department of Health, Education, and Welfare.
15. Hellison, D.: Humanistic physical education, Englewood Cliffs, N.J., 1973, Prentice-Hall, Inc.
16. Kennedy, M. M., and Danielson, L. C.: Where are unserved handicapped children? Educ. Train. Ment. Retarded 13:408-413, December 1978.
17. Mann, P. H., editor: Mainstream special education, Proceedings of the University of Miami conference on special education in the great cities, 1976, Bureau of the Handicapped, U.S. Office of Education, U.S. Government Printing Office.
18. Mewett, F. M.: Mainstreaming the handicapped: concept and fact, Third national conference on physical activity, Long Beach, Calif., 1974, Office of the Los Angeles County Superintendent of Schools, Division of Special Education.
19. Meyers vs. Nebraska, 262 U.S., 390, 399-401, 1923.
20. One in eleven handicapped adults in America: a survey on 1970 U.S. census data, Washington, D.C., 1970, U.S. Government Printing Office.
21. Program for handicapped: a clarification of terms, J. Health Phys. Ed. Rec. 42:64, September 1971.
22. Rusk, H. A.: Rehabilitation medicine, ed. 4, St. Louis, 1977, The C. V. Mosby Co.
23. Schiffer, C. G., and Hunt, E. O.: Illness among children, Washington, D.C., 1963, U.S. Department of Health, Education, and Welfare.

24. Stafford, G. T.: Sports for the handicapped, Englewood Cliffs, N.J., 1947, Prentice-Hall, Inc.
24a. Stafford, J., Congressional Record **121:**10961, 1975.
25. Stone, A.: Mental health and law: a system in transition, Washington, D.C., 1976, U.S. Department of Health, Education, and Welfare.
26. U.S. Department of Health, Education, and Welfare, Regulations for the Rehabilitation Act of 1973, Federal Register (May 4) 1977, **42:**22676-22702.
27. U.S. 94th Congress, Public Law 94-142 (November 29) 1975.
28. Wolfensberger, W.: Principles of normalization, Toronto, 1972, National Institute on Mental Retardation.
29. Wyatt vs. Stickney, 344 F. Suppl. 387 (M.D., Ala. 1972) affirmed 503 F. 2d 1305 (Fifth Circuit Court), 1974.

RECOMMENDED READINGS

Daniels, A. S., and Davies, E. A.: Adapted physical education, ed. 3, New York, 1975, Harper & Row, Publishers.
Kirk, S.: Educating exceptional children, Boston, 1962, Houghton-Mifflin Co.
Tilford, C. W., and Sawrey, J. M.: The exceptional individual, Englewood Cliffs, N.J., 1967, Prentice-Hall, Inc.

2

Individual development

This chapter is primarily concerned with the factors in personal development that are pertinent to the field of adapted physical education. Physical educators, particularly those teachers concerned with the exceptional individual, must have an understanding of the typical and atypical factors relevant to growth and development. Such kowledge provides the instructor with a sound rationale for following certain procedures and applying particular techniques.

Various meanings have been attached to the terms *growth, development,* and *maturation* by numerous authorities. Therefore, to provide the student with a common understanding, the following definitions are given. *Growth* refers to change in an individual's bodily structure and function. It implies a quantitative change in height, weight, and girth that can be assessed by the employment of some anthropometric techniques. *Development* is a general term indicating the process by which an individual attains maturity.[31] *Maturation* refers to the innate anatomical and physiological bodily changes that are predetermined by heredity.[8]

EARLY GROSS MOTOR DEVELOPMENT

The typical unborn fetus is a unique entity undergoing a complex process of orderly cell division. This cell division develops into different types of tissue that ultimately develop into organs and organ systems that become a coordinated complex of physiological functions. Physical development and maturation usually follow a predictable pattern, occurring from the center of the body outward (proximodistal) and from the head downward (cephalocaudal).

At first, the fetus within the mother displays movement that is random. Gradually, however, there occurs immature control of the head, then the arms, and, finally, the legs. The infant's movement control both before and after birth follows a similar pattern of development.[14] Generally speaking, from gross undefined and uncoordinated behavior, the human infant gradually acquires complex behavior skills that continue throughout life.

The newborn is mainly dominated by primitive reflexes. Many of the reflexes seen in the infant directly after birth are designed to sustain life; for example, the rooting reflex, in which the infant's head turns when the cheek is tactually stimulated, is present in order that milk may be obtained from the breast. Other survival reflexes are breathing, yawning, coughing, sneezing, and sucking. The central nervous system matures slowly, starting with the spinal cord and ending with the higher brain centers. The infant's early development is controlled by the spinal cord. Each developmental milestone (e.g., lifting the head, sitting, and walking) is dependent on the maturation of the nervous system (Fig. 2-1). The primitive postural reflexes are designed so that eventually the individual will function effectively in the upright posture. From a completely grounded, helpless organism, the normal infant develops viable and efficient movement capabilities in the upright bipedal posture.[15,16]

Infants seek ultimate movement independence in order to move freely and explore the environment. In the beginning, infants are almost completely dominated by the downward force of gravity; with increased strength and muscle control, they force themselves upward until they can balance and propel themselves on their small feet. When in the upright posture, the hands are free to feel, to explore, and to learn from a variety of experiences that are limited only by receptivity, the extent of exploration, and the experiential richness of the environment. Full physical, mental, and emotional development can only occur when there is a constant variety of experiences provided by the environment.[36]

From relatively uncontrolled and purposeless movement behavior, the newborn prepares for the next big event by squirming, thrashing out, moving the head, rolling, and kicking. The ability to transport the body over a terrain evolves from the infant's early random movement and the rolling over, crawling, and creeping activities. Purposefully transporting the body forward stems from the infant's pushing with the legs at the same time that he or she is pulling and reaching with the arms.

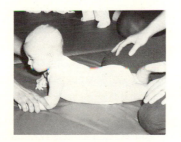

Fig. 2-1. An infant gaining head control. (Courtesy of California State University, Audio Visual Center, Long Beach, Calif.)

Although in the beginning movements are highly unsophisticated, each new movement skill serves as a building block to a more complex skill. The concept that each new skill stems from and is built on a less complex skill can be applied to almost every learning situation that may be encountered by the child.

From the beginning locomotor skill of crawling infants gradually gain enough maturation and courage to raise themselves to a four-point posture.[13] When the infants posess the ability to effectively balance on the hands and knees, the locomotor skill called creeping can be executed. Maturation and experience lead children to pull themselves from a four-point posture to the precarious two-point bipedal, or upright, position. Infants accomplish something outstanding when they can bring themselves to their knees and finally rise to balance unsteadily on the two small surfaces provided by the feet. Normally, it takes a development period of up to 14 months in order for infants to achieve the upright position (Table 2-1).[18,27,29]

Table 2-1 presents normal developmental characteristics of fundamental motor patterns and skills and indicates specific tasks that are paired with chronological age expectancies. By utilizing this chart, one can judge which activities and tasks can be done by a child of a specific age, which activities a child cannot be expected to master, and which activities can be introduced at the child's present level of educational performance. Furthermore, by comparing the child's performance with chronological age expectancies, one can determine developmental delays among the handicapped on fundamental motor patterns and skills. The identification of such delays constitutes one procedure for determining the unique educational needs of a specific child.

Tables 2-1 to 2-4 indicate chronological age expectancies of specific motor behaviors. There is considerable conflict with respect to the ages at which several behaviors occur. Furthermore, in many instances the specific conditions for acquiring the data are not available. It is well established that there are age ranges in which the behaviors may appear and still indicate normal development; for example, walking behavior may occur between 11 and 15 months and still indicate normal development. The test conditions to obtain data on the de-

Table 2-1. Gross motor development

Age	Major events
1 month	Prone, rotates and slightly lifts head. Prone, raises chin 2 inches. Prone suspension, head stays in line with abdomen. Prone, crawling movements with legs. Thrusts arms in play. Rolls to back when placed on side. Lag of head when assisted to sitting. Holds head up for 3 seconds when sitting. Supine, kicks and waves legs. Shows tonic neck reflex.
2 months	Prone, lifts head 45 degrees. Sitting, some neck control. Turns from side to back. Pushes self with arms and lifts chest. Prone suspension, plane of head beyond plane of trunk.
3 months	Prone, crawls. Holds head steady for 5 seconds. Prone, raises chest. Limb posture in flexion. Supine, bilateral activity at midline. Supine, limb and trunk posture symmetrical. Prone, pelvis is flat when plane of face is 45 to 90 degrees. Sitting, head held mostly up. Sitting, back mostly rounded. Prone, lifts head 90 degrees.
4 months	Head steady when sitting. Attempts to right self when tilted. Bears some weight on feet. Bilateral leg extension with back arching. Prone, lying head in midline. Pulls to sitting, head lags at first. Sitting, head forward but steady. Sitting, back shows lumbar curvature. Prone, chest up with arm support. Rolls over. Exhibits swimming action when placed on stomach.
5 months	Reaches out with each hand. Stands by holding on to a support. Prone, supports on one forearm, reaches for toy with other. Pulls self to sitting position, no head lag. Head stable when in sitting position.
6 months	Bears weight on the feet. Crawls backwards. Stands holding on to a support. Reaches forward with extended arms to be picked up. Lifts legs and rolls prone to supine. Weight bearing on both arms and hands (full extension). Sits alone unsupported for 8 seconds. Sits when hands are on floor to stabilize balance.
7 months	Rolls from back to stomach. Crawls (arms).
8 months	Supports weight on feet. Steps when supported under arms. Crawls forward 5 feet. Pivots from prone position. Sits in balance for 1 minute. Adjusts posture to reach. Pulls self to standing. Bears whole weight on legs when supported. Sits with hands free for manipulation. Sits and pulls self forward. Lifts head and shoulders from supine position. Bounces three times when supported in standing position.
9 months	Pulls self to feet. Stands by holding on to a support. Creeps on hands and knees over a 2-inch-high obstacle. Stands unsupported for 1 minute. Moves from prone to sitting position. Sits unsupported for 10 minutes. Adjusts posture to reach. Leans forward and recovers. Walks holding on to furniture. Stands holding on to a support and lifts one foot. Prone, pulls self forward 5 feet. Pivots 180 degrees on abdomen while in a prone position, coordinates arms and legs. Pulls self to sitting position holding on to object. Scoots on floor on the buttocks. Log roll, three times.
11 months	Creeps by using hands and feet. Leans sideways and recovers. Pivots to pick up object. Lowers self to floor by holding. Moves to sitting from prone position. Stands momentarily. Recovers object on floor from sitting position. Moves in circular pattern when sitting. Creeps with one foot flat on floor. Alternating stepping movements with support.
1 year	Stands alone. Hurls ball. Shuffles on buttocks with use of hands. Walks, one hand held. Rolls a ball forward from a sitting position. Crawls over 6-inch barrier. Creeps, hands and soles contact the floor. Climbs stairs on hands and knees.
13 months	Moves from back lying to standing position. Crawls over 4-inch barrier. Extends arm at the elbow joint when throwing.
15 months	Creeps upstairs. Ascends 8-inch steps, marks time. Stoops and recovers. Walks alone. Rolls ball forward with hands from sitting. Crawls over barrier pillows 6 inches high. Assumes kneeling position without support. Climbs stairs on hands and knees. Picks up object. Stands alone. Walks backwards.
18 months	Ascends stairs, marks time. Jumps in place. Walks sideways 10 feet. Pulls an object on a string. Log rolls. Throws ball from standing position. Walks backwards.

Table 2-1. Gross motor development—cont'd

Age	Major events
24 months	Begins to rotate wrist horizontally. Walks backwards. Squats on floor. Throws object overhead. Jumps from 12-inch box with one foot leading. Jumps forward 4 inches. Ascends four 8-inch steps, marks time. Kicks 9-inch ball 3 feet. Bounces 3-inch ball 4 feet. Seats self. Runs 8 feet.
27 months	Jumps up and down with both feet. Balances on one foot for 1 second. Ascends ladder, marks time. Rolls 9-inch ball while sitting. Bounces 9-inch ball 3 feet. Throws 6-inch ball 5 feet. Throws 3-inch ball 7 feet. Stands on tiptoes with hands on hips for 3 seconds. Walks backwards without looking for 10 feet.
30 months	Stands on tiptoes for 1 second. Moves from standing to sitting position. Moves from sitting to standing position. Catches 6-inch ball from a distance of 4 feet. Balances on one foot for 3 seconds. Broad jumps 5 inches. Descends four 6-inch steps, marks time. Jumps from an 11-inch box. Takes one step on a beam 2 inches wide. Walks backwards for 10 feet in a path of 12 inches. Stands on tiptoes for 3 seconds. Stands on one foot for 1 second. Throws 3-inch ball 8 feet. Rolls 9-inch ball from sitting position. Bounces 9-inch ball 3 feet. Throws 9-inch ball 4 feet. Takes running steps on toes. Jumps from 18-inch elevation with one foot leading.
36 months	Catches 6-inch ball thrown from distance of 5 feet three out of three times. Descends four 7-inch steps, marks time. Balances on one foot for 3 seconds. Broad jumps distance of 10 inches. Jumps from 12-inch box. Ascends ladder (12-inch rungs), marks time. Jumps over obstacle 3 inches high. Bounces 3-inch ball 4 feet. Catches 3-inch ball from a distance of 4 feet. Jumps on both feet four steps. Rides tricycle 10 feet. Catches 9-inch ball with arms and body. Jumps in place. Jumps down from 18-inch elevation.
42 months	Stands on one foot for 5 seconds. Walks upstairs, alternates feet. Throws tennis ball 5 feet. Jumps ten steps. Bounces 3-inch ball 6 feet. Catches 3-inch ball thrown from a distance of 5 feet. Walks 10-foot by 1-inch line without stepping off. Jumps and lands on balance from a height of 18 inches. Descends ladder, marks time. Performs arrhythmical skip. Rides tricycle. Hops on one foot. Jumps over a rope less than 20 cm high.
48 months	Performs somersault. Walks downstairs, alternates feet. Throws 6-inch ball 9 feet. Bounces 6-inch ball 6 feet. Catches 6-inch ball from a distance of 6 feet. Hops on preferred foot six steps. Jumps off and lands on feet from a 28-inch height. Catches $16\frac{1}{4}$-inch ball with elbows in front of body. Balances on one foot for 4 to 10 seconds. Broad jump 8 to 10 inches. Running broad jump 23 to 33 inches.
54 months	Throws 3-inch ball 12 feet. Catches 3-inch ball from a distance of 4 feet. Hops on one foot 9 steps. Broad jumps 22 inches. Catches 9-inch ball with hands and body. Hops on one foot for 4 feet.
5 years	Throws 3-inch ball 13 feet. Catches 3-inch ball from a distance of 5 feet. Hops on one foot 12 steps. Skips 10 steps. Broad jumps 30 inches. Descends ladder (12-inch rungs) alternates feet. Somersaults over 6-inch object. Walks line with heel to toe. Throws 9-inch ball 12 to 13 feet. Catches bounce pass three or four times out of five. Kicks soccer ball through the air 8 to 11 feet. Steps while throwing.
6 years	Stands with heel to toe. Runs 50 yards in 12 seconds. Marches in rhythm. Throws 4-inch ball 25 feet. Hops in pattern. Kicks 6-inch ball 10 feet. Walks on tiptoes 12 inches, heels do not touch. Walks a beam 4 inches wide, 8 feet long. Bounces and catches tennis ball four times in a row. Jumps 12-inch hurdle. Hops 50 feet in 11 seconds. Broad jumps 35 inches. Gallops steady rhythm. Skips well. Jumps and reaches (boys 4 feet, girls $3\frac{1}{2}$ feet)

Table 2-2. Fine motor development

Age	Major events
1 month	Grasp reflex present. Drops rattle immediately when placed in hand. Eyes fixate on object held at midline. Follows object to midline. Swipes at object. Symmetrical eye movements.
2 months	Swipes at objects. Reflex grasp. Involuntary release. Follows dangling toy 180 degrees. Tracks ball 180 degrees. Retains rattle for 15 seconds. Manipulates 6-inch ring attached to a string. Grasps object upon contact. Attempts to reach for dangling ring.
3 months	Plays with own fingers. One- and two-arm control. Looks alternatively at object and hands. Brings hands in front of body. Waves arms at interesting object. Symmetrical arm movements. Follows past midline.
4 months	Plays with hands. Moves hands to object. Reaches for object. Picks object up with hand. Hands come to midline. Grasps rattle. Hands predominantly open. Visually tracks 180 degrees. Plays with rattle longer than 1 minute. Hands come together 50 percent of the time. Intentional grasp of object. Hands approach the midline when reaching for an object.
5 months	Reaches for object. Transfers object from hand to hand. Fixation during distraction. Crumples large piece of paper.
6 months	Reaches for object. Transfers object from hand to hand. Visually tracks to midline. Begins to rotate wrist horizontally. Ulnar palmar grasp.
7 to 8 months	Grabs object with palm. Unilateral lead in reaching. Transfers object from hand to hand. Radial palmar grasp. Rotates wrists when manipulating object. Grasps with thumb and finger when picking up cube. Grasps bead with thumb and tip of middle or index finger.
9 to 10 months	Plays with fingers. Puts object into container. Holds two 1-inch cubes in one hand. Bangs two cubes together at midline. Holds object bilaterally. Reciprocal reach. Removes $1/4$-inch peg from board. Claps hands together at midline. Brings two objects together at midline while manipulating. Picks up block with thumb and index and middle finger. Grasps bead with thumb and tip of index and middle finger. Grasps with forefinger. Advertent release of objects.
11 months	Strings seven 1-inch beads in 2 minutes. Arm rotation. Opposed pinch. Begins to release object. Neat pincer grasp. Places three cubes in cup.
12 months	Mature grasp. Places block in box. Squeezes. Eyes track object 78 inches away. Incidental marks with pencil. Pulls pegs from board one by one. Releases rather than drops object. Pokes at object with index fingers. Secures pellet with pincer grasp over hand grasp. Turns pages of book. Opens hinged box. Picks up two cubes in one hand. Grasps with forefinger and thumb.
13 months	Makes incidental marks with crayons. Dumps pellet from bottle. Places pellets in bottle with 4-inch opening.
15 months	Dumps pellets from container. Pulls $1/4$-inch pegs from board one by one. Holds two cubes in one hand. Builds tower of two 1-inch blocks. Turns pages of a storybook one by one. Grasps with approximate adult ability.
18 months	Pincer grasp. Builds tower of two 1-inch blocks. Inserts pellet in bottle with 1-inch opening. Places five $1/4$-inch pegs in boards.
24 months	Transfers object from hand to hand. Tracks to midline. Strings three $5/8$-inch beads. Makes a vertical mark. Builds tower of four blocks. Stirs.
27 months	Opens and closes scissors. Holds crayons with fingers. Draws horizontal line. Demonstrates an H stroke.
30 months	Builds tower of eight blocks. Snips with scissors. Strings five 1-inch beads.
3 years	Builds a tower of ten blocks. Copies circle. Copies square. Uses spoon. Cuts 6-inch paper in half. Strings five $1/2$-inch beads.
$3^1/_2$ years	Stacks six blocks. Copies cross.
4 years	Holds pencil with pincer grasp. Cuts 2-inch triangle in 45 seconds. Copies bridge of three squares.
$4^1/_2$ years	Places nine pellets in a bottle in 25 seconds. Cuts squares and circles within $1/4$-inch lines. Puts paper clip on paper. Creases paper. Cuts 6-inch square within $1/4$ inch lines in 45 seconds.
5 years	Connects dots 8 inches apart. Cuts 8-inch straight line with no more than $1/4$ inch deviance. Places ten $1/8''$ pellets in box in 25 seconds. Colors within lines.
6 years	Carries glass 8 feet without spilling liquid. Opens and closes safety pin. Builds pyramid of three blocks. Copies printing.

Table 2-3. Adaptive behavior

Age	Major events
3 months	Swallows soft foods.
6 months	Lifts head.
7 to 8 months	Chews bananas and bread. Feeds self cracker. Lifts cup with two hands.
9 months	Plays pat-a-cake. Holds own bottle.
11 months	Chews and swallows. Laces own shoes. Stirs with spoon. Feeding (drooling under control).
13 months	Finger feeds. Chews in circular manner.
15 months	Brings food to mouth. Climbs onto chair 16 inches high. Places pellet in cup.
18 months	Sucks and uses straw. Chews solid foods. Drinks from cup. Removes socks. Turns page in book. Unzips zipper.
24 months	Examines objects. Searches for hidden objects. Lifts cup. Unwraps paper covering. Takes off shoelaces. Turns doorknob. Unscrews 3-inch lid. Drinks from glass in one hand. Uses spoon in fist. Removes unfastened garment.
27 months	Eats with fork. Unbuttons large buttons. Turns doorknob.
30 months	Removes pull-down garment. Removes shoes. Unbuttons front buttons.
3 years	Uses spoon. Sits on toilet. Turns faucet on and off. Removes socks. Snaps in front. Turns crank handle. Unscrews 1-inch lid. Uses fork in fist. Puts on shoe.
3½ years	Winds up toy. Buttons series of five buttons.
4 years	Puts on socks. Puts on and fastens belt. Sorts dissimilar objects (nuts and bolts). Zips zipper.
4½ years	Copies circle. Holds fork in fingers.
5 years	Buttons ½-inch buttons. Uses knife to spread.
6 years	Ties bow. Sweeps with broom. Drives nail. Erases pencil marks. Dials telephone. Sorts items by shape, size, and color.

velopment of the motor behavior are varied. Thus, compilation of researchers' data to profile the motor development of young children is difficult.

The information presented in Tables 2-1 and 2-2 reflects the views of several researchers.* In an attempt to synthesize the developmental data, it was sometimes necessary to interpolate the development of behavior between reported ranges of age. The tables do, however, provide general expectations for the acquisition of specific motor behaviors with respect to chronological age.

FINE MOTOR DEVELOPMENT

Besides transportation skills, effective object manipulation is highly important to the child's ultimate learning and physical development. Efficient object control stems from the child's ability to grasp and release an object at will. In the early days following birth, the infant reflexively grasps when pressure is applied to the palm of the hand. Gradually, the infant gains the ability to close and open the hand as desired. In the beginning, pur-

poseful manipulation is performed by the child first with the palms of the hands and later with the fingers. Mature manipulation does not occur until about the sixteenth month of life, at which time the thumbs can be used in opposition (Table 2-2).[27]

All early behavior is dependent on the complex interweaving of visual, tactile, auditory, manipulative, and gross motor functions. It should also be noted that the senses of smell, taste, sight, hearing, and touch, taken together with the ability to move, provide the means by which the human organism learns about and makes adaptations to the environment (Table 2-4). All senses act independently and in combination with one another to process and store information. A person who is deprived of adequate sensory experiences often has problems reaching full maturation and development that may carry throughout the individual's lifetime.

The proper coordination of the six pairs of eye muscles must take place before the child can adequately focus on objects. Inadequate coordination of both eyes may lead to problems in total body coordination as well as later difficulty in learning. The eyes are important to the child's normal devel-

*See references 2, 6, 7, 9, 14, 16, 17, 19, 20, 21, 35, 39, 40, and 41.

Table 2-4. Early normal developmental social characteristics

Age	Major events
0	Responds to sounds. Responds to persons. Responds to brightly colored objects.
4 weeks	Shows awareness of persons. Searches for nipple. Regards persons' faces.
8 weeks	Smiles when talked to. Shows excitement when being approached by adult. Looks for source of sounds.
12 weeks	Likes to be around persons. Anticipates being fed. Tenses muscles when about to be lifted. Plays with own fingers.
16 weeks	Shows pleasure with certain toys. Laughs with persons. Plays with hands. Recognizes bottle. Is aware of self in mirror.
20 weeks	Plays peekaboo. Smiles at familiar person. Shows displeasure when toy is taken away. Inspects own hands.
24 weeks	Smiles at image in mirror. Wants to be talked to. May fear strange persons.
28 weeks	Makes noise to gain attention. Explores objects. Pats own image in mirror.
32 weeks	Watches persons. Says "da da" and "ma ma." Uncovers toy.
36 weeks	Brings arms in front of face. Uses fingers to feed self from dish. Defends own possessions. Drinks from cup with some spill. Responds to questions.
40 weeks	Plays pat-a-cake. Likes to play. Looks at pictures in book. Responds to "no, no."
52 weeks	Puts everything into mouth. Jabbers with expression. Imitates words. Plays nursery games.
64 weeks	Exhibits solitary play. Drops things from crib and high chair to gain attention. Cooperates in dressing. Plays ball. Speaks two words.
16 months	Carries personal things. Indicates when diapers are wet. Identifies common clothes.
18 months	Demonstrates side-by-side play. Is very possessive of own things. Imitates scribbling. Follows simple directions.
21 months	Makes two-word sentences. Makes basic wants known. Identifies objects in picture.
24 months	Holds and hugs doll. Pulls off own clothes.
27 months	Imitates other children's play. Indicates need to go to toilet.
30 months	Avoids specified dangers.
36 months	Takes turns.
42 months	Plays with another child.
48 months	Plays highly structured games. May have imaginary playmate. Is very aggressive in play. Washes and dries hands. Cooperates in play.
5 years	Dresses without help. Plays in group of three.

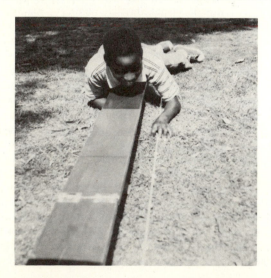

Fig. 2-2. Mastery of each level of development sets the stage for the next. Incomplete development may require programming at lower levels. (Provided through Unit on Programs for the Handicapped, American Alliance for Health, Physical Education, Recreation, and Dance.)

Table 2-5. Early normal developmental characteristics: language and communication

Age*	Major events
0	Exhibits undifferentiated birth cry.
4 weeks	Watches person moving. Makes demand cry. Makes throaty cry.
8 weeks	Attends to person's voice. Shows discomfort. Gurgles. Coos.
12 weeks	Makes different sounds when touched or played with. Tenses when lifted. Shows vital or differentiated crying when cold, uncomfortable, or hungry.
16 weeks	Turns head to sound of voice. Recognizes mother. Laughs. Experiments with voice.
20 weeks	Turns to sounds. Shows displeasure. Responds to voices.
24 weeks	Responds to anger. Displays nonrhythmical crying. Babbles.
28 weeks	Squeals. Makes "M-m" sound. Smiles at mirror. Demands attention. Tries to imitate speech.
32 weeks	Combines babbling and gestures. Combines two syllables. Displays rhythmical babbling.
36 weeks	Cries to gain attention.
40 weeks	Understands "no." Waves bye-bye. Looks for hidden object. Imitates sounds. Says "da-da" and "ma-ma."
44 weeks	Shakes head "no." Says one word. Imitates new sounds. Listens to words. Anticipates playing pat-a-cake.
48 weeks	Knows own name. Indicates personal desires. Commands through gestures.
52 weeks	Knows names of objects. Shows likes and dislikes. Imitates words. Possesses three-word vocabulary. Anticipates being scolded. Responds to "Give it to me."
64 weeks	Points to things wanted. Shows variety of emotions. Possesses five-word vocabulary.
18 months	Knows three body parts. Imitates talking. Possesses 10-word vocabulary. Hums and sings to self. Uses words to indicate wants.
21 months	Tries to follow directions. Knows five body parts. Leads adult to object. Exhibits great curiosity. Connects three or four words. Possesses 20-word vocabulary.
24 months	Follows simple commands. Refers to self by name. Knows how some objects work. Names most objects played with. Imitates parents' speech. Expresses two- or three-word sentences.
27 months	Repeats two numbers. Knows three prepositions. Names most common objects in home. Uses plurals.
30 months	Identifies objects by use. Knows the number "one." Knows simple songs and rhymes.
36 months	Gives full name. Knows own sex. Identifies at least two objects from picture. Answers simple questions. Talks in simple sentences.
42 months	Counts to three. Follows simple verbal directions. Knows the concepts of longer and heavier. Can tell a story.
48 months	Uses conjunctions. Understands prepositions. Makes five- and six-word sentences. Names the colors "red," "blue," and "yellow." Possesses 800-word vocabulary. Gestures with entire body. Forms sentences.
5 years	Expresses mature articulation. Asks "Why?" Can define six words. Explains composition of materials.

*The ages at which the major events noted here occur are approximate.

opment of body balance, postural awareness, spatial awareness, and self-image.

The sense of touch is the most mature sense that infants have at birth. A variety of information about themselves and surroundings comes to the infants through their tactile sense. Infants and young children must have a rich backlog of touch experiences in order to develop maximally.

A variety of movement experiences is necessary to adequately stimulate the kinesthetic system. Body movement stimulates sensory organs that are located in the muscles, tendons, and joints as well as within the ear. A keen awareness of movement is necessary for the acquisition and maintenance of good posture, the ability to effectively deal with spatial relationships, and the ability to initiate synchronous motor patterns.[9]

Hearing and vocal language are synonymous to the human organism. The fetus begins to hear about 5 weeks after conception. After birth, the infant should be provided with a rich sound environment in order to acquire sound discrimination and sound identification for vocal communication (Table 2-5).

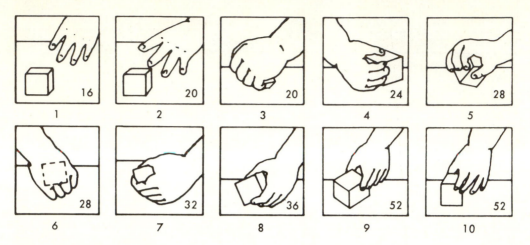

Fig. 2-3. Developmental progressions in grasping. (From Halverson, H. M.: Genet. Psychol. Monogr. **10:**107-286, 1931.)

For the child's ultimate development, there must occur an effective processing of information through the senses. It is speculated that, from the time of conception, the human being is continually processing information and gaining a backlog of experiences that will be used for future behavior.[4] It is imperative that the child be able to recognize, identify, and discriminate between different stimuli in order that behavior is accurate and effective according to individual requirements. Accurate perception and normal responses are necessary for normal behavior.*

NORMATIVE SCALES FOR DIAGNOSIS AND PROGRAMMING

Numerous researchers in growth and development have studied the chronological occurrence of motor behaviors on a normative continuum. These include Gesell (1954), Bayley (1951), Guttridge (1939), Wild (1938), and Wellman (1937). Most authorities classify behaviors according to the gross and fine motor domain. Gesell indicates that gross motor development proceeds in two directions: the cephalocaudal and proximodistal directions. Knowledge of the directions of development provides valuable information for developmental diagnosis of and subsequent programming for

*See references 6, 10, 18, and 29.

Table 2-6. Cephalocaudal cycles of development*

Age (weeks)	Condition
0 to 29	Trunk in contact with supporting surfaces
30 to 42	Alternate flexion of legs
49 to 56	Movement to upright position in attempt to gain control over gravitational forces while standing
50 to 60	Full trunk extension and upright postural control, bilateral flexion and extension of legs

*From Rarick, G. L.: Motor development during infancy and childhood, Madison, Wis., 1954, University of Wisconsin.

young children who are in the early stages of development. Such information indicates which behaviors are part of the learner's repertoire and which have yet to be developed Fig. 2-3. There may be some exceptions to the cephalocaudal and proximodistal principles, since there may be head-to-foot and shoulder-to-hand sweeps that are appropriate to advancing levels of maturity. These exceptions, however, do not impair the validity of the principle.

Motor development scales provide guidelines for curriculum construction and subsequent formulation of instructional objectives. Developmental

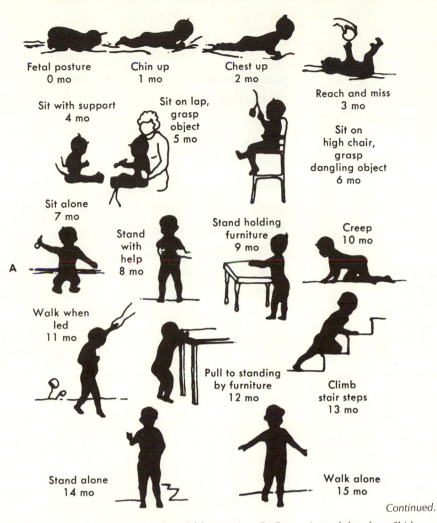

Fetal posture
0 mo

Chin up
1 mo

Chest up
2 mo

Reach and miss
3 mo

Sit with support
4 mo

Sit on lap,
grasp
object
5 mo

Sit on
high chair,
grasp
dangling object
6 mo

Sit alone
7 mo

Stand
with
help
8 mo

Stand holding
furniture
9 mo

Creep
10 mo

Walk when
led
11 mo

Pull to standing
by furniture
12 mo

Climb
stair steps
13 mo

Stand alone
14 mo

Walk alone
15 mo

A

Continued.

Fig. 2-4. A, Developmental sequence in bipedal locomotion. **B,** Comparison of data from Shirley and from California infant growth study on median age of first passing of certain motor items. (**A,** From Shirley, M. M.: The first two years: a study of twenty-five babies, vol. II, Intellectual development, Minneapolis, 1933, University of Minnesota Press; **B,** From Bayley, N.: Monogr. Soc. Res. Child. Dev. **1:**1-26, 1935.)

principles can be utilized in the formulation of curricula. One such principle is that children develop from the head to the foot (cephalocaudal). Rarick[8] indicates that there are definite cycles the child passes through in which he or she gains control over the axial skeleton in a cephalocaudal manner (Table 2-6).

Shirley's[9] developmental scales indicate the sequence that leads to bipedal locomotion. Such information provides a guide to programming in order to assist cephalocaudal development. The chronological age norm associated with developmental progressions gives opportunities for the determination of acceleration rates as well as devel-

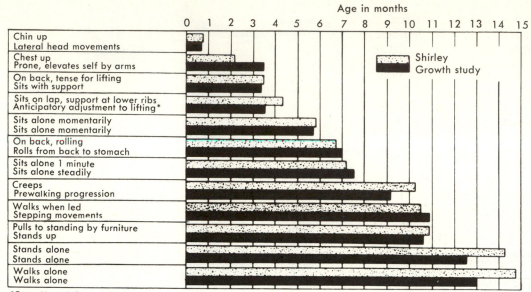

*From Mental Growth Series.

Fig. 2-4, cont'd. For legend see p. 33.

SERVING POPULATIONS VIA DEVELOPMENTAL PRINCIPLES

opmental lags of the children who have been assessed in these sequences (Fig. 2-4).

The direction of development (cephalocaudal and proximodistal) is most relevant to children at preschool ages and particularly to the motor development of those who are developmentally in the first year of life. Therefore, children who can benefit most from the application of these developmental principles are normal children up to 1 year of age, handicapped infants, and profoundly mentally retarded children who have not developed beyond the first year of life according to chronological norms.

Humans are by nature gregarious, needing stimulation from other persons to reach their full growth and development. From the first time the child smiles at a parent to the time he or she plays with other children, socialization is necessary for the development of the child's self-concept and emotional stability. From the egocentricity of infancy, the side-by-side play of the toddler, and the cooperative play of the young child, there gradually emerges the ability to give and take graciously, to follow, to lead, to interact in many social situations, and, finally, to effectively compete in life under rigid rules of personal conduct.[3]

PHYSICAL GROWTH

Physical growth is an extremely complex phenomenon that has a multitude of sensitive, interdependent variables. An individual's growth and development are affected mainly by heredity, prenatal factors, disease, and the environment.[24] The genetic plan of each cell provides the foundation for the potential size of an individual. However, ultimate growth can be adversely altered or can exceed its natural potential through the influence of nutrition, exercise, and general health. For example, the person who eats beyond his or her maintenance requirements will exceed the weight level that heredity has set. Similarly, continued heavy weight lifting with low repetition, as conducted by many football players, will often produce a large bulky musculature, modifying considerably a person's natural inherited tendencies.

Many prenatal factors can adversely affect the growing individual. Maternal conditions such as malnutrition, defective implantation, Rh incompatibilities, diabetes, or contraction of rubella or syphilis during the very early development of the unborn infant may alter the ultimate growth and development of the fetus, as may drug addiction or heavy cigarette smoking.

Diseases of all types can result in significant hindrance of normal growth. Infections, for example, may prevent proper weight gain. A bedridden individual may fail to develop normally because of lack of exercise and fresh air. Motor development may also be impaired as the result of disease, compounded by inactivity and the lack of opportunity for proper skill development. Metabolic and endocrine gland disorders can directly and indirectly affect the growth process.

Increasingly, environmental factors are identified as being the primary etiological factor in many growth and development problems. Poor living standards, together with inadequate health care and diet, constitute one of the major causes of mental retardation and deficient physical growth. Child neglect and lack of parental love also produce climates in which full maturation cannot be reached.

Accurate assessment of normal physical development is difficult because different parts of the body grow at different rates and at varied periods in life. Consequently, age and general height and weight charts serve only as estimates of a child's stage of development. A method that has proved of some benefit to the educator is the Wetzel grid. This type of system provides the teacher and parent with a simple direct means for calculating a child's growth progress.

Conventionally, a child's physical growth has been compared with the corresponding *age means* of height or weight or as derived from samples (even as small as 100 or fewer subjects) and ethnic origin. Apart from comparing a child's own weight and height with the *mean* of a group to which he or she never belonged, judgment of growth in terms of weight or height is precarious at best, considering what is at stake and what the serious limitations of such procedures really are. The Wetzel grid,[32] on the other hand, avoids all such handicaps by providing, instead, a fixed parameter—a universal and accurate standard for measuring and appraising the body *size* and *shape* (build) and the *direction* and *speed* of human physical development. These estimates are distribution free and independent of the original units of measurement as well as of ethnic and sample variability. The grid's applications to pediatrics, school health, and physical education have often been described (Fig. 2-5). Its principles, too, have been confirmed by worldwide data, including the very first observations of Quetelet in 1831. Yet the severest test of validity and reliability, of course, resides in the fact that the grid *predicts* the *preferred paths* of healthy development as observed in today's children.

Typical children display considerable variation in height and weight throughout their growing years. The rate of growth in height increases and decreases as the individual matures. With the exception of the adolescent growth spurt, at age 10 to 12 years for girls and age 12 to 14 years for boys, the rate of height increase decelerates at a continual rate. The most dramatic height increase occurs as the individual matures in the pubescent period of life. Weight, in contrast to the development of height, is less predictable, having a number of fluctuations in most individuals' lifetimes. Because of the wide divergence in factors affecting weight, it is difficult to predict. As an example, muscle growth increases from the 30% that is normal in childhood to almost 40% during adolescence. Commonly, children who mature early tend to be heavier than those who mature late. Similarly, the longer period of growth of children maturing late results in proportionally longer legs as compared to the trunk. Abnormal weight gain and obesity during the pubescent period may cause both physical and personality development problems that can adversely affect individuals throughout their lives.

Structural changes

A number of methods are employed to assess the maturational state of an individual. Many use age, height, and weight, whereas others use anthropometric measurements such as skeletal breadth or body circumferences. However, the most accurate assessment is made by x-ray examination of dental and skeletal osseous development.

The most obvious methods of indicating skeletal

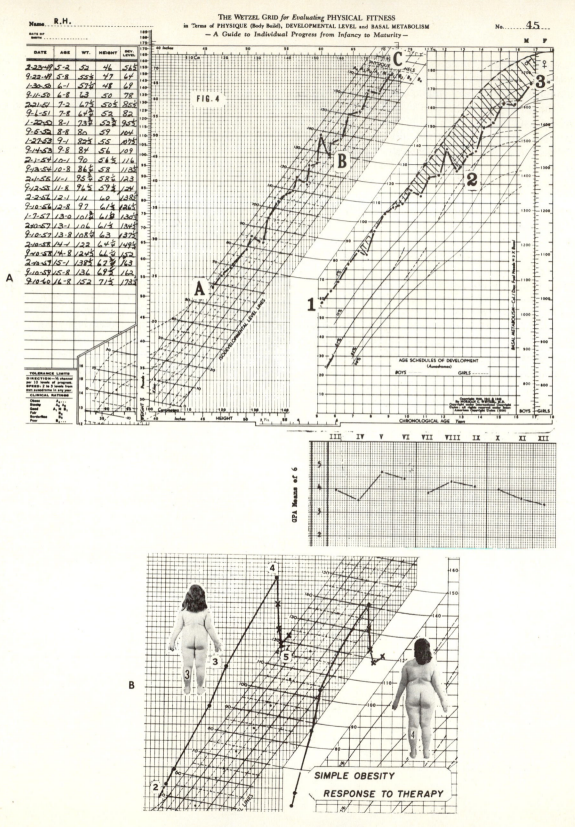

Fig. 2-5. For legend see opposite page.

maturity are through observing long bone growth and through x-ray study of carpal ossification. Anatomically, the long bone consists of a shaft known as the *diaphysis;* at each end of its shaft is the *metaphysis*. An epiphyseal cartilaginous plate, termed the *epiphysis*, separates the metaphysis from the end of the long bone. Growth of the long bones occurs by the laying down of osseous tissue at the metaphysis, which pushes the epiphyseal plate up, extending bone length. Gradually, during adolescence and early adulthood, through the influence of hormones, particularly thyroxin, the diaphysis and the epiphysis reach maturity by joining together in an ossified unit (Fig. 2-6).

The carpal index has been proven one of the most valid and reliable growth measures. Through x-ray examination, the child's stage of development can be detected. Carpal bones do not begin to show ossification until 2 to 3 years of age and complete epiphyseal closure does not occur until late adolescence.

Before maturation, during the period when bones are predominantly cartilaginous and have active epiphyseal growth centers, they are subject to stresses and trauma that may result in various structural deviations. This is a crucial period for injuries incurred by engaging in vigorous and traumatic sports activities. *Postural deviations occurring at this time may later develop into permanent structural changes, whereas diseases of the growth centers or of the epiphysis may result in disability and deformity.*

Postural adjustment

Good posture is that quality in which the body segments such as the head, trunk, pelvis, and lower limbs are in proper muscular and skeletal balance. Dynamically speaking, this means that the body is used in the most effective way with the least amount of strain placed on its supporting structures. Proper segmental alignment provides protection against acute injury or gradual deformity. The musculoskeletal system of the newborn child is extremely pliable and is subject to molding by the forces of gravity. Ossification and bone rigidity occur slowly with mineral salts, primarily calcium and phosphorus, replacing cartilaginous tissue. Muscle growth is associated with skeletal maturation. As the child uses his or her body, the musculoskeletal system is developed. Julius Wolff's law of functional adaptation, developed in 1876, clearly describes the influence of stress on the supporting structures of the body. It is stated as an "early change in the form and the function of bones, or in their function alone, . . . followed by certain definite changes in their internal architecture, and equally definite changes in their external conformation, in accordance with mathematical laws." Wolff's law indicates that the pull of gravity, coupled with muscle contraction, serves to inhibit or stimulate the growth rate of bones, depending on the degree and duration of the stress.

One of the greatest stresses placed on the musculoskeletal system is gravity. Ideally, the body should react against gravity by aligning its segments so that there is as little stress as possible. Constant faulty positioning of the young body can result in permanent structural deformities and asymmetry. Therefore the developmental process must be considered as playing an integral part in the posture of the child. The two most important changes that can be attributed to early posture are the development of the vertebral curvature and the transition of the center of gravity.

Fig. 2-5. A, Long-term (11-year) Wetzel grid record based on semiannual measurements of weight and height routinely made in the School Health Program, Shaker Heights, Ohio. *AB,* "Good growth" gradually but definitely changing to "early growth failure," with change in direction along *AB* and "slowdown" along *1-2*. These trends became even worse along *BC* and *2-3*. Note, too, the continuing drop-off in growth potential average (GPA). **B,** Characteristic direction and speed trends in childhood obesity clearly confirmed by the accompanying photos at points *3* and *4*, respectively. Section *4-5* shows the response (return to the Channel A_3A_4 boundary and to the "less advanced auxodrome expected from the first two observations"). (**A,** By permission of Newspaper Enterprise Association, Cleveland, Ohio, 1965, from special reprint of a paper by Hopwood, H. H., and Van Iden, S. S.: J. School Health **35:**337, 1965; **B,** From Wetzel, N. C.: Don't take growth for granted, Cleveland, Ohio, 1961, Newspaper Enterprise Association.)

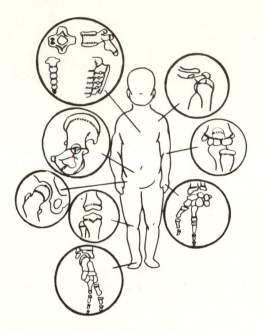

Fig. 2-6. Bones and their epiphyses. Carpal bones are often used as an index to determine the degree of ossification that has occurred at a particular age. Their development occurs between 2 and 18 years of age.

Because of the fetal position, in which the head and legs are placed in toward the trunk, the spine is forced into a single convex curve. In adjusting to the efforts at raising its head while in the supine position and, later, in attempting to crawl, the infant begins to develop the anterior cervical curve. Progressing through the stages of sitting, standing, and, eventually, walking, a compensatory anterior lumbar curve develops in response to the gravitational force and the various musculoskeletal demands. However, it is not until late childhood that the mature vertebral curves occur. Adaptation of the spine to the stress of the upright posture is reflected in the increased size of the posterior aspect of the lumbar vertebrae and their thick intervertebral discs. The ilopsoas muscle serves to maintain the lumbar curve and the inclination of the pelvis and is one of the main stabilizers of the upright posture.

As the child develops posturally, there also occurs a lowering of the center of gravity, which gradually permits greater mobility in the upright position, freeing the upper extremities for fine motor activity. Lowering the center of gravity affords the child better balance and mobility.

Characteristically, the infant displays structural weaknesses until adjustment to the upright position has been accomplished. In preparation for locomotion, the child goes through various developmental periods such as sitting, crawling, creeping, and standing, which prepare him or her for the next stage. In standing and walking during the early years, the infant often displays many normal postural characteristics that in later life may be deemed abnormal, for example, flat feet, knock-knees, pronated ankles (bearing weight on the inner side of the foot), and a pointing of the toes outward for a wider base of support. Many parents and educators become needlessly alarmed at the posture of small children when, in reality, it is normal for that particular maturational level. As the child develops strength and motor control, these postural adaptations usually give way to normal alignment. However, failure at adaptation may cause postural deviations that will eventually need to be corrected by professional help. Without proper balance, nutrition, sleep, relaxation, exercise, habit formation, and a general feeling of well-being, various postural asymmetries may occur to affect the individual adversely the rest of his or her life. The prevention of severe postural anomalies is of concern to all those who deal with children (Chapter 9).

Good postural adjustment, in reality, means good body mechanics and efficiency in the use of the body.[12] This is especially important to individuals requiring an increased conservation of energy, for example, those suffering from cardiorespiratory problems or chronic musculoskeletal disorders.

REFLEX MATURATION

Whereas growth was earlier defined simply as the increase of body size, motor development is best characterized as the process by which individuals, through maturation and experience, acquire management of their bodies. It is commonly accepted that as individuals grow, they become involved with integrating various segmental and random movements into complex patterns of motor behavior. From the very beginning, children are reacting to their environments with primitive reflexes

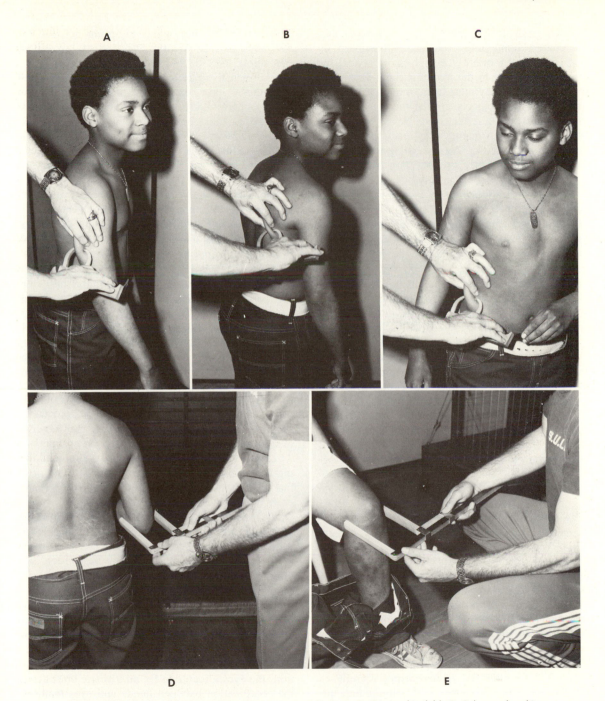

Fig. 2-7. Skin fold and biepicondylar diameter measurement. **A,** Tricep skin fold. **B,** Subscapular skin fold. **C,** Suprailiac skin fold. **D,** Humerus diameter. **E,** Femur diameter. (Courtesy of California State University, Audio Visual Center, Long Beach, Calif.)

that will gradually diminish as higher nervous system centers come into command.[16] Newborn infants attempt to orient themselves in space and time and to adjust to the many physical forces imposed on them. They must learn to manipulate both their bodies and objects around them. The more specialized a cell, a tissue, or an organ system, the longer the period of maturation. This is particularly evident in nerve tissue. As myelinization of nerves occurs phylogenetically in the young organism, it is generally followed by an improvement of motor ability. At birth, the infant's lower brain centers are well developed as compared to the cerebral cortex. Reflexes such as sucking, swallowing, yawning, and sneezing are present at birth. However, reflexes such as grasping when the palm of the hand is touched, the *startle* reflex, and the Babinski reflex (extension of the great toe and flexion of the other toes in response to stroking the plantar aspect of the foot) disappear as development progresses.

Fiorentino[16] divides normal reflexive development into the following three levels: the *apedal* (or spinal and/or brain stem) level with motor response of supine and/or prone lying; the *quadropedal* (or midbrain) level with a postural response of crawling and sitting; and the *bipedal* (or cortical) level with allowance for the action of standing and/or walking. If the normal sequential development of reflex maturation is disrupted because of neurological dysfunction, there often occurs delayed sensorimotor integration, for example, children who are diagnosed as having cerebral palsy may retain many reflexes that would normally have been replaced by the inhibiting functions of a higher neurological level.

Although reflex classification systems vary slightly, there is general agreement that a group of primitive reflexes appears and should disappear during the first year of life. These early reflexes assist the child in assuming an upright posture in preparation for ambulation. Until primitive reflexes appear in a child's neuromotor repertoire, lifting the head, rolling from supine to prone, and sitting cannot be accomplished. When primitive reflexes persist beyond the first year of life, automatic, unwanted flexion and extension of the limbs contribute to jerky, clumsy-looking movement patterns.

A second set of reflexes that facilitate maintenance of equilibrium begins to appear between the ages of 6 and 18 months and persists throughout life unless their development is inhibited in some way. When these reflexes fail to develop affected individuals have extreme difficulty maintaining balance, particularly while moving at medium and fast speeds and when attempting to change direction. Because these children do not make automatic postural adjustments when their center of gravity moves beyond their base of support, they tend to fall easily.

Because abnormal reflex development and concomitant equilibrium problems can have such a pervasive effect on efficient perceptual and motor functioning, the importance of careful evaluation in this area cannot be overemphasized.

Normal infants have rudimentary control of the head and neck in the first 4 to 6 months; then, during the seventh month, they begin to roll over from the stomach to the back. Sitting up, moving on all fours, and creeping occur in the first 7 months. With skeletal and neuromuscular maturity, children progress from crawling and creeping to the upright posture and then, between the ninth and eighteenth months, to taking independent steps.

In the early stages of walking, the young child walks with toes outward to provide a wider base of support. As strength is increased, the feet begin to realign to a straighter position. By the age of 3 or 4 years most children have acquired a mature walking habit. A wide number of variations to the original walking pattern occurs in the next 2 to 3 years, each requiring successively greater skill, for example, standing on one foot, running, climbing up and down stairs, jumping and hopping, riding a tricycle and a scooter, skipping and galloping, jumping over something, and kicking an object. All these skills can be excuted by the normal youngster by the age of 5 or 6 years.

The upright position of the human body frees the hands for fine coordinated activity. The use of the hands in prehension stems from the early grasping reflex. Purposeful manipulation by the hands can take place only when the thumb develops opposition, the eyes are able to fix on a single object, and the coordination between hands and eyes matures. Shirley[39] described the maturational sequence of hand development as (1) reaching and missing an object; (2) reaching and touching an object; (3)

reaching, grasping, and holding an object; and (4) reaching, grasping, and manipulating an object.

The rudimentary patterns of throwing, catching, and striking objects can be seen in early childhood, but a number of years is required before these become competent skills. However, proficiency in these movements is seen in typical children between the ages of 6 and 7 years. A lack of proficiency in these basic motor skills may eventually cause difficulty in engaging in play activities.

Sex difference in movement behavior is apparent early in life. From an early age, boys can be noted to perform better than do girls in most types of motor activities, which is more indicative of cultural influences than differences in physical potential. This difference gradually becomes greater during adolescence. Because of the dramatic changes in bodily proportions and functions, the pubescent boy develops increased strength, leverage, and stamina, which aid in all motor skills. Girls also go through marked physiological changes, which result in broad hips, narrow shoulders, and a low center of gravity, all of which tend to cause difficulty in improvement in motor skills. Many of the differences between adolescent girls and boys in performance have been attributed to body structure; however, social aspects are also important. In the last few years, girls' participation in vigorous physical activity has increased considerably. Since this increased interest, physical activity for girls has become more socially acceptable. In addition, there are fewer indications of sexual differences in physical performance than once were thought to exist.

As the typical child grows and matures, the motor abilities develop in an orderly and continuous manner from the simple to more complex. In this way, the child is better able to adapt to more complex problems in the environment that can be solved at present levels of motor ability. However, the instructional procedures implicit in delivering physical education for the handicapped through the Individual Education Program accommodate children at their ability levels. Consequently, the major problem for the teacher, in relation to the developing child, is to help the child engage in activities that are appropriate for his or her particular developmental level. Oxendine[33] describes readiness for motor activities as dependent on maturation, phys-

ical development, and specific prerequisites of learning. Children who, as a result of some physical, mental, or environmental factor, fail to develop motor skills appropriate for their maturational levels must be reached at their present levels of educational performance.

Children who become ill or who receive inadequate nutrition become less active in order to conserve their energies. Evidence indicates that prolonged inactivity and lack of movement experiences results in physical deterioration and motor retardation in the young. Besides affecting musculoskeletal functions, such inactivity also diminishes neural stimulation. Hebb[23] indicated that inadequate physical and mental stimulation of humans and animals results in a breakdown of their total behavior. Whether the child is typical or atypical (normal or handicapped), motor development is a factor of maturation and involves the individual's ability to modify his or her behavior for varying situations. Although a physical or mental disability may create distinct retardation of motor responses, every opportunity for a great diversity of movement experiences must be afforded the child. Only by being able to make a wide variety of movement responses can the growing child face the numerous challenges of internal bodily functions and the external demands of the environment. Each challenge, when surmounted, provides the child with a backlog of useful tools for overcoming additional and more complex problems in the future. Competency in physical play is of the greatest importance for a child's self-esteem and positive self-concept. Children (especially boys) who have poor motor ability find themselves left out of peer activities. Involuntary exclusion from play, whatever the reason, may cause the child to have feelings of devaluation.

With the growing awareness of the developmental needs of handicapped children has come the realization that motor proficiency tests are neither adequately evaluating the problem nor providing sufficient information for program planning. It is more apparent that information regarding child growth and development should be applied in planning and administering physical education programs. Disregard for principles of physical and motor development makes teaching less efficient. Children must be taught at their present levels of educational performance, otherwise they may become frustrated and use awkward movements to compensate for the inability to function at desired levels.

There can be physical growth without corresponding motor learning. Such learning is achieved through experience and experimentation with movements and patterns of movements. Physical education planned on the basis of sensorimotor experiences would be highly structured, developmental in nature, and seeking improvement in other areas through motor training.

FUNDAMENTAL MOTOR PATTERNS AND SKILLS

Whoever coined the phrase *first things first* said a great deal in a few words. The development of fundamental motor patterns is of paramount importance to the development of specific and more complex skills and therefore should not be overlooked in physical education programs.

It was the intent of legislation for education of the handicapped that all children should have the opportunity to learn to use their bodies appropriately and to develop motor skills. One of the prerequisites for efficient movement is the development of fundamental motor patterns. A child who is unable to perform the fundamental movement patterns will have difficulty developing the more specific motor skills that are used for recreation.

Although there may be disagreement among authorities as to what the characteristics of a fundamental motor skill are, for the purpose of this discussion fundamental motor patterns are those movement patterns that are, for the most part, inherent in the development of all children. Fundamental motor skills, on the other hand, are more specific and are prerequisite to specific sport skills. The fundamental motor patterns are usually less complex than are fundamental motor skills, and often the fundamental motor patterns give rise to the fundamental skills. Discrimination between the two concepts is especially relevant for programs of

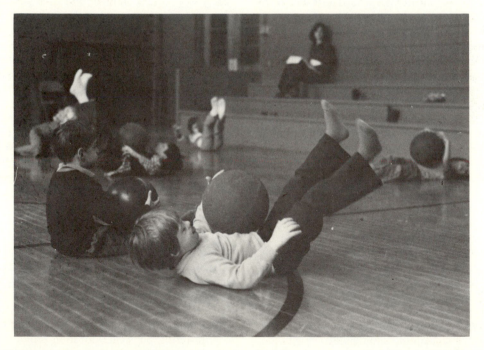

Fig. 2-8. Fundamental motor patterns that require bending. (Courtesy of Julian Stein, American Alliance for Health, Physical Education, Recreation, and Dance, and Project PERMIT, Tennessee Technological University, Cookeville, Tenn.)

physical education of younger and more severely handicapped children because it enables the teacher to focus on the specific aspects of development. To assist the reader in distinguishing between motor patterns and motor skills, lists of behaviors of both categories are provided below.

Fundamental motor patterns

1. *Balancing:* Innervation of one side of the body against the other to maintain body equilibrium against the forces of gravity
2. *Bending:* Flexion, extension, abduction, adduction, circumduction, rotation, eversion, inversion, and utilization of all the dimensions of movement of each joint of the body.
3. *Bouncing:* Short bipedal jumps involving a series of small jumps
4. *Climbing:* Using arms and legs to raise the body against the gravitational force
5. *Crawling:* Developmental pattern involving alternate use of opposite hand and leg to move in a prone position
6. *Creeping:* Pattern of locomotion in which the individual propels himself or herself on hands and knees
7. *Crouching:* Flexion of ankles, knees, hips, and trunk
8. *Falling:* Acceptance of force as a result of gravitational pull
9. *Galloping:* Running with a leap interpolated after every other stride
10. *Hanging:* Resistance of weight against gravitational pull with arms or legs fixed and supported by an object
11. *Holding:* Exerting enough upward force against an object to balance gravity's pull so that the object has no vertical motion
12. *Hopping:* Propulsive force exerted by one foot, followed by landing on same foot
13. *Jumping:* Propulsive force exerted by one or two feet, but both feet contact the ground simultaneously
14. *Landing:* Acceptance of loss of kinetic energy when contacting a surface
15. *Leaping:* Propulsive force made by one foot with the landing made on the other
16. *Lifting:* Overcoming the gravitational force of an object by employing external resistance of muscles of the body

17. *Pulling:* Overcoming a resistance so that an object will move toward the body
18. *Pushing:* Overcoming a resistance in a direction away from the body
19. *Reaching:* Movement of arms away from the medial aspect of the body and over head
20. *Rising:* Raising the center of gravity
21. *Rocking:* Rhythmic transfer of center of gravity
22. *Rolling:* Imparting motion to an object with an underhand movement so that it travels along a horizontal surface
23. *Running:* Locomotion in which a flight phase is generated (from continuous movement)
24. *Skipping:* Continuous movement in which a hop is followed by a leap
25. *Starting:* Overcoming inertia of the body at rest by a muscular contraction
26. *Stooping:* Hip, knee, and ankle flexion that lowers the center of gravity over the base
27. *Stopping:* Overcoming the inertia of the body while it is in motion to bring it to a rest
28. *Stretching:* Maximum movement of a joint
29. *Striking:* Using an implement to hit an object
30. *Swinging:* To-and-fro movement with the body suspended from a fixed object (body parts and object can also swing)
31. *Touching:* Tactile stimulation to hand rendering it possible to discriminate the texture, size, and shape of an object
32. *Trotting:* Slow run in which there is a flight phase
33. *Walking:* Continuous locomotor movement with the body in an upright posture involving a swing phase, contact, double support, and propulsion sequence that gives the body a linear direction

Fundamental motor skills

1. *Carrying:* Exploration of lifting weights relative to base of support and experimentation with muscle groups most capable of coping with objects carried by the body
2. *Catching:* Executing the complicated match between hand and eye in an attempt to control an external moving object
3. *Dodging:* Ability to stop and change direction relative to visual or auditory cue
4. *Dribbling:* Matching hand and eye or foot and

eye, while moving the entire body, in order to control a ball bouncing or rolling on the floor

5. *Hitting:* Swift contact by hand with an external object (implement not used)
6. *Kicking:* Matching foot and eye so that leg and foot may exert force to propel an object
7. *Passing:* Propulsive force given to an object held in hands (many times a graded response)
8. *Pivoting:* Transference of weight to one foot with angular velocity applied so as to move body around a fixed point
9. *Punching:* Hitting with no preliminary movement
10. *Tagging:* Reaching and touching while running activities
11. *Throwing:* Imparting force to an object held in the hand and releasing it to give it desired direction or distance
12. *Tossing:* Short throw with graded impetus
13. *Tumbling:* Continuous transfer of weight from one part of the body to the other in a smooth fashion
14. *Twisting:* Rotation of a body part or the total body
15. *Vaulting:* Transfer of weight and center of gravity from feet to hands to feet in a continuous direction

Fundamental motor skills can often be thought of as having the characteristic of qualitative motor performance, which requires hand/eye or foot/eye coordination, manual dexterity, or refined body coordination. Fundamental motor skills usually take longer, to reach optimal levels of proficiency than do the fundamental motor patterns.

Although each physical educator may have his or her own classification system for the fundamental motor patterns and skills, the movements of handicapped children should be comprehensively reviewed so that their motor needs can be programmed in a systematic fashion.

PSYCHOSOCIAL IMPLICATIONS

To understand the atypical individual adequately, the physical educator must become sensitive to the innumerable psychological and sociological factors that interact within each person. To explain human behavior fully as it relates to exceptionality would be an extremely difficult task.

Therefore this section is intended to survey some of the more relevant psychosocial areas that relate to the handicapped person.

A handicap could be considered any encumbrance or disadvantage that makes personal goals more difficult to attain than if the disability were not present. If this concept is accepted, it can be speculated that most persons are handicapped in some manner. It should be apparent to all that whether one wears glasses, is a member of an ethnic minority, or is unable to continue to work because of paralysis, *an individual's psychological reaction to a disability is personal, unique, and relative to his or her social environment.* In other words, an individual with a particular disability must not be expected to act in a prescribed manner, nor must handicapped persons in general be expected to cope differently with life's problems than the nonhandicapped population.[5]

One must recognize that the person who is handicapped by a disability must adjust not only to his or her own limitations but also to the demands of society. Because of the numerous adjustments required of the severely disabled, psychological problems may be more frequent and serious than with individuals who are not handicapped.[11] However, there is no guarantee that because an individual is mentally, physically, or emotionally disabled he or she will react differently than a person who does not have such a disability.

Individual adaptation

Man's adaptation and adjustment to the stresses of life are dependent on individual personality. Allport[1] broadly defined personality as "what a man really is." More descriptively, personality is "the dynamic organization within the individual of those psychophysical systems that determine his unique adjustments to his environment." This definition implies that personality is ever changing. The total human organism is in a constant state of flux. To acquire a healthy or positive adjustment to life, an individual must constantly be able to interact with the environment. The well-adjusted person is realistic in the requirements placed on self and the environment.

Adaptation by the individual begins at conception and continues throughout life. In the primary years, life's problems are resolved through the method of trial and error. As successes and failures are gradually incurred, the individual builds a backlog of ways of handling various psychosocial problems. The exceptional individual may be denied many of life's experiences. Placed frequently in new psychological situations, handicapped persons may find coping with their disabilities difficult and may resort to numerous adjustment mechanisms to alleviate the psychological pain. However, whether this adjustment is healthy or unhealthy is primarily dependent on how the individual has met the primary psychological growth stages, which include (1) *dependence and deprivation,* (2) *autonomy and discipline,* (3) *sexual development,* and (4) *management of aggression.*[42]

The first 6 months of a child's life represent a time of complete dependence, in which primary concern is satiation of the immediate biological needs. Unsuccessful efforts to fulfill personal needs may result in a denial of reality. This early period helps to establish foundations for later behavior and determines whether the individual learns to trust or mistrust the immediate surroundings. If personal requirements are satisfied without undue duress, there is a good chance the individual will develop self-confidence and a positive self-concept, whereas a constant struggle to satisfy basic needs may lead to personal discontent and an environmental mistrust. Janov[25] describes the primary needs of the infant as those of being "fed, kept warm and dry, . . . held and caressed, and . . . stimulated."

As the child emerges from the helpless period, he or she gradually seeks independence. Increasingly, the child strives to control the immediate surroundings. As successful authority is gained over the environment, self-confidence is also gained. However, a constant thwarting of desired independence, as experienced by many disabled children, may eventually lead to discouragement and feelings of devaluation. With the second and third years of life, the individual stores a milieu of experiences and explores the new vistas of movement and speech. This also becomes a time for learning discipline. Through the imposition of guidelines and rules, the child learns behavior control. Complete freedom of expression produces within the individual unruly behavior, whereas a

lack of adequate freedom produces fears and a rigidity of personality. Therefore, the right amount of discipline and freedom becomes a subtle matter of creating or establishing a firm, but loving and accepting, environment.

Sexual development is of primary importance to the total personality of an individual. Most authorities concur that sexual needs are apparent from earliest childhood. Feelings of affection, jealousies, and desires for bodily contact and caresses are basic to personality development. It is not until puberty, coupled with its obvious physiological changes, that the powerful sexual motive often presents overt problems of adjustment. Changes of body structure and the development of secondary sex characteristics, together with a newly acquired sex drive, serve to create unique conflicts for the individual. The individual views himself or herself and others in a new perspective. Peer acceptance becomes uppermost in the thoughts and actions of the adolescent. The turmoil of adolescence becomes an extremely crucial period for the handicapped person, when he or she must face the added burden of the impairment and perhaps the depressing realization that love of the opposite sex, courtship, and marriage may be difficult or impossible.

The maturing individual must also cope with aggression, a general term referring to the emotion of anger or hostility that stems from frustration. The seeds of aggression and its attending anxiety are sown early in a child's life when the attempts at environmental control are thwarted. Psychologists have described three basic ways that persons manage their anger or aggression: (1) *directing anger toward the environment,* (2) *directing anger toward the person,* and (3) *coping with anger in socially acceptable ways.* Depending on in individual personality and circumstances, the venting of anger can be rational or irrational, overt or covert. Misplaced hostility acted out on society may become expressed in violence, prejudice, or bigotry. Also, a fear of the consequence of acting out anger may become inverted to a feeling of self-hate that may be manifested, in its most severe state, in self-annihilation. A healthy ability to cope with anger requires an understanding of its cause, an acceptance of its presence, and the ability to direct it into acceptable channels of expression. Anger is one of the most difficult emotions to manage because of its numerous social implications. As a result, handicapped persons could feel threatened by acting out normal anger because of their extreme dependency on others or, on the other hand, they may strike out in retaliation against a world that has caused them much pain and unhappiness. Aggression for handicapped children may also take the form of tantrums as a means of gaining attention or of controlling the environment.

Social development follows closely the other factors of personal development already mentioned. Man is a *social being,* with much of his success based on how well he gets along with others. Basically, the involvement of the individual in group situations emerges slowly from self-centeredness to the gregariousness of the teenager.

The family

The family has a great influence on the total lifestyle of the disabled child. Children who have severe or prolonged disabilities often are delayed in normal growth and development. Their life experiences are limited, with childhood extending far beyond the normal period. Long suffering often results in a preoccupation with the self and an emotional dependency on parents. Through the family and parental influences, personality strengths and weaknesses are forged to form adaptive mechanisms against the psychosocial stresses of life. Children have a tendency to view their disabilities in the same manner as do their parents. If parents regard them unrealistically, then the children fail to understand their limitations. Kessler[26] described the most common parental attitudes as oversolicitude, rejection, pushing the children to succeed beyond their abilities, and inconsistency in behavior toward the children.

The impact of an abnormal child on the family defies generalizations. Each child and each family presents an individual set of problems, requiring individual solutions. Any meaningful assessment of the impact of an abnormal child on the family requires an understanding of the family members as people—how they feel, how they live, their hopes and aspirations, their fears, their [religious] beliefs, their cultural, social, educational, and economic background.[26]

Ideally, genuine love, warmth, and acceptance of their handicapped child on the part of the parents are the most important factors for the development of a well-adjusted personality.

Of great importance to the parents of a disabled child are the problems of overprotection, dependence, and independence. As is the case with most children, the disabled child needs to develop independence wherever possible. Overprotection or extended help, especially when the child is very capable, confines and narrows growth possibilities. The feeling of dependency can be both a frightening and a depressing experience.[5]

Many stresses and strains can be experienced in a family with a disabled child. The husband and wife may feel guilt and remorse for having this child. Anger and frustration may be displaced and vented on the child or siblings. Brothers and sisters may feel deprived of the attention of the parents, sensing that they are relegated to second place in the hearts and minds of the parents. Kohut stated:

It is not surprising, then, that well children become bitter and vent their anger on the abnormal child. In some instances, children act out the underlying hostility and anger felt by parents. . . . Older children are sometimes ashamed of an abnormal brother or sister. . . . Also, some will wonder if the disability is inherited and how this will affect their chances for marriage.[28]

No matter what the disability, the handicapped child must have responsibilities within the scope of his or her particular capabilities and must be depended on to carry them out. Praise and acknowledgment must follow each new accomplishment; however, caution must be taken that a parent does not become oversolicitous and overindulgent. A child who becomes too much the center of attention, or egocentric, fails to experience the pleasure that comes from sharing with others.

The school

Because of the limited opportunities for experiencing social situations, the disabled children may find school difficult. Cruickshank[11] indicated that handicapped children very often find difficulty in verbalizing or communicating frustration, self-consciousness, and disappointment. The children often hesitate in new social situations, wondering whether they will be accepted, pitied, patronized, praised, rejected, or ignored. Therefore, feelings of inferiority may crop up when the children attempt new things or suddenly find themselves in competitive situations with normal children. It is extremely important that exceptional children be accepted by their peers. Family acceptance is vital for healthy psychological adjustment. A positive self-concept is largely attributable to the attitudes of peers and how they relate to exceptional children. A concerted effort must be made by schools and teachers to help normal children understand and accept their atypical schoolmates.

The National Easter Seal Society for Crippled Children and Adults offers the following list of suggestions to aid the relationship between nondisabled and disabled persons:*

1. First of all remember that the person with a handicap is a person. He is like anyone else, except for the special limitations of his handicap.
2. A disability need not be ignored or denied between friends. But until your relationship is that, show friendly interest in him as a person.
3. Be yourself when you meet him.
4. Talk about the same things as you would with anyone else.
5. Help him only when he requests it. When a handicapped person falls, he may wish to get up by himself, just as many blind persons prefer to get along without assistance. So offer help but wait for his request before giving it.
6. Be patient. Let the handicapped person set his own pace in walking or talking.
7. Don't be afraid to laugh with him.
8. Don't stop and stare when you see a handicapped person you do not know. He deserves the same courtesy any person should receive.
9. Don't be overprotective or oversolicitous. Don't shower the handicapped person with kindness.
10. Don't ask embarrassing questions. If the handicapped person wants to tell you about his disability, he will bring up the subject himself.
11. Don't offer pity or charity. The handicapped person wants to be treated as an equal. He wants a chance to prove himself.
12. Don't separate a disabled person from his wheelchair or crutches unless he asks it. He may want them within reach.
13. When dining with a handicapped person, don't offer help in cutting his food. He will ask you or the waiter if he needs it.

14. Don't make up your mind ahead of time about the handicapped person. You may be surprised at how wrong you are in judging his interests and abilities.
15. Enjoy your friendship with the handicapped person. His philosophy and good humor will give you inspiration.

Self-esteem

How handicapped children view themselves as persons is extremely important to their total psychosocial adjustment. Children construct a sense of uniqueness and exclusiveness from the responses they elicit from other persons. If, for the most part, others' reactions are affirming, then a positive self-perception is acquired. If, however, a negative response is elicited, a variety of defense mechanisms may be used unconsciously by disabled persons to protect themselves against threats to self-esteem and the feelings of pain and anxiety.

The sense of personal worth or self-esteem is attained by individuals from their earliest strivings for autonomy and independence. A feeling of competence comes from accomplishing intended goals. However, when failure becomes the predominant experience, individuals develop a low self-evaluation. How persons value themselves is predominantly determined by society. Acquisition of feelings of personal worth begins with the family, expands to the playground and the school, and, subsequently, encompasses total experience.

Early group acceptance and self-esteem stem almost solely from one's appearance and ability to engage actively in play. Children who deviate considerably in looks and actions may find denial of group membership. Without active participation within the group, handicapped children may find personal adjustment difficult. Because opportunities for peer approval and recognition may be lacking, the courage to face many of life's problems fails to develop.

Atypical children soon become aware that others consider them different, treat them differently, and hold different expectations of them. They soon realize that society places a high premium on an attractive appearance and a normal body. Cruickshank[11] described the disabled as being in an extremely untenable position in society. The disabled are denied the satisfaction of being disabled; to be accepted by society, they must continually strive to

*From When you meet a handicapped person. By permission of the National Easter Seal Society for Crippled Children and Adults, Chicago.

overcome their handicaps, often with minimal success. Such social pressures may cause psychological problems of adjustment and adaptation. Experiencing prejudice, discrimination, and lack of status, children perceive themselves as less worthy and capable individuals. To the disabled, society may serve only to produce emotional distress, conflict, and development of a defense system.

Physique is one of the most important factors in the total development of personality. It is primarily through exploring and discovering the functions of the body that children conceptualize themselves as distinct persons. Body image has been described as the way in which individuals picture their bodies or, in other words, it is a system of ideas and feelings that the individuals have about their physical structure. Wittreich and Grace[43] incorporated the concept of body image into expectation of present and future behavior by stating that ''in every percept, or in every act, the individual is making some prediction as to what his body can do.''

Physically or mentally handicapped children may be denied the many experiences that can be derived from movement. Lacking a positive body image, the children may consider themselves marginal persons, rejected from the mainstream of life.

The well-adjusted person uses defense mechanisms moderately without jeopardizing personal identity or a positive self-concept. A sense of being a distinct person in society requires an understanding and acceptance of the self with its strengths and its weaknesses. Various qualities such as physical makeup, temperament, mental abilities, and special abilities, are reflected in behavior, affecting the individual's outlook on life and unique perception of self.

Reaction to sudden physical loss

The individual who suddenly receives a severe physical disability must face many crucial psychosocial adjustments. Because the body is an integral part of a person's total personality, any alteration in its function or appearance constitutes a threat to the total organism. The ultimate adjustment to a recent handicapping condition is dependent on the individual's mental health at the time the condition occurs. Ideally, the person with a handicap should not only fully acknowledge limitations but, above all, be realistically aware of his or her personal attributes and capabilities. In doing so, the individual shows the ability to adapt to new situations and to grow to become a more positively functioning person. The experienced teacher or therapist in a well-planned program of adapted physical education can do much to help the handicapped individual adjust satisfactorily to limitations and to environments.

A developmental point of view seems most essential to program planning for disabled children. It takes as its point of departure the child's basic nature and needs. It acknowledges the racial implications that determine sequences and the distinctive growth patterns of each individual child. Because of the great variability in the motor skills of the generic handicapped population, this philosophy seems particularly applicable. A perceptiveness of growth appears most indispensable for accurate guidance in establishing programs in physical education and recreation. It demands that the teacher be alert to the growth needs of the child and be able to answer the follwoing questions: ''How does the child grow?'' ''How does the child learn?'' and ''How does the child advance from stage to stage as he or she matures?'' These three questions are really one: ''How can the tremendous heterogeneity in needs among the handicapped population be met?''

Programs should intervene, assist, direct, postpone, encourage, and discourage many turns of development. They should create the most favorable conditions for self-regulation and self-adjustment.

It is necessary to remember that growth is a unified process and that the forces affecting one phase of development make an imprint on others as well. There is no step in the growth process that can be bypassed without consequence to subsequent development.

It becomes apparent that there should be a reduction in the tendency to adhere to chronological and mental age norms and scales. Rather, the child should be viewed in terms of maturity. The disabled child's behavior is a result of a composite of factors that cannot be defined adequately by chronological or mental age alone. The lable *handicapped* tells little about the needs, characteristics, motor abilities, and limitations of the child. A diagnosis should be made of each child regarding motor and physical characteristics and subsequent plans should be implemented to meet the defined needs.

REFERENCES

1. Allport, G. W.: Personality: a psychological interpretation, New York, 1937, Holt, Rinehart & Winston, Inc.
2. Ames, L. B.: The sequential patterns of prone progression in the human infant, Genet. Psychol. Monogr. **19:**411-460, 1937.
3. Ansubel, D. P.: Theory and problems of adolescent development, New York, 1954, Grune & Stratton, Inc.
4. Arnheim, D. D., and Sinclair, W. A.: The clumsy child: a program of motor therapy, ed. 2, St. Louis, 1979, The C. V. Mosby Co.
5. Baldwin, C. P., and Baldwin, A. L.: Personality and social development of handicapped children. In Psychology of the handicapped child, Washington, D.C., 1974, U.S. Department of Health, Education, and Welfare.
6. Bayley, N.: Manual for the Bayley Scales of Infant Development, New York, 1969, The Psychological Corporation.
7. Bleck, E., and Nagel, D. A.: Physically handicapped children: a medical atlas for teachers, New York, 1975, Grune & Stratton, Inc.
8. Cratty, B. J.: Movement behavior and motor learning, Philadelphia, 1967, Lea & Febiger.
9. Cratty, B. J.: Perceptual and motor development in infants and children, New York, 1970, Macmillan Publishing Co., Inc.
10. Cratty, B. J.: Perceptual-motor behavior and educational processes, Springfield, Ill., 1969, Charles C Thomas, Publisher.
11. Cruickshank, W., editor: Psychology of exceptional children and youth, Englewood Cliffs, N.J., 1966, Prentice-Hall, Inc.
12. Cureton, T. K., Jr.: Physical fitness appraisal and guidance, St. Louis, 1947, The C. V. Mosby Co.
13. Damon, A.: Adult weight gain, accuracy of stated weight and their implications for constitutional anthropology, Am. J. Phys. Anthropol. **23:**307-311, 1965.
14. Espenschade, A. S., and Eckert, H. M.: Motor development, Columbus, Ohio, 1967, Charles E. Merrill Publishing Co.
15. Fiorentino, M. R.: Normal and abnormal development, Springfield, Ill., 1972, Charles C Thomas, Publisher.
16. Fiorentino, M. R.: Reflex testing methods for evaluating C.N.S. development, ed. 2, Springfield, Ill., 1970, Charles C Thomas, Publisher.
17. Folio, M., and DuBose, R. F.: Peabody developmental motor scales, rev. experimental ed., IMRID, Behavioral Science Monograph, serial no. 25, Nashville, Tenn., 1974, George Peabody College.
18. Frankenberg, W. K., and Dodds, J. B.: The Denver Developmental Screening Test, J. Pediatr. **71:**181-191, 1967.
19. Gesell, A., et al.: The first five years of life, London, 1950, Methuen and Co. Ltd.
20. Guttridge, M. V.: A study of motor achievements of young children, Arch. Psychol. **244:**1-17, 1939.
21. Halverson, H. M.: Studies of the grasping responses of early infancy, J. Genet. Psychol. **51:**371-449, 1937.
22. Heath, B. H., and Carter, J. E.: A modified somatotype method, Am. J. Phys. Anthropol. **27:**57-74, 1967.
23. Hebb, D. O.: The mammal and his environment, Am. J. Psychiatry **3:**826-871, 1955.
24. Hughes, J. G.: Synopsis of pediatrics, ed. 5, St. Louis, 1979, The C. V. Mosby Co.
25. Janov, A.: The primal scream, New York, 1970, Dell Publishing Co., Inc.
26. Kessler, J. W.: The impact of disability on the child, J. Am. Phys. Ther. Assoc. **46:**153-159, 1966.
27. Knobloch, H., and Pasamanick, B.: Gesell and Amatruda's developmental diagnosis, 1974, Harper & Row, Publishers.
28. Kohut, S. A.: The abnormal child: his impact on the family, J. Am. Phys. Ther. Assoc. **46:**160-167, 1966.
29. Koontz, C. W.: Koontz Child Developmental Programs training activities for the first 48 months, Los Angeles, 1974, Western Psychological Services.
30. LeWinn, E. B.: Human neurological organization, Springfield, Ill., 1969, Charles C Thomas, Publisher.
31. Logan, G. A.: Adaptations of muscular activity, Belmont, Calif., 1964, Wadsworth Publishing Co., Inc.
32. Montoye, H. I., editor: An introduction to measurement in physical education, Indianapolis, 1970, Phi Epsilon Kappa Fraternity.
33. Oxendine, J. B.: Psychology of motor learning, New York, 1968, Appleton-Century-Crofts.
34. Parnell, R. W.: Somatotyping by physical anthropometry, Am. J. Phys. Anthropol. **12:**209-239, 1954.
35. Rarick, L.: Motor development during infancy and childhood, Madison, 1954, University of Wisconsin.
36. Roach, E. G., and Kephart, N. C.: The Purdue perceptual-motor survey, Columbus, Ohio, 1966, Charles E. Merrill Publishing Co.
37. Sheldon, W. H.: The varieties of human physique, New York, 1940, Harper & Row, Publishers.
38. Sheldon, W. H., Hartl, E. M., and McDermott, E.: Varieties of delinquent youth, New York, 1949, Harper & Row, Publishers.
39. Shirley, M. M.: The first two years: a study of twenty-five babies, Minneapolis, 1931, University of Minnesota Press.
40. Wellman, B. L.: Motor performance of preschool children, Child Educ. **13:**311-316, 1937.
41. Wellman, B. L., and McCaskill, C. L.: Study of common motor achievements at the preschool age, Child Dev. **9:**141-150, 1938.
42. White, R. W.: The abnormal personality, New York, 1964, The Ronald Press Co.
43. Wittreich, W. J., and Grace, M.: Body image development, Unpublished progress report to the Office of Naval Research, 1955.
44. Wright, B. A.: Physical disability—a psychological approach, New York, 1960, Harper & Row, Publishers.

RECOMMENDED READINGS

Baldwin, A. L.: Theories of child development, New York, 1967, John Wiley & Sons, Inc.
Barker, R. G.: Adjustment to physical handicap and illness: a survey of the social psychology of physique and disability, New York, 1953, Social Science Research Council.

Bayley, N.: The development of motor activities during the first three years, Soc. Res. Child Dev. Monogr. **1**:1-26, 1935.

Fisher, S., and Cleveland, S. E.: Body image and personality, ed. 2, New York, 1968, Dover Publication, Inc.

Garrett, J. F., and Levine, E. S.: Psychological practices with the physically disabled, New York, 1962, Columbia University Press.

Ginott, H. G.: Between parent and child, New York, 1965, Macmillan Publishing Co., Inc.

Kephart, N. C.: The slow learner in the classroom, Columbus, Ohio, 1964, Charles E. Merrill Publishing Co.

Telford, C. W., and Sawrey, J. M.: The exceptional individual, Englewood Cliffs, N.J., 1967, Prentice-Hall, Inc.

3

Factors in perceptual-motor development

Perception enables persons to accurately interpret events and information so that they may respond in meaningful ways. Before engaging in meaningful physical activity persons must accurately assess the information that is relevant to task performance. This chapter will discuss the perceptual-motor abilities that are prerequisites to acquiring motor skills for purposeful leisure and community living. Sport skills are developed through directive practice. However, sport skills can be learned efficiently only if essential prerequisite perceptual abilities have been developed. Thus, it is important to make a clear distinction between sport skills and activities designed to develop prerequisite perceptual abilities. Examples of sport skills are dribbling and shooting in basketball; serving, setting, spiking, and digging in volleyball; and fielding, hitting, and catching in baseball. All of these specific sport skills require practice. However, the attainment of levels of proficiency is dependent on prerequisite perceptual abilities such as hand-eye coordination, timing, kinesthetic motor awareness, balance, and rhythm. Perceptual abilities enable persons to learn sport skills, are fairly resistant to forgetting, and are acquired through participation in varied motor activities. Sport skills, on the other hand, are acquired through practice, have little transfer to the learning of other skills, and are retained less well than are perceptual abilities.

The development of proficient sport skills and academic tasks is dependent on the presence of perceptual abilities associated with specific tasks. It is meaningful to those who implement physical education programs to understand the relationship between perceptual abilities and specific motor skills to be taught to handicapped children. The teacher with knowledge of the perceptual abilities required for each sport skill can gain valuable information about why children have difficulty in learning a specific skill.

Legislation for education of the handicapped requires that instruction of educational tasks be at the present level of the child's educational performance. The identification of perceptual abilities is essential for determining present levels of educational performance on specific tasks. For instance, two severely handicapped persons may have difficulty in ascending stairs: one person may have impaired balance that prevents appropriate and safe ascent, whereas the other may have visual problems that prevent appropriate placement of the feet on the steps. In each case the programming would be different. Thus, it is necessary to observe and analyze the perceptual abilities of each person so that programming can be directed toward the perceptual deficits. Procedures for analyzing tasks will be discussed in Chapter 4.

FUNDAMENTAL MOTOR PATTERNS AND SKILLS AND PERCEPTUAL-MOTOR DEVELOPMENT

Kephart,[13] Ayres,[2] and Frostig[8] indicate that visuomotor activity is a prerequisite to the development of cognitive skills. Motor activity that enhances the development of perceptual abilities involves fundamental motor patterns and skills that require visuomotor experience.

Perception enables one to establish a relationship with the environment. Skillful movement will be severely impaired in the presence of a perceptual deficit that is related to a specific sport skill. It is an established fact that perceptual abilities can be developed for most persons. Thus, once the perceptual abilities have been identified as deficient in a specific sport or academic task, meaningful programming can be planned.

Perception enables persons to identify objects and interpret events; thus, it assists in learning. There is a growing awareness in the field of physical education that perceptual abilities differentiate poor and proficient performers of some motor tasks. Therefore, the perceptual development of children cannot be overlooked. Task-oriented programs that are sequentially constructed to develop perceptual abilities are important to adapted physical education programs as well as programs for normal children. *

Normal perception is essential to the efficient learning of sport and academic skills. A person must accurately perceive symbols that form words before meaning can be attached to the words. There is evidence that fulfillment of sensorimotor

*See references 3, 10, 12, and 13.

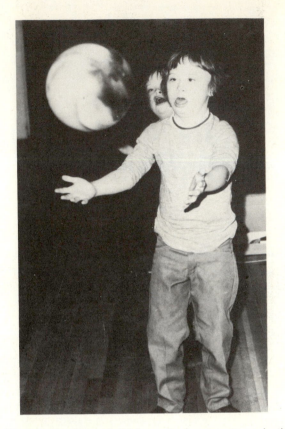

Fig. 3-1. Handicapped children who function at preschool cognitive and motor levels learn to focus attention on a ball and track with their eyes.

prerequisites may assist in the development of cognitive abilities.

Reading is one of the highest cognitive abilities, requiring many perceptual functions; consequently, children younger than 5 years usually do not read well. Perceptual-motor development training programs are desirable for school-age children who function at preschool levels of development. These programs are particularly valuable to children who have delays in perceptual development (Fig. 3-1).

PERCEPTUAL-MOTOR DEVELOPMENT AND THE DISABLED

There is a need for perceptual programs for disabled children because perception is required for many of the learning activities that are required by

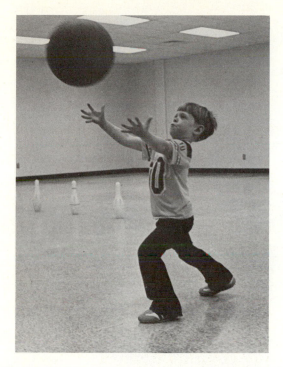

Fig. 3-2. Catching a ball requires ocular tracking and hand eye coordination. (Courtesy of the Special Education Early Childhood Intervention Program, University of Kansas, Lawrence.)

the schools. Normal children develop perception when movement experiences are paired with auditory, visual, and tactile information. Children who are physically, mentally, or emotionally impaired may be limited in perceptual ability and may require some form of perceptual training (Fig. 3-2). Mentally retarded children, for example, are limited in the ability to use sensory information and past experience to solve problems. The basic components of the perceptual process that are involved in solving motor problems require assessment and treatment in the case of each learner (whether handicapped or normal). Approximately 20% of the normal population could benefit from perceptual training to use sensory information better and, consequently, to solve problems more efficiently.

Frequently, handicapped children are limited in their ability to physically explore the environment; thus, they have difficulty developing perception. Depending on the nature of the handicap, adapta-

tion may be necessary to compensate for the sensate deficit. The following are examples of such adaptations:

1. Blind children must learn to perceive objects through audition or touch.
2. In physical activities, the blind can receive verbal or braille instruction or manual guidance.
3. To receive instruction, deaf children must refine their vision in order to develop skill in lipreading.
4. Physically handicapped children may have had limited motor experience and therefore may not have developed coordination between their senses and movements; thus adaptation may be needed (Fig. 3-3).
5. Slow learners or children with minimal brain injuries often are deficient in all areas of perception.

The physical educator's failure to consider the impact of the handicapped child's limited perceptual capability on his or her total development severely limits the possibility of enhancing that development.

Perceptual development vs. perceptual adaptation

There are two possible ways of dealing with perceptual impairments of handicapped children so that they may interact effectively in their environments: one is through participation in activities that will facilitate perceptual development; the other is to modify the environmental demands to enable children to participate in physical activities even though they lack the perceptual prerequisites. Age, comprehension level, and extent of neuromotor impairment all enter into the decision of whether a developmental or adaptational program should be attempted with children who have perceptual difficulties. In some cases the answer is clearcut. For example, we change visual cues to auditory cues for the blind child; in so doing we adapt the environmental demands to enable the child to participate more fully. In other cases the decision is not so easily made. In general, the younger the child, regardless of neuromotor impairment and comprehension level, the more promising the developmental approach; the older the child, the less effective the results from an excellent developmental pro-

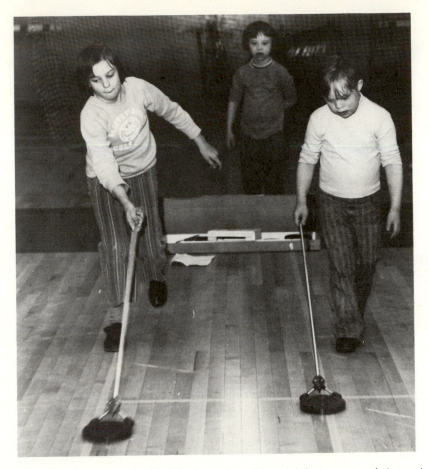

Fig. 3-3. Handicapped children move their bodies and shuffleboard disks in space as their eyes inspect.

gram. Because of a tendency to compensate for perceptual impairments, older children may benefit more fully from an adaptive approach than from a developmental approach.

Section 504 makes note of the concept of *reasonable accommodation*.[17] In a related sense, the adaptation of the environment to a handicapped child's perceptual problem so that he or she may successfully participate in activities with the nonhandicapped is a form of reasonable accommodation. Such accommodation, of course, is to be undertaken if it does not cause undue hardship on those persons who are to implement the program.

The focus of this chapter will be directed toward procedures for development of perceptual abilities. Other chapters specify procedures for adapting the environment so that handicapped children with perceptual and sensory deficits may successfully participate in physical activities in regular physical education class.

PERCEPTUAL DEVELOPMENT

Children need primary perceptual-motor experiences in order to master higher-order perceptual-motor skills. The instructor must assess the learner's present abilities and select tasks that will enhance perceptual-motor functioning.

It is accepted that early perceptual learning is

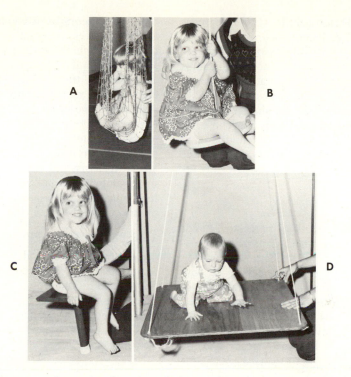

Fig. 3-4. Assisting sensory integration through vestibular stimulation. **A,** Swinging and twisting in a net. **B,** Bouncing and turning on a swing. **C,** Balancing on a "T" stool. **D,** Maintaining balance on a platform swing. (Courtesy of California State University, Audio Visual Center, Long Beach, Calif.)

provided through differential movement experiences.* Early in development, a child moves his or her body in fundamental motor patterns, gaining strength and mobility as a consequence. As the child's body moves from object to object the pairing of eye functioning with muscular movement enables the child to structure objects visually in space and to determine their spatial relationships to the self. For instance, if a child sees a table that is 15 feet away, the visual placement of the table from the child has been developed through a visuomotor match. This match results from repeated comparisons of motor movements with eye functioning: the child perceives the table as large when he or she is close and small when he or she is far away. As the child moves toward the table, he or she perceives it as becoming larger and larger; the child can accurately measure the distance to the ta-

ble only through a comparison of the distance covered with the enlarging of the image. Thus, the confirmation of objects in space, as perceived by the eye, is the result of movement experiences paired with visual experiences. Kephart[13] has indicated that movement enhances the development of vision and contributes to interpretation of visual objects in space.

Perceptual development is cumulative in that the utilization of each additional motor experience provides opportunities for the person to seek more and varied experiences. Engaging in new experiences greatly expands motor capability; thus, perceptual-motor capability increases in almost geometric proportions. On the other hand, stereotyped motor activity may contribute to a lag in perceptual development because of the lack of new developmental experience. "Furthermore, handicapped children who lag in early motor development may be afflicted with maldevelopment in the social and emo-

---

*See references 2, 11, 12, and 16.

tional spheres.''[18] These aspects of development are interrelated, and deficiency in motor development may adversely affect other aspects of development such as the social and/or emotional factors. Society has expectations of a child at each level of development; therefore, if the individual is unable to fulfill the expectancies of a certain age, particularly in the areas of self-help skills, psychosocial stresses may arise. Furthermore, if a child is incapable of accurately perceiving reality, then his or her adaptability to the environment is adversely affected.

Educational approaches

There are several systems of perceptual-motor training. Among them are those proposed by Frostig and Horne,[9] Dunsing and Kephart,[6] and Ayres.[2] The Frostig approach is primarily concerned with visual-perceptual skills as they relate to reading, and the purpose of the training is to achieve skills related to these particular ends. Frostig also incorporates gross motor behavior in her program of educational remediation.[8] Kephart[13] poses training based on a theory of perceptual-motor development that emphasizes the child's orientation to the environment. Kephart's concern is with learning problems in which the perceptual process is incomplete. Therefore, in training the child, he frequently returns to basic motor patterns and motor experiences that enable one to attain adequate relationships between one's body and the environment in a spatial-temporal context. Ayres,[2] on the other hand, proposes a neurophysiologically based program intended to assist the child with a learning disorder in developing normal sensory integration through techniques that stimulate the tactile, vestibular, and proprioceptive systems (Fig. 3-4).

THE PERCEPTUAL PROCESS

Perception has been defined as the meaning that is attached to objects and events that occur in the environment. Therefore, accuracy in the interpretation of what is perceived by an individual will be directly related to the quality of a motor response. For instance, if a handicapped child playing basketball cannot accurately judge the distance to the

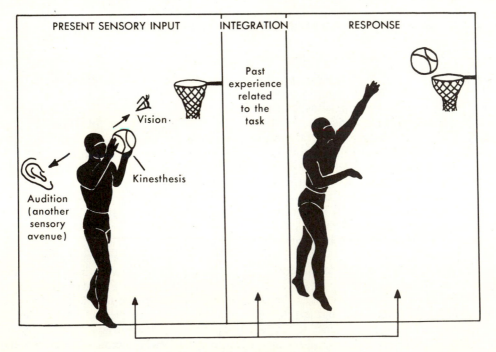

Fig. 3-5. Model of perceptual process.

basket, the chances for successful shooting are reduced. A successful basketball player must also be able to determine how much force is required to shoot the ball into the basket. If the player cannot judge this distance accurately and coordinate enough force to make the shot, the task success will be impaired. Another example might be the golfer's attempt to put a ball into a hole. If he or she cannot ascertain the appropriate force to be applied to the ball through the club head, the possibility of task success will be reduced. If a disabled softball player cannot perceive the speed of a thrown ball and determine where it is in relation-

ship to the bat as it approaches the plate, he or she will not be able to hit the ball effectively. Fundamental motor skills and sport skills involve the interpretation of stimuli to which a response is to be made. Impaired perception will detract from the pupil's ability to perform motor tasks in a great many spheres of physical activity.

Perceptual development involves opportunities in activities to interpret visual objects, auditory symbols, and kinesthetic events so that an individual may behaviorally adapt by making the desired responses. In essence, perceptual development relies upon memories of past experiences for the

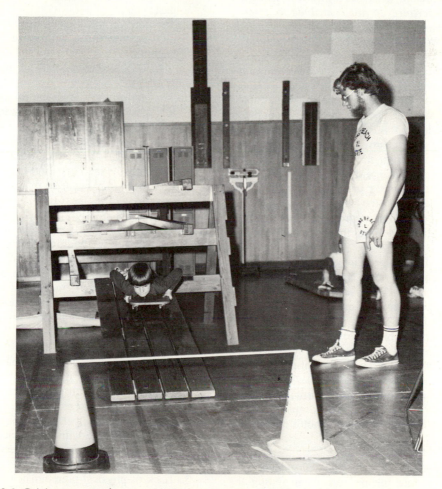

Fig. 3-6. Gaining perceptual-motor experiences. (Courtesy of California State University, Audio Visual Center, Long Beach, Calif.)

interpretation and solution of present problems. In its simplest form, the perceptual process involves interpreting current sensory information, which is associated with a specific context and integrated with past experience and to which a response is made. Information is provided regarding the appropriateness of the response and is then fed back to the participant for storage. Thus, prior experience is utilized in solving current motor problems. A perceptual development training program seeks to establish a background of varied but similar experiences for the learner so that he or she may solve other similar problems in the future. One should note that *redundant activities within the learner's behavioral repertoire do not contribute to perceptual development*. For example, if a child can efficiently walk a beam 4 inches wide there is little value in performing the activity again, for he or she is not struggling to extend the behavioral repertoire. However, if the child falls off the beam or if he or she must struggle with the balancing mechanism to stay on the beam, then the assumption could be made that this particular experience is outside of his or her current behavioral repertoire. Information regarding the consequences of not properly equating innervation of one side of the body to the other would probably be provided as the child moves down the balance beam. Such an experience would be in accord with the perceptual development that involves the balancing mechanism.

Perceptual development involves a greater variety of instructional experiences than does the acquisition of specific motor skills. The selection of such experiences should be precise. With the selection of the precise activity, a new experience should be provided for the learner. Therefore, similar but not identical elements must be part of the composition of tasks in the perceptual-motor development training program (Fig. 3-6). The purpose of perceptual development is to provide a broad base of varied motor experiences to enable skillful performance of specific complex motor tasks.

Analysis of skill proficiency

Four components of the perceptual process must be operative before the performer can master the desired tasks. Shooting a basketball will be used as an example of a skill to be analyzed. The four components are the following:

1. The learner must be able to perceive or conceptualize the outcome of the desired response.

    EXAMPLE: The ball must pass through the basket.

2. The learner must make a response relevant to current sensory input as it relates to past experience.

    EXAMPLE: The learner must be aware of the distance to the basket and remember the amount of force that was given to the ball when shooting from similar distances in the past.

3. The learner must compare consequences of the response made with those of the desired response.

    EXAMPLE: Did the ball go into the basket? If not, why?

4. The learner must store the information, using it to perform better the next time, remembering the new experience so that it can be used to improve subsequent performances.

    EXAMPLE: The learner must remember the outcomes of the shots and the conditions under which they occur so that performance can be corrected the next time.

Such a model provides a basis for determining the deficiency in task performance by a learner who has a disabling condition. For example, if the defined task is to hit a softball and the performer (impaired or normal) cannot hit the ball, the question that must be asked, in light of the perceptual process model, is "why?" The reasons for failure to achieve mastery of the tasks may include the following:

1. Inability to interpret current stimuli.

    EXAMPLE: The performer may fail to determine the speed or direction of the ball or the location in which it is to be hit.

2. Inappropriate past experience.

    EXAMPLE: The performer may not have had prior experience with such space-time predictions as when the ball will meet the bat to hit it properly.

3. Lack of physical prerequisites of the task.

    EXAMPLE: The performer may not be

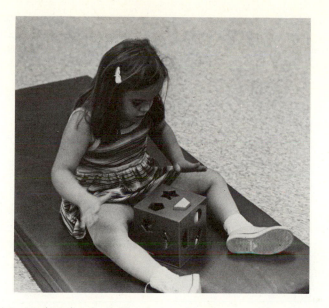

Fig. 3-7. This activity involves the visual, kinesthetic and haptic senses. (Courtesy of the Special Education Early Childhood Intervention Program, University of Kansas, Lawrence.)

strong enough or coordinated enough to move the bat with sufficient speed to hit the ball.

4. Inability to anticipate the desired response because of inappropriate use of feedback.

   EXAMPLE: The performer may misinterpret feedback or may fail to remember prior performances. He or she will then repeat the same mistakes.

Any combination of the reasons mentioned above may be a deterrent to learning.

Application of a perceptual-process model

The application of a perceptual process model enables an instructor to identify precisely the deficiencies of a handicapped learner. For instance, if a child had problems batting a ball, there are several reasons why the learner may fail. Application of the perceptual-process model would explore the following possibilities:

1. It may be that the visual mechanism is at such a low level of development that the oculomotor muscles cannot track the ball well enough for the learner to master the task. If

this is the case, the learner has not developed the prerequisites for achieving task success. Therefore, developmental programs are needed to establish better functioning of the oculomotor mechanism before the ball can be hit with the desired proficiency. Prior experiences related to oculomotor movement have failed to develop the eye to the point where performance is consistent. Therefore, sequential tasks of oculomotor ability related to the skill to be taught are in order.

   EXAMPLE: Use a larger ball and throw it slowly so that the eye can track the object.

2. If the child, because of lack of strength development, is incapable of moving the bat fast enough, a strength development program might be a prerequisite to task mastery.

   EXAMPLE: Throw a ball from a greater distance or use a lighter bat. In addition, the child may perform special developmental exercises to develop sufficient strength.

3. Inappropriate functioning of the feedback mechanism may be a deterrent to learning. The pupil may be unable to accurately inter-

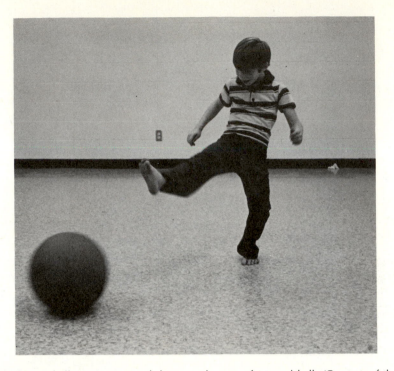

Fig. 3-8. Kicking a ball requires a match between the eyes, foot, and ball. (Courtesy of the Special Education Early Childhood Intervention Program, University of Kansas, Lawrence.)

pret and rectify errors that have occurred before or, because of prior task failures in similar learning situations, may tend to repress information that may assist in task mastery.

EXAMPLE: Arranging successful experience with stronger reinforcement for hitting the ball may be added to the process. This may better activate use of the feedback mechanism. Hitting a ball suspended on a string or from a batting T may also be effective.

4. The child may be unable to make a connection between the consequence of the motor act and the conditions under which the motor act took place.

EXAMPLE: Feedback is expressed by the distance and direction the ball travels as a result of being hit by the child. Therefore, the adaptation to facilitate feedback for this specific task is the introduction of a large, light ball. With the application of relatively little force the ball travels a considerable distance.

The projection of the ball provides feedback that is connected by the child with the motor response and the conditions under which the ball is projected. Therefore, the size of the ball enables the child to be repeatedly successful and provides positive feedback in terms of the distance that the ball travels as a result of the efforts. The input conditions and the hitting response may be retained better because of the strong, positive feedback.

The interpretations of information may be made progressively more difficult by a reduction of the size of the ball, or heavier bats could be introduced gradually into the activity. Eventually, the child might be able to hit a ball using a bat that approximates one used in a conventional softball game.

Generalizing perceptual-motor experience

With few exceptions, perceptual-motor development training programs indicate that training activities are specific to the skill that has been practiced.

There is a need to explore a generalized activity experience that might be transferred to perceptual-motor skills other than those that have been practiced. Therefore, the nature of the perceptual-motor experience consists of searching for a reservoir of motor experiences that, hopefully, will facilitate learning of a broad group of skills.

ASSESSMENT OF AND ACTIVITIES FOR SPECIFIC PERCEPTUAL DEFICITS

Specific components of perceptual-motor structure have been hypothesized by Dunsing and Kephart.[6] Such a classification system of perceptual components enables the identification of specific traits to be developed within the framework of the visuomotor structure. Thus, once the specific weaknesses are identified, activities that develop these areas may be paired with measured needs for the treatment of handicapped children. Furthermore, through the generation of a profile of specific perceptual abilities it is then possible to select appropriate activities to enhance the visual-perceptual development of a specific child.

There are several types of perceptual-motor assessments, all of which yield different kinds of data. Two types of data result from tasks that are observed for qualitative performance: one type involves observational assessment of the patterns of movement from which the subject's perceptual-motor deficit is inferred; another type involves behavioral performance that can be quantified, and the resulting score can then be used to compare the pupil's skills with the performance characteristic of his or her chronological age. Whatever form testing takes, it is essential that activities that constitute the program be directly related to assessment and that the specific child's present level of educational performance be considered before prescriptive activity is implemented (Chapter 4).

Types of perceptual inputs during physical activity

There are essentially three types of sensory input utilized in physical activity: visual, kinesthetic, and aural. All senses are used to some degree in the performance of motor activity; however, in a given task, one or two forms of input may predominate over the others.

Vision refers to sensation interpreted by the eye and to the meaning that is attached to the interpretation of the event. Visual skill is particularly important in those activities involving projectiles (Fig. 3-9).

Kinesthesis is the awareness of the position, direction, and extent of movement of the limbs and of the whole body. Closely associated with kinesthesis is the vestibular mechanism, which is found in the inner ear. This mechanism informs the body of its rate of movement and its position in space; hence, it is particularly important in activities that involve changes in body position, such as gymnastics. Kinesthesis is a prerequisite for refined skills requiring precise movement and accuracy. The utilization and development of these senses in handicapped children is essential for gaining motor control.

Audition refers to the reception of sound by the ear and its interpretation by the auditory center in the brain. Many activities in the physical education curriculum rely on audition, especially rhythms.

Specific activities in the physical education curriculum may be associated with the reception of information through specific sensory avenues. The knowledge of the relation of sensory input to activity is important because it assists the teacher in progressive selection of activities and facilitates more accurate pairing of the difficulty of the task with the ability level of the child. The following are examples of pairing sensory avenues of reception with motor tasks:

1. Development of kinesthetic awareness is obtained through participation in motor experience. Programs of this nature would include activities that involve gross motor movements, such as beam walking and movement exploration activities, or precise tasks that require accuracy.
2. Visual development in physical education may occur through developmental programs that involve looking at objects as well as catching and throwing them. Examples of such activities are ball games in which eye-hand coordination is developed.
3. Auditory development can be effected by rhythm programs in which auditory inputs are paired with motor movements.
4. Perceptual development programs can be made more complex by requiring more elab-

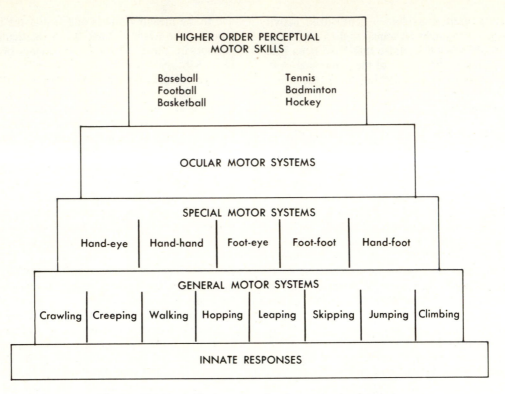

Fig. 3-9. The hierarchical sequence for visuomotor development.

orate integration of sensory input with motor output. The following are examples of visual-kinesthetic movements:

a. Qualitative movements in catching or hitting projectiles require kinesthetic perception for proper application of force and appropriate positioning of limbs. Activities become more complex when the eyes must track objects that involve distance-time ratios.

b. Auditory-kinesthetic movements occur in the more elaborate dances and floor exercise routines such as gymnastics.

c. Rhythmical gymnastics may involve throwing and catching balls to music and engaging the body in qualitative movement; thus, there is expression of the integration of all senses.

Regardless of the nature of the act performed, it is important to be aware of the complexities of per-ceptual inputs and the expected responses so that the degree of task difficulty can be matched to the level of the handicapped child's ability. Appropriate selection of activities is essential to perceptual development for these activities and the instruments that help each child progress.

HIERARCHY OF PERCEPTUAL DEVELOPMENT

Getman[12] has provided information that suggests a hierarchy of motor behavior that serves as prerequisite functions to the acquisition of higher-order visual activities. This is of great significance to the physical educator, since classifying children according to their abilities makes it easier to select appropriate activities for them.

A normal child is born with innate responses that appear to be the initial bases from which motor responses will develop. Established innate responses are interwoven with the first random movement and later with the basic locomotor patterns such as crawling, creeping, walking, hopping, skipping, and jumping that all humans acquire in developing visuomotor potential.

Use of the visuomotor developmental levels

Knowledge of the visuomotor levels of development provides information to the physical educator as to what general types of programming are acceptable for specific individuals who are to respond to perceptual-motor development programming. If there is gross failure of persons who are attempting to succeed on a visuomotor task such as ball catching there would obviously be a need for activity that is related to the specific problem. However, when the nature of visuomotor development is considered, as purported by Getman[12] and Kephart,[13] it becomes apparent that the prerequisite to precise hand-eye coordination, which ball catching requires, is extensive experience with fundamental motor patterns such as walking, running, hopping, and skipping. It is theorized that such activity enables the prerequisite visual skills for ball catching to be developed as a result of the child moving in the environment while making visual assessments. The visual development that results from experience in fundamental motor patterns and skills then provides the underpinning for the more complex visual tasks such as ball catching and other tasks involving projectiles. Therefore, a productive approach to visual development for a child deficient in ball-catching skills might be activity that involves fundamental motor patterns. This, however, is not to say that the child should not be participating in tasks that involve projectiles that are at his or her present level of educational performance.

If a child is unable to track with precision projectiles approaching at varying distances and speeds in such activities as tennis, badminton, baseball, and basketball and thus fails to perform the tasks successfully, then some type of instructional intervention is needed. Again, there would be an obvious need for activities that relate to the specific task that the child is unable to master. For instance, responding to a slowly rolling ball is less difficult than trying to catch a thrown ball because gravity plays an uncontrollable role once the projectile is airborne. On the other hand, a rolling ball can easily be controlled at the ability level of the child with respect to the speed at which the ball is rolled. But as the nature of the development of the visuomotor system is studied in light of previously mentioned theory, it becomes apparent that prerequisites for precise oculomotor tracking, which is a central part of the ball-catching skill, may not be fully developed for the acquisition of such tasks. Thus, it would be hypothesized that corollary programming of such a nature should accompany the acquisition of such complex tasks that are at an appropriate level for the child. Such a notion would indicate that a child who has problems mastering tasks that require high-level oculomotor abilities should be exposed to hand-eye, foot-eye, and hand-hand types of activities for which time and space variables are not essential for task success; or, as Getman[12] would say, the special motor systems must be developed before the oculomotor systems. (See Fig. 3-9 for the levels of visuomotor development.)

Most of the tasks that appear at each of the levels of visuomotor development can be sequenced to reach each learner at his or her ability level. Although it is suggested that tasks to be taught be analyzed and be presented to the learner at the present level of educational performance, it is also suggested that there be a general developmental structure for acquiring efficient visuomotor behavior.

Reflex development levels

Although reflex classification systems vary slightly, there is general agreement that a group of primitive reflexes appears and should disappear during the first year of life. These early reflexes assist the child in assuming an upright posture in preparation for ambulation. Until primitive reflexes appear in a child's neuromotor repertoire, lifting the head, rolling from supine to prone, and sitting cannot be accomplished. When primitive reflexes persist beyond the first year of life, automatic, unwanted flexion and extension of the limbs contribute to jerky, clumsy-looking movement patterns.

A second set of reflexes that facilitate maintenance of equilibrium begins to appear between the ages of 6 and 18 months and persists throughout life unless development is inhibited in some way. When these reflexes fail to develop, affected individuals have extreme difficulty maintaining bal-

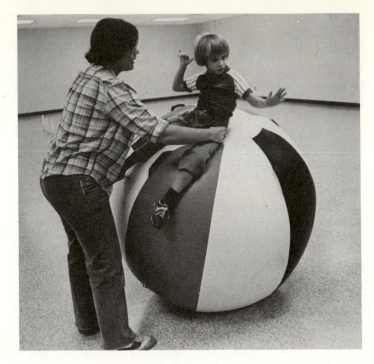

Fig. 3-10. Large ball is used to provide experiences to enhance optical righting. (Courtesy of the Special Education Early Childhood Intervention Program, University of Kansas, Lawrence.)

Table 3-1. Primitive and equilibrium reflex development

Reflex	Age	Age inhibited	Effect on movement patterns
Primitive reflexes			
Flexor withdrawal	Birth	2 month	Uncontrolled flexion of leg when pressure is applied to sole of foot.
Extensor thrust	Birth	2 month	Uncontrolled extension of leg when pressure is applied to sole of foot.
Crossed extension 1	Birth	2 month	Uncontrolled extension of flexed leg when opposite leg is suddenly flexed.
Crossed extension 2	Birth	2 month	Leg adducts, and internally rotates and foot plantar flexes when opposite leg is tapped medially at level of knee (scissor gait).
Asymmetrical tonic neck	Birth	4-6 months	Extension of arm and leg on face side or increase in extension tone; flexion of arm and leg on skull side or increase in flexor tone when head is turned.
Symmetrical tonic neck 1	Birth	4-6 months	Arms flex or flexor tone dominates; legs extend or extensor tone dominates when head is ventroflexed while child is in quadreped position.

Data from Fiorentino, M. R.: Reflex testing methods for evaluating C.N.S. Development, Springfield, Ill., 1970, Charles C Thomas, Publishers.

Table 3-1. Primitive and equilibrium reflex development—cont'd

Reflex	Age	Age inhibited	Effect on movement patterns
Symmetrical tonic neck 2	Birth	4-6 months	Arms extend or extensor tone dominates; legs flex or flexor tone dominates when head is dorsi-flexed while child is in quadreped position.
Tonic labyrinthine supine position	Birth	4 months	Extensor tone dominates when child is in supine position.
Tonic labyrinthine prone position	Birth	4 months	Flexor tone dominates in arms, hips, and legs when child is in prone position.
Positive supporting reaction	Birth	4 months	Increase in extensor tone in legs when sudden pressure is applied to both feet simultaneously.
Negative supporting reaction	Birth	4 months	Marked increase in flexor tone in legs when sudden pressure is applied to both feet simultaneously.
Neck righting	Birth	6 months	Body rotates as a whole in the same direction the head is turned.
Landau reflex	6 months	3 years	Spine, arms, and legs extend when head is dorsi-flexed while child is held in supine position; spine, arms, and legs flex when head is ventro-flexed while child is held in supine position.
Equilibrium reflexes			
Body righting	6 months	Throughout life	When child is in supine position and initiates a full body roll there is segmented rotation of the body (i.e., head turns, then shoulders, then pelvis)
Labyrinthine righting 1	2 months	Throughout life	When child is blindfolded and held in prone position head raises to a point where child's face is vertical.
Labyrinthine righting 2	6 months	Throughout life	When child is blindfolded and held in supine position, head raises to a point where face is vertical.
Labyrinthine righting 3	6-8 months	Throughout life	When child is blindfolded and held in an upright position and is suddenly tilted right head does not right itself to an upright position.
Labyrinthine righting 4	6-8 months	Throughout life	Same as labyrinthine righting 3, but child is tilted to left.
Optical righting 1	2 months	Throughout life	Same as labyrinthine righting 1, but child is not blindfolded.
Optical righting 2	6 months	Throughout life	Same as labyrinthine righting 2, but child is not blindfolded.
Optical righting 3	6-9 months	Throughout life	Same as labyrinthine righting 3, but child is not blindfolded.
Optical righting 4	6-8 months	Throughout life	Same as labyrinthine righting 4 but child is not blindfolded.
Amphibian reaction	6 months	Throughout life	While child is in prone position with legs extended and arms extended overhead, flexion of arm, hip, and knee on same side can be elicited when pelvis on that side is lifted.
Protective extensor thrust	6 months	Throughout life	While child is held by pelvis and is extended in air, arms extend when the child's head is moved suddenly toward the floor.

Continued.

Table 3-1. Primitive and equilibrium reflex development—cont'd

Reflex	Age	Age inhibited	Effect on movement patterns
Equilibrium—supine position	6 months	Throughout life	While child is supine on a tiltboard with arms and legs suspended if the board is suddenly tilted to one side, there is righting of the head and thorax and abduction and extension of the arm and leg on the raised side.
Equilibrium—prone position	6 months	Throughout life	Same as equilibrium supine except child is prone on tiltboard.
Equilibrium—quadreped position	8 months	Throughout life	While child balances on all fours if suddenly tilted to one side, righting of head and thorax and abduction-extension of arm and leg occur on raised side.
Equilibrium—sitting position	10-12 months	Throughout life	While child is seated on chair if pulled or tilted to one side, righting of head and thorax and abduction-extension of arm and leg occur on raised side (side opposite pull).
Equilibrium—kneeling position	15 months	Throughout life	While child kneels on both knees if suddenly pulled to one side, righting of the head and thorax and abduction-extension of the arm and leg occur on the raised side.
Hopping 1	15-18 months	Throughout life	While child is standing upright if moved to the left or right, head and thorax right and child hops sideways to maintain balance.
Hopping 2	15-18 months	Throughout life	While child is standing upright if moved forward, head and thorax right and child hops forward to maintain balance.
Hopping 3	15-18 months	Throughout life	While child is standing upright if moved backward, head and thorax right and child hops backward to maintain balance.
Dorsiflexion	15-18 months	Throughout life	While child is standing upright if tilted backward, head and thorax right and feet dorsiflex.
See-saw	15 months	Throughout life	While child stands on one foot another person holds arm and free foot on same side. When arm is pulled forward and laterally, head and thorax right and held leg abducts and extends.
Simian position	15-18 months	Throughout life	While child squats down if tilted to one side, head and thorax right and arm and leg on raised side abduct and extend.

ance, particularly while moving at medium and fast speeds and when attempting to change direction. Because these children do not make automatic postural adjustments when the center of gravity moves beyond the base of support, they tend to fall easily.

Because abnormal reflex development and concomitant equilibrium problems can have such a pervasive effect on efficient perceptual and motor functioning, the importance of careful evaluation in this area cannot be overemphasized. Categories of reflex, expected ages of appearance, and resulting effects on movement patterns are presented in Table 3-1.

Interestingly enough, as important as equilibrium reflexes are, they do not always serve the skilled performer. Some of these reflexes actually veto certain movement behaviors that are essential to task mastery of complex skills. When such cir-

Table 3-2. Mature reflexes that interfere with motor skill performance

Task	Reflex	Inhibition of reflex
Forward somersault	Protective extensor thrust: arms straighten, head thrusts up as head moves to ground.	The child must tuck the head and chin to chest and give with the arms to transfer the weight evenly from the neck down the spine.
Two-footed standing broad jump	Equilibrium reactions: the movement of the posturing mechanism outside of the base is vetoed. Thus the center of gravity must be maintained over the base.	When the child jumps, the body is projected up rather than out. The posturing mechanism is difficult to project outside of the base. Posture must be projected in front of the base.
Back dive or half gainer	Righting reflex: the head rights instead of being held back. The chin is away from the chest.	The child lands on the water on the back instead of head first. Head must be held back.

cumstances occur in the teaching of a skill the teacher must take steps to inhibit these reflexes. Examples of skills and a list of reflexes that interfere with skill acquisition are given in Table 3-2.

It is important that teachers keenly observe the learner during instructional tasks to determine which reflexes must be inhibited. If such reflexes are present and the performer is unable to inhibit them, steps must be taken to rectify these problems. The techniques of stimulus prompting and response prompting are detailed by Becker, Engelmann and Thomas.[4] Such procedures, when appropriately applied to the reflexes, result in inhibition and should enhance the skill development of the handicapped learner.

It is important to assess the reflexes that need to be inhibited or facilitated for the purpose of assisting a learner to acquire a motor skill. Therefore, it is suggested that reflexes be assessed as a part of the task analysis of the specific skill that is the target of instruction. The process of task analysis will be described in greater detail in Chapter 4.

Locomotor system

It is through the development of the locomotor system that the one gains the capability to explore first oneself and later oneself in relation to the environment. Through locomotion, the concept of distance between objects and the self is formulated by moving the body from object to object. This helps the individual to gain experience in calculating differences in size by moving toward and away from specific objects. The locomotor system thus serves as the integrating factor between vision and object. However, when the child initially tends to the skill itself and fails to interpret the complex arrangement of environmental objects, visual development progresses at a slower rate. If this is the case, the child cannot effectively use information provided to the eye regarding his or her movements to and from objects. Therefore, for vision to develop further, the eye must be freed from the locomotor skills themselves. It is necessary for these locomotor patterns to be built in as subroutines where little or no attention is on the locomotor skill itself, but primary attention is on the environment. For example, a disabled child will often focus attention on the placement of the feet as he or she walks. Vision is thus being directed to executing the walking skill, not to orienting the body to the environment as the child moves among objects. The integration of the visual mechanism with the locomotor skill of walking increases the possibility that combined hand-eye activity will take place while the child is in locomotion. The basic locomotor patterns included in this unit are to roll, creep, walk, run, slide, gallop, jump, hop, and skip. Ability to use these patterns is necessary before a child can begin to explore the environment. Through such exploration higher-level concepts such as body image and spatial awareness are developed. Also, participation in active games and sports is dependent on basic movement pattern capabilities.

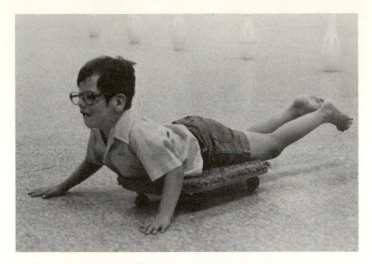

Fig 3-11. Body control and righting of the head are necessary for efficient propulsion of the scooter. (Courtesy of the Special Education Early Childhood Intervention Program, University of Kansas, Lawrence.)

Development of locomotor patterns can be accomplished when learners achieve basic levels of strength, endurance, flexibility, and postural reflex control. Behavioral objectives included in this unit presume that appropriate fitness levels are present; therefore, the teacher may want to review the strength, endurance, and flexibility status of each learner before beginning this unit.

In most cases, activities to promote dynamic balance include practice in the specific locomotor pattern being attempted; however, when the possibility exists that persisting primitive reflexes such as positive or negative supporting reactions could be interfering with the learner's ability to perform, then activities to eliminate the primitive reflexes are suggested.

A list of behavioral objectives for various activities is given below. In some instances more than one behavioral objective has been included. In each of those cases the objectives have been sequenced developmentally with the easier goals listed first, followed by more difficult accomplishments (see Figs. 3-12 to 3-14).

BEHAVIORAL OBJECTIVES

1. *Roll lying on mat with arms at side*
   a. Complete three full body rolls with head and shoulders turning first, followed by hips, with legs turning last. (Note: If knees are the first body part to turn, a body-righting reflex may be present and should be inhibited before expecting the learner to accomplish the task correctly.)
2. *Creep (on floor or mat on hands and knees)*
   a. Move forward 10 feet on hands and knees using right arm and left leg in unison and left arm and right leg in unison. (Note: If the learner moves forward by hopping knees up to hands or by moving arm and leg on the same side in unison, the task has not been completed satisfactorily.)
3. *Walk (in tennis shoes or barefoot)*
   a. Walk forward 10 feet swinging right arm forward with left leg and left arm with right leg. (Note: An efficient walking pattern consists of placing the heel on the floor first, followed by passing body weight over the outer border of the foot, and finally pushing off with the ball of the foot. The feet should point straight ahead. Developmentally delayed individuals sometimes have a tendency to use a shuffling walking pattern and/or walk with the head down. If either or both of these occur, thigh strength may be inadequate and/or depth perception may not be fully developed.)
   b. Walk forward 10 feet between two lines 2 feet apart moving alternate arm and leg in unison.
   c. Walk forward 10 feet on a line 2 inches wide on the floor.

d. Walk forward 10 feet on a board 4 inches wide raised 2 inches from the floor.

e. Walk forward 10 feet on a board 2 inches wide raised 2 inches from the floor.

5. *Run (in tennis shoes or barefoot)*

a. Run forward 25 feet alternating opposite arm and leg with free movement in the arms and head held up. (Note: A run differs from a walk in that during the run there are periods when neither foot is touching the floor. If the learner appears to run in a clumsy manner, observe closely to note if there appears to be any unusual stiffness or exaggerated flexion in the legs. Marked stiffness or flexion could be an indication that primitive negative or positive supporting reflexes are persisting.)

6. *Slide (in tennis shoes or barefoot)*

a. Slide sideways 15 feet to the right. (Note: A slide consists of moving the body sideways by transferring body weight from one foot to the other while keeping the same lead foot.)

b. Slide sideways 15 feet to the right.

c. Slide sideways 15 feet to the right while staying between two lines placed 12 inches apart.

d. Slide sideways for a distance of 15 feet to the left while staying between two lines placed 12 inches apart.

7. *Leap (in tennis shoes or barefoot)*

a. Complete a series of five leaps without stopping. (Note: A leap consists of taking off on one foot and landing on the other. A leap differs from a run in that during the leap the lead leg is fully extended in front of the body, and the time the body is airborne is longer than the time the body is in the run.)

8. *Gallop (in tennis shoes or barefoot)*

a. Gallop forward 15 feet keeping the same lead foot. (Note: A gallop consists of combining a leap on the lead foot with a step on the trailing foot.)

b. Gallop forward 25 feet alternating lead feet every 5 feet.

9. *Jump (in tennis shoes on a nonskid surface)*

a. Jump once using both feet together for the take-off and landing. (Note: The learner should flex the hips and knees to provide thrust for the take-off and then again to absorb the shock of the landing. If marked tension or flexion of the legs is noted during the landing, it could be an indication that primitive negative or supporting reflexes are persisting.)

b. Jump once using both feet together for the takeoff and landing, and maintain balance upon landing.

c. Jump half his or her own height using both feet together for the takeoff and landing and using arms in unison.

d. Initiate a series of six jumps in a row using both feet together.

10. *Hop (in tennis shoes or barefoot)*

a. Hop on one foot once without touching the free foot to the floor. (Note: If marked tension (extension) or flexion of the hopping leg or free leg is noted during the takeoff or landing it could be an indication that primitive negative or supporting reflexes are persisting.)

b. Hop 6 feet without stopping or touching the free foot to the floor.

11. *Skip (in tennis shoes or barefoot)*

a. Skip 20 feet with the head up and free movement of legs and arms. (Note: A skip consists of a step and a hop on one foot followed by the same pattern with the other foot. The learner must be able to hop before being expected to skip.)

Special motor systems

Locomotor systems also serve the development of hand-eye, hand-foot, hand-hand, eye-foot, and foot-foot relationships (Fig. 3-12). One must assume that when a child reaches the stage of development in which the feet and hands function independently of vision, locomotion functions at a subroutine level, thus enabling vision to be directed toward specific tasks involving greater refinement of the hand and the eye (Fig. 3-13). Ball activities requiring hand manipulation or kicking activities involving the eye and the foot all contain this particular dimension of perceptual-motor structure. It is during this period that the hand and the eye become paired. Actual information from the hand provides the eye with data so that vision can be refined and can accurately structure objects in space. Authorities have hypothesized that 20% of vision consists of focusing light onto the retina and that 80% consists of the development of interpretation. Vision refers both to sensation interpreted by the eye and to the meaning attached to it. When hand and eye as well as foot and eye are coordinated with locomotor patterns functioning at subroutine levels, the prerequisites to the next level of development are fulfilled.

Oculomotor development

After perceptual information has been provided to the brain via hand-foot experience, there even-

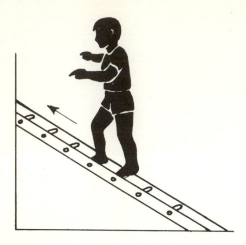

Fig. 3-12. Foot-eye coordination and anteroposterior balance.

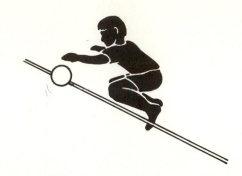

Fig. 3-14. Locomotor and hand-eye coordination. This task involves jumping back and forth across a line while bouncing a ball.

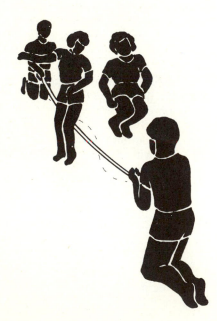

Fig. 3-13. Rhythm and locomotion. The rope is moved back and forth so that the child must raise both feet at the same time and transfer her weight.

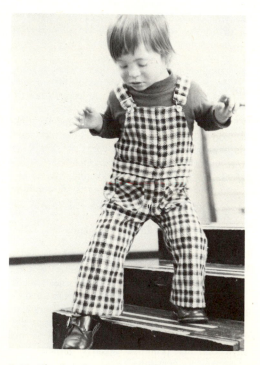

Fig. 3-15. The handicapped child learning to walk down stairs.

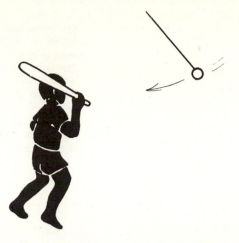

Fig. 3-16. Gaining oculomotor control. The child strikes a ball as many times as possible with a bat as it swings toward him.

tually develops an autonomous capability to identify and track visual stimuli without the aid of kinesthetic movements. This has been labeled the "ocular-motor level of development."[12] Functioning at this level in sport skills involves projectiles that make it necessary for the eye and brain to track objects and interpret speed, direction, and spatial positioning appropriately. Although there are other progressive steps that lead to more elaborate perceptual structures, oculomotor development is perhaps the highest level of functioning applicable to activities found in physical education.[12]

It is essential for the implementation of perceptual-motor development training programs that the physical educator be aware of the hierarchical levels of visuomotor development. Once the hierarchical structure of visual development is established as a frame of reference, curricula that take into account the development of visuomotor perception can be constructed, programs can be conducted, handicapped children can be tested for appropriate placement of the hierarchy, and activities can be selected in accord with the needs of specific pupils (Fig. 3-16).

Ocular control

Ocular control includes the ability to visually fixate on stationary objects and moving objects and to perceive the location of the objects in space. Until a learner has developed control over the move-

ment of the eyes, attention span is limited, visual comprehension is difficult, and movement efficiency (including hand-eye coordination) is next to impossible.

Two aspects of visual development that contribute to ocular control are refractive and orthoptic vision. Good refractive vision is dependent upon visual acuity, that is, freedom from nearsightedness, farsightedness, astigmatism, and factors that contribute to blindness. Sound orthoptic vision is determined by the capability of the eyes to move in perfect unison.

Individuals who have refractive visual problems do not see objects clearly at near and/or far points. The object of their visual attention may be blurred or distorted because light rays entering the eye do not strike the retina at appropriate points to permit clear, sharp vision. Orthoptic (eye alignment) problems distress depth perception. For us to perceive the exact placement of objects in space light rays should enter each eye at the same point. When one eye is misaligned from the other, depth perception deteriorates. If the misalignment is severe, such as in the case of the "lazy eye," an individual has impaired depth perception. Such an individual cannot judge where a moving object is, has difficulty descending stairs, and misjudges the placement of targets.

Persons who tend to squint the eyes, hold the head close to the page, jumble material being copied from the chalkboard, complain of frequent headaches, blink excessively, or have a tendency for the eyes to water should be referred to a visual developmental specialist for a complete refractive and orthoptic visual exam. When the problems have been corrected or assurance is given that no refractive or orthoptic problems exist, ocular control activities may be used.

BEHAVIORAL OBJECTIVES FOR OCULAR CONTROL

1. *Fixation (seated in a chair facing a seated evaluator)*
   a. Fixate with both eyes on an object held 18 inches in front of nose at eye level for 10 seconds.
   b. Fixate with the right eye on an object held 18 inches in front of nose at eye level for 10 seconds. (Note: cover the left eye with your hand or a 3- by 5-inch card.)
   c. Fixate with the left eye on an object held 18 inches in front of nose at eye level for 10 seconds. (Note: Cover the right eye with your hand or a 3- by 5-inch card.)

   (Note: Any tendency to turn the head to one side, to blink excessively, or for the eyes to water could be an indication that the learner needs to be referred to a visual developmental specialist for a refractive and orthoptic visual exam.)
2. *Ocular alignment (depth perception) (seated in a chair facing a seated evaluator)*
   a. Fixate on an object held 18 inches in front of nose at eye level without moving right eye as left eye

is covered for 3 seconds. (Note whether the right eye moves and in what direction.)
   b. Fixate on an object held 18 inches in front of the nose at eye level without moving the left eye as the right eye is covered for 3 seconds. (Note whether the left eye moves and in what direction.)
   c. Fixate on an object held 18 inches front of the nose at eye level without moving the right eye for 3 seconds as the right eye is uncovered. (Note whether the right eye moves as it is uncovered and in what direction.)

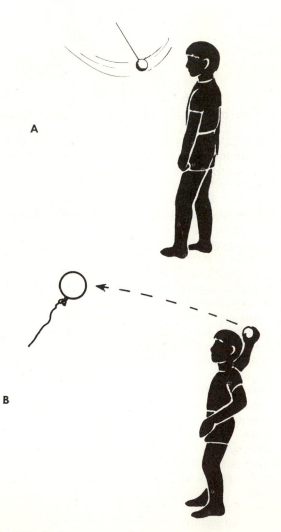

Fig. 3-18. Ocular tracking and distance duration. **A,** Tracking a moving ball. **B,** Throwing a sponge rubber ball at a descending balloon.

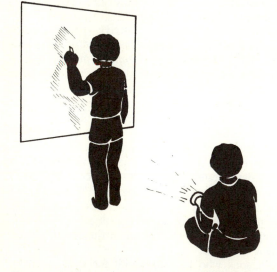

Fig. 3-17. Producing a movable image with a flashlight.

d. Fixate on an object held 18 inches in front of the nose at eye level without moving the left eye for 3 seconds as the left eye is uncovered. (Note whether the left eye moves as it is uncovered and in what direction.)

3. *Convergence-divergence (seated in a chair facing a seated evaluator)*
   a. Visually follow with both eyes an object moved slowly from 18 inches directly in front of the nose at eye level to 4 inches from the eyes (midpoint) and back to 18 inches (Note whether the eyes move equally without jerking.)

4. *Visual tracking (seated in a chair facing a seated evaluator)*
   a. Without moving the head, visually pursue with both eyes an object held 18 inches from the eyes as the object is moved in the following patterns: a 12-inch square, a 10-inch circle, a 10-inch X, and a 12-inch horizontal line.
   b. With the left eye covered, visually pursue with the right eye without moving the head an object held 18 inches from the eyes as the object is moved in the following patterns: a 12-inch square, a 10-inch circle, a 10-inch X, and a 12-inch horizontal line.
   c. With the right eye covered, visually pursue with the left eye without moving the head an object held 18 inches from the eyes as the object is moved in front of the face in the following patterns: a 12-inch square, a 10-inch circle, a 10-inch X, and a 12-inch horizontal line.
   (Note: During all tracking tasks note any tendency for the eyes to jump when the object moves across the midline of the body, to jump ahead of the object, to jerk while pursuing the object, to water, or to blink excessively. The watering and/or excessive blinking could be an indication of visual stress and such cases should be referred to a visual developmental specialist for a refractive and orthoptic visual examination.)

Body image

Body image is the perception of the relationship of body parts to external objects and the position of the body to gravitational forces. With the progressive acquisition of motor ability and movement experience as a result of vestibular and kinesthetic exploration, there is a concomitant development of spatial knowledge. This contributes to an awareness of the body and the development of body image. The growth and development of body image give a person a perceptual set or a stable platform for the reception of visual images from the outside world. Sensations received by the nervous system are based on this perceptual set; consequently, this results in a need to test body image experiences to see which parts will fit into the perceptual whole or into a particular time frame. Authorities believe that the developmental aspects of body image involving the integration of body parts with sensation mature at the age of approximately 7 years in normal children. Handicapped children often lag in body image development.[11]

The development of body image is a prerequisite to the development of vision. Impaired body image may produce impaired visual perception, and a lack of awareness of one's bodily functions and capabilities impairs optimal use of the visual sense.

Kephart[13] and Barsch[3] have hypothesized components of the body image that develop through qualitative movement. These are as follows:

1. *Kinesthetic motor awareness:* Awareness of what the motor capabilities are and the ability to elicit motor responses.
2. *Verticality:* Awareness of the vertical alignment of the body's segments.
3. *Laterality:* Internal awareness of two sides of the body.
4. *Directionality:* Ability to relate the body to objects and to space (space-time-body relationships).

Kinesthetic motor awareness

Kinesthetic motor awareness has been reported to be an important component of the development of body image. According to Dunsing and Kephart,[6] movement input is stored by the systematic gathering of initial information that is a result of

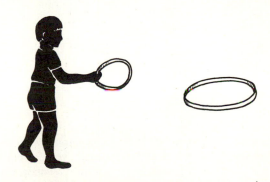

Fig. 3-19. Developing kinesthetic motor awareness and oculomotor tracking by throwing a ring through a hoop.

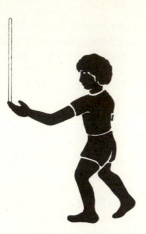

Fig. 3-20. Gaining kinesthetic motor awareness and the ability to conduct oculomotor tracking by balancing a wand on the index finger while running as far as possible.

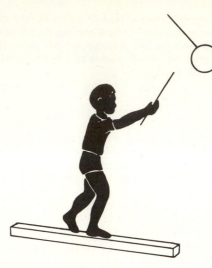

Fig. 3-21. Engaging in oculomotor tracking and laterality by standing with one foot ahead of the other on the balance beam. A ball is swung so that the child must track laterally with the eyes. He tracks the ball with the point of the wand as it moves back and forth.

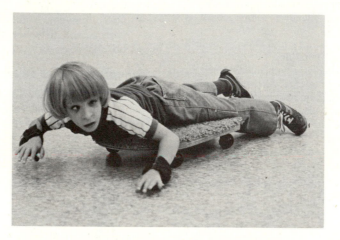

Fig. 3-22. Movement on a scooter provides information about the amplitude of force applied through the limbs of the body. (Courtesy of the Special Education Early Childhood Intervention Program, University of Kansas, Lawrence.)

movement exploration. This storage provides feedback data that are associated with movement output. The term given to this is *motor awareness*. Thus motor awareness enables the body to interpret motor data and to predict motor capability based on past experience.

Kinesthetic motor awareness is important in the development of vision because it is the central avenue through which motor movements are interpreted and paired with visual images. Stated another way, it is the means of assessing the relationship between energy expenditure and time lapse in order to judge distance visually. Kinesthetic motor awareness is essential in accurately establishing the relationships between visual objects and oneself (Fig. 3-19).

Kinesthetic motor awareness is also essential in executing higher-order complex skills that require the application of force. For instance, refined kinesthetic motor awareness is necessary in putting a golf ball, bunting a baseball, shooting a basketball, or executing a dropshot in tennis or badminton. If motor awareness is inaccurate in terms of the precise amount of force that must be applied in various game activities requiring striking, the performer may have difficulty mastering these skills (Fig 3-20).

Verticality

Another proposed construct that is part of the perceptual-motor structure is verticality. It has been hypothesized that this construct aids in erection of the body on the vertical axis and thus contributes to visual assessment of objects along vertical axes.[3] Vision is therefore used to identify objects accurately on a vertical continuum. Impairment of this factor would make it difficult for a child to perform many complex tasks; for example, in batting, the child might hit over or under a projectile.

Laterality

Laterality is an important construct in the cognitive development of children. Barsch[3] indicates that laterality is related to the structuring of symbols and objects in space on a lateral coordinate. It appears to be an internal awareness of the rightness and leftness of the body. This construct is purported to be developed through participation in lateral tasks of balance (Fig. 3-23).

Static balance. Static balance is the ability to maintain equilibrium in a variety of positions under various environmental conditions. Individuals need to be able to hold their balance to perform other tasks. One of the first static balance developmental milestones is the ability to hold the head up. Until an infant can lift and hold the head in an upright position, control over other movements of the head and body are not possible. Advanced static balance control is believed necessary before high levels of fine and gross motor control can occur.

Static balance is accomplished through develop-

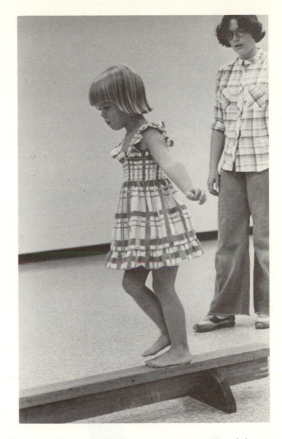

Fig. 3-23. Walking on a beam. The movement of the arms from side to side develops laterality. (Courtesy of the Special Education Early Childhood Intervention Program, University of Kansas, Lawrence.)

ment of strength, inner ear (vestibular) maturation, and postural reflex control.

Directionality

Spatial-temporal relationships are inseparable; however, for the purpose of this presentation five components relevant to an individual's perception of space and time are postulated. The constructs of the organization of space and time are distance duration, time, space, synchrony, and rhythm.

Distance duration. Distance duration is concerned with the perception of distance movement of objects or the body through space in a given period of time. This results from the movement of a projectile, which may be one's own body, to and from objects as the projectile covers a specified

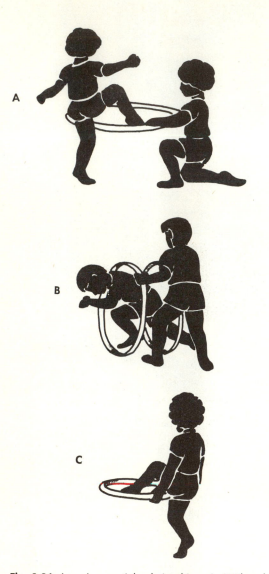

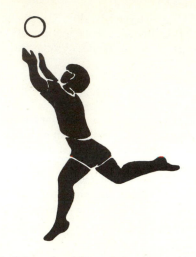

Fig. 3-25. Gaining the ability to judge distance duration and oculomotor tracking by throwing a ball into the air and running to catch it.

Fig. 3-24. Learning spatial relationships. **A,** With a hoop held level so that it is off the ground, the child steps over the front edge of the hoop and pulls it over the head without touching the body. **B,** With two hoops held apart and vertical to the ground, the child crawls through the hoops without touching them. **C,** With the hoop held in front of the belt area, the child swings it like a jump rope and jumps through it each time it comes around.

distance in a specified time. Perceptual judgments of persons' and objects' movements in relationship to distance and time are essential to mastering almost every game activity in the physical education curriculum. For example, when passing the ball to a receiver, a football player must predict with precision the length of time it will take the ball to reach a specified spot so that the receiver will not have to slow down to receive the ball. The passer must also accurately judge the speed of the receiver in relationship to the length of time the ball will be in the air. Any deficiency in distance-duration perception will hinder task mastery. Also, a diver or a gymnast must perceive specific points in time at which a tucking or twisting action is to be executed. With practice, the distance-duration component within a specific task may become a subroutine. A baseball batter must be able to predict the speed of the ball and anticipate the precise time it will arrive at the most advantageous spot to hit it with the bat. In addition, the batter must know how fast the bat should be swung to hit the ball at the optimal spot. Therefore, without perception of the distance-duration construct it is difficult to perform complex tasks that call for time-space interpretations of objects external to oneself. Acquisition of this ability is particularly essential in sports involving projection.

Time. Although time and space are inseparable,

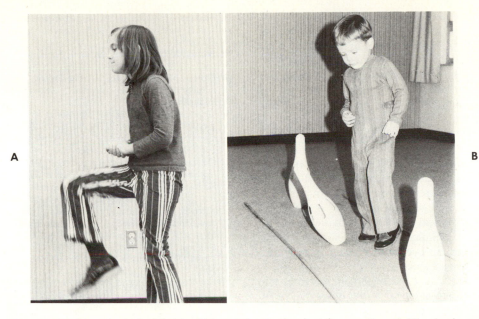

Fig. 3-26. Synchrony in rhythm. **A,** Marching and clapping hands at the same time. **B,** Weaving in and out of the bowling pins is difficult without synchrony of movement.

some motor activities are more heavily dependent upon predicting the occurrence of an event at a specific time. An example of an activity that would be highly time oriented would be rhythmical activities. An auditory stimulus is provided by music or a beat, and the body must make certain movements at precise time intervals. Spatial perception is thus less important than temporal perception. If a child has difficulty judging responses in relation to time intervals, then his or her motor performance will not be rhythmical.

Visual time is another component of the total time structure that must be interpreted by the senses. Visual time is concerned with the inspection of objects and then with the prediction of where an object will be at a specific moment. In physical activity, this is essential because a response must be made at specific time intervals for successful participation in many tasks. Thus, motor activity provides the opportunity for structuring the general developmental components of visual and auditory time. If a pupil cannot interpret time intervals visually, kinesthetically, and auditorially, then difficulty may be encountered in higher-order perceptual-motor tasks.

Space. Space is another perceptual component

that must be interpreted by the visual mechanism. Children who have problems relating the body kinesthetically to objects interpreted by vision will not perform well in tasks requiring these spatial relations. A hitter who swings at an object too soon exhibits inaccurate perception of space; since the person has not accurately interpreted the ball's spatial relations to the bat, he or she may fail to hit it. While learning to play, many elementary school baseball outfielders will stand still long after the ball has been hit and, consequently, will not make the catch; they may move toward the ball only a short time before it falls to the ground. Children who perform in this manner may be improperly relating the ball to themselves and to space.

Synchrony. Synchrony, also, is a component of the time-space structure. It is concerned with the transformation of one motor act into another in a time block and is designed to obtain proficient muscular control for a specific purpose. It occurs in many gross motor acts and also in refined motor tasks. Examples of motor tasks that involve synchrony include the following:

1. Starting and stopping a gross motor pattern.
2. Running a zigzag line or moving between objects and changing direction.

3. A springboard dive, such as a forward somersault half-twist. The somersault is one discrete action from which direction and body position must be transformed into the half-twist. Many gymnastics tasks include this perceptual-motor component. Synchrony is also common to fine motor skills such as prehensive manipulation of objects.

Rhythm. Synchrony is the disruption of rhythmical activities and its transformation into other movements. Rhythm involves similar repetitive motor acts performed in approximately equal time blocks.[3] Dance, requiring the learner to pair body movements with regular beats, is an obvious example of rhythmical activity. Activities such as walking and swimming are rhythmical also, in that repeated movement cycles must occur in sequence within equal time blocks.

Although synchrony and rhythm appear to be antithetical, both are essential to the development of a broad base of activities that enable the learner to adapt efficiently to the environment (Fig. 3-26).

SUMMARY

The development of perceptual ability is of critical importance to handicapped children, for it is closely associated with skill learning. If cues in the environment cannot be interpreted accurately, motor response will be less efficient. Inasmuch as most handicapped children have some perceptual deficiency and given that perception can be developed, it is the responsibility of physical educators to include perceptual-motor development opportunities in their curricula.

REFERENCES

1. Arnheim, D. D., and Sinclair, W. A.: The clumsy child: a program of motor therapy, ed. 2, St. Louis, 1979, The C. V. Mosby Co.
2. Ayres, A. J.: Sensory integration and learning disorders, Los Angeles, 1973, Western Psychological Services.
3. Barsch, R. H.: Achieving perceptual-motor efficiency, Seattle, 1967, Special Child Publications.
4. Becker, W. C., Engelmann, S., and Thomas, D. R.: Teaching: a course in applied psychology, Chicago, 1971, Science Research Associates, Inc.
5. Cratty, B. J.: Perceptual and motor development in infants and children, New York, 1970, Macmillan Publishing Co., Inc.
6. Dunsing, J., and Kephart, N. C.: Motor generalizations in space and time. In Hellmuth, J., editor: Learning disorders, Seattle, 1965, Special Child Publications.
7. Fiorentino, M. R.: Reflex testing methods for evaluating C.N.S. development, ed. 2, Springfield, Ill., 1970, Charles C Thomas, Publishers.
8. Frostig, M.: Movement education: theory and practice, Chicago, 1970, Follett Publishing Co.
9. Frostig, M., and Horne, D.: The Frostig program for the development of visual perception. Chicago, 1964, Follett Publishing Co.
10. Gearheart, B. R.: Learning disabilities: educational strategies, ed. 2, St. Louis, 1977, The C. V. Mosby Co.
11. Gesell, A., and Amatruda, C. S.: Developmental diagnosis, ed. 3, New York, 1975, Harper & Row, Publishers.
12. Getman, G. N.: Visuomotor complex in the acquisition of learning skills, Seattle, 1965, Special Child Publications.
13. Kephart, N. C.: Motor aids to perceptual training, Columbus, Ohio, 1968, Charles E. Merrill Publishing Co.
14. Kiphard, E. J., and Leger, A.: Basic psychomotor education, Flottman, Gutersloh, 1975, West Germany.
15. Muller, H., et al., editors: Motor behavior of preschool children, Schorndorf, Germany, 1975, Hofmann.
16. Piaget, J.: The psychology of intelligence, Totowa, N.J., 1967, Littlefield, Adams & Co.
17. U.S. Department of Health, Education, and Welfare, Regulations for the Rehabilitation Act of 1973, Federal Register **42:**22676-22702 (May 4) 1977.
18. Wundelich, R. C.: Learning disorders, Phys. Ther. **47:**700-708, 1969.

RECOMMENDED READINGS

Ball, T. S., Itard, S., and Kephart, N. C.: Sensory education—a learning interpretation, Columbus, Ohio, 1971, Charles E. Merrill Publishing Co.
Falik, L. H.: The effects of special perceptual-motor training in kindergarten on second grade reading, J. Learning Disabilities **2:**325-329, 1969.
Frostig, M.: Visual perception, integrative functions, and academic learning, J. Learning Disabilities **5:**1-15, 1972.
Hammill, D. D., and Bartel, N. R.: Teaching children with learning and behavior problems, Boston, 1975, Allyn & Bacon, Inc.
Hammill, D. D., Goodman, L., and Wiederholt, J. L.: Visual-motor processes: what success have we had in training them? The Reading Teacher **27:**469-478, 1974.
Kirk, S. A., and Kirk, W. P.: Psycholinguistic learning disabilities: diagnosis and remediation, Urbana, Ill., 1972, University of Illinois Press.
Lerner, J. W.: Children with learning disabilities, Boston, 1971, Houghton Mifflin Co.
Mann, L.: Perceptual training: misdirections and redirections, Am. J. Orthopsychiatry **40:**30-38, 1970.
Myklebust, H. R., editor: Progress in learning disabilities, New York, 1971, Grune & Stratton, Inc.
Turner, R. U., and Fisher, D.: The effects of a perceptual-motor training program upon the readiness and perceptual development of culturally disadvantaged children, ERIC ED 041 633, Washington, D.C., 1970, U.S. Government Printing Office.
Waugh, K. W., and Bush, W. J.: Diagnosing learning disorders, Columbus, Ohio, 1971, Charles E. Merrill Publishing Co.

4

Individual Education Program

Education is a lifelong process that relates to overall human development. Children grow and develop physically, mentally, socially, and emotionally along rather predictable paths. Allowing for individual differences, a teacher can thus use behavior as an observable indication of development. Such information can be used in a viable process for delivering educational benefits to handicapped children. The application of the developmental concept to instruction implies that benefits to be delivered to handicapped children should be specified in terms of behavioral characteristics in order to determine where students *are* within a hierarchical sequence of objectives, where they *should be* at present, and where they *might be* at a specified point in time as a result of some instructional intervention. (This approach to instruction is the basis of legislation and court decisions of the 1970's.)

LEGISLATION

The philosophy that education is for individual development and is a right of every child is implicit in the historic 1972 consent decree of the United States District Court for the Eastern District of Pennsylvania in the case of *PARC etc. vs. Commonwealth of Pennsylvania et al.* (Civil Action No. 71-42). Whereas this court action was directed at the inclusion of all children in the educational process, other judicial rulings as well as legislation in many states require the mainstream education of handicapped children.

P.L. 94-142[19] clearly indicates the right of handicapped children to appropriate physical education. The expectations are that physical education for the handicapped person should be designed to maximize the developmental potential of the person through mastery of functional leisure and domestic skills that lead to self-sufficiency in the community. The act itself, as well as its legislative history, is clear about the kinds of discrimination the Congress finds offensive. In so legislating P.L. 94-142 and other related enactments, Congress exercised its power under the Fourteenth Amendment to provide access to the educational benefits due each handicapped child in the United States. Thus, there is provision for equal protection under the law for handicapped children to acquire meaningful skills through physical education. The law reads as follows:

(16) The term ''special education'' means specially designed instruction, at no cost to parents or guardians, to meet the unique needs of a handicapped child, including classroom instruction, instruction in physical education, home instruction, and instruction in hospitals and institutions.

(19) The term ''individualized education program'' means a written statement for each handicapped child developed in any meeting by a representative of the local educational agency or an intermediate educational unit who shall be qualified to provide or supervise the provision of specially ''designed'' instruction to meet the unique needs of handicapped children, the teacher, the parents or guardian of such a child, and, whenever appropriate, such child, which statement shall include (A) a statement of the present levels of educational performance of such child, (B) a statement of annual goals, including short-term instructional objectives, (C) a statement of the specific educational services to be provided to such child, and the extent to which such child will be able to participate in regular educational programs, (D) the projected date for initiation and anticipated duration of such services, and appropriate objective criteria and evaluation procedures and schedules for determining, on at least an annual basis, whether instructional objectives are being achieved.

Although all components of the Individual Education Program are important and interdependent, the aspect that will receive most discussion in this chapter is *present level of educational performance,* which is extended by the acquisition of the *short-term instructional objective,* which thus ignites the developmental process. The definitions of these two essential terms are as follows: *present level of educational performance* means the present level from which short-term instructional objectives are formulated; *short-term instructional objective* means an activity performed by the pupil, described in specific, objective, and measurable terms, that is an intermediate step and extends the

present level of educational perfromance toward annual goals. There must be a relationship between the two concepts that provides the criteria for measurement of development.

TASK ANALYSIS AND THE INSTRUCTIONAL PROCESS OF THE INDIVIDUAL EDUCATION PROGRAM

It has been indicated by the courts that all children have the right to advance their capabilities to learn and develop. Thus, a zero reject by the public schools of severely handicapped children has been incorporated into P.L. 94-142. The instructional procedures that were found to be productive have since been incorporated into the instructional process of the Individual Education Program of P.L. 94-142. Thus, two questions immediately come to mind. First, how are these instructional procedures conducted? Second, do these procedures indeed work?

Implicit in the implementation procedures of teaching motor tasks to handicapped persons is the technical utilization of an instructional process. In a general manner, Gold[8] defines *task analysis* as all of the activity that results in there being sufficient power for the learner to acquire the task. Simply stated, task analysis involves observing a learner performing an educational task (preevaluation), identifying what the learner can and cannot do (present level of educational performance), breaking the instructional content into teachable units that are targets of instruction (short-term instructional objectives), and proceeding to teach those aspects of instruction that are presently unlearned. Using these procedures, handicapped persons can at least engage in the process of continuous learning. Thus, the instructional procedures are conducted as outlined by Congress for implementation of the Individual Education Program.

Regarding the effectiveness of the procedures, consider Gold,[8] who, in 20 trials, taught a person who was legally blind and deaf, physically handicapped, and mentally retarded (I.Q. of 28) to assemble a 14-part Bendix bicycle coaster brake. Keep in mind that the bicycle coaster brake assembly is a motor task and has similar prerequisites of motor behavior that can be generalized to many tasks in the physical education curriculum.

Gold's productive paper also provides insight for training personnel to conduct instructional strategies for those who use task analysis. In the study mentioned above, Gold did not conduct the study himself; rather, three trainers who received 2 days of training conducted the instruction to 22 moderately, severely, and profoundly retarded blind and deaf-blind persons.

The work of Gold[8] and Bellemy[2] indicates that there can be little question that the instructional technology of the nature that Congress had in mind is available to conduct programming.

Task analysis and readiness

The old belief that children simply did not learn because they were not ready does not apply in education today. In the past, the view was prevalent that readiness was a precondition for learning, with which we all can agree. However, according to this view, activities are presented by the teacher to the children on a trial and error basis. Those activities that are rejected by the children indicate that they are not ready to learn those specific tasks. Tasks to which the learners attend are at their readiness levels. For the most part, this approach is based on the intuition of the teacher with respect to pairing appropriate activities to the ability levels of the children. However, to a greater extent the development of the children is left to chance.

Task analysis and use of the instructional process of the Individual Education Program control the learning readiness of children because task activities reach them at their present levels of educational performance. Handicapped children are not provided with appropriate education unless instruction reaches them at their present levels of educational performance. If the instructional level is far above the children's abilities, they will not learn the specific tasks. Because of the frequency of discrepancy between instructional levels and ability levels, Congress addressed this issue when it outlined the Individual Education Program. It specified that every Individual Education Program is to reflect present levels of educational performance. This implies that when educational tasks are taught to handicapped children the limits of the children's capabilities should guide the selection of meaningful developmental activities. Thus, the readiness

factor is systematically controlled with the process of task analysis and programmed instruction.

Individual Education Program in the least restrictive environment

The handicapped child is entitled to an Individual Education Program in the least restrictive environment that is designed to meet his or her unique needs. A full preevaluation[19] should indicate unique needs by comparing actual performance with behaviors required for self-sufficiency in leisure motor skills in a specific community. Partial lists of norm-referenced tasks appear in Tables 2-1, 2-2, and 2-3 and may apply to preschool children who are thought to be handicapped. In addition, assessment must also be made of the capabilities of handicapped children to appropriately employ the strategies and to conform to the rules of the games that are taught in the physical education curriculum.

Arbitrary and capricious judgments by school officials that deny handicapped children the Individual Education Program in physical education without a substantiating data base from assessment of comprehensive curricula are unwarranted.

Meeting the unique needs of the handicapped individual

An axiom often heard among educators is that of meeting the unique needs of the student. In the past, such a phrase was vague to say the least. However, current diagnostic and instructional procedures enable educational needs to be met through precise measures. Communication through measured data is so precise that the school and the parents can assess the ongoing development of the child on the specific tasks prescribed in the Individual Education Program.[8,16,17] Indeed, instructional procedures at present are so specific that the courts have declared, based on expert testimony, that all handicapped children can learn if the unique needs or objectives are precisely identified and careful learning strategies are employed. Thus, meeting the unique needs of handicapped children has been incorporated by Congress into the definition of special education.[19]

The courts have requested documentation of educational outcomes for the handicapped as a result

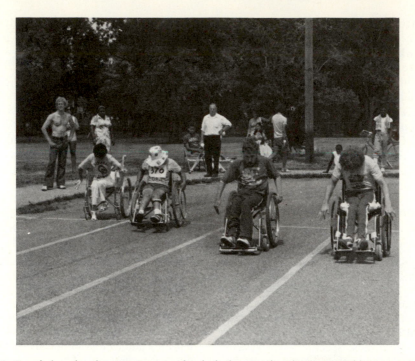

Fig. 4-1. Knowledge of each person's present level of educational performance enables management of equitable competition. (Provided through Unit on Programs for the Handicapped, American Alliance for Health, Physical Education, Recreation, and Dance.)

of education and training, and in so doing they have raised the question of whether children are receiving educational benefits as a result of programming. As has already been mentioned, measurable data must provide valid information that handicapped children are receiving *real*—not *imagined*—benefits. Implicit in statutes is that progress must be measured objectively and that there is a rationale for implementation of specific programming. The rationale for the establishment of a *need* (a goal or objective) to which programming is directed is derived from evaluation of the child's performance on educational tasks as compared with normative standards. If there is a discrepancy between the child's performance and a normative standard and if it represents a developmental delay, then it can be said that the child has a unique need on that specific task. Thus, the identification of developmental delays on specific tasks constitutes the identification of a unique need.

Once the need has been determined by assessing the child on educationally relevant tasks, goals for attaining mastery of the tasks are included in the Individual Education Program. Group teaching in which all children perform the same task is of little value in meeting the unique needs of handicapped children.

Unique needs can be developed in another sense. A need may not necessarily be a deficit, but rather it may be a task that would further develop an interest of a child. An interest in a strength area may be identified by the child, parents, or the school. Further development of the skill may enable greater participation and may enhance the individual's satisfaction. The development of such skills can be utilized in intramural and interscholastic competition and can provide opportunity for participation in the community.

Unique needs are considered those properties of the individual that pose some limitation of func-

Table 4-1. Misconceptions about special education

Misconception	Conditions under which assumption is valid
Special education is a classroom where handicapped children are educated.	Not unless they receive specially designed instruction to meet their unique needs that includes the contents of the Individual Education Program of Section 602(19) of P.L. 94-142.
Handicapped children receive special education.	Special education is their entitlement, but they are not receiving special education unless the instruction is specially designed to meet their unique needs and includes the contents of the Individual Education Program of Section 602(19) of P.L. 94-142.
Handicapped children do not receive special education in the regular class.	Special education is their entitlement, but they are not receiving special education unless the instruction is specially designed to meet their unique needs and includes the contents of the Individual Education Program of Section 602(19) of P.L. 94-142.
Regular classroom teachers do not administer special education to handicapped children in the regular class.	It is the entitlement of every handicapped child to receive special education regardless of educational placement. However, they do not receive special education unless the instruction is specially designed to meet their unique needs and includes the contents of the Individual Education Program of Section 602(19) of P.L. 94-142.
Nonhandicapped children in the regular class do not receive special education.	They may receive special education if the instruction is specially designed to meet their unique needs and includes the contents of the Individual Education Program of Section 602(19) of P.L. 94-142.
Special education teachers who are certified deliver special education.	Certified special education teachers should deliver special education services. However, they do not unless they provide specially designed instruction that includes the contents of the Individual Education Program of Section 602(19) of P.L. 94-142.

tioning in the school or the community. They indicate discrepancy between performance and normative expectations on tasks in the physical education curriculum. Furthermore, needs that are unique to the individual are not determined by arbitrary judgments. Indeed, they are determined by precise, objective measurement procedures employed by highly trained professionals on educationally relevant motor behaviors. Judicious instructional decisions are made from these data to effect ongoing, measured development of the child.

The enactment of P.L. 94-142 requires new procedures for instructing handicapped children. Consider the design of this legislation as indicated in the following passage:

The Senate Bill and House amendments add a new definition to the Education of the Handicapped Act of *special education*. The definitions are identical . . . [and] additionally specify that the instruction is to meet the unique needs of the handicapped child as set forth in the *individual education program of such child*.[4]

An analysis of the new definition indicates that educational personnel who work with the handicapped must focus on the delivery of educational service through implementation of the Individual Education Program. Indeed, implementation of the Individual Education Program *is* special education. Thus, the central focus of this chapter is on the implementation aspects of the Individual Education Program (or, stated another way, *special education*), of which physical education is a part.

Special education is an instructional process

Special education is a process in which there is specially designed instruction that meets the unique needs of children and that is conducted as set forth in the Individual Education Program, section 602(19) of P.L. 94-142. Inasmuch as physical education is an integral part of special education, it is desirable to alleviate misconceptions about special education. There are several invalid assumptions about special education and the instruction of handicapped children. P.L. 94-142 has made these previous assumptions conditional. The assumptions and conditions are listed in Table 4-1.

Special education is not a place where handicapped children are taught nor a place where special education teachers instruct. It is a specific instructional process of the Individual Education Program, section 602(19) of P.L. 94-142. It has been indicated that the Individual Education Program must provide written statements that indicate specially designed instruction to meet the unique needs of handicapped children and that include statements of present levels of educational performance, annual goals, and short-term instructional objectives.

Equally effective education

Section 504 of the Rehabilitation Act of 1973[18] specifies that no handicapped person shall be denied benefits from programs receiving federal assistance. Inasmuch as institutions of public education receive federal funds, they must provide educational benefits to handicapped children. Not only must handicapped children benefit from their education, but it is to be as effective as that provided to the nonhandicapped. Section 504 indicates that for education to be equally effective, it must afford handicapped persons equal opportunities to attain the same results, gain the same benefits, or reach the same levels of achievement as their nonhandicapped peers. To be equally effective, however, an aid or service need not produce equal results. Each must merely afford an equal opportunity to achieve equal results. This process is intended to encompass the concept of equivalent (as opposed to identical) services and to acknowledge the fact that, to meet the individual needs of handicapped persons to the same extent that the corresponding needs of nonhandicapped persons are met, adjustments or accommodations to regular programs or provisions of different programs may sometimes be necessary. *Equal treatment and equal opportunity, thus, are not synonymous.* In fact, equal treatment of handicapped persons can be discriminatory. Equality of opportunity for every handicapped person is the key consideration in this process.

In the case of *Lau vs. Nichol*,[12] the Supreme Court ruled that the provision of schooling in the English language alone to children from non–English-speaking families was tantamount to the denial of schooling altogether and that hence it was illegal. Regarding equally effective programs, Supreme Court Chief Justice Berger wrote in response to a unanimous court decision:

Congress has now required that the posture and conditions of the . . . seeker be taken into account and the criterion of services may not provide equality of opportunity merely in the sense of the fable which offers milk to the fox in a long-necked pitcher and the stork in a shallow pitcher, but must provide the vessel in which the milk is proffered be one all seekers can use.[12]

Equally effective service (physical education for the handicapped) should provide for accommodation of the individual as needed to attain maximum

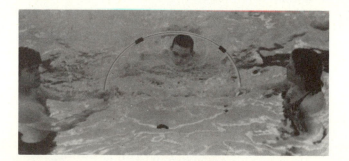

Fig. 4-2. Hierachies for swimming involve the distance that the individual can swim, distance over time, and the degree to which the body assumes a horizontal position. The submerged lower portion of the hoop provides feedback to the swimmer regarding horizontal positioning of the body. (Courtesy of Carolyn Williams, Handicapped Swim Program, Slipperty Rock State College, Slippery Rock, Penn.)

program benefits. This implies that there be compensatory aids, services, or adjustments in regular programs. Thus, in physical education, individualization of instruction provides accommodation and is essential for equally effective services to the handicapped.

The theme of consideration for the individual again was sounded in the case of *Fredrick vs. Thomas*,[9] in which the Eastern District Court of Pennsylvania ruled that the placement of a learning disabled child in a regular class with no provision for individual accommodation was tantamount to no education at all and may even have been harmful. It is clear that handicapped children placed in regular class must participate in Individual Education Programs that meet their unique needs.

MAINSTREAMING

The concept of mainstreaming is predicated on the application of the developmental concept, which implies that each individual is unique with respect to specific abilities. Since the abilities of each individual are at different developmental levels, the developmental concept cannot be applied unless there is individualization of instruction. If individualization of instruction is practiced, there is less need for homogeneous grouping, allowing handicapped children to be educated in the mainstream of education.

Modern educational technology has made the implementation of the developmental process feasible for each child through attainment of instructional objections. These objectives are organized in prerequisite order to form programmed instruction. Thus, the application of the developmental process involves the establishment of a sequence of hierarchical instructional objectives. Current legislation clearly indicates that there must be a direct relationship between assessment and programming and that there must be precise and continuous monitoring of all behaviors as an individual progresses through these sequences en route to mastery of specific tasks.

Mainstreaming vs. restrictive environment

It is fallacious to assume that handicapped and nonhandicapped children can be taught in two separate groups in a regular physical education class.

Stigmatizing handicapped children in front of their peers by magnifying differences between them and nonhandicapped children restricts their opportunities to function in a normal setting.

Handicapped children are receiving physical education in the least restrictive environment when there is individualized instruction for all of the children who are in a specific class. The procedures for conducting the Individual Education Program for all children are not new. The technology for such a system was developed in the 1960's and was employed in many school districts. However, problems at that particular time included the systematic curriculum that extended from kindergarten through grade 12 and inadequate personnel preparation to conduct the curriculum. However, with the advent of P.L. 94-142, deficiencies in the total individualized system have been rectified. Thus, the implementation of the Individual Education Program in the least restrictive environment can be effectively conducted only if all children in a specific class receive an Individual Education Program.

All handicapped children are to profit from a Individual Education Program conducted in the regular class. A prerequisite to participation in such a class is to teach learners to use self-instructional procedures and an evaluative, task-analyzed, hierarchically structured curriculum. Once these behaviors are learned, it is possible for the children to learn without direct input and feedback from the teacher. Thus, under such conditions, the teaching of handicapped persons does not restrict the learning of normal children who are also progressing at their own rates. Therefore, analysis of tasks to formulate instructional hierarchies enables measured and systematic organization of education to maximize developmental potential. Prearranged, task-analyzed motor behavior that is the target of instruction promotes accountability of the measured educational progress of each child. Such programmed instructional materials enable measurement of the degree of competence when instruction starts (content-referenced measurement). From this point in the task-analyzed activity, meaningful skills can be taught. However, trained teachers are needed to implement such instructional materials. Such a system can facilitate evaluation of teacher performance in relationship to the outcomes of the learner.

DEVELOPMENTAL CONCEPT OF EDUCATION
Hierarchy and developmental tasks

Hierarchies developed from task analyses facilitate the ordering of instructional activities for the purpose of development. A hierarchy is a continuum of ordered activities in which a task of a lower order and of lesser difficulty is prerequisite to acquisition of a task of greater difficulty. Progress from one task to another in a hierarchy serves as a measure of student development and answers three vital, educationally relevant questions: (1) What is the student's present level of educational performance? (2) What short-term instructional objectives should be provided to extend the present level of educational performance or development? (3) How much development has already occurred? Task analysis therefore is a valuable tool for the development of instructional hierarchies.

The application of the developmental concept to education was an attempt by the United States Office of Education to promote the accountability of the measured educational progress of each child. It has as its central concern the development of instructional procedures that involve the following factors:

1. *Curricula* that provide learning experiences that state educational progress in terms of developmental concept and from which diag-

nosis of the unique needs of children is possible
2. *Trained teachers* to implement the curricula
3. *Evaluation procedures* that are addressed to individual teacher competency, curricula quality, and pupil competency

Individualizing instruction

Procedures employed in applying developmental concepts to individualized instruction vary greatly from traditional instruction designed to teach groups. Table 4-2 compares the essential differences between these two instructional approaches.

Programmed instruction

Modern trends call for the individualization of instruction; however, as typical children begin formal education during the fifth year of life, they usually have developed the capability to begin to direct some of their own learning. With the acquisition of self-directing and self-evaluating skills students are freed from dependency on the teacher. The possibilities for unlimited instructional input and feedback become a reality. It is at this point in development that self-instructional and self-evaluative learning materials in the form of programmed instruction should be introduced into the educational schema. One major goal of an individualized instruction system is to develop a communication system between the student and teacher by which they can become as independent of one another as possible. The teacher's ultimate primary role is one

Table 4-2. Traditional approach versus the Individual Education Program approach to instruction

Traditional approach	IEP approach
Teachers design curricula according to their experience in areas of intended interest.	There must be measurable predetermined objectives to be taught by teachers.
Teachers develop their own curricula within framework of guidelines. Assessment instruments are at discretion of teachers.	There must be programmed materials or behavioral inventories that indicate what a child can and cannot do prior to program implementation so that progress can be made toward goals.
Teachers' skills are a composite of their particular learning experiences.	There must be specifically trained teachers with competencies that will enable reproducibility of curricula to to provide measurable learning results.
Lesson plans tend to be general and follow guidelines.	Lessons of teachers must be so specific that they are reproducible by another person.

of guiding and managing instruction according to the student's individual needs and learning characteristics. This approach enables the teacher to cope with heterogeneous groups of children and to accommodate large numbers of children in the same class without sacrificing instructional efficiency. In order to implement such a program, however, three major factors must be taken into consideration: (1) programming must be constructed on the basis of scientific principles,[2,3,6] (2) learners must be trained in specific behaviors,[7] and (3) learning principles must be applied through the use of programmed curricula.

The most expeditious way to manage an average-sized class in a public school, using the individualized developmental approach, is through the use of instructional objectives that shift learning conditions to create developmental task sequences. Prearranged instructional objectives take the form of self-instructional and self-evaluative programs that are appropriate for typical children and for atypical children. However, for the child who cannot self-instruct and self-evaluate, task analysis and pattern analysis will facilitate development. The child functioning at a low level and the child who strives to reach upper limits of development for competitive purposes will need special types of programming and thus specific attention by instructors when the teacher-student ratio is low. Self-instructional and evaluative materials composed of prearranged objectives provide opportunities for students to develop skills at their own rates. Thus, when such materials and procedures are introduced to handicapped and nonhandicapped persons who participate in regular class, they all have opportunities to maximize their developmental potential. An adapted list of characteristics for such a program has been suggested by Lindvall and Bolvin[13] and appears below.

1. Definition of the objectives the students are expected to achieve must be clear and specific.
2. Objectives must be stated in behavioral terms.
3. Objectives must lead to behaviors that are carefully analyzed and sequenced in a hierarchical order so that each behavior builds on the objectives immediately preceding and is prerequisite to those that follow.
4. Instructional content of a program must consist of a sequence of learning tasks through which a student can proceed with little outside help and must provide a series of small increments in learning that enable the student to proceed from a condition of lack of command of behavior to a condition of command of behavior.
5. A program must permit the student to begin at the present ability level and allow him or her to move upward from that point.
6. A program must allow each student to proceed independently of other students and learn at a rate best suited to his or her own abilities and interests.
7. A program must require active involvement and response on the part of the student at each step along the learning sequence.

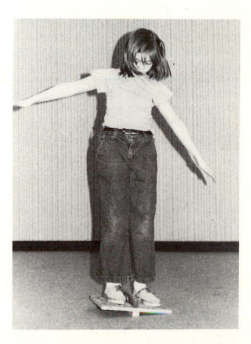

Fig. 4-3. Equipment that relates to a program. Balance sticks are different widths. The board can be turned to the other side for a more difficult task; the eyes can be used in a different way; constraints can be placed on movement of the arms. To form either a less or more difficult sequence, activities can be constructed to that one is a required prerequisite to another.

8. A program must provide immediate feedback to the student concerning the adequacy of his or her performance.
9. A program must be subjected to continuous study by those responsible for it and should be regularly modified in the light of available evidence concerning the student's performance.
10. A program must accommodate the ability range of many students, thus enabling continuous progress.

Preevaluation of children

Content measurement refers to information of the learner's present level of educational performance in classroom instruction prior to initiation of programming. Preevaluation through content measurement links data from assessment with classroom instruction. The overall goal of such an instructional procedure is to enable measured learning of each child, handicapped or not, along developmental continua. Preevaluation information secured through content measurement is essential to indicate measured educational progress of students. Some preevaluation techniques are as follows:

1. Preevaluation data on motor development tasks as measured against *normative developmental scales* with suggested techniques for subsequent programming based on task analysis and knowledge of the *principles of development*
2. Preevaluation data obtained through task analysis of *skills from behavioral inventories*
3. Preevaluation data obtained through the placement of the individual in *hierarchical learning curricula* that take the *form of programmed instruction*

INSTRUCTIONAL OBJECTIVES

The instructional objective is a specific, predetermined learning experience that, if mastered, extends development. Instructional objectives take several forms. The purpose of this discussion is to establish objectives in relationship to the total instruction process.

Objectives occur at different levels of curricular development and must be appropriate for the ability level of a specifically diagnosed individual (Fig. 4-4). They require an assessment of the learner in relationship to what he or she can and cannot do. In the event that mastery of a specific behavior is not possibly by a learner, the question is asked, "What prerequisites are needed for this individual to achieve mastery of this task?" This question, once answered, is restated until the student's present level of performance is determined and the appropriate instructional objective is determined. A sequence of prerequisite activities thus

---

General objective: Develop the elbow extensors and arm flexors with *push-up* activity.

SPECIFICATION OF CONDITIONS	RATIONALE
1. Straighten back and hips to 180 degrees.	Bending either part of body reduces length of resistance arm and decreases degree of difficulty of task.
2. Place hands shoulder width apart on floor.	Spreading hands wider than shoulder width increases difficulty of task.
3. Tuck chin against sternum.	Raising head while performing tends to bend the back and shorten resistance arm.
4. Touch forehead to floor.	Touching forehead indicates starting and ending position of push-up.
5. Straighten arms to 180 degrees.	Straightening arms indicates degree of movement of arms (will count as one repetition).
6. Support weight on hyperextended toes, which rest on floor.	Supporting weight indicates the point of the fulcrum to control length of resistance arm.

provides a chain of instructional events that leads the learner from lower to higher levels of mastery within the instructional content. The utilization of this instructional process requires that detailed records be kept on each learner so that one can understand where he or she is in a learning activity sequence. The mastery of one objective is the prerequisite that gives rise to a more complex objective, making development progressive (see Chapter 18).*

The instructional objective must incorporate four concepts: (1) it must possess an action, (2) it must establish conditions under which actions occur, (3) it must establish a criterion for mastery of a spe-

---

*See also assignments 29 and 30 in Crowe, W. C., Arnheim, D. D., and Auxter, D.: Laboratory manual in adapted physical education and recreation, St. Louis, 1977, The C. V. Mosby Co.

cific task, and (4) it must lie outside the child's present level of educational performance.

The action concept

The action aspect of the instructional objective indicates what the learner will do in the execution of the task. It is important that the action take a verb form.

It is necessary to specify the conditions under which the action of the instructional objective is to occur. This is particularly necessary when programming instruction to preserve developmental sequences that lead to goals and objectives. The specification of the movement to be demonstrated is most important in preserving the hierarchical elements of a programmed activity. An example of conditions from which an instructional objective can be developed is provided on p. 88.

The violation of any of the conditions that make up an instructional objective render it inappropriate and a deterrent to measured development. If the conditions are not specified, there can be little agreement as to the capability of a student and thus

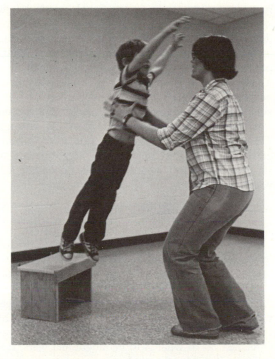

Fig. 4-4. Persons learn body control when they are airborne. (Courtesy of the Special Education Early Childhood Intervention Program, University of Kansas, Lawrence.)

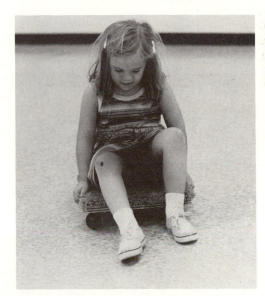

Fig. 4-5. The measure of this task is the distance that the scooter can be moved over a given period of time. (Courtesy of the Special Education Early Childhood Intervention Program, University of Kansas, Lawrence.)

as to the appropriate selection of a developmental activity. It should be noted that specified conditions of the objective channel development of the individual in the hierarchy (Fig. 4-5).

Criterion for mastery of a specific task

The criterion for mastery of a specific task indicates when students have mastered assigned instructional objectives and indicates pupil progress. It serves notice that one prerequisite has been mastered. Criteria for task mastery can take several different forms, as may be seen in the following examples:

1. Number of repetitions (10 repetitions)
2. Number of repetitions over time (20 repetitions in 15 seconds)
3. Distance traveled (8 feet on a balance beam without falling off)
4. Distance traveled over time (200 yards in 25 seconds)
5. Number of successive trials without a miss (four times in a row)

6. Specified number of successful responses in a block of trials (three of five)
7. Mastery of all the stated conditions of the task
8. Number of degrees of movement (flexibility in degrees of movement in starting and terminal positions)

There are other forms of measurement for the criterion of mastery. The intent of the criterion of mastery is to objectively communicate to all parties concerned when the task has been mastered. This is important to the learner for the following reasons: (1) it is immediately reinforcing, (2) it provides an immediate target of performance mastery, and (3) it acts as an indicator of readiness to be assigned more advanced tasks (Fig. 4-6).

It should be noted that objectives are not valid unless they are directed at the acquisition of behaviors that lie outside the current repertoire of an individual's capability. The intent of the instructional process is to add new behaviors; therefore, a prerequisite for stating an instructional objective is to assess each learner on a continuum of activities to determine what he or she can and cannot do. Hierarchies are important for the construction of appropriate instructional objectives. Once a behavior on a hierarchy can be mastered by an individual, all behaviors falling below it are not worthy of being considered instructional objectives for that person (thereby reducing the amount of initial testing). Therefore, the hierarchically structured learning curriculum must be considered a very efficient instructional instrument in managing accountable educational data.

Acceptable and unacceptable instructional objectives

There are three central features essential to fulfilling the developmental systems model of instruction through instructional objectives: (1) there must be justification that the objectives are relevant to the learner, (2) objectives must possess the capability of being reproduced when implemented by independent instructors, and (3) there must be an agreement as to what is to be taught and when it is to be mastered by the student.

The unacceptable instructional objectives and goals presented in Table 4-3 are discussed in more detail in the following outline:

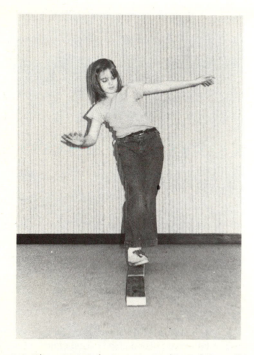

Fig. 4-6. The criterion for mastery in this task is walking 8 feet, the length of the 4-inch-wide balance beam.

1. Run as fast as you can.
   CONDITIONS: The condition of distance or other environmental arrangements such as hurdles and nature of the course are not specified.
   CRITERION: An objective distance over measured time is not in the objective. The perception *as fast as you can* is subjective. Players or students may think that they are running as fast as they can. The coach or teacher may evaluate the performances differently.
2. Walk on a balance beam without falling off.
   CONDITIONS: The width of the balance beam makes the task more or less difficult. It is not specified. The position of the arms and utilization of the visual mechanism are other conditions that affect performance.
   CRITERION: The distance to be traveled and distance over time are not specified.
3. Swim to the end of the pool.
   CONDITIONS: The type of stroke is not specified.
   CRITERION: Swimming pools are different lengths. The behavior in the performer's pool cannot be generalized to another pool.

Effective utilization of instructional objectives

There has been considerable controversy concerning the use of instructional objectives. Concerns that have been indicated by critics include the following: (1) instructional objectives are difficult to manage, (2) they take too much time, (3) they require too much testing, (4) more important aspects of instruction that cannot be measured are not stressed, and (5) they impersonalize instruction. Many of these concerns are well founded; however, with the effective management of programmed instruction and the proper utilization of instructional objectives, an accounting of measured learning and a systematic revision of the instructional processes can be achieved.

Task analysis

There are several techniques for the analysis of abilities that are the basis for the instructional ob-

Table 4-3. Acceptable and unacceptable objectives

Action	Condition	Criterion
Acceptable objectives		
Run	1 mile	In 5 minutes 30 seconds
Walk	A balance beam 4 inches wide, heel to toe, eyes closed, and hands on hips	For 8 feet
Swim	Using the American crawl in a 25-yard pool for 50 yards	In 35 seconds
Unacceptable objectives		
Run		As fast as you can
Walk	On a balance beam	Without falling off
Swim		To the end of the pool

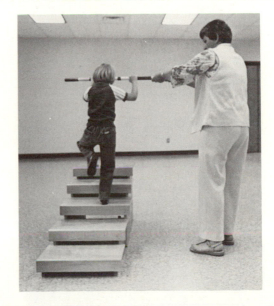

Fig. 4-7. A stick held by the child serves as a prompt to assist the child in ascending stairs. (Courtesy of the Special Education Early Childhood Intervention Program, University of Kansas, Lawrence.)

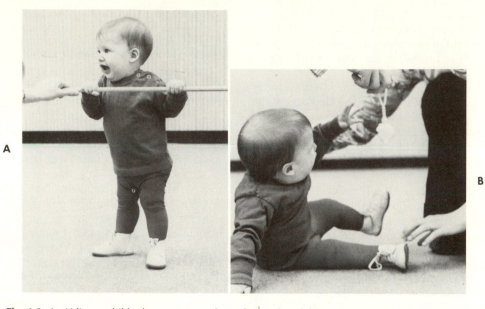

Fig. 4-8. A, Aiding a child who cannot stand erectly. **B,** This child needs greater balance to maintain a sitting position. Through task analysis of sitting, it can be seen that the placement of the hand indicates that balance is a prerequisite to the sitting behavior. Task analysis can start with any skill at any level of development.

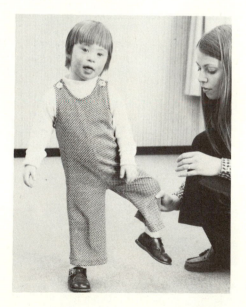

Fig. 4-9. Development of the balance mechanism should start early. A handicapped child 33 months of age begins a balance program.

jective of a specific learner. Some of these procedures involve (1) analysis of higher-order skills or abilities that require open-ended development for leisure activity or vocational pursuits, (2) analysis of a skill or task to serve as a prerequisite for engaging in a more complex task, (3) acquisition of a behavior within the pattern of a skill, and (4) analysis of behaviors through inventory of subtasks to determine needed prerequisite behaviors. Whatever the procedure, the instructional objective is usually the result of an analysis of higher-order tasks that lead to present tasks for instruction. It then becomes necessary to perform task analysis to determine the prerequisite behaviors that lead to the attainment of higher-order objectives (Figs. 4-7 and 4-8).

Examples of task analysis to formulate instructional objectives (terminal objectives)
Example A

I. Correct reversals of a child in visualizing letters or symbols such as *b* and *d* by activating the lateral balancing mechanisms. This will establish internal lateral perception, which is expressed externally with the child's vision.

A. *Task analysis*
  1. Relate problem to development of laterality (internal awareness of right and left).[11]
  2. Place in a lateral balance program (operational description of laterality).[11]
  3. Diagnose current level of the learner's ability to balance (Fig. 4-9).
B. *The task*
  Balance in a heel-to-toe position on a stick 1 inch wide for 5 seconds with eyes closed and hands on hips. (This is assuming that the child has not mastered this task.) This instructional objective would be derived through preevaluation of the present level of educational performance with subsequent determination of appropriate activity.

Example B

I. Demonstrate the ability to stand in an upright position.
  A. *Task analysis*
    List all behaviors prerequisite to standing:
    1. Control of the thoracic extensors of the spine
    2. Control of the lumbar extensors of the spine
    3. Muscular strength in the hips and knees
    4. Counterbalance of gravitational forces to maintain balance
  B. *The task*
    After assessment for a hypothetical learner, a subtask might be to sit erect with legs extended and hands on the floor beside the hips for 10 seconds. (Many programs need to be constructed to achieve this goal.)

Task-analyzed, preplanned activities and programmed instruction that lead to goal tasks contribute to efficient instructional management. Preplanned activities that enable continued development of the individual through attainment of short-term instructional objectives are implicit in P.L. 94-142. Inasmuch as the short-term instructional objectives are the cornerstones of development, it does not make sense that they should be selected intuitively. Indeed, to provide maximal opportunity for development, activities should be related to behavioral task analysis or hierarchical programmed instruction.

Congress has specified that there should be frequent monitoring of a handicapped child's progress throughout the school year so that appropriate steps can be taken to resolve problems in educational progress.[5] In the event that a child is not progressing as he or she should be, opportunities for correction of instructional errors are provided within

a reasonable length of time.[3,5,6] The preplanned activities from task analysis and programmed instruction enable adequate monitoring for a handicapped child's progress throughout the school year[6] because of the specificity of what is to be taught. Furthermore, preplanned activities enable the parent to take part in the process.[5] There are several distinct ways in which preplanned activities help children learn. Programmed instructional objectives function as follows:

1. They assist teachers with evaluation of the curriculum so that it may be revised to facilitate the child's learning at a subsequent time.
2. They structure behavior so that there are interrelationships between activities. This facilitates development.
3. They can introduce scientific validity to curriculum materials. This enhances accountability and assists refinement of measures that indicate the child's educational progress.
4. They enable employment of procedures that indicate limits of the child's current functioning on a specific task.
5. They provide opportunities for the child to become a self-directed learner and to have an Individual Education Program in the regular class without undue attention.
6. They enable a comparison between where the child *is* in the sequence and where the child *should be* based on chronological age expectancies.
7. They provide information about the strengths and weaknesses of the child so that relevant instructional decisions can be made to meet unique needs.
8. They enable communication with the parents so that instructional programming may be continued in the home.
9. They free the teacher from curriculum construction so that he or she may manage individualized instruction.
10. They facilitate the monitoring of the instructional delivery system.
11. They enable evaluation of instructional techniques through knowledge of measurable learning outcomes.
12. They enable the child to progress continuously when the instructional setting is

changed and facilitate the coordination of efforts between the physical educator and those who provide related services.

13. They guide the revision process when changes are made in the Individual Education Program.
14. They expedite the attainment of goals of the Individual Education Program.
15. They assist with appropriate allocation of responsibility, time, facilities, and other resources among professionals.
16. They enable placement of the handicapped child in regular class where he or she can work independently on the Individual Education Program.
17. They enable the systematic application of principles of learning to behavioral analysis.

Selection of appropriate curricular tasks

Data indicated on the Individual Education Program must be capable of measuring the learning of each student along a developmental continuum (or of measuring the acquisition of skills not yet mastered in a behavioral inventory). The development of curricula is based on building blocks that consist of short-term instructional objectives that are discrete and unambiguous. The developmental in-

structional approach cannot be studied separately from the total curriculum. The application of the Individual Education Program can yield accountable learning results (data) for each learner, whether handicapped or not. This can be accomplished through behavioral inventories, task-analyzed curricula, programmed instruction, or comparison of abilities along a developmental continuum.

Incorporation of learning principles in the curriculum

Once target behaviors have been identified, it is possible to apply known learning principles to enable the learner to acquire new behaviors. However, without programmed curricula to which assessment can be linked, there is little opportunity for the application of learning principles.

Sequential hierarchical curricula, mastered and unmastered,[1] tend to keep instructors informed as to which behaviors lie outside the current repertoire of each child. Behavioral inventories are more difficult to interpret in the management of pupil information because one behavior may not be prerequisite to the acquisition of another. The charting of progression becomes much more difficult as the complexity of behavioral acquisition increases. The objective specification of what is to be learned pro-

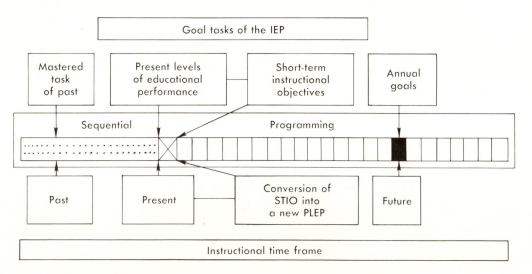

Fig. 4-10. Instructional process of the Individual Education Program.

vides immediate feedback to the learner as to whether or not the task has been mastered. This enables self-reinforcement through known task mastery so that instruction can be directed toward the positive aspects of task mastery.

The intent of curricula designed to implement the Individual Education Program is to allow reproducibility of the results achieved by the learner. The specification of such programming as well as implementation procedures that allow for instructional reproducibility have several positive features, namely:

1. External evaluators can provide information on the procedures employed by the teacher and the results achieved by learners.
2. Evaluation, followed by revisions of implementation in the training of teachers, may be tested empirically.

3. Incorporation of suggestions from other teachers using the same or similar instructional materials may be employed to improve instructional efficiency.

Placement profile

The placement profile sheet describes the strengths and weaknesses of each student on all instructional tasks indicated by preevaluation data. Utilizing the information received on each child, the teacher then selects those programs or tasks that are of highest priority to a particular child. The placement profile may also indicate the amount of time or the emphasis to be placed on specific tasks as compared with other tasks (Fig. 4-11).

The placement profile sheet should contain the following information:

1. A vertical listing of the programs

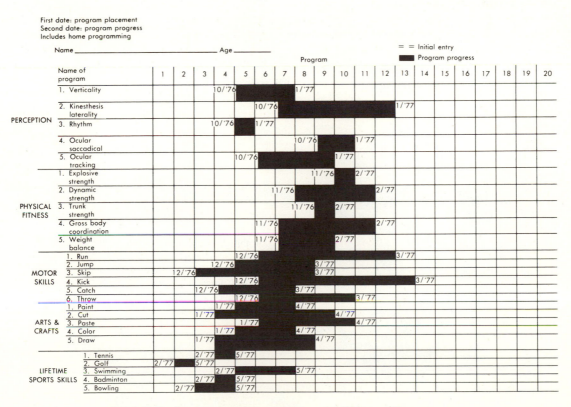

Fig. 4-11. Profile sheet for shifting criterion and shifting condition programs.

Program domain: Perceptual-motor

Justification of program: Two balls of different resiliency are dropped simultaneously (a 1-inch hard rubber ball with great resiliency and a 2-inch sponge rubber ball with less resiliency). This imparts variance in the height of the rebound and develops identification of different rates of speed of moving objects. The increment of distance between the balls that are dropped increases the span of perception that is important in sport, academic, and vocational skills.

Components developed by the program: Span of perception, hand-eye coordination

Type of program: Shifting criterion

Materials needed: Yardstick, 1-inch Superball, 2-inch sponge rubber ball

Communication code: Pictorial symbols:

Equipment layout: Sufficient space to perform the task

Description of task: Place a yardstick on the floor in front of the body and drop the two balls on the floor so that the distance between the landing points of the balls can be measured. Arms start in front of shoulders and gradually increase in width during the ball drop.

Measurement system: Distance between the dropped balls

Task specifications:
1. The balls must be dropped from shoulder height.
2. The balls must be caught in the hands.

Fig. 4-12. Ball drop test, an example of a shifting criterion program.

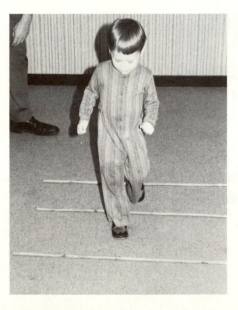

Fig. 4-13. In this shifting criterion program, the task, requiring that sequentially longer steps be taken, lengthens the stride and requires more efficient utilization of the balancing mechanism. The program is designed so that sequentially the sticks are moved a greater distance apart until the desired alteration in gait occurs.

2. The numbers or measures of the program objectives indicated horizontally at the top of the page
3. The pupil's name
4. The student's birth date to compute the age (to make comparison with normative data)
5. A graph of the entry level on each element of the program
6. The date on which each child entered the program

TYPES OF PROGRAMS USING THE DEVELOPMENTAL PROCESS

A program is built around a conceptual model of a skill that is analyzed into prerequisites. Four types of programs can be used with this in mind. The *criterion shifting program* utilizes sequential instructional objectives in which the standards of performance are continually raised. The *condition shifting program* allows sequential behaviors to emerge through shifting the conditions of the instructional objective from a lesser to a greater difficulty. The *task analysis program* uses analysis of subtasks of a behavior in which there is a relationship of one specific subtask to another. The *subjective movement analysis program* uses subjective analysis of movement behavior that is dependent on temporal-spatial relationships of elements of movement for such activities as running, jumping, and throwing.

Name of program: Broad jump

Program domain: Physical and motor

Justification of program: The broad jump is a significant program because it is (1) a normative measure for the construct of explosive strength and (2) a skill at the preschool levels that has the capability of measuring the phylogenetic development of the child. Therefore it is an important development task at most levels of development. Furthermore, it is a basic task that may be generalized into many aspects of sport skill performance. At the preschool levels of development, it involves (1) bilateral development, which later has implications for binocular fusion in the development of vision, and (2) elaboration of the posturing mechanism through its projection in front of the base.

Components developed by the program: Explosive strength
Type of program: Shifting criterion
Materials needed: Yardstick
Communication code: Pictorial symbols:

Equipment layout: There is a restraining line behind which the jump must be executed. Markers may be placed on the floor by the performer to indicate target distances that are to be attempted, commensurate with ability.

Criterion measure: Acquire a performance baseline on the jump and then require the pupil to jump 1 inch farther. The base level of performance should be determined for each child. The criterion measure for any jump for a specific child would be a specified distance indicated by the instructor above the base level, yet within the child's range of success in the near future.

Task specifications:
1. Place feet behind starting line.
2. Measure from the tip of the toe of the foot closest to the starting line.
3. Land on two feet.
4. Feet cannot move after they land.

Fig. 4-14. Broad jump test, an example of a shifting criterion program.

Criterion shifting program

Fig. 4-12 illustrates an example of the criterion shifting program. In the ball drop, the wider the distance between the two dropped balls (which must be caught simultaneously on the rebound), the greater is the degree of difficulty. The smaller the area of focus, the more attention can be paid a specific aspect of a given environment.

Criterion shifting programs may be developed from an instructional objective. The task specifications of the objective are taught and remain during the subsequent execution of the tasks. However, the criterion is shifted to make the standard of performance more or less difficult. It is likely that persons in such programs will practice the skill and record the best performance. If such a procedure is employed, learning principles (see Chapter 16) are violated and the end result is inefficient learning of the task at higher levels of performance (Fig. 4-13).

The following is a sample of the elements of a criterion shifting program. These aspects are contained in this type of program:

Name of program: Communicates the behavioral description of performance

Program domain: Classifies the program by major goals of instruction

Components developed: Specify the worth of the program in achieving major goals

Table 4-4. Suggested measures for specific ability traits

Ability trait	Criterion
Strength	Increasing number of repetitions above present level
Speed	Decreasing time it takes to run specified distance
Endurance	Increasing number of push-ups over specified time
Balance	Increasing length of time one can balance
Flexibility	Increasing range of motion of specific joint
Power or explosive strength	Increasing distance one can jump
Vision	Increasing span of vision on specific task

Type of program: Specifies the program as (1) shifting condition, (2) shifting criterion, (3) task analysis of a skill, (4) pattern analysis, or (5) developmental scale programming

Materials: Materials needed to conduct the program

Communication code: Symbols that enable persons who are nonreaders to participate in the program

Equipment layout: Suggestions for management of the instructional area

Measurement: Way in which the activity is measured

Task specifications: Specifications of the conditions (Fig. 4-14)

Criterion shifting programming provides the strongest type of measurement and thus unequivocally accountable data on the progress of children. However, its application to various types of tasks is limited. It is applicable to conversion of deficient ability prerequisites, as is suggested in Table 4-4.

Tasks that are most amenable to criterion shifting programs are those that relate to ability structures.

Condition shifting program

Condition shifting programs have utility when teaching skills. The conditions of a model behavior are stated. From this model, task hierarchies are constructed and programs are formulated. Using bowling as an example, conditions such as the performer's distance from the pins, the distance apart that the pins are set, and the size of the ball can be changed to structure the task to fit the child's level of ability (Fig. 4-15).

The strength of condition shifting programming lies in the following:

1. There is variation in activity that tends to hold pupil interest.
2. There are subsequent activities with respect to difficulty that, if constructed appropriately, include something for most learners.
3. There is accommodation for children who function at low levels of development.
4. This form of curriculum facilitates the introduction of desired elements representing ability traits to be integrated into the activity of the program. More than one specific trait can be developed in a single activity.

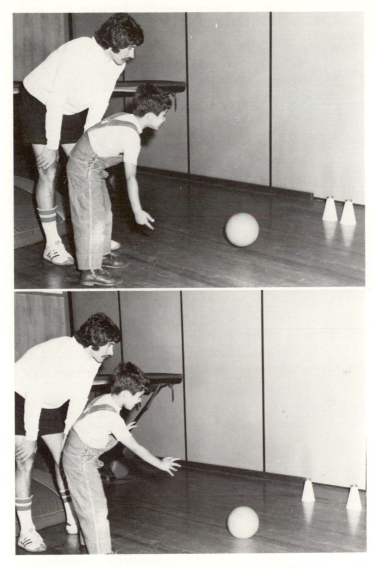

Fig. 4-15. A condition shifting program. In this bowling program, the hierarchies are (1) the bowler's distance from the pins, (2) the distance apart the pins are set, (3) the number of pins that are knocked down, and (4) the number of pins that are set up and that are required to be knocked down. These variables can be manipulated. (Courtesy of California State University, Audio Visual Center, Long Beach, Calif.)

Goal: Demonstrate the ability to square dance to *Marching through Georgia* without error and subject to the criterion of mastery of all subtasks.

SQUARE DANCE	CRITERION FOR MASTERY
1. Locate your partner.	Find partner within 2 seconds after the call indicates to do so.
2. Place your hand on your partner's hip.	Extend arm, place hand on hip, and with other hand grasp palm of partner's hand.
3. Place your inside foot next to your partner's.	Make sure the outer portion of your foot touches the outer portion of your partner's foot.
4. Pivot on the inside foot and push off with the outside foot.	Make at least three pivots and no more than five pivots to one revolution.
5. Release your partner.	Take no longer than 2 seconds after the command.

Example of a short-term instructional objective: Pivot on the inside foot and push off with the outside foot so there are at least three and no more than five pivots for each clockwise turn.

NOTE: This behavior could be broken down further as a physical or motor prerequisite that needs to be fulfilled before mastery of the task can be achieved. If the instructional objective reaches the developmental level of the learner, all children (handicapped or not) can be included in the instructional process.

Goal: Execute the basic skill of the standing broad jump appropriately as defined by a conceptual model.

BROAD JUMP	CRITERION FOR MASTERY
Prepare for jump.	1. Retract arms at least parallel with torso at take-off.
	2. Flex knees and hips between 45 and 90 degrees at takeoff and arms at 45-degree angle to jumping surface.
	3. Keep arms straight and in line with torso.
Take off.	4. Maintain knees extended to 180 degrees.
	5. Maintain hips extended to 180 degrees.
	6. Maintain ankles extended to 135 degrees.
	7. Hold body at 45-degree angle to floor.
Sustain flight.	8. Retract arms behind body before feet strike ground.
Make a landing.	9. Thrust arms forward so balance is maintained.
	10. Make legs reach forward and stay straight.
	11. Flex legs and hips to cushion landing.

Example of a short-term instructional objective: Flex knees and hips between 45 and 90 degrees at takeoff.

NOTE: This objective is stated in terms of an analyzed behavior that is part of the total movement pattern, not in terms of the outcomes of behavioral performance, which involves the total integration of the task.

5. The profiling procedure is not difficult.
6. Stick figures that represent the enactment of instructional objectives of the program enable nonreaders to engage in self-instructional activity.
7. The units of gain can be computed in the program to indicate educational progress.
8. Pupils are aware of the progress that they are making in the program.

Task analysis program

Many physical education activities require a chain of tasks, all of which must be mastered to perform a routine. This type of curricular activity is best instructed through task analysis. Specific behaviors that are different from other behaviors in a routine are isolated for analysis. An assessment is then made to determine which behaviors in a routine have been developed to the point where successful participation by the handicapped person may be achieved. Those behaviors that are deficient receive further programming until all the behaviors in the instructional routine are mastered.

Examples of task analyses of a square dance routine and the standing broad jump are provided on p. 100.

Task analysis is a procedure that can be applied to determine the appropriate selection of activity to attain goals. The analysis can begin at any level, with any stated instructional objective, and asks the question, "To accomplish this behavior, what prerequisites must the learner be able to perform?" For each behavior so identified, the same question is asked; thus, a hierarchy of objectives based on testable prerequisites is generated. The behavior can begin at any level and always specifies prerequisite components, according to Glaser and Nitko.[10] The task analysis is an essential tool for deriving

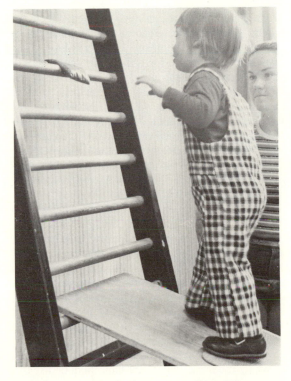

Fig. 4-16. A task analysis of a mature walking skill.

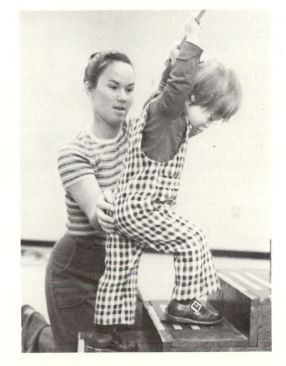

Fig. 4-17. An activity to develop stair-climbing skills through task analysis.

Criterion performance measure: Demonstrate the ability to feed yourself with a spoon in a socially accept-able manner.

FEEDING BEHAVIOR	CRITERION FOR MASTERY
1. Sit in chair at table.	Hold the head and trunk erect with no support to the back.
2. Grasp the spoon.	Use a pincer grasp, with the spoon resting on the third finger.
3. Scoop the food.	Scoop from $^3/_4$ to 1 teaspoonful.
4. Move the food to the mouth.	Do not spill the food.
5. Accept the food from the spoon.	Move all the food from the spoon into the mouth.
6. Move the food to where it can be chewed.	Keep the tongue in the mouth as the food is moved through the chewing mechanism.
7. Chew the food.	Utilize the teeth and make at least three chews.
8. Swallow the food.	Keep the head in an erect position.
9. Return the spoon to the dish to repeat the process.	Look toward where the next intended bite of food will come from.

---

instructional objectives for severely handicapped children. Task analysis is especially appropriate in the development of self-help skills that involve motor development (Figs. 4-16 and 4-17).

Task analysis of self-help skills

The development of self-help skills that will assist severely handicapped persons in independent self-fulfilling living are of the utmost importance. A task-analyzed curriculum may be developed through analyzing the ability prerequisites of various skills. Once the prerequisites have been identified, the child is assessed on each behavior prerequisite to the analyzed skill. From this assessment, a profile of acquired and unacquired behaviors is derived. Subcurricular areas that need development are identified. Thus, instruction may proceed from this assessment. The boxed material above presents a task analysis of a feeding skill with prerequisite behaviors of mastery identified for the learner and appropriate programming suggested to facilitate the development of the feeding skill.

Task analysis of locomotor skills

Severely handicapped persons are often nonambulatory or cannot move with efficiency in their en-vironments. Therefore, an essential prerequisite for gaining greater independence is the development of a more appropriate means of locomotion. The goals and objectives for locomotor patterns will vary depending on the developmental level of the child. Basic movement skills include rolling, crawling, creeping, and walking. Locomotor skills of a higher order (running, hopping, skipping, galloping, and leaping) are often outside the capabilities of severely handicapped persons (Fig. 4-18).

Task analysis can be applied to locomotor development. If a person cannot walk, an anatomical analysis might indicate deficient movement prerequisites at hip, knee, and ankle joints in relation to the ability areas of flexibility, strength, and endurance. An evaluation of each ability trait can then be made at each joint. It is not uncommon for a child to possess a deficient gait as a result of loss of range of motion in the ankle, knee, or hip. Table 4-5 presents a sample evaluation of assessment of a walking behavior. This table provides information on the specific areas in which strength, flexibility, and endurance deficiencies may occur. However, coordination problems must be determined by other methods. The table may be used to assess the prerequisites of flexibility, strength, and endurance required at the hip, knee, and ankle for

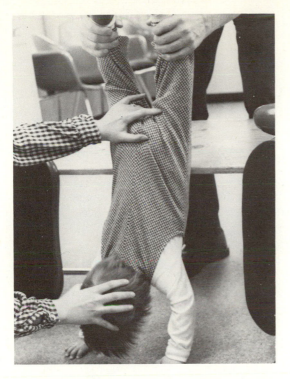

Fig. 4-18. One of the tasks that a learner must perform as a result of a task analysis of the forward roll is to move to a tuck position when the trunk is in a inverted position. A prompting procedure is employed to break up a reflex so that the child can assume the tuck position to eventually perform a modified forward roll.

Table 4-5. Assessment of walking

Anatomical part	Flexibility	Strength	Endurance
Hip	90 degrees	Kneeling or standing	Can stand erect for 7 seconds
Knee	25 degrees	Cannot support weight (stand)	
Ankle	20 degrees	Cannot support weight (stand)	

minimum walking. If a prerequisite is deficient at any joint in flexibility, strength, or endurance, specific programming should be introduced.

Subjective movement analysis program

Kinesiologists study movement patterns objectively through cinematographical analysis and the computer. However, for patterns such as throwing, running, jumping, and kicking, the information, more often than not, is of a subjective nature. Setting short-term objectives for students from patterns is difficult. Information of this type provides little feedback to the learner. However, the outcomes of performance as a result of the pattern are of significance to the learner. Thus, subjective movement analysis has limited utility for the Individual Education Program when learners must self-evaluate. Furthermore, it is not uncommon for students to show improvement in the mechanics of a skill with little improvement in performance. The temporal-spatial relationships of the components of the movement pattern may be as important as the pattern itself in acquiring behavioral results. It is not uncommon for one aspect of a movement pattern to reflect improvement while other aspects of the movement pattern reflect regression. For instance, many persons are unable to project their bodies at a 45-degree angle when performing the two-footed standing broad jump. Often, when there is alteration of the pattern so that the body is projected closer to the 45-degree angle, there is compensation for control of the balancing mechanism by failure to extend at the hips and knees in optimal fashion at takeoff. Thus, it is difficult to accurately determine performance gains from subjective description of movement patterns. The pattern is the wherewithal to optimum performance.

A descriptive analysis of movement patterns is useful for identifying deficiencies in prerequisite movements that prevent skill mastery. For instance, if a person does not rotate the hips while attempting to throw a ball, specific training for hip rotation may be a part of the training separate from the throwing pattern. When the hip rotation deficiency is rectified, increased performance toward a model pattern will result.

Application of learning principles

The curriculum for the severely handicapped child in motor development should be composed of hierarchical, sequential behavioral objectives. With

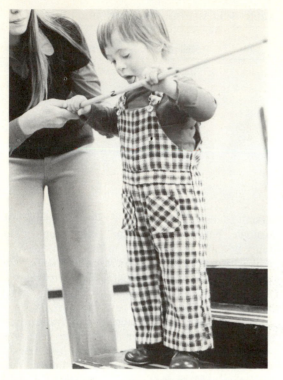

Fig. 4-19. The stick held by the implementor is a prompt that can assist the child in learning to walk up and down stairs.

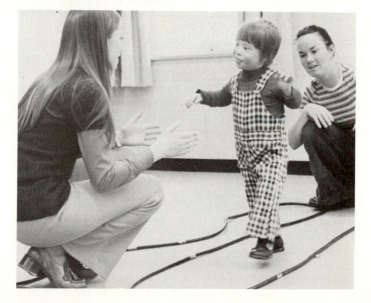

Fig. 4-20. The designed pathway where child is to walk can be narrowed. Thus, the walking behavior can be shaped. An implementor waits to apply the learning principle of immediacy of reinforcement when the child walks the pathway without touching the boundaries.

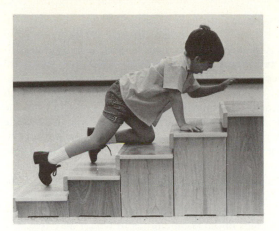

Fig. 4-21. Fundamental motor patterns may be generalized to other movement patterns. The child has generalized the specific skill of creeping to climbing the stairs. (Courtesy of the Special Education Early Childhood Intervention Program, University of Kansas, Lawrence.)

the formulation of behavioral objectives, there is the need to teach new behaviors. Thus, it becomes imperative that learning principles be appropriately applied to the learners if they are to progress properly in the developmental continuum. Some aspects of the learning principles that may assist in the development of appropriate behaviors are as follows:

1. *Application of shaping procedures:* Determining the specific sequence of steps that are small enough to enable the child to be successful and yet progress toward the target behavior.
2. *Prompting procedure:* Assisting the child in the response so that he or she may be successful.
3. *Fading the prompt:* Using the minimum amount of prompt necessary.
4. *Reinforcement component building:* Pairing neutral and positive reinforcers, then fading the positive reinforcer so that a transfer to the neutral reinforcer occurs.
5. *Identification of reinforcers:* Determining that a consequence of the performance will strengthen desired behaviors.
6. *Application of learning principles:* Practicing a sequence of (a) reward immediately; (b) reward after, not before; and (c) reinforcement

of the correct behavior, being fair, honest, and clear. In addition to these principles, there are several others that can be applied to programming.

It is necessary to apply learning principles to make the instructional processes come alive. The learning process is an essential part of the total delivery system for the severely handicapped child (Figs. 4-19 and 4-20).

Component building

An important instructional technique to apply when working with a severely handicapped child is to build the components of the operant learning system. The components of the learning system that need to be built are a greater number of stimulus properties to which the learner may respond and a greater number of responses that may be used as reinforcers for the child. The procedure of building the components of the learning system involves the pairing of a positive stimulus and a neutral stimulus to elicit a response. After repeated pairing, the positive stimulus may be withdrawn; it is hoped that a transfer of the positive stimulus to the previously neutral stimulus occurs. The same procedure may be used in building a reinforcer. In the case of building response capability, manual movement of the body can be applied and, through the physical prompting and fading procedure, motoric function can be developed in the child. With the capability of building stimulus, response, and reinforcement capacities for an existing response repertoire, it may then be possible for all children to learn instructional tasks that lie within their grasp. Therefore, appropriate programming for the severely handicapped child consists of appropriate selection of objectives through task analysis and the proper application of learning principles to ensure that the objective will be achieved.

Use of the systems approach

There appears to be increased emphasis on the employment of a systems approach to education for the handicapped. Inasmuch as handicapped children possess limited capabilities systematic instruction is a critical factor in furthering their motor development. A systems approach involves a solution to a large problem. The optimal motor development of handicapped children is a large problem.

To solve this problem, all the components that are brought to bear on the problem need to be identified, isolated, and developed through controls. Some of these components of the instructional process are the following:

1. Developmental curriculum
2. Assessment instruments
3. Programming of the child in the curriculum
4. Application of learning principles
5. Training of personnel
6. Management of personnel with learners
7. Home training programs

When these components have been identified and developed, it is then necessary to establish relationships among the system components, as follows:

1. The diagnostic instrumentation and the program
2. The curriculum and the needs of the learner
3. The program in the school and the program in the home
4. The training of implementation personnel for the school and for the home
5. The application of learning principles among personnel
6. The management formats to interface personnel, pupils, and the curriculum
7. The program continuity for the child among teachers (so that progress of the child may be continuous)

SUMMARY

Federal and state laws require that handicapped children receive Individual Education Programs in physical education. Individual Education Programs make provision for handicapped children to receive the best instructional and behavioral technology available. The function of the Individual Education Program is to meet those unique needs in motor skills that will maximize the developmental potential toward self-sufficient living in the community. To achieve such an outcome, a full preevaluation of educational needs for self-sufficient living in leisure motor skills of physical education must be conducted. The efficient system of continuous development of individuals during their total school experience is to follow the progress of the children through data recorded on task-analyzed or pro-grammed curricula. The sequential objectives of the task to be learned through the programming/task analysis will not ensure that handicapped children attain the desired skills. Rather, behavioral technology must be applied to instruction of specific objectives that are programmed into small teachable components and are presented to the learners. Programmed materials make it possible for the handicapped to self-instruct and self-evaluate so that they will be able to learn tasks that meet their unique needs. Furthermore, they may learn at their own rates and involve parents in the program as they move toward meaningful leisure motor skills that they utilize in an independent manner in the communities in which they live.

REFERENCES

1. Auxter, D. M.: Perceptual-motor development programs for an individually prescribed instructional system, Slippery Rock, Pa., 1971, Slippery Rock State College.
2. Bellamy, G. T., Peterson, L., and Close, D.: Habilitation of the severely and profoundly retarded: illustrations of competence, Education and Training of the Mentally Retarded **10**(3):174-186, 1975.
3. Congressional record (June 18) 1975, p. S10974.
4. Congressional record, Senate Report No. 94168 (Education for All Handicapped Children Act), (June 2) 1975, p. 10, 11.
5. Congressional record, (June 18) 1975, p. S10960.
6. Congressional record, (June 18) 1975, p. S10977-10978.
7. Gagne, R. W.: Learning hierarchies, Educ. Psychol. **6**:1-9, 1968.
8. Gold, M.: Task analysis: a statement and example using acquisition and production of a complex assembly task by the retarded blind, Institute for Child Behavior and Development, University of Illinois at Urbana-Champaign, 1975.
9. Fredrick vs. Thomas, 419 F. Supp. 960, 1976.
10. Glaser, R., and Nitko, A. J.: Measurement in learning and instruction. In Thorndike, R. L., editor: Education measurement, ed. 2, Washington, D.C., 1970, American Council on Education.
11. Kephart, N. C.: The slow learner in the classroom, Columbus, Ohio, 1961, Charles E. Merrill Publishing Co.
12. Lau vs. Nichol, **414**:563, 1974.
13. Lindvall, C. M., and Bolvin, J. D.: Programmed instruction in the schools: an application of programming principles in individually prescribed instruction, Sixty-sixth Yearbook of the National Society of the Study of Education, Chicago, 1967, University of Chicago Press.
14. Miller, R. A.: Task description and analysis. In Gagne, R. M., editor: Psychological principles in system development, New York, 1962, Holt, Rinehart & Winston, Inc.
15. Miller, R. B.: Analysis and specification of behavior for training. In Glaser, R., editor: Training research and education, Pittsburgh, 1962, University of Pittsburgh Press.

16. Nitko, A. J.: Problems in the development of criterion referenced tests: the IPI Pittsburgh experience, Unpublished working paper, Pittsburgh, 1975.
17. Resnick, L. G.: Task analysis and the instructional design: some cases from mathematics, Unpublished working paper, Pittsburgh, 1975.
18. U.S. Department of Health, Education, and Welfare, Federal register **42**:22676-22702, (May 4) 1977.
19. U.S. Department of Health, Education, and Welfare, Federal register, vol. 4, (August 23) 1977.

RECOMMENDED READINGS

Barsch, R. H.: Achieving perceptual-motor efficiency: an approach to learning, Seattle, 1967, Special Child Publications.

Broer, M. R.: Efficiency of human movement, Philadelphia, 1960, W. B. Saunders Co.

Bunn, J. W.: Scientific principles of coaching, Englewood Cliffs, N.J., 1977, Prentice-Hall, Inc.

Espenschade, A. S., and Eckert, H. M.: Motor development, Columbus, Ohio, 1967, Charles E. Merrill Publishing Co.

Gallahue, D. L., Werner, P. H., and Luedke, G. C.: A conceptual approach to moving and learning, New York, 1975, John Wiley & Sons, Inc.

Gesell, A.: The ontogenesis of infant behavior. In Carmichael, L., editor: Manual of child psychology, ed. 2, New York, 1954, John Wiley & Sons, Inc.

Getman, O. D.: The visuomotor complex in the acquisition of learning skills. In Hellmuth, J., editor: Learning disorders, vol. 1, Seattle, 1965, Special Child Publications.

Glassow, R. B., and Kruse, P.: Motor performance of girls age 6 to 11 years, Res. Q. **31**:426-433, 1960.

Green, B. F.: A method of scalogram analysis using summary statistics, Psychometrics **21**:79-88, 1956.

Guttman, L. A.: Basis for scaling quantitative data, Am. Sociol. Rev. **9**:139-150, 1944.

Guttridge, M. V.: A study of motor achievements of young children, Arch. Psychol. **244**:1-178, 1939.

Halverson, H. M.: An experimental study of prehension in infants by means of systematic cinema records, Genet. Psychol. Monogr. **10**:107-286, 1931.

Halverson, H. M.: Studies of the grasping responses of early infancy, J. Genet. Psychol. **51**:371-449, 1937.

Hay, J. G.: The biomechanics of sports techniques, Englewood Cliffs, N.J., 1973, Prentice-Hall, Inc.

Hendrickson, H.: The vision development process. In Wold, R. M., editor: Visual and perceptual aspects for the achieving and underachieving child, Seattle, 1969, Special Child Publications.

Hirst, C. F., and Michaelis, E.: Developmental activities for children in special education, Springfield, Ill., 1973, Charles C Thomas, Publisher.

Kibler, R. J., Barker, L. L., and Miles, D. T.: Behavioral objectives and instruction, Boston, 1970, Allyn & Bacon, Inc.

Lingoes, J. C.: Multiple scalogram analysis: a set theoretic model for analyzing dichotomous items, Educ. Psychol. Measurements **23**:501-524, 1963.

McCaskill, C. L., and Wellman, B. L.: A study of common motor achievements at preschool ages, Child Dev. **9**:141-150, 1938.

Miller, D. I., and Nelson, R. C.: Biomechanics of sports, Philadelphia, 1973, Lea & Febiger.

Nelson, R. C.: Biomechanics four, Baltimore, 1974, University Park Press.

Plagenhoef, S.: Patterns of human motion, Englewood Cliffs, N.J., 1971, Prentice-Hall, Inc.

Popham, W. J., editor: Instructional objectives, Skokie, Ill., 1969, Rand McNally & Co.

Resnick, L. G., and Wang, M. C.: Approaches to the validation of learning hierarchies, Paper presented at the Eighteenth Annual Western Regional Conference on Testing Problems, San Francisco, May 1969.

Stephens, B.: Training the developmentally young, New York, 1971, John Day Co., Inc.

Taber, J. I., Glaser, R., and Schaefer, H. H.: Learning and programmed instruction, Reading, Mass., 1965, Addison-Wesley Publishing Co., Inc.

Wellman, B. L.: Motor achievements of preschool children, Childhood Educ. **13**:311-316, 1937.

Wild, M. R.: The behavior pattern of throwing and some observations concerning its course of development in children, Res. Q. **9**:20-24, 1938.

PART TWO

Key teaching and therapy skills

Part Two of the text is designed to help the reader understand the therapy skills that can be used with all types of handicapped persons of all age levels. Exercise, relaxation, fitness, nutritional status, and adapted sports and games are presented in this section.

5

Exercise therapy programs

Selection □ Assignment □ Teaching

Remedial exercises play an important part in the adapted physical education program. In fact, carefully selected special exercises properly executed by students in regular physical education classes can do much to prevent bodily malalignment and to aid in the correction of deviations in posture, muscular imbalance, weak musculature, and poor general physical fitness. The values of performing regular exercises, when properly taught and assigned in the correct amount, are stated and substantiated in numerous texts on medicine, physiology of exercise, and physical education.

In general, exercise improves muscular strength and tone, can increase flexibility, produces increased efficiency in circulation and respiration, strengthens the heart muscle, and helps educate or reeducate the neuromuscular systems of the body so that we sit, stand, and move more effectively. When properly performed, exercises can aid in the correction of body deviations that are related to the neuromuscular joint systems and may aid in certain cardiorespiratory conditions.

THERAPEUTIC EXERCISE

The values of regular and therapeutic exercise have been established for many years. Since World War II, when such concepts as the need for early ambulation and preoperative and postoperative exercise programs were reinforced, to the present time, during which great stress is being placed on cardiovascular fitness for both the normal and the handicapped individual, there has been an increase in the acceptance of the value of exercise.

The following are selected factors that are important to therapeutic exercise:

1. Strength
   a. Muscle strength is increased with use and decreased with disuse.
   b. Muscle size increases (hypertrophy) with use and decreases (atrophy) with disuse.
   c. Heavy resistance increases muscle strength and size more rapidly than does light resistance (the overload principle).

d. Isotonic exercises (involving muscular contraction and movement of a joint) increase strength, promote circulation and cardiovascular endurance, and maintain joint flexibility.

e. Isometric exercises (involving muscular contraction, but no movement of the joint) increase strength and economize in the time spent in exercising, but contribute little to cardiovascular fitness and joint flexibility.

f. DeLorme's Progressive Resistance Exercises (PRE) provide a system for exercising using the isotonic principle.[6,7] This method employs the use of 10 repetition maximums (RM). The student selects a weight or any resistance that he or she can lift maximally 10 times in bouts or sets of three employing the following system: (1) first bout, 10 repetitions (reps) using one half the 10 RM load; (2) second bout, 10 reps using three fourths the 10 RM load; and, finally, (3) third bout, 10 reps using the full 10 RM load. There are many variations of the DeLorme method depending on the special requirements of the participant. If greater strength is needed, more resistance and fewer repetitions should be used in each bout; conversely, if greater muscle endurance is needed, less resistance and more repetitions should be employed.

g. The Hettinger-Müller research provides a system for exercises using the principle of isometric exercises.[11] Their work, although considered controversial by some researchers, has provided a rationale for using isometrics in the development of strength. They suggested that a single isometric contraction held for 6 seconds and executed once a week at three fourths the maximum effort will develop strength. This concept has direct implications for persons who are recumbent and are not allowed isotonic movements, for the prevention of atrophy of a part, and for those persons who may be subdeveloped and debilitated. Ordinarily, some modification of the procedure is employed when it is used in the adapted physical education class.

h. Great strength is unnecessary in a muscle if proper balance is not maintained between antagonistic muscles.

i. Strength is wasted if proper muscle, fascia, and joint flexibility is not maintained.

2. Flexibility

a. Flexibility is maintained with normal use and is decreased with disuse.

b. Body efficiency and grace are reduced as flexibility is decreased.

c. Immobilized joints or restricted joint actions for long periods of time (consequences of casts, braces, or disuse) result in loss of flexibility.

d. Stretching exercises are most effective when performed slowly and when aided by the pull of gravity.

e. Sudden, rapid motions to induce stretch (bouncing or jerking against the muscles to be stretched) induce the *stretch reflex,* which causes the affected muscle to tighten, and are thus less effective and may cause tearing.

f. Actively contracting the muscle groups antagonistic to those that are being stretched aids flexibility through *reciprocal inhibition* (causes relaxation of the stretched muscle and is thus more effective for increasing flexibility).

g. The use of principles of proprioceptive neuromuscular facilitation (PNF) to aid in stretching programs is receiving an increased acceptance by physical educators, therapists, and athletic training personnel. Kabat,[8] Knott and Voss,[9] and others have used the findings of Sherrington[12] to suggest methods of application of PNF to the areas of therapeutic exercise including stretching. These areas need further study by physical educators and therapists so that applicable facets of PNF can be applied to their work in therapeutic exercise, neuromuscular development, motor development and behavior, and motor learning to facilitate movement patterns of normal and handicapped persons. The general technique used in stretching exercises involves an active stretch of the affected muscle group *(stretch)* accompanied by an active contraction of the antagonistic muscle group. This helps to determine the maximum stretch possible at this time. This is followed by a strong isometric contraction of the muscle group being stretched *(hold)* (resistance is provided by the subject, or if the subject is unable to provide this resistance because of pain, lack of flexibility, or lack of strength, it may be provided by a partner, teacher, or therapist). This is followed 3 to 6 seconds later *(relax)* by another active stretch of the muscle group as described in No. 1, above *(stretch).* Each repetition of this technique should increase the flexibility of the muscle group involved. The rationale for the isometric contraction of a given muscle group, inserted between two active stretches of this same group, is that the isometric contraction activates the proprioceptice centers and Golgi tendon organs located in the muscles and tendons, allowing for a more complete release when the next stretch is instigated. A short delay (3 to 6 seconds) may be necessary for this relaxation phase to take place. The subject, partner, teacher, or therapist can feel this release mechanism and then have the subject begin the active contraction of the antagonistic muscle group. This technique is not easy to master and may be more complex if diagonal and rotary elements are added to the stretch pattern.[9] A clear verbal description—followed by close supervision of the excercise with hands-on guidance and resistance provided by a teacher or therapist if available—should provide for an exact performance and the desired results. These exercises are illustrated in Fig. 5-1.

3. Relaxation
   a. Relaxation principles and techniques are described in Chapter 6.
4. Endurance
   a. Endurance is increased when the rate of performance of an activity is increased.
   b. Endurance is developed by increasing the number of times an activity is performed.
   c. As endurance is increased, the rate and the number of repetitions must be increased to continue improvement.
   d. Endurance may be general (total cardiovascular system in the body).
   e. Specific (muscular) endurance is obtained through repetitious exercises for selected muscle groups.
   f. General (cardiovascular) endurance involving the total body is obtained by such activities as jogging,[1] walking, swimming, circuit training,[10] rope skipping, and bicycling.

To be effective for prevention or correction of body weakness or malalignment, exercises must be scientifically based, accurately taught, and properly learned. They must then be *practiced regularly*. Additional information on strength, endurance, and flexibility is found in Chapter 7.

Choice of exercises

The following points should be considered in the development or choice of an exercise:
1. What is the purpose of the exercise?
2. Does it accomplish that purpose?
3. Does it violate any principles of sound body mechanics?
4. What are the main joints involved?
5. What are the main muscle groups involved?
6. Is the exercise primarily for flexibility, strength, endurance, or coordination?
7. Is the intensity of the exercise mild, moderate, or vigorous?
8. What elements of danger are involved? What cautions should be remembered in assignment and execution of the exercise?
9. Is the exercise good for more than one disability?
10. Can you measure student progress through this exercise?

Assignment of exercises to students

Since individuals have different needs and different problems, the students' exercise programs will be most effective if they are designed specifically for them. Persons who qualify for programs mandated by P.L. 94-142 must have written Individual Education Programs. Some important factors to consider in the selection of exercises for the students are the following:
1. What are the medical diagnosis and the recommendation of the physician?
2. What factors were discovered through physical education testing (posture and body mechanics examinations, fitness tests, neuromuscular tests, and perceptual-motor assessment)?
3. What are the interests of the students?

Selection of exercises for the individual should further consider the following points:
1. The type and extent of warm-up exercises needed should be considered; they should loosen, stretch, and warm up the parts to be concentrated on in the regular exercise workout.
2. All the areas to be exercised should be considered so that, when possible, exercises that aid two or more areas or conditions can be used and so that an exercise that may aid one condition, but may aggravate another, will not be used.
3. Exercises should be progressive, starting with stretching and loosening, then light active exercises, and, as the condition of the student permits, performance of active and resistive exercises, using the overload principle.
4. The sequence of exercises should be from one body area to another. When all of the prescribed areas have been exercised once, they may be exercised a second and third time either by repeating the exercise program or by having more advanced exercises assigned by the instructor. Thus, a student can work a part of the body vigorously, then allow a rest period for that body area while exercising other body areas, returning to each body area with additional exercises later in the exercise period.
5. Relaxation may be an important part of the ex-

ercise program. If so, it should be scheduled as part of the workout. The student should be taught the techniques of progressive relaxation (Chapter 6).

6. The student should have a written exercise program showing progression, sequence, repetitions, resistance used, and the goal toward which he or she should work as the semester progresses. A more detailed explanation of the use of an exercise record card is presented later in this chapter, as is information about meeting special requirements for persons in Individual Education Programs.

7. Proper breathing during exercise in important. Holding the breath—especially during heavy lifting or vigorous exercises in which the handi-capped person is straining to perform—should be done with an *open throat,* accompanied by either inhalation or exhalation. This prevents intra-abdominal strain that can result in a hernia, helps to prevent the pooling of blood in the abdominal area when the breath is held during heavy lifting and strain activities, and prevents closing off the carotid artery, which may cause the Valsava effect. Regular breathing, like rhythmic isotonic exercise, promotes normal and increased flow of the blood through the cardiovascular system.

Teaching of exercises

If an exercise is worth doing, it is worth doing well. Thus, instruction must be clear and the stu-

Fig. 5-1. A, Stretch-hold-relax-stretch technique for thigh adductor muscle group. **B,** Stretch-hold-relax-stretch technique for quadriceps muscle group. **C,** Stretch-hold-relax-stretch technique for hip extensor muscle group.

Hip adductor stretch (stretch-hold-relax-stretch) *(Fig. 5-1, A)*
Starting position: Sitting, soles of feet together, elbows inside knees, hands clasped in front of body.
1. Stretch adductor muscles by actively pulling the knees down and apart as far as possible with the hip abductors. Keep the soles of the feet together and the heels as close to the buttocks as possible. Hold 3 seconds. Relax. (This should establish your starting *stretch maximum*).
2. Pull knees toward the rigidly held elbows maximally executing an isometric contraction. Hold 3 seconds. Relax 3 to 6 seconds.
3. Pull heels closer to crotch (soles together) and repeat active stretch as in No. 1. Hold 3 seconds. Relax.
4. Repeat No. 2 with a strong isometric contraction of the hip adductors.
5. Repeat No. 3.

Quadriceps stretch (stretch-hold-relax-stretch) *(Fig. 5-1, B)*
Starting position: Prone, left knee flexed to 90 degrees, thighs together.
1. Stretch anterior thigh muscles actively by contracting vigorously with the knee flexors (hamstrings). Hold 3 seconds. Relax.
2. Reach back with the left hand, grasp the left ankle. (If this is impossible the teacher, therapist, or partner may substitute the proper resistance). Hold the ankle in position as a strong isometric contraction (toward extension) is executed with the anterior thigh muscles. Hold 3 seconds. Relax 3 to 6 seconds.
3. Actively stretch as in No. 1, increasing the range of motion in knee flexion.
4. Repeat No. 2 with an isometric contraction of the quadriceps group.
5. Repeat No. 3.

Hip extensor (hamstring) stretch (stretch-hold-relax-stretch) *(Fig. 5-1, C)*
Starting position: Supine, legs straight and together, arms down by the sides of the body.
1. Lift right leg to point of tightness (knee straight) for an initial active stretch. Hold 3 counts. Relax.
2. With the leg in the same position, isometrically contract the hamstring group using the antagonistic quadriceps group as resistance or, if possible, have a teacher, therapist, or partner offer firm resistance to hip extension and knee flexion. Hold 3 seconds. Relax 3 to 6 seconds.
3. Repeat active stretch as in No. 1 for increased motion. (Be sure the other leg remains on the ground and straight.)
4. Repeat No. 2 executing a firm isometric contraction.
5. Repeat No. 3.

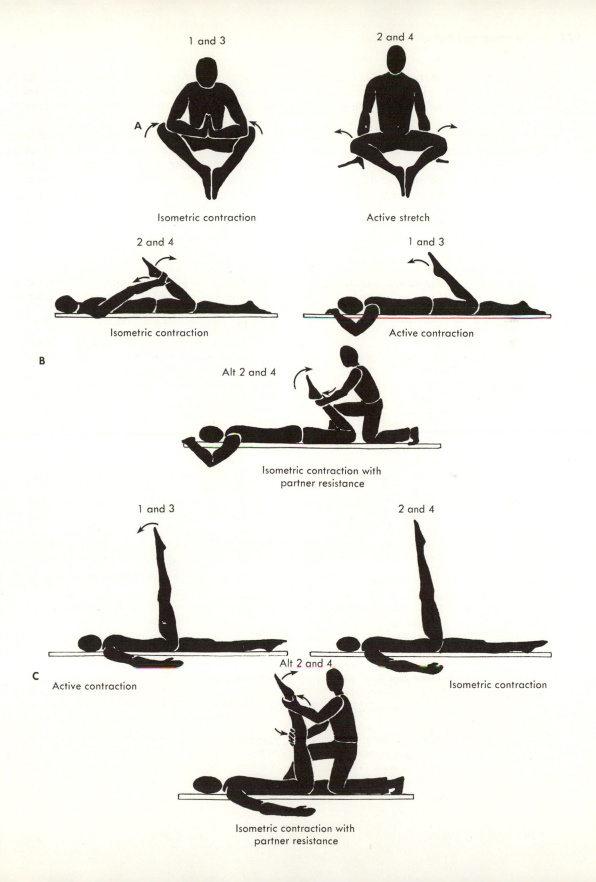

1 and 3

A

Isometric contraction

2 and 4

Active stretch

2 and 4

Isometric contraction

1 and 3

Active contraction

B

Alt 2 and 4

Isometric contraction with partner resistance

1 and 3

C

Active contraction

2 and 4

Isometric contraction

Alt 2 and 4

Isometric contraction with partner resistance

dents must be motivated to want to exercise and exercise correctly. Effective teaching of each exercise should help toward this end. Some points to be considered in teaching special exercises are the following:

1. An accurate demonstration and verbal description should be given by the teacher. Teach the *why* of the exercise as well as the *how* so that the students understand the reason for doing an exercise and doing it correctly.

2. The demonstration-explanation should take the students through each exercise step by step, that is, starting position, first move, second move, etc. The cadence or speed, the number of repetitions, the amount of resistance, and the precautions to observe in performing each particular exercise must be explained.

3. Important points about an exercise and the exercise pogram should be reviewed during the semester.

4. The instructor should observe the students' performance and make corrections frequently throughout the year.

5. Students should be given a reference for each exercise, that is, a written description and pictures or diagrams (Figs. 5-2 and 5-7 through 5-43). This will enable them to learn each exercise more accurately and to review their performance periodically throughout the school year.

6. The instructor should test the students and correct their exercise techniques by observing their performance. Demonstrations and written or verbal quizzes can be given to check the students on knowledge and performance of exercises and exercise programs, reasons for assignment of particular exercises, and special values of each exercise.

7. It is desirable to limit the number of exercises taught at one time to three or four. More than this may serve to confuse the students.

Points to stress in doing a program of exercises include the following:

1. Do each exercise exactly right. The correct number of repetitions and the amount of resistance used are also important. The number of repetitions and/or the amount of resistance used should be steadily increased during the semester. Muscular endurance can be increased. If strength and muscle size are the major objectives, repetitions may be reduced and the amount of resistance used may be steadily increased. The DeLorme system previously discussed is a plan that will promote both muscular strength and endurance, yet it is a safe procedure to use in a rehabilitation setting.

2. Warm up and stretch first; then exercise and develop the desired parts.

3. In posture development programs, progress from recumbency exercises (to gain control of body segments with the aid of gravity) to sitting, then standing, and, finally, resistance exercises in which greater body control is necessary to perform the exercise properly.

4. Do exercises vigorously, hold correct positions momentarily, then relax and repeat. By using these techniques, both isotonic and isometric principles are used in the execution of an exercise.

5. Keep all body segments in good alignment throughout the exercise program, especially when resistive exercises are performed. This will help to reduce strain.

6. Complete the exercise program by *cooling down,* gradually reducing the intensity of the exercises to prevent blood engorgement in the muscles.

7. Keep an accurate record of performance (Fig. 5-47), including the sequence in which exercises are done, the number of repetitions, and the amount of resistance used. (This should be recorded by the student at least once each week and can be checked periodically by both the student and the teacher to note the progress being made.)

Correct positioning is essential for the proper execution of a particular exercise. Fig. 5-3 provides a key to standardizing therapeutic exercise starting positions.

Intensity of exercises

Exercises should be prescribed in terms of how vigorous they are. Two methods often used to consider and to describe the intensity of an exercise are discussed in the following paragraphs.

One classification of exercises, which grades them from easy to difficult, lists them as passive,

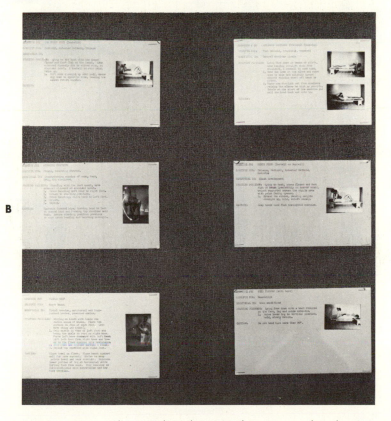

```
                    EXERCISE INSTRUCTION CARD

EXERCISE # 42  WINDMILL LYING

SPECIFIC FOR:  Abdominals and Hipflexors

BENEFICIAL IN:  Low back and Hamstring stretch

STARTING POSITION:  Lying on back with arms extended
                    to the side at shoulder level,
                    palms up.
              1.  Curl to sitting position
                  spreading the legs and
                  keeping arms at shoulder
                  level; palms up.  Sit tall.
              2.  Twist body & touch right
                  hand to left toe.  Keep
                  knees straight.
              3.  Twist body & touch left
                  hand to right toe.  Keep
                  knees straight.
              4.  Curl back down to starting
                  position; repeat exercise.

CAUTION:  1.  Make stretch a slow, controlled movement
          2.  To relieve intra-abdominal strain,
              breathe out while sitting up and curling down.
```

Fig. 5-2. Exercise instruction cards. **A,** Each card contains the name, number, description, and illustration of an exercise. **B,** Bulletin board displaying exercise cards for students to study and to check their performance.

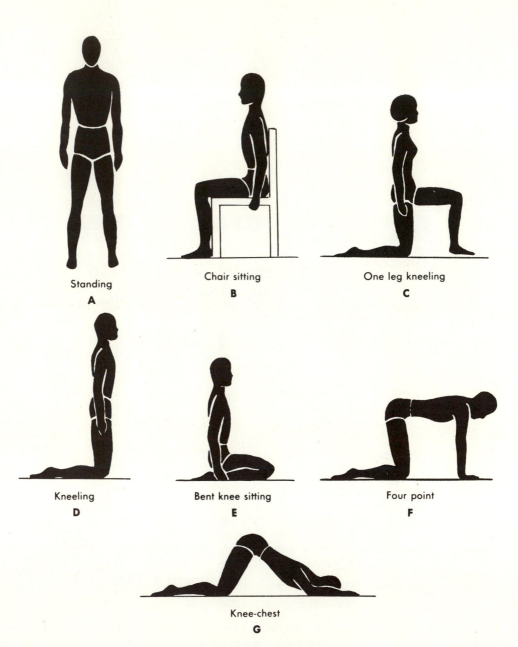

Standing
A

Chair sitting
B

One leg kneeling
C

Kneeling
D

Bent knee sitting
E

Four point
F

Knee-chest
G

Fig. 5-3. Exercise positions.

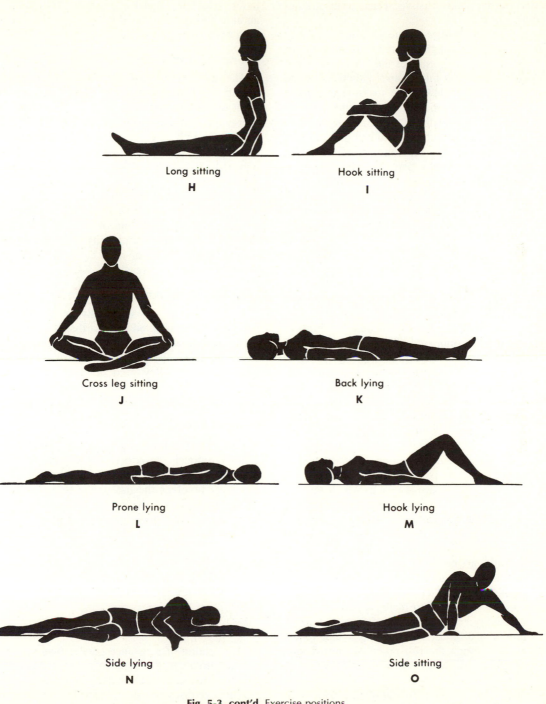

Long sitting
H

Hook sitting
I

Cross leg sitting
J

Back lying
K

Prone lying
L

Hook lying
M

Side lying
N

Side sitting
O

Fig. 5-3, cont'd. Exercise positions.

assistive, active, and resistive. These terms are defined as follows:

1. A *passive exercise* is one in which the body part is put through the range of motion for the student. This enables the student to maintain joint flexibility and produces some movement of the muscle mass. The student should be conscious of the attempted movement and should think about and try to execute the movement. The student may do passive exercises by moving the affected part with an unaffected part, a pulley arrangement, or other types of special exercise equipment. Passive exercises may also be performed for the student by the teacher, a therapist, or another student, using a *partner* system (Appendix I).

2. An *assistive exercise* is one in which the body part is moved for the student but in which the student assists in the movement to the extent of his or her ability. Thus, neuromuscular patterns are learned or relearned, muscle fibers are developed, and flexibility is retained or improved. These exercises may be performed as described in paragraph 1.

3. An *active exercise* is one in which the student moves the body part and usually works against the counterforces of gravity. Many types of calisthenic exercises exemplify this type of action. Strength is developed, neuromuscular patterns are improved, and flexibility is maintained. Retention or restoration of normal function is the desired result.

4. A *resistive exercise* is one in which the student exercises against some form of resistance. This may include the use of weights, springs, pulleys, dynamic tension, another person, water, or friction. The student strives to build greater strength in weak or subpar musculature than would normally be accomplished using active exercises. The student must be cautioned to increase resistance progressively, to exercise body parts through proper neuromuscular pathways, and to exercise through the full range of normal joint flexibility while engaged in resistive exercises.

Another similar plan for grading exercise in terms of difficulty is to consider the exercise in relation to gravity, that is, exercising with gravity as an aid, with gravity ruled out, against gravity, and with resistance greater than gravity.

Gravity as an aid in exercising

The easiest form of exercise is one in which gravity is used to assist the student in the movement of a body part. Examples of this type of exercise are those in which a body part is moved against the pull of gravity by good musculature, by a pulley, or by another person. The part is then helped in its return to the starting position by the weak musculature working with the assistance of the pull of gravity. The student must make a conscious effort to use the weak muscles, othrwise the exercise may become one of lengthening contraction of the already strong muscles and neglect of the muscles in need of mild exercise. More harm than good may then result.

Gravity ruled out

Ruling gravity out is usually accomplished by supporting the affected part so that it can be exercised without the interference of the pull of gravity. Supporting the part in a pool or ultilizing the support of a pulley or of another person allows the student to exercise the desired muscles with minimum interference from gravitational pull.

Against gravity

Antigravity exercises are more vigorous than the types previously described and involve the use of the affected parts against the pull of gravity. Standing erect involves the use of the extensor muscles of the body in opposition to the pull of gravity. Many of our traditional calisthenic exercises are of the antigravity type, either in their main movement or in the positions held by the other body segments to permit this main movement. Lifting the arms overhead while in the standing position or doing a sit-up or a leg-raise while recumbent exemplifies this type of exercise.

Resistance greater than gravity

Application of resistance greater than the pull of gravity involves the same principles described in the previous section on resistive exercise.

The exercises to be assigned to students in an adaptive physical education class must be chosen with great care regarding the difficulty involved in execution and the amount of work required. They must be graded carefully so that development occurs and improvement is made, but so that strain and injury are avoided. A safe number of repetitions for most exercises would be enough to involve a good workout for the affected muscles without undue fatigue or strain and without assuming an undesirable body position to accomplish the movement. This is often the case when a student tries to do too many repetitions or use too much resistance. Symptoms of overexercising, such as fatigue that lasts more than 5 hours, soreness the next day, or decreased range of motion the next day, may indicate a need for reexamination of the exercise program.

Students in an adapted physical education class who are assigned active or resistive exercises should be limited to 12 to 15 repetitions of the exercise (properly done) before progressing to a more difficult exercise or to the use of greater resistance. This minimizes the chance of strain or injury.

For the most part, it is wise to be conservative and careful in the assignment of the number of repetitions and the amount of resistance used by a student in the initial workout program. The teacher can easily increase the dosage as soon as the student's capacity for exercise has been determined.

EXERCISES FOR POSTURE CORRECTION

The assignment of exercises for the correction of body posture is largely a matter of selecting the proper exercises to develop certain antigravity muscles (see Fig. 9-34) and to enable the student to realign body parts by stretching and developing the proper antagonistic muscle groups. Proper neuromuscular patterns must be developed and the proprioceptive centers reeducated to enable the student to obtain the feeling of well-balanced sitting, standing, and moving postures. Attention must be given both to the assignment and to the execution of exercises so that the body is not placed in positions of poor alignment and strain. Each exercise that is performed should contribute to the proper alignment of the body or one or more of its parts.

EXERCISES FOR REHABILITATION

The 40 key exercises described in the next section of this chapter can also be used as a nuclear set of exercises for rehabilitation of a variety of pre- or postoperative conditions or for therapeutic exercise programs to be assigned following illness, accident, or injury. (See discussion of exercise assignment information, pp. 123 to 125.) To the exercises that are suggested for the rehabilitation of these special conditions, teachers or therapists can add others selected from other chapters of this text, from their own experience, or from standard texts covering these conditions. Exercise programs for special areas are discussed in other chapters; for example, the foot, ankle, and knee (Figs. 10-6 through 10-10), the hip and back (Figs. 10-15 through 10-17), and the shoulder (Figs. 10-19 through 10-22) are discussed in Chapter 10; exercises for tension reduction are given in Chapter 6; exercises for low vitality and fitness are contained in Chapter 7; exercises for chronic musculoskeletal disorders such as amputation, arthritis, hip afflictions, and spinal disabilities are discussed in Chapter 11; and exercise programs for cardiovascular problems are discussed in Chapter 12.

Muscle strength assessment procedures

To obtain assessment information that must be used to determine an individual's present level of educational performance several test procedures might be used. The number of repetitions of a given exercise with or without resistance could be measured. The strength of muscle groups could be measured using a standard manual technique[5] or objective measurements could be made with various types of dynamometers or the cable tensiometer.[2] Data thus gathered would help determine the specific activity level of the muscles measured. Based on this level of performance, behavioral objectives could be written and a program of activities and exercises could be planned to enable the student to meet prescribed goals as mandated for persons participating in programs under regulations of P.L. 94-142.

An example of such a procedure using the manual muscle-testing technique of Daniels, Williams, and Worthingham[5] would include the following for a person assigned to adapted physical education with partial paralysis of the right quadriceps muscle group.

1. *Muscle testing.* The results of the test indicate that the student has "fair-minus" use of

the quadriceps, which means that the person has near normal range of motion against gravity but that no added resistance can be overcome. This represents the present level of educational performance.

2. Based on this information and observation of the performance of the individual during the test procedures, annual goals and specific performance objectives can now be written.

GOAL: To walk without a limp and to run without assistance by the end of the school year.

PERFORMANCE OBJECTIVES: (a) Lift a 10-pound sandbag strapped to the ankle from a 90-degree angle to a 180-degree angle while seated as in exercise No. 18, Fig. 5-21, to be accomplished by the end of the sixth month of instruction; (b) execute 10 one-quarter deep knee bends with the partial support of the parallel bars by the end of the fifteenth week; (c) kick a soccer ball on the fly an additional 10 feet by the end of each 6-week period; and (d) walk-run 50 yards further each 2 weeks for a 16-week period.

EVALUATION: The performance objectives can be measured by the student, the parent, and the instructor.

EXERCISE ASSIGNMENT SYSTEM

Since the problems and needs of students in an adapted physical education class are different, each student must have a program of exercise that is based on his or her needs and interests. Classes of adapted physical education may include 25 to 35 students, making individual assignment of and instruction in exercises a difficult problem. Persons in P.L. 94-142 programs must have written Individual Educational Programs and specific objectives and goals to be achieved annually.

The following system of exercise assignment and technique of instruction is planned to facilitate assignment of individual exercise programs for individuals or for groups.[3] These 40 exercises should form the nuclear group to be used for all types of cases found in an adapted physical education program, whether the student needs rehabilitation of body parts, improvement in physical fitness, attention to body mechanics, or an exercise program for some particular type of disability. Individual teachers or therapists will wish to add exercises to this series, strengthening areas of special need in their program. These 40 exercises were selected from a set of 105 exercises that we have used extensively for the past 25 years.

The system consists of:

1. A list of exercises, each with a name and a number, arranged according to the type of exercise performed or the type of equipment used. (See Section I, which follows immediately.)

2. An exercise assignment sheet that further categorizes the exercises into groups that can be assigned for some 50 special conditions, graded as to whether they are for a specific condition or for general value. They are further differentiated for use as flexibility exercises or developmental exercises. (See Section II.)

3. Forty key exercises, described and illustrated. Since they have been chosen to include exercises for all parts of the body (both as stretches and as strengtheners), they can serve as the base of a set to be used by classes in adapted physical education. (See Section III.)

4. Information on how to organize the class to allow for the selection of the proper exercises for each student, how to assign the exercises properly, how to work out proper progressions, and how to teach each student the individual exercise program using a small group method is presented in the section on selection of an exercise program for each student, which follows Section III.

Section I □ FORTY KEY EXERCISES FOR ADAPTED PHYSICAL EDUCATION

1. Supine stretch
2. Leg crossover
3. Windmill sitting
4. Neck, back, and shoulder flattener
5. Breaking chains
6. Neck flattener at mirror
7. Abdominal curl
8. Mad cat
9. Knee-chest curl
10. Bicycle
11. Heel cord stretch
12. Foot circling
13. Building mounds
14. Foot curling
15. Knee rotator
16. Quadriceps setting

17. Foot drag
18. Knee extension with boot
19. Tense and stretch
20. Elbow side falling
21. Horizontal ladder
22. Crosslegged stretch (modified from Billig)
23. Side stretch (Billig)
24. Head tilt (Billig)
25. Four-count wall weight
26. Shoulder rotator (wall weight)
27. Arm curl
28. Arm press
29. Chin lift
30. Toe lift
31. Arm crossover
32. Shoulder shrug
33. Towel wringing
34. Gripper
35. Wrist machines
36. Back stoop falling
37. Push-up
38. Chin-up or pull-up
39. Jumping jack with variations
40. Rope skipping

Section II □ EXERCISE ASSIGNMENT INFORMATION

Basic warm-up exercises

1. Supine stretch
2. Leg crossover
3. Windmill sitting
10. Bicycle
39. Jumping jack with variations
40. Rope skipping

Exercises for postural divergencies

Total body conditions

(S)*   *Sway*   Body sways, leans, and tilts are total body con-
(L)   *Lean*   ditions often resulting from some other
(T)   *Tilt*   deviation. The correction of this deviation will often result in the elimination of the sway, lean, or tilt. Since the conditions may also be caused by carelessness, habit, and faulty body mechanics, the student should be made conscious of correcting total body malalignment as he or she corrects special deviations and improves total body fitness. Correcting total body alignment also necessitates the reeducation of the proprioceptive centers. Special symmetrical exercises that can be done to improve body alignment and thus correct a sway, lean, or tilt include the following:

    No. 1, supine stretch; No. 4, neck, back, and shoulder flattener; No. 3, windmill sitting; No. 6, neck flattener at mirror; No. 21, horizontal ladder; No. 25, four-count wall weight; No. 39, jumping jack with variations.

    Exercises performed in front of a mirror aid the student to see and feel correct body alignment.

---

*Letter abbreviations are for those conditions shown in Fig. 5-46 on the posture examination card and described in Chapter 9 and shown in Figs. 9-34, *B,* and 9-35.

Head and neck conditions

(F)   *Forward head:* No. 24, head tilt (stretch); No. 4, neck, back, and shoulder flattener; No. 5, breaking chains; No. 6, neck flattener at mirror; No. 29, chin lift.

(T)   *Head tilt:* No. 24, head tilt (stretch); No. 4, neck, back, and shoulder flattener; No. 5, breaking chains; No. 6, neck flattener at mirror.

Chest conditions

(F)   *Flat chest:* No. 4, neck, back, and shoulder flattener; No. 5, breaking chains; No. 6, neck flattener at mirror; No. 25, fourcount wall weight; No. 28, arm press; No. 31, arm crossover; No. 29, chin lift; No. 21, horizontal ladder.

(H)   *Hollow chest:* same as flat chest unless especially prescribed by a physician.

(P)   *Pigeon breast:* Prescription by physician.

Shoulder conditions

(F)   *Forward or round shoulders:* No. 1, supine stretch; No. 4, neck, back, and shoulder flattener; No. 5, breaking chains; No. 6, neck flattener at mirror; No. 29, chin lift; No. 25, four-count wall weight; No. 21, horizontal ladder.

(L)   *Low shoulder:* No. 1, supine stretch; No. 5, breaking chains; No. 6, neck flattener at mirror; No. 21, horizontal ladder; No. 32, shoulder shrug; No. 29, chin lift.

Knee conditions

(K)   *Knock-knee:* No. 10, bicycle; No. 15, knee rotator; No. 14, foot curling; No. 17, foot drag.

(HK)   *Hyperextended knee:* Develop hamstring muscles; work on leg alignment at mirror to develop a balance of pull between quadriceps and hamstring muscle groups; No. 10, bicycle; No. 17, foot drag.

(BK)   *Bent knee:* No. 2, leg crossover; No. 3, windmill sitting; No. 16, quadriceps setting; No. 18, knee extension with boot.

Pelvic deviations

(L)   *Lateral tilt:* Prescription by physician.

(R)   *Rotated pelvis:* Prescription by physician.

(T)   *Anteroposterior pelvic tilts:* Forward and backward.

(F)   *Forward pelvic tilt:* No. 3, windmill sitting; No. 2, leg crossover; No. 4, neck, back, and shoulder flattener; No. 8, mad cat; No. 7, abdominal curl; No. 9, knee-chest curl; No. 5, breaking chains; No. 6, neck flattener at mirror.

(B)   *Backward pelvic tilt:* Supine—double leg lift; prone—back arching; prone—double leg lifts; No. 36, back stoop falling; No. 25, four-count wall weight (with low back hyperextended).

Spinal deviations

(Ky)   *Kyphosis:* No. 1, supine stretch; No. 4, neck, back, and shoulder flattener; No. 5, breaking chains; No. 6, neck flattener at mirror; No. 25, four-count wall weight; No. 29, chin lift.

(Lo)   *Lordosis:* No. 3, windmill sitting; No. 2, leg crossover; No. 22, crosslegged stretch; No. 4, neck, back, and shoulder flattener; No. 8, mad cat; No. 7, abdominal curl; No. 9, knee-chest curl; No. 5, breaking chains; No. 6, neck flattener at mirror.

(F)   *Flat:* See exercises for backward pelvic tilt.

(Sc)   *Scoliosis:** Symmetrical exercises: No. 1, supine stretch; No. 4, neck, back, and shoulder flattener; No. 3, windmill sitting; No. 6, neck flattener at mirror; No. 25, four-count wall weight; No. 29, chin lift; No. 38, chin-up or pull-up. Asymmetrical exercises: No. 1, supine stretch; No. 21, horizontal ladder; No. 20, elbow side falling; No. 19, tense and stretch.

Abdominal conditions

(Pt)   *Ptosis:* No. 3, windmill sitting; No. 2, leg crossover; No. 6, neck flattener at mirror; No. 8, mad cat; No. 7, abdominal curl; No. 9, knee-chest curl.

Foot conditions

(L)   *Longitudinal arch:* No. 10, bicycle; No. 11, heel cord stretch; No. 12, foot circling; No. 15, knee rotator; No. 14, foot curling; supination board or balance beam.

(M)   *Metatarsal arch:* No. 10, bicycle; No. 11, heel cord stretch; No. 12, foot circling; No. 13, building mounds.

(P)   *Pronated ankles:* No. 10, bicycle; No. 12, foot circling; No. 15, knee rotator; No. 14, foot curling; supination board or balance beam.

(TT)   *Tibial torsion (prescription of physician):* No. 10, bicycle; No. 12, foot circling; No. 15, knee rotator; No. 14, foot curling.

Exercises for specific body areas and conditions
Foot and ankle

No. 10, bicycle; No. 11, heel cord stretch; No. 12, foot circling; No. 13, building mounds; No. 30, toe lift; No. 39, jumping jack with variations; No. 40, rope skipping (Chapter 10).

Knee

No. 10, bicycle; No. 16, quadriceps setting; No. 18, knee extension with boot; No. 39, jumping jack with variations; No. 40, rope skipping (Chapter 10).

Shoulder

For general conditions: No. 5, breaking chains; No. 6, neck flattener at mirror; No. 26, shoulder rotator (wall weight); No. 25, four-count wall weight; No. 32, shoulder shrug; No. 28, arm press; No. 31, arm crossover; No. 29, chin lift; No. 33, towel wringing; No. 37, push-up; No. 38, chin-up or pull-up; No. 21, horizontal ladder.

For postdislocation: No. 26, shoulder rotator (wall weight) (Chapter 10).

Hand, wrist, and elbow

No. 33, towel wringing; No. 35, wrist machines; No. 40, rope skipping; No. 29, chin lift; No. 27, arm curl; No. 37, push-up; No. 38, chin-up or pull-up; No. 28, arm press; No. 31, arm crossover; No. 21, horizontal ladder (Chapter 10).

---

*With approval of physician.

Low back and sacroiliac

For low back stretch and development of abdominal group; No. 4, neck, back, and shoulder flattener; No. 3, windmill sitting; No. 2, leg crossover; No. 22, crosslegged stretch; No. 7, abdominal curl; No. 9, knee-chest curl (Chapter 10).

Weak back

For low back and hip extensor development: No. 1, supine stretch; No. 4, neck, back, and shoulder flattener; No. 5, breaking chains; No. 6, neck flattener at mirror; No. 25, four-count wall weight; No. 32, shoulder shrug; No. 29, chin lift; prone back arches (Chapter 10).

Balance and coordination

No. 6, neck flattener at mirror; No. 25, four-count wall weight; No. 39, jumping jack with variations; No. 40, rope skipping; supination board or balance beam.

General muscle tone

No. 3, windmill sitting; No. 2, leg crossover; No. 7, abdominal curl; No. 10, bicycle; No. 25, four-count wall weight; No. 27, arm curl; No. 28, arm press; No. 31, arm crossover; No. 30, toe lift; No. 40, rope skipping.

Dysmenorrhea

No. 1, supine stretch; No. 22, crosslegged stretch; No. 23, side stretch; No. 8, mad cat; No. 7, abdominal curl; No. 9, knee-chest curl; No. 6, neck flattener at mirror. (See Chapter 17 for complete discussion and for additional exercises.)

Exercises for special muscle groups
Erector spinae

No. 1, supine stretch; No. 4, neck, back, and shoulder flattener; No. 3, windmill sitting; No. 25, four-count wall weight; No. 29, chin lift; No. 20, elbow side falling; No. 19, tense and stretch; prone back arches; No. 36, back stoop falling.

Abdominals

No. 4, neck, back, and shoulder flattener; No. 3, windmill sitting; No. 2, leg crossover; No. 8, mad cat; No. 7, abdominal curl; No. 9, knee-chest curl; No. 5, breaking chains; No. 6, neck flattener at mirror; No. 20, elbow side falling.

Rhomboid and trapezius

No. 4, neck, back, and shoulder flattener; No. 5, breaking chains; No. 6, neck flattener at mirror; No. 21, horizontal ladder; No. 25, four-count wall weight; No. 32, shoulder shrug; No. 29, chin lift; prone back arches with hands in small of back.

Pectoral

No. 3, windmill sitting; No. 26, shoulder rotator (wall weight); No. 28, arm press; No. 31, arm crossover; No. 33, towel wringing; No. 37, push-up; No. 40, rope skipping; No. 21, horizontal ladder.

Latissimus

No. 21, horizontal ladder; No. 25, four-count wall weight; No. 33, towel wringing; No. 38, chin-up or pull-up; No. 40, rope skipping; No. 5, breaking chains; No. 6, neck flattener at mirror.

Deltoid

No. 4, neck, back, and shoulder flattener; No. 5, breaking chains; No. 6, neck flattener at mirror; No. 25, four-count wall weight; No. 28, arm press; No. 31, arm crossover; No. 29 chin lift; No. 37, push-up.

Biceps brachii

No. 40, rope skipping; No. 27, arm curl; No. 29, chin lift; No. 33, towel wringing; No. 38, chin-up or pull-up; No. 35, wrist machines.

Triceps

No. 28, arm press; No. 31, arm crossover; No. 37, push-up; No. 33, towel wringing; No. 25, four-count wall weight.

Forearm muscles

No. 27, arm curl; No. 33, towel wringing; No. 40, rope skipping; No. 35, wrist machines; No. 38, chin-up or pull-up; No. 28, arm press; No. 31, arm crossover; No. 29, chin lift; No. 21, horizontal ladder; No. 37, push-up.

Hip extensors

No. 10, bicycle; prone single and double leg lifts; No. 25, four-count wall weight; No. 40, rope skipping.

Hip flexors

No. 3, windmill sitting; No. 2, leg crossover; No. 9, knee-chest curl; No. 18, knee extension with boot.

Knee extensors

No. 10, bicycle; No. 16, quadriceps setting; No. 18, knee extension with boot; No. 39, jumping jack with variations; No. 40, rope skipping.

Knee flexors

No. 7, foot drag; No. 9, knee-chest curl; No. 10, bicycle.

Gastrocnemius and soleus

No. 12, foot circling; No. 11, heel cord stretch; No. 22, cross-legged stretch; No. 30, toe lift; No. 39, jumping jack with variations; No. 40, rope skipping.

Section III □ DESCRIPTIONS OF 40 KEY EXERCISES FOR ADAPTED PHYSICAL EDUCATION

1. Supine stretch *(Fig. 5-4)*

Specific for: General loosening and stretching of body

Beneficial in: Lateral curvatures of spine, kyphosis, forward shoulders, and low shoulder

Starting position: Lying on back on mat with legs extended:

1. Extend arms overhead and reach as far as possible; stretch so that heels reach down the mat as far from hands as possible. Do not arch the back.
2. Relax right leg and left arm and stretch crossways so that left heel and right hand are maximum distance apart. Repeat with opposite arm and leg.
3. Relax completely after each stretch and repeat as many times as required.

2. Leg crossover *(Fig. 5-5)*

Specific for: Low back and hip extensor stretch, warm-up and development of hip flexors, and abdominals

Starting position: Lying on back, arms extended at shoulder level, palms facing upward, heels pointed:

1. Flex left leg at hip to lift heel to rest on toes of right foot.
2. Twist body to right, bringing left foot across to floor, pause and stretch; then, keeping knee straight, slide foot toward right hand, stretch and return. (Keep heel pointed and legs straight.)
3. Do the same for right leg.

3. Windmill sitting *(Fig. 5-6)*

Specific for: Back stretch, hamstring stretch, and warm-up

Beneficial in: Abdominals and shoulder girdle

Starting position: Sitting on mat with arms extended sideward at shoulder level, palms up, legs spread wide apart, ankles plantar flexed:

1. Twist to right and bend forward with trunk so that fingers of left hand touch toes of right foot; stretch and hold. (Do a slow, controlled stretch.) Keep both legs straight.
2. Return to starting position and sit tall; then swing to left and repeat the exercise.
3. To increase the stretch of the back of the leg dorsiflex the ankle.

4. Neck, back, and shoulder flattener *(Fig. 5-7)*

Specific for: Forward head, cervical lordosis, kyphosis, forward shoulders, and lordosis

Beneficial in: Pelvic tilt

Starting position: Lying on back, knees drawn up, arms at sides with palms down:

1. Inhale and expand chest as nape of neck is forced to mat by stretching tall and pulling chin toward chest.
2. At the same time, flatten small of back to mat by tightening abdominal and buttocks muscles.
3. Check with fingers to see if neck and back are flat on mat. Exhale.
4. As it becomes easier to flatten back, the exercise may be made more difficult and more beneficial by gradually extending legs until the low back cannot be maintained in a flattened position.

5. Breaking chains *(Fig. 5-8)*

Specific for: Forward shoulders

Beneficial in: Kyphosis, flat chest, forward head, lordosis, and shoulder development

Starting position: Standing, with back against corner of post or sharp edge of corner of a room, feet 6 inches apart; place fists together in front of chest with elbows at shoulder level:

1. Imagine you are breaking a chain by strenuously pulling fists apart, keeping elbows at shoulder level, pinching shoulder blades together. Inhale.
2. Tuck pelvis and press low back as close to wall as possible.
3. Hold position 10 seconds.
4. Relax and exhale.

Caution: Keep abdomen and buttocks tight and maintain body in starting plane during the exercise; when lordosis

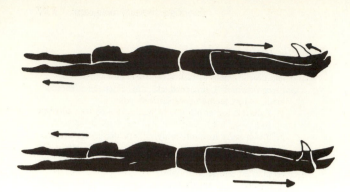

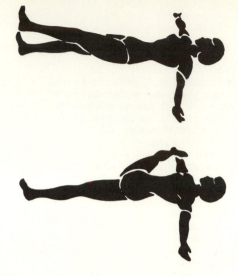

Fig. 5-4. No. 1, Supine stretch.

Fig. 5-5. No. 2, Leg crossover.

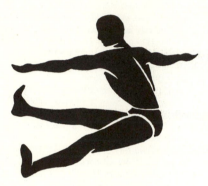

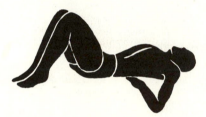

Fig. 5-6. No. 3, Windmill sitting.

Fig. 5-7. No. 4, Neck and back flattener.

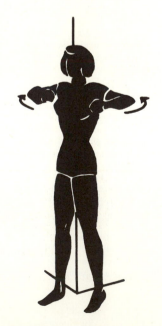

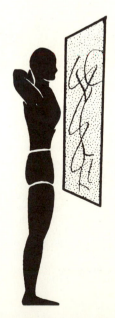

Fig. 5-8. No. 5, Breaking chains.

Fig. 5-9. No. 6, Neck flattener at mirror.

is present, the exercise may be done in sitting position with legs crossed in tailor's position.

6. Neck flattener at mirror (*Fig. 5-9*)

Specific for: Forward head, kyphosis, forward shoulders, lordosis, and shoulder development

Beneficial in: Total anteroposterior postural deviations

Starting position: Standing tall in front of mirror, head up, chin in, elbows extended sideward at shoulder level, fingertips behind base of head:

1. Draw head and neck backward vigorously as fingers are pressed forward for resistance and elbows are forced backward (flattening upper back). Inhale.
2. Flatten low back by tucking the pelvis by tightening the abdominals and hip extensors.
3. Hold; exhale; return to starting position. (Student can stand facing the mirror or with side of body toward mirror to check body position and to correct either anteroposterior or lateral posture deviations.)

7. Abdominal curl (*Fig. 5-10*)

Specific for: Ptosis (protruding abdomen), lordosis, and developing and shortening abdominals

Beneficial in: Forward pelvic tilt

Starting position: Lying on back, elbows at side of body and bent at 90 degrees, knees flexed, feet flat on floor:

1. Keep lower back flat on mat and, starting with head, curl body slowly forward and up to a 45-degree angle, lifting vertebra by vertebra off mat.
2. Uncurl slowly and with control.

Note: In all leg raising or trunk raising from the backward lying position, the student should exhale or count aloud as legs or trunk are raised to relieve intra-abdominal pressure and strain.

8. Mad cat (*Fig. 5-11*)

Specific for: Lordosis and abdominal muscles

Beneficial in: Dysmenorrhea, arms, shoulders, shoulder girdle, and low back stretch

Starting position: Kneeling on all fours:

1. Hump lower back by tightening abdominal and buttocks muscles and drop head down while inhaling.
2. Lean forward by bending arms until forehead touches floor; keeping back humped, exhale and return to starting position.

9. Knee-chest curl (*Fig. 5-12*)

Specific for: Ptosis, lordosis, and developing abdominal strength

Beneficial in: Development of hip flexors and stretch of spinal extensors

Starting position: Lying on back with knees bent at right angles, feet flat on floor, arms straight out from shoulders, elbows bent 90 degrees, palms up:

1. Bring knees toward chest while pulling with abdominal muscles and curl spine segment by segment off floor or mat; try to touch knees to chest or shoulders; hold, then uncurl to starting position.

Caution: See note on proper breathing for this exercise under description of exercise No. 7.

10. Bicycle (*Fig. 5-13*)

Specific for: General warm-up of foot and leg (for development and stretch)

Starting position: Lying on back, elbows at side of body, flexed at 90 degrees:

1. Bring knees to chest and roll up so that weight of body rests on shoulders and neck; place hands under hips for support and peddle on an imaginary bicycle with a large peddle sprocket.
2. Stress full motion in hip, knee, and ankle; alternately point toe and then heel to increase flexibility of foot

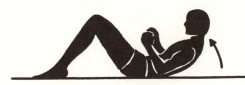

Fig. 5-10. No. 7, Abdominal curl.

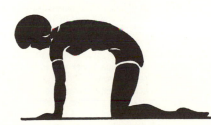

Fig. 5-11. No. 8, Mad cat.

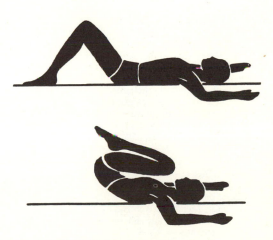

Fig. 5-12. No. 9, Knee-chest curl.

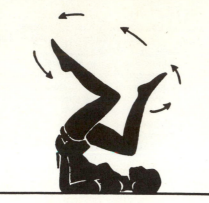

Fig. 5-13. No. 10, Bicycle.

and ankle. Do slowly for increased flexibility, then rapidly for warm-up.

Caution: Those with arthritis of spine and cardiac problems should not roll up into inverted position on back of neck.

11. Heel cord stretch *(Fig. 5-14)*

Specific for: Stretch heel cord and back of leg

Beneficial in: Arms, shoulders, and shoulder girdle

Starting position: Standing at arm's length from wall, body inclined slightly forward, back flat, feet toed in slightly with hands on the wall, shoulder high and shoulder width apart, elbows slightly bent:

1. Bend arms until chest nearly touches wall. (Keep body in straight line; keep heels on floor to obtain heel cord stretch.)
2. Progressions: position self as before. Move feet back an inch or so, keeping heels on floor, and repeat exercise.

Note: Heel cord stretch board with back flattened against wall may be used as an advanced exercise.

12. Foot circling *(Fig. 5-15)*

Specific for: Metatarsal arch and toe flexors

Beneficial in: Flexibility and strength of foot and ankle and longitudinal arch

Starting position: Having removed shoes and socks, sitting on bench and fully extending knees, with toes pointed and heels resting on a towel on floor or mat:

1. With toes flexed, circle foot inward.
2. Circle foot upward extend toes.
3. Circle foot outward extend toes.
4. Circle foot downward, while flexing toes, making full circle with foot and ankle; then repeat movements several times; rest. Value lies in obtaining full motion in each direction.

Caution: This exercise is contraindicated (never used) in hammer toes.

13. Building mounds *(Fig. 5-16)*

Specific for: Metatarsal arch and toe flexors

Beneficial in: Flexibility and strength of intrinsic muscles of feet and Morton's toe

Starting position: Sitting on bench, feet directly under knees, toes placed on end of towel:

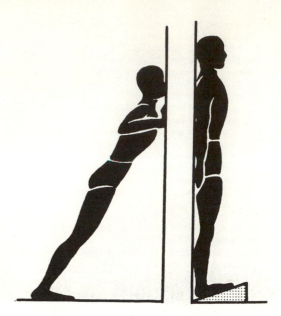

Fig. 5-14. No. 11, Heel cord stretch.

1. Grip towel with toes and pull toward body, building a mound; pull with toes of both feet working together or pull alternately; heels must remain firmly on floor during exercise and pull on towel should be made to maximum toe flexion.
2. Repeat movements until end of towel or weight is reached.
3. When towel is to be flattened, shove its end back to former position with foot.
4. A weight may be placed on end away from body to increase resistance; when five repetitions can be done correctly, add more weight.

14. Foot curling *(Fig. 5-17)*

Specific for: Longitudinal arch, tibialis posterior muscle, and pronated ankle

Beneficial in: Tibial torsion

Starting position: Sitting tall on bench with thigh horizontal to floor, place left heel forward of knee about 6 inches, bring toes of right foot to rear and outside of left heel to serve as a brace; fold a towel lengthwise in thirds and place one end next to outside of left foot, extended to left:

1. Lift and turn foot to left, then press ball of foot forcibly on towel and rotate lower leg and foot to the right, pulling towel inward.
2. Repeat until towel is completely pulled across.
3. When exercise can be repeated five times, add a weight to far end of towel to add resistance.

Note: Do not substitute thigh adductors or rotators to pull towel across. Keep ball of foot and toes firmly on towel while pulling towel medially.

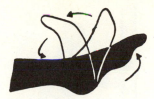

Fig. 5-15. No. 12, Foot circling.

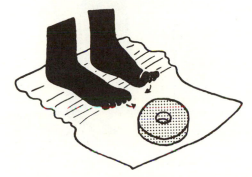

Fig. 5-16. No. 13, Building mounds.

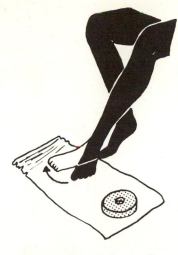

Fig. 5-17. No. 14, Foot curling.

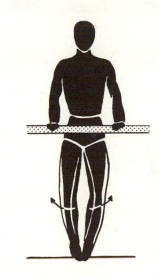

Fig. 5-18. No. 15, Knee rotator.

15. *Knee rotator* *(Fig. 5-18)*
    Specific for: Knock-knees and tibial torsion
    Beneficial in: Pronated ankle and longitudinal arch realignment
    Starting position: Standing, holding onto stall bars, back of chair, etc., heels 3 inches apart, big toes together, with weight toward outside of feet:
    1. Flex knees slightly and rotate knees outward vigorously as if to bring heels together against friction of the floor (but do not let them move); keep whole forepart of foot on floor so that a high, long arch is formed and kneecaps face outward.
    2. Hold this position for 10 seconds.
    3. Relax the foot and leg muscles by walking in place.
    4. Repeat the exercise.

16. *Quadriceps setting* *(Fig. 5-19)*
    Specific for: Stabilizing the knee anteriorly
    Beneficial in: Stabilizing knee joint and improving muscle tone of the quadriceps muscle group (pre- and postoperatively)
    Starting position: Standing with feet pointed straight ahead, one leg slightly in front of the other with the knee straight, but not locked (may be done in sitting position if necessary):
    1. Extend knee of front leg well backward.
    2. Tense and raise kneecap. Hold.
    3. Relax muscles, allowing kneecap to drop to regular position.
    4. Gradually increase amount of weight on foot.

Caution: When leg is tensed, hold contraction for a few moments and then relax muscles; more advanced exercises may include stair and hill climbing, running on smooth surfaces, and rope skipping.

17. *Foot drag* *(Fig. 5-20)*
    Specific for: Reeducation of muscle groups, stabilizing knee and ankle joints, and improving muscle tone of whole leg and thigh
    Starting position: Standing erect, feet pointed straight forward, knees slightly flexed, weight mostly on right foot:
    1. Apply mild pressure to floor with bottom of left foot;

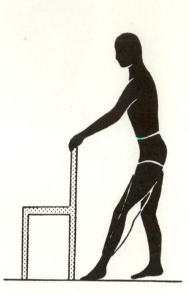

Fig. 5-19. No. 16, Quadriceps setting.

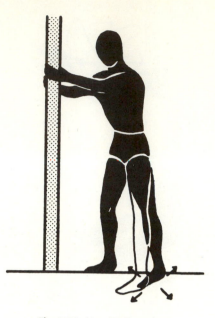

Fig. 5-20. No. 17, Foot drag.

then push it forward and backward, left and right and diagonally to form an X to greatest range of movement; cease movement at point of pain.
2. Circle foot clockwise and counterclockwise.
3. As condition improves, increase resistance by placing more weight on dragged foot.

Caution: Keep knees slightly bent and toes straight forward at all times, thus lessening strain on knee joint. Wear rubber-soled shoe to increase friction.

18. Knee extensor (with boot) *(Fig. 5-21)*
Specific for: Strengthening quadriceps muscle group
Beneficial in: Improving muscle tone of anterior thigh and hip flexors (if step 3 is added)
Starting position: Sitting on plinth or high bench with knee flexed and a weight on foot (boot or sandbag, *foot supported*):
1. Extend knee to straighten leg.
2. Hold, then lower slowly to supported position.
3. To increase strength of hip flexors, add the following movement: raise entire leg above horizontal, tensing leg muscle, sitting tall; lower slowly.

Caution: Be sure that exercise is done very slowly to ensure maximum development of whole front of thigh; climb stairs on every occasion, walk uphill, do road work on smooth surface. Exercises on a Universal Gym or with special isotonic exercise machines can be substituted.

19. Tense and stretch *(Fig. 5-22)*
Specific for: Scoliosis
Beneficial in: Torsion of trunk and low shoulder
Starting position: Standing tall (facing a mirror if possible):
1. Raise arm vertically over head, opposite from the way in which the spine curves (right arm for a left C sco-

liosis); rotate other hand and arm outward and vigorously press it into side of body (left arm for a left C scoliosis).
2. Hold position for 10 seconds. Lower arms to sides and assume normal position.
3. Repeat exercise required number of times.

Caution: Be certain that back is maintained in straight position without twisting trunk; stand tall; do not let shoulders sag.
Note: Give only on prescription of physician unless exercise is done symmetrically, that is, to both sides.

20. Elbow side falling *(Fig. 5-23)*
Specific for: Scoliosis and development of lateral flexors of trunk
Starting position: Resting on side toward convex side of spinal curve:
1. Rest on elbow toward curve; extend opposite arm, shoulder height, to side and lift hip completely off floor; hold with body support on forearm and side of foot.
2. Lower hip to floor and rest.
3. Repeat.

Caution: Back must be in horizontal plane with neck, head, and back straight; upper leg may be placed in front of supporting leg for better balance.
Note: Give only on prescription of physician unless exercise is done symmetrically by doing the same exercise while resting on the opposite side of the body.

21. Horizontal ladder *(Fig. 5-24)*
Beneficial in: Total body stretch, scoliosis curves in spine, kyphosis and forward shoulders, low shoulder, and development of shoulder girdle muscles

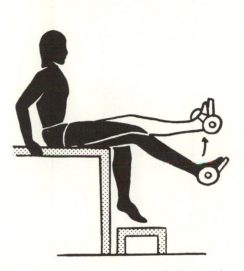

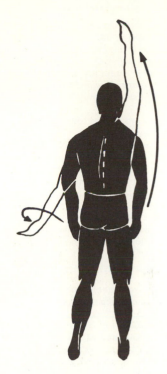

Fig. 5-21. No. 18, Knee extensor (with boot). A leg press machine or quadriceps machine can also be used for this exercise.

Fig. 5-22. No. 19, Tense and stretch. Dotted line indicates improved alignment resulting from exercise done in *keynote* position illustrated.

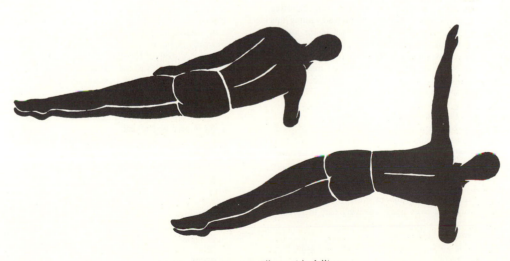

Fig. 5-23. No. 20, Elbow side falling.

Note: This exercise should be specified for each individual by the instructor; it may include climbing, hanging, stretching, swinging, etc. If horizontal ladder is mounted with one end higher than the other, asymmetrical exercises can be given for low shoulders, scoliosis, etc.

22. *Crosslegged stretch (modified from Billig)* *(Fig. 5-25)*

Specific for: Stretch of lower back, back of leg, and heel cord

Beneficial in: Lordosis and bent knees

Starting position: Standing on affected leg with knee fully extended, about 20 inches from and with back to stall bars, chair, or bench, reach back and rest hand of affected side on stall bars for balance:

1. Then, with knee flexed, twine opposite leg tightly around front of affected leg; foot is placed in tiptoe position on floor, back of and to the outside of heel of affected leg.
2. Free hand is placed on opposite shoulder and, from this position, student bows forward at hips, reaching for heel of crossed-over foot with elbow, at the same time dropping entire heel from tiptoe position to floor.
3. Execute five controlled stretches. Hold each stretch for 10 seconds; relax and repeat on opposite side (see also Fig. 5-1).

23. *Side stretch (Billig)* *(Fig. 5-26)*

Specific for: Mobilization of hip and pelvis

Beneficial in: Dysmenorrhea (Chapter 17)

Starting position: Heels and toes together approximately upper-arm's distance from and with side to wall:

1. Place elbow against wall at shoulder level, elbow slightly ahead of line of shoulders, with forearm and hand resting on wall; heel of opposite hand is placed in back of hip joint (behind greater trochanter).
2. Keep shoulders in line with the elbow perpendicular to wall; do not allow them to shift forward. Keep knees completely extended and locked; strongly contract abdominal and gluteal muscles while shifting hips slightly forward and in toward wall, aiding this by pressure of the outside hand; push inside hip toward a point directly below hand that rests on wall.
3. Force the sideward and forward shift of hips toward wall far enough to produce a stretch on muscles and ligaments. Hold stretch position for 10 seconds. Repeat on opposite side.

24. *Head tilt (Billig)* *(Fig. 5-27)*

Specific for: Neck muscle stretching

Beneficial in: Muscle relaxation, remediation of neck strain, and muscle tension

Starting position: Seated in a chair with hand on one side firmly grasping back leg of chair; head and neck are tilted laterally 45 degrees in the opposite direction:

1. Retract chin maximum distance possible and hold retracted (pulled in) throughout stretch.
2. Place free hand over head, covering ear, to forcibly continue tilt.
3. Pull to stretch, hold 10 seconds.
4. Repeat this stretching three times on each side three times daily.

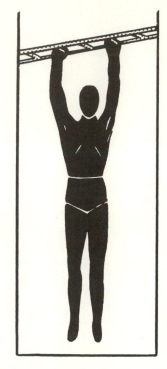

Fig. 5-24. No. 21, Horizontal ladder.

25. *Four-count wall weight* *(Fig. 5-28)*

Specific for: General conditioning of shoulders and upper back, kyphosis, and forward shoulders

Beneficial in: General fitness, back and hamstring flexibility, and abdominal strength

Starting position: Standing facing wall weights, holding handles straight forward at shoulder level:

1. Pull handles to toes, keeping legs and arms straight.
2. Return to starting position and pull handles back beyond sides of hips.
3. Return and pull handles out to side at shoulder level.
4. Return and pull handles straight overhead.
5. Return and repeat.

Caution: Keep body straight and tall throughout exercise: *do not* use more weight than can be handled while body is maintained in a good anteroposterior alignment; breathe freely.

26. *Shoulder rotator (wall weights)* *(Fig. 5-29)*

Specific for: Shoulder dislocation, pectoral muscles, and subscapularis

Beneficial in: General shoulder strength

Starting position: Standing with side toward wall weights, back straight and feet shoulder distance apart; grasp one or both handles with hand that is nearest weights:

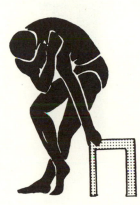

Fig. 5-25. No. 22, Crosslegged stretch (modified from Billig).

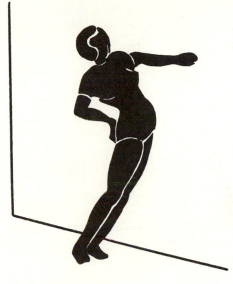

Fig. 5-26. No. 23, Side stretch (Billig).

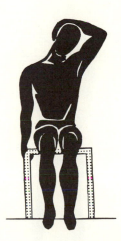

Fig. 5-27. No. 24, Head tilt (Billig).

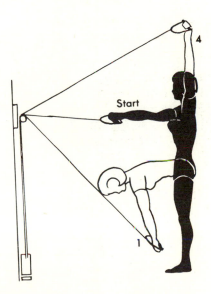

Fig. 5-28. No. 25, Four-count wall weight.

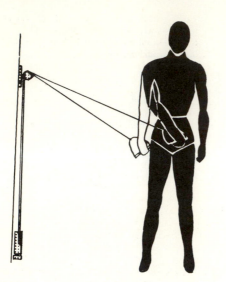

Fig. 5-29. No. 26, Shoulder rotator (wall weights).

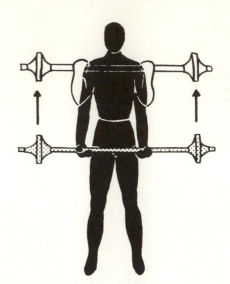

Fig. 5-30. No. 27, Arm curl (barbell or dumbbell).

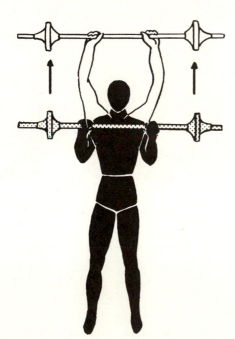

Fig. 5-31. No. 28, Arm press (barbell or dumbbell).

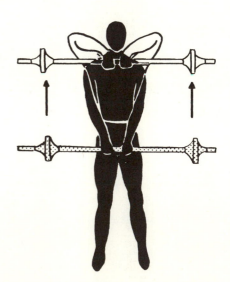

Fig. 5-32. No. 29, Chin lift (barbell or dumbbell).

1. Pull handle across in front of body with hand at hip level, elbow fully extended, body stationary.
2. Rotate arm inward (medial rotation) as far as possible as it is brought across body; hold; return.

27. *Arm curl (barbell or dumbbell)* (*Fig. 5-30*)
Specific for: Biceps, brachialis, and brachioradialis
Beneficial in: Forearm and shoulder muscles
Starting position: Standing or sitting, weights held in front of body at thigh level, palms turned away from body:
1. Flex arms, keeping elbows close to, but not against sides, bringing weights to chest; hold and return slowly; reverse curl; repeat as described, except palms turned toward body in starting position.
2. Breathe freely.

28. *Arm press (barbell or dumbbell)* (*Fig. 5-31*)
Specific for: Triceps and deltoid
Beneficial in: General shoulder girdle and forearms
Starting position: Standing or sitting, palms facing away from body, weights at chest level:
1. Extend arms overhead; hold; lower slowly to back of neck. Extend arms; hold; return to starting position.
2. Stand tall with head up and chin in; do not arch low back excessively or strain to press too heavy a weight.
3. Breathe freely.

29. *Chin lift (barbell or dumbbell)* (*Fig. 5-32*)
Specific for: Deltoid, biceps, trapezius, and levator
Beneficial in: Erector spinae and forearm muscles
Starting position: Standing or sitting, hands held close together, weights at thigh level, palms facing body, arms fully extended:
1. Inhale as you raise elbows upward and backward until

weights touch chin; hold; exhale as weights are returned slowly to starting position.
2. Stand tall; raise elbows as high as possible; keep low back and abdomen flat.

30. *Toe lift* (*Fig. 5-33*)
Specific for: Ankle extensors (gastrocnemius, soleus)
Beneficial in: Heel cord stretch
Starting position: Standing, with weights supported by hands at back of neck, place toes and balls of feet on block of wood, mat, or other material raised $1\frac{1}{2}$ to 2 inches higher than heels:
1. Stretch lower leg muscles and heel cord.
2. Raise up on forefoot until heels are higher than support and ankles are completely plantar flexed.
3. Hold; lower and repeat.
4. Keep body straight and stand tall throughout exercise.
Note: Leg press bar may be substituted.

31. *Arm crossover (dumbbells)* (*Fig. 5-34*)
Specific for: Pectoral, anterior deltoid, and triceps muscles
Beneficial in: Muscles of arm and shoulder girdle and stretch of anterior shoulder muscles
Starting position: Lying on back with knees flexed and feet flat on bench or plinth, arms extended directly out to either side at shoulder level, a dumbbell in each hand, palms up; let gravity stretch the anterior shoulder muscles:
1. Lift arms straight up (forward) over body, cross and bring them down to opposite sides, bending elbow; return slowly, straightening elbow and then returning to starting position.
2. Exhale as arms cross; inhale as arms are stretched down and back.

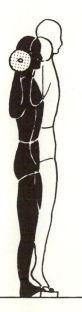

Fig. 5-33. No. 30, Toe lift.

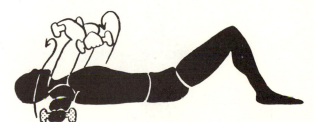
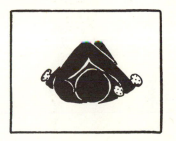

Fig. 5-34. No. 31, Arm crossover (dumbbells).

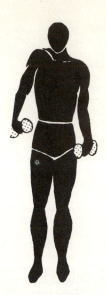

Fig. 5-35. No. 32, Shoulder shrug (barbells or dumbbells).

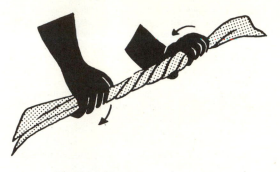

Fig. 5-36. No. 33, Towel wringing.

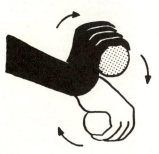

Fig. 5-37. No. 34, Gripper.

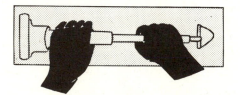

Fig. 5-38. No. 35, Wrist machines.

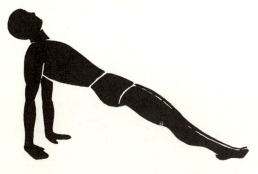

Fig. 5-39. No. 36, Back stoop falling.

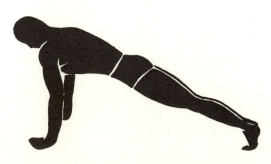

Fig. 5-40. No. 37, Push-up.

32. **Shoulder shrug (barbell or dumbbell)** *(Fig. 5-35)*
    Specific for: Low shoulder, forward shoulders, trapezius, rhomboids, and levator
    Starting position: Standing or sitting with arms at sides, palms facing body, weight held at thigh level, arms fully extended:
    1. Roll shoulders forward, upward, backward as you inhale; hold.
    2. Exhale while returning to starting position.
    Caution: Keep head up, chin in, and back straight; watch body alignment and shoulder position in mirror to check on body alignment.

33. **Towel wringing** *(Fig. 5-36)*
    Specific for: Entire arm and shoulder strength
    Beneficial in: Development of rotation of forearm and strengthening of entire arm, shoulder girdle, and grip strength
    Starting position: Standing or sitting; fold towel lengthwise in four layers to avoid tearing:
    1. Hold elbows close to sides and grasp near center of towel with both hands.
    2. Twist towel as if wringing water from it, first in one direction and then in the other.
    3. Repeat five times.
    Caution: Keep arms at sides, wring towel vigorously, and squeeze hard as if wet to obtain proper wrist action; keep shoulders back; sit or stand tall.

34. **Gripper** *(Fig. 5-37)*
    Specific for: Strengthening hand and forearm
    Beneficial in: Improving muscle tone of all flexor muscle groups and decreasing joint limitations
    Starting position: Either sitting or standing while grasping rubber doughnut, tennis ball, handball, or sponge ball:
    1. Squeeze doughnut or ball hard while tensing upper arm; while gripping, rotate wrist one direction and then the other; relax, repeat.
    2. Advanced exercise: Use spring hand gripper.

35. **Wrist machines** *(Fig. 5-38)*
    Specific for: Flexion, extension, abduction, adduction, rotation, and combinations of these wrist movements
    Beneficial in: Hand and shoulder conditions
    Note: Various types of wrist machines available from commercial manufacturers enable the student to exercise with progressively greater amounts of resistance (Fig. 20-15); special exercise equipment can also be improvised by the instructor.

36. **Back stoop falling** *(Fig. 5-39)*
    Specific for: Development of spinal and hip joint extensors, shoulder girdle, and arm strengthening
    Starting position: Sitting on mat with legs extended and hands (palms down, fingers pointing toward feet) on mat just behind buttocks:
    1. Extend arms and shoulders and straighten body, keeping head back, chin in, and back flat so that weight is supported on heels and hands.
    2. Hold; return to starting position.
    3. Add alternate leg raises to increase difficulty of this exercise and involve hip flexors.

37. **Push-up** *(Fig. 5-40)*
    Specific for: Shoulder girdle, anterior deltoid, triceps, and pectoral strength
    Beneficial in: General conditioning and abdominals
    Starting position: Lying face down with hands palms down on the mat directly beneath shoulders:
    1. Push up by extending arms with body straight so that weight is supported on hands and toes.
    2. Return only far enough to touch chest to mat and then push up again.
    3. Keep head back, but chin in.
    4. Modified push-ups are recommended as a lead-up skill (use knees, not toes for lower body support).

38. **Chin-up or pull-up (stall bar or horizontal bar)** *(Fig. 5-41)*
    Specific for: Biceps, brachialis, and latissimus
    Beneficial in: Shoulder girdle and pectoral, hand, wrist, and forearms
    Starting position: Hanging on top rung facing stall bars, palms toward wall:
    1. Keep body straight and relaxed while flexing arms to raise chin to top bar. (Horizontal bar may be used.)
    2. Modified pull-up on stall bars: Ease weight on arms by climbing bars with toes; then slowly lower body under control.
    Note: Do not swing or kick to aid in pull.

39. **Jumping jack with variations** *(Fig. 5-42)*
    Specific for: General body warm-ups, cardiovascular fitness
    Beneficial in: Improving coordination, rhythm, and timing
    Starting position: Standing tall, arms down at sides:
    1. Jump, spreading feet apart sideways while arms are swung sideward and hands brought together overhead (arms remain straight throughout).
    2. Return to starting position. Variations:
       a. Spread feet forward and backward instead of sideways.
       b. Spread feet forward and backward, alternating left foot forward, then right foot forward.
       c. Alternate spreading feet sideways, then forward and backward, etc.
       d. Bring hands together in front of body at shoulder level, arms straight (in coordination with various foot movements).
       e. Bring hands together behind buttocks (in coordination with various foot movements).
       f. Employ various combinations and patterns of these foot and hand movements.
       g. Employ various rhythms: slow, medium, fast, etc.; teacher leads first, then allows student to experiment with new patterns and rhythms. All of these variations can be done to music.

40. **Rope skipping** *(Fig. 5-43)*
    Specific for: General body warm-up and improving endurance and strength
    Beneficial in: Improving balance, coordination, and rhythm
    Starting position: Standing, one end of jumping rope held in each hand, with rope adjusted so that it is slightly longer than necessary to enable student to jump through

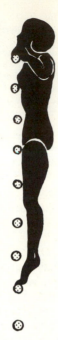

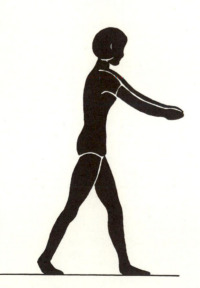

Fig. 5-41. No. 38, Chin-up or pull-up (stall bar or horizontal bar). Figure shows modified chin-up with toes on lower stall bar to help lift body.

it and have it clear the head at the top of its swing. Variations:

1. Vary foot patterns to go with each swing of the rope: jump on both feet, jump on one foot only, jump on alternate feet (like running in place with one foot ahead of the other, stepping through each swing of the rope so that both feet are used during each turn).

2. Jump as in step 1, but perform two foot movements to each turn of the rope, then three movements, etc.

3. Employ hand and arm variation: turning rope once to each foot pattern, progressing to three or four turns for the advanced student; turning rope backward and performing various foot patterns. (See Chapter 8 for additional information on rope skipping.)

SELECTION OF INDIVIDUAL EXERCISE PROGRAM

The selection of the proper exercises for students in the class must be based on needs and interest. The needs are determined as a result of the physician's examination and recommendations (Figs. 5-44 and 18-1), the posture and body mechanics screening examination (Figs. 5-45 and 5-46), and any other assessment data available (physical fitness tests, tests previously performed on the student by the instructur or physical therapist, etc.). The interest of students can be ascertained from a written questionnaire or oral consultation. Consid-

Fig. 5-42. No. 39, Jumping jack with variations.

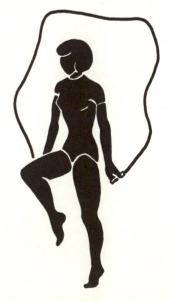

Fig. 5-43. No. 40, Rope skipping.

erable responsibility can be placed on students in secondary school and college in this respect. All these data are recorded on the form for the Individual Education Program and/or on the adapted physical education appraisal form. Methods that have been used successfully with Individual Education Programs and with classes in adapted physical education are edscribed in detail in the following paragraphs and in Chapters 18 and 19.

Orientation procedures
Individual orientation

After the students' assessments have been completed and the Individual Education Programs, annual goals, performance objectives, program activities, and motivational techniques have been planned, the instructor will meet with the students to begin the instructional process. The most severely handicapped persons will have completely individualized programs with methods and teaching strategies chosen to help them reach intermediate and terminal objectives and to make progress toward their stated goals. An orientation session should be planned to acquaint the students with these procedures including, when appropriate, the findings of the assessments and an interpretation of how the activities and/or exercises should contribute to progress. After this type of foundation has been laid, the teaching of the activity programs should begin. Forms for recording this type of information are found in Fig. 5-45 and in Chapters 18 and 19.

Group and class orientation

After the completion of the physical examination, posture screening, fitness, perceptual-motor, and other types of diagnostic assessments, an orientation session is conducted for the students in the adapted physical education class. Departmental and class rules and regulations, general findings relative to the physical examination and other examinations (and what they mean to the students), and the types of activity programs available to the students should be explained. The adapted physical education appraisal form, containing general information about the students' medical, postural, and fitness conditions, should be in the hands of the students during this orientation period so that they can relate the orientation information to their own needs for the special exercise and activity programs offered in the adapted class (Figs. 5-45 and 5-46).

After this general orientation session, the students should make a list, in order of importance, of those things that *they* want to concentrate on during the coming semester (individual objectives). (Programs for young children and severely handi-

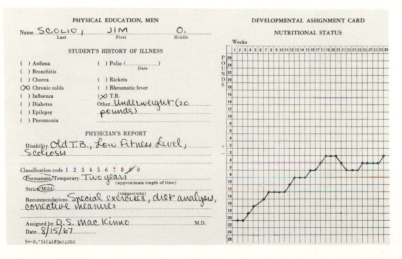

Fig. 5-44. Permanent record card including student's history of illness, physician's report, and body weight graph.

NOTE: This section of card should be folded down when it is placed in the permanent file. Keep straight for Kardex.

SMITH, JUDY

UNIVERSITY OF CALIFORNIA, LOS ANGELES
Department of Physical Education • Developmental Division
CASE ANALYSIS

Disability Old rheumatic fever, cardiac, poor ant.-post. posture, over weight

Physician's Recommendations Modified exercises and activities

Code Classification X 2 3 4 5 6 7 8 9 0
(Health Service)

Other conditions kyphosis 2°, lordosis 3°, ptosis 2°, back knees 2°

Duplicate conditions: 1 2 3 4

RESULTS AND DISPOSITION

Date entered Developmental Jan. 30, 1980 Date discharged

Results by semesters:	①	2	3	4	Other
Disability corrected					
Disability improved					
Preventive program	✓				
To Reg. Phys. Educ.					
Temporary assignment					
Left school					
Remarks					

NUTRITIONAL STATUS	Freshman		Sophomore		Junior		Senior		Other
Semester	1	2	1	2	1	2	1	2	
Age (Yrs.–Mos.)	18-7								
Height (Inches)	66								
Pelvic (Width cm.)	32.5								
Chest (Width cm.)	30.1								
Weight (Normal)	150 lbs								
Weight (Actual)	190 lbs								
Weight (Variation) ±	40 lbs								

FOLLOW UP EXAMS	DATES CHECKED	* RESULTS		EXAMINATION	DATES CHECKED	* RESULTS
Blood Pressure				Spine		
Heart				Tracings	2/5/80	
Cardiogram	2/5/80			Flexible Rule		
Others				Anthropometric (Specify) Abdominal Girth		
X-ray				1.	2/5/80	34"
Photography				2.		
Posture				3.		
Special				4.		
Foot				Nutritional		
Tracings				Diet Analysis	2/5/80	
Pedograph				Basal Metab.		
Others				Others		
Joint Measurements						
Calipers						
Goniometer						
Tracings						

CODE USED ON CARD
1° = Noticeable–Slight—(Brown tab)   1st Exam = Black
2° = Moderate—(Blue tab)   2nd Exam = Orange
3° = Severe—(Red tab)   3rd Exam = Green
* Results of Follow-up examinations.   4th Exam = Purple

Fig. 5-45. Adapted physical education case analysis (front side).

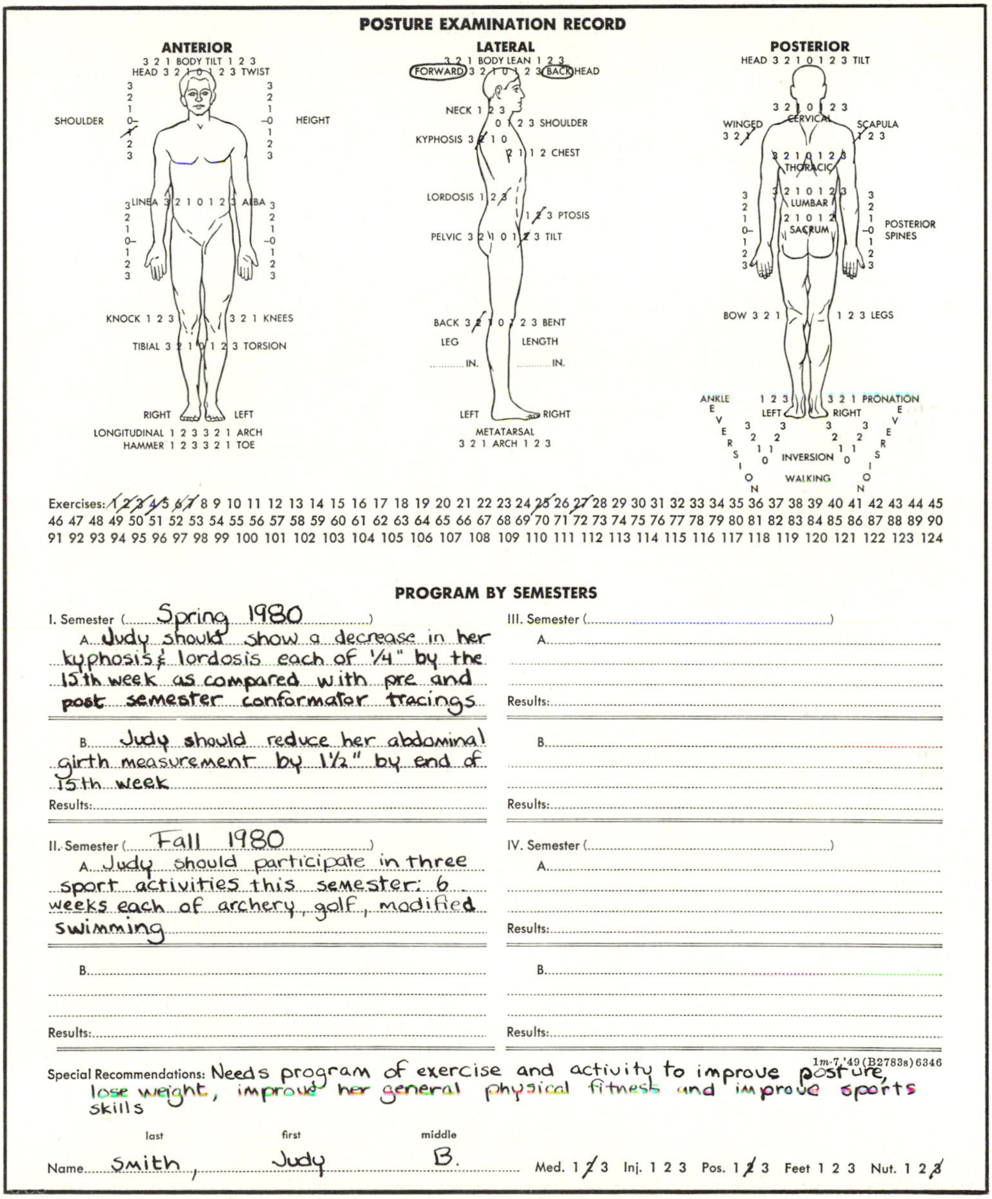

POSTURE EXAMINATION RECORD

ANTERIOR

3 2 1 BODY TILT 1 2 3
HEAD 3 2 1 0 1 2 3 TWIST

SHOULDER 0

HEIGHT

LINEA 3 2 1 0 1 2 3 ALBA

KNOCK 1 2 3   3 2 1 KNEES

TIBIAL 3 2 1 0 1 2 3 TORSION

RIGHT   LEFT

LONGITUDINAL 1 2 3 3 2 1 ARCH
HAMMER 1 2 3 3 2 1 TOE

LATERAL

3 2 1 BODY LEAN 1 2 3
(FORWARD) 3 2 1 0 1 2 3 (BACK) HEAD

NECK 1 2 3
0 1 2 3 SHOULDER

KYPHOSIS 3 2 1 0

2 1 2 CHEST

LORDOSIS 1 2 3

1 2 3 PTOSIS

PELVIC 3 2 1 0 1 2 3 TILT

BACK 3 2 1 0 1 2 3 BENT

LEG   LENGTH

.... IN.   .... IN.

LEFT   RIGHT

METATARSAL
3 2 1 ARCH 1 2 3

POSTERIOR

HEAD 3 2 1 0 1 2 3 TILT

3 2 1 0

WINGED   CERVICAL   SCAPULA
3 2 1   1 2 3

3 2 1 0 1 2 3
THORACIC

LUMBAR

2 1 0 1 2 3
SACRUM

POSTERIOR
SPINES

BOW 3 2 1   1 2 3 LEGS

ANKLE 1 2 3   3 2 1 PRONATION
E   LEFT   RIGHT   E
V   3   3   V
E   2   2   E
R   1   1   R
S   1   1   S
I   INVERSION   I
O   WALKING   O
N   N

Exercises: 1 2 3 4 5 6 7 8 9 10 11 12 13 14 15 16 17 18 19 20 21 22 23 24 25 26 27 28 29 30 31 32 33 34 35 36 37 38 39 40 41 42 43 44 45 46 47 48 49 50 51 52 53 54 55 56 57 58 59 60 61 62 63 64 65 66 67 68 69 70 71 72 73 74 75 76 77 78 79 80 81 82 83 84 85 86 87 88 89 90 91 92 93 94 95 96 97 98 99 100 101 102 103 104 105 106 107 108 109 110 111 112 113 114 115 116 117 118 119 120 121 122 123 124

PROGRAM BY SEMESTERS

I. Semester (_Spring 1980_)

  A. Judy should show a decrease in her kyphosis & lordosis each of ¼" by the 15th week as compared with pre and post semester conformater tracings.

  B. Judy should reduce her abdominal girth measurement by 1½" by end of 15th week

Results:

II. Semester (_Fall 1980_)

  A. Judy should participate in three sport activities this semester: 6 weeks each of archery, golf, modified swimming

  B.

Results:

III. Semester (...........................)

  A.

Results:

  B.

Results:

IV. Semester (...........................)

  A.

  B.

Results:

Special Recommendations: Needs program of exercise and activity to improve posture, lose weight, improve her general physical fitness and improve sports skills

1m-7,'49 (B2783s) 6346

Name _Smith_ , _Judy_ _B._
   last   first   middle

Med. 1 2 3   Inj. 1 2 3   Pos. 1 2 3   Feet 1 2 3   Nut. 1 2 3

Fig. 5-46. Adapted physical education case analysis (back side).

Exercise objective	No.	Exercise name	Rec. Reps./Resist.	Weeks 1	2	3	4	5	6	7	8	9	10	11	12	13	14	15
Warm up	2	Leg cross over																
	3	Windmill sitting	5 min.															
	10	Bicycles																
Dysm.	22	Cross-legged stretch	15 each side															
	23	Side stretch	5 each side															
	8	Mad cat	10															
Ky. 2°	4	Neck, back and shoulder flat	8															
	6	Neck flat at mirror	8															
	29	Chin lifts	12/15 lbs.															
Pron. 3°	12	Foot circling	10															
	15	Knee rotator	8															
	14	Foot curling	5 ea./1 lb.															
Low fit.	7	Abdominal curl	8															
	25	Four count wall wts.	12/3 wts.															
	28	Arm press	12/20 lbs.															

CALIFORNIA STATE UNIVERSITY, LONG BEACH
ADAPTED PHYSICAL EDUCATION EXERCISE CARD
Sect. No. 5 Date _____
Name Jill Jones Disabilities Dysmenorrhea, Low physical fitness
Posture deviations Kyphosis 2°, Pronated feet and ankles 3

Weekly grades

Fig. 5-47. Exercise assignment card.

capped persons are planned for them by the instructor or therapist.) These are reviewed with the students by the instructor so that important items are not missed and so that the conditions selected by the students are given the proper priority. Some adjustments and changes may need to be made at this time. The final choices, listed in the order of their importance, constitute the objectives of the students for the coming semester in the adapted physical education class (Fig. 5-47). The objectives should be stated in behavioral or performance terms so that the students and instructor know exactly what the students must do to successfully accomplish the objectives. This should help in making student, instructor, and program evaluations and in arriving at a mark or grade for each person in a school situation.

For example, a 16-year-old boy assigned to an adapted physical education class (or to a therapist) for a special program for asthma, for kypholordosis, and for rehabilitation of a postoperative knee condition might have the following performance objectives:

For asthma
1. Demonstrate that he can walk/run 1 mile in 6 minutes by the end of the fifteenth week.
2. Show his ability to exhale vigorously using three different techniques to encourage forced exhalation while blowing a Ping Pong ball 5 feet across the top of a table by the end of the tenth week.

For kypholordosis
1. Show a decrease of at least $1/4$ inch in each of his two curves as measured on the conformator by the end of the fifteenth week.
2. Write one paragraph each on the correction of kyphosis and lordosis, including information on gravitational pull, flexibility, and muscle development necessary to effect a correction of each condition. This assignment is to be judged and evaluated by the instructor for accuracy and completeness as compared with information given in a specified standard text.

For postoperative knee condition
1. Demonstrate the ability to perform the knee extensor exercise (No. 18) correctly, making 15 repetitions with 15 pounds of resistance by the end of the eighth week.
2. Increase the girth of the affected thigh to at least that of the unaffected one by the end of the fifteenth week.

ASSIGNMENT OF INDIVIDUAL EXERCISE PROGRAMS

Persons who are participating in programs mandated P.L. 94-142 must have Individual Education Programs planned by an appropriate committee and approved by parents and the school or agency.

The Individual Education Program for each person must be based on proper assessment procedures, have annual goals, and have definite performance objectives written as described earlier in this chapter.

Although the instructional program may have to be highly individualized for the most severely handicapped, it may range from one-to-one instruction to group instruction of several handicapped persons with similar types of problems or to assignment to regular physical education classes where individuals can reach their program objectives in the least restrictive environment (mainstreaming). The essential factor is that each individual is placed in the most appropriate situation to meet the unique needs listed in the Individual Education Program.

An example of an Individual Education Program for a profoundly handicapped person in a special education setting might include the following:

ASSESSMENT: Tests indicate that the person is unable to roll over from prone to supine and supine to prone positions.

GOAL: To be able to roll over in the supine position from right to left and left to right.

OBJECTIVES: To develop sufficient total body strength, endurance, and flexibility to perform rolling activities and to develop the necessary skills and patterns of coordination to be able to roll from front to back and from back to front.

PROGRAM PLANS: To teach the subject exercises and activities designed to develop strength, endurance, and flexibility based on the unique needs found in the assessment.

EVALUATION: To retest to find whether the subject has met the stated objectives.

Individual exercise programs for classes

The priority list of needs and interests (objectives) worked out by the student and the teacher, together with the results of all the assessment examinations and the recommendations of the physician, enables the teacher to plan an individual activity program. Since the teacher has available all the necessary information, this can be done in the office or home prior to the next meeting of the class. This enables the student to start on an individual exercise or activity program at the earliest possible time.

The mechanics of this operation can be simplified for the teacher by having the student do some of the basic clerical work. As soon as the student

and teacher have agreed on the student's objectives, the student can write them in the proper place on the exercise or activity card (Fig. 5-47). The rest of the information needed on the card can also be filled out (name, disability, etc.) by the student so that it is ready for the teacher to write in the assigned exercises.

Using the exercise assignment information (pp. 123 to 125), the teacher then selects the exercises that will best meet the needs and interest of each student, listing these in proper order on the exercise card. A suggested starting dosage (repetitions, resistance, time, etc.) should also be recorded in the first column of the card by the instructor. An exercise program, which would require approximately 30 minutes, should include from 10 to 12 exercises. Since persons teaching adapted physical education full time may have as many as five classes of 25 students each, they may find it necessary during their first session of exercise program planning to limit the number of exercises for each student to one or two key exercises for each of the conditions listed. Other exercises can then be added to the program when the teacher has more time after the first class meeting. This basic exercise program can be modified and the number of repetitions and the amount of resistance can be adjusted by the instructor as the exercises are being taught and again throughout the year as the student finds that the suggested program is too easy or too difficult.

TEACHING OF EXERCISE PROGRAMS

Students should report to class dressed for activity on the class period after the orientation and planning period previously discussed. They should be given their exercise cards, which list their individual exercise programs and suggest a starting number of repetitions for each exercise. To enable all the students to learn these exercises quickly and to facilitate teaching a variety of individual exercises to a group of 25 students, the following system of organization for the class has proved successful:

1. The instructor first teaches four or five exercises that have been most frequently assigned as warm-up exercises. Students do only those exercises assigned on their exercise cards. They sit and observe or practice an exercise

already learned while exercises not on their cards are being taught to others in the group.

2. By a quick show of hands (or by compiling the information while assigning the exercises), the teacher can determine how many students have each of the 40 key exercises on their exercise card. Usually 10 or 12 of the key exercises will appear on a majority of the students' exercise cards. These exercises are taught in the order of frequency of assignment as soon as the warm-ups have been learned. Other exercises are similarly taught until the instructor comes to the special exercises assigned to only one or two students. By then, most of the class will have learned the majority of their exercises and thus can be engaged in their workouts while the instructor teaches the excercises that are assigned less frequently.

3. When all the students have learned their complete programs, attention should be given to doing the exercise routine in the proper sequence. The usual order is as follows: (a) warm-up exercises; (b) the first exercise assigned under the first condition (objective), which is usually either the least difficult exercise or a stretch exercise; (c) the first exercise assigned under the second condition, and so on, until the first exercise for each of the areas has been completed; (d) the student then proceeds to the second exercise in each area (a more difficult exercise), until all exercises are completed, thus allowing for concentration on one body area at a time, followed by a rest period for each body area while another is being exercised; (e) if there is additional time after completing an exercise program, the student can go back and review certain key exercises that are of special *value* or can repeat exercises that are of special *interest*. No exercise should be attempted by the student unless it is included on the exercise card.

4. Students can also check the written descriptions and study the diagrams of the exercises, which should be posted on the bulletin board or made available to the students for study. This will enable them to do the exercises correctly and to better understand what each exercise is designed to do (Fig. 5-2).

5. After all the exercises have been taught, the teacher should circulate from student to student to check on correct performance of exercises, to further explain how and why the exercise is done, to add to or change exercise programs when necessary, and to evaluate and grade the students on their performance.

This individual method of exercise assignment and instruction and other methods of class or group assignment and instruction are discussed in Chapter 19. Explanations of other special exercises and systems of organizing exercise programs for selected disabilities are found in the chapters in which particular disabilities are discussed. The reader should consult the index for exercise and activity programs for specific conditions. Chapters 4, 6, 7, 9, 10, 11, 12, and 13 and the appendix include such materials.

EXERCISES IN WATER

There are many advantages to including aquatic exercises and activities in an adapted physical education program. Aquatic exercises are discussed in this section, whereas aquatic activities, games, and sports are covered in Chapter 8. Some of the special values of offering a unit in swimming and water therapy include the following:

1. Often exercises that cannot be done elsewhere can be performed in the water, since it is quite easy to rule out the effect of gravity and therefore exercises can be more accurately graded according to their severity.

2. Students who have the support of the water or who use floating devices while walking or swimming in water reduce the amount of pressure on joints and are able to walk and perform activities in water before attempting to do so against the pull of gravity in the exercise room.

3. Swimming provides good all-around exercise for musculature.

4. Swimming provides a release of tension and may even promote relaxation if the water is sufficiently warm (82° to 86° F in a regular pool and 90° to 100° F in a therapeutic pool).

5. Swimming activities are generally fun for all

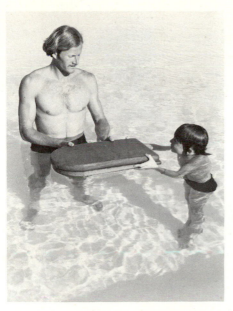

Fig. 5-48. Walking with aid of buoyancy, kickboards, and instructor. (Courtesy of California State University, Audio Visual Center, Long Beach, Calif.)

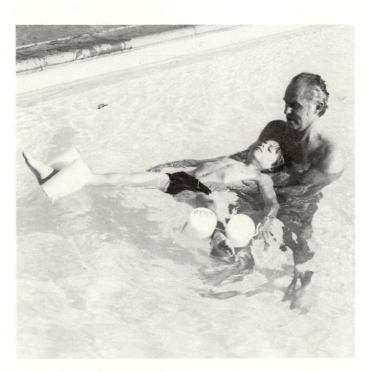

Fig. 5-49. Hip abduction and adduction with instructor and flotation support. (Courtesy of California State University, Audio Visual Center, Long Beach, Calif.)

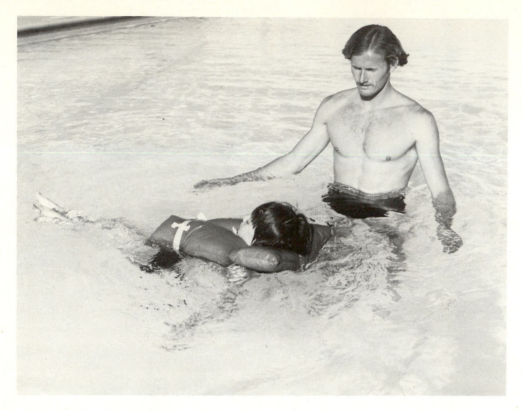

Fig. 5-50. Life jacket as a flotation support. (Courtesy of California State University, Audio Visual Center, Long Beach, Calif.)

students, but they are especially desirable for students in the adapted physical education program, since they can be adapted for almost any disability, thus providing physical and skill development not possible in many other types of physical activities.

The buoyancy of the body and its parts in water makes many types of movements and activities much easier in water than under the direct influence of gravitational pull. A person standing in water up to the chin has minimal weight to bear and can stand and walk much earlier in the rehabilitation period than would be possible out of the water. Walking in progressively shallower water, using support as needed, is an excellent activity to lead up to locomotion activities in the ward, the clinic, and the gymnasium. Walking forward, backward, and sideways using different patterns of movement will help build the muscle strength, body balance, and coordination necessary for locomotion.*

The therapist or teacher should carefully consider the changes that must be made in assigning therapeutic exercises in water as contrasted with exercises for similar body parts used in the ward or gymnasium. Each person and each of the limbs must be considered individually, for they will have different degrees of buoyancy. The body as a whole may float, but the legs and arms *individually* may be less buoyant and may sink unless supported.

---

*For suggested activities and exercises, see Assignment 12 in Crowe, W. C., Arnheim, D. D., and Auxter, D.: Laboratory manual in adapted physical education and recreation, St. Louis, 1977, The C. V. Mosby Co.

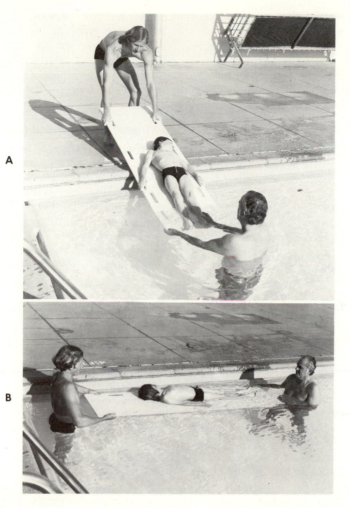

Fig. 5-51. Assisting with pool entry. **A,** Sliding method. **B,** Lifting method. (Courtesy of California State University, Audio Visual Center, Long Beach, Calif.)

If a progressive resistance exercise (PRE) system is to be effected in water, factors such as buoyancy and water resistance must be carefully considered; for example, if a passive exercise is desired for the hip flexors and the patient's legs are nonbuoyant, he or she should be placed near the surface of the pool in the prone position so that the weight of the leg will pull it down into the flexed position. If the legs are buoyant, however, the patient should assume a half-sitting supine position to allow buoyancy to lift the leg to the surface and cause the hip joint to flex.

If a mildly active exercise is desired, the student should be placed on the side with the leg supported by the clinician, a tube, or a buoy. The leg can then be slowly flexed and extended from the hip by the student without the influence of either buoyancy or gravity. The same movement can become a more active exercise by increasing speed. A resistance exercise will result if the tube or buoy on the ankle is retained, the student is turned face down (prone), and hip flexion is performed against the resistance of the flotation device. Resistance can be made greater by increasing the amount of buoyant material used at the ankle or by increasing the speed of leg movement.

There are ways to increase or decrease resistance in water. Resistance is reduced if a part is moved slowly through the water and if it is as streamlined as possible (presents its narrowest side). Resistance is increased by presenting broad surfaces of the body to the water, by wearing rough, absorbent materials on a part (a sweat suit), and by increasing the speed of the movement (the resistance increases according to the square of the speed: a movement that is twice as fast creates a resistance four times as great).

Adjustments similar to those described earlier can be made to enable a person to exercise all body segments using progressive resistance exercise techniques. A series of exercises that can be modified by using these techniques is presented in the *Laboratory Manual in Adapted Physical Education and Recreation,* as previously mentioned.

Types of support for aquatic exercises

Many types of support can be given to maintain the student in a given position while he or she performs the exercise program. Some of these include a water plinth, a support table, the parallel walking bars (in a therapeutic pool), the steps, the ladder, the gutter, a large kickboard, a water mat, and the therapist, the teacher, the aide, or another student in a regular pool. Most areas of the body can also be exercised quite specifically by the more advanced swimmer while he or she is floating or maintaining either a vertical or a horizontal position in the pool with minimal finning or sculling motions.

Materials that can be used as flotation devices for the limbs include life jackets; inner tubes (from trucks, cars, bicycles, or wheel toys); styrofoam rings, tubes, and squares with ropes or straps for attachment; water mats; and kickboards of various types and sizes.

Persons representing many different types of disabilities will benefit from a well-planned aquatic exercise program. For many it is important to have the water as warm as 90° to 95° F, if possible, and to have protection from the cold when entering and leaving the pool. The outside temperature should be 5° warmer for the aged, for persons with arthritis, for those with spinal cord injuries or cerebral palsy, and for persons in relaxation programs. With other types of disabilities and for younger and more active persons, temperature is not as critical, but in most cases the disabled person will be more comfortable and relaxed and the attention span will be longer if the person does not become chilled.

Swimming as a general therapeutic activity

Swimming generally accepted strokes such as the crawl, elementary backstroke, breaststroke, and sidestroke is an excellent way to promote general cardiovascular fitness and to develop the general musculature of the body. Whether this is good for persons with various types of disabilities should be carefully decided by the physician, the therapist, and the physical education teacher. To have persons with already weak musculature swim the regular strokes commonly taught in our school and recreation programs may develop already strong musculature to the detriment of those muscles that most need to be developed. Students should be carefully studied to see if special therapeutic exercises are needed or if they should be taught to swim one or more of the traditional swimming strokes, possibly with some modification of the standard technique, so that swimming as an activity will not negate the advantages of the rehabilitation program.

Severely handicapped persons may have to be lifted into and out of the pool. Hospitals often have electric lifts. In school and recreational pools, teachers, clinicians, and recreation leaders may have to improvise their own procedures. Safety and patient comfort must be considered (Fig. 5-51).

REFERENCES

1. Bowerman, W. J., and Harris, W. E.: Jogging, New York, 1967, Grosset & Dunlap, Inc.
2. Clarke, H. H.: Application of measurement to healthe and physical education. New York, 1967, Prentice-Hall, Inc.
3. Crowe, W. C., et al.: Developmental syllabus, Unpublished, University of California at Los Angeles, 1950.
4. Crowe, W. C., Arnheim, D. A., and Auxter D.: Laboratoratory manual in adapted physical education and recreation, St. Louis, 1977, The C. V. Mosby Co.
5. Daniels, L., Williams, M., and Worthingham, C.: Muscle testing, Philadelphia, 1965, W. B. Saunders Co.
6. DeLorme, T. L.: Restoration of muscle power by heavy resistance exercises, J. Bone Joint Surg. 27:645-667, 1945.
7. DeLorme, T. L., and Watkins, A. C.: Progressive resis-

tance exercises, New York, 1951, Appleton-Century-Crofts.

8. Kabat, H. Proprioceptive facilitation in therapeutic exercise. In Licht, S., editor: Therapeutic exercise, ed. 2, New Haven, Conn., 1961, Elizabeth Licht, Publisher.

9. Knott, M., and Voss, D. E.: Proprioceptive neuromuscular facilitation, New York, 1968, Harper & Row, Publishers.

10. Morgan, R. E., and Adamson, G. T.: Circuit training, New York, 1958, Sportshelf and Soccer Associates.

11. Müller, E. A.: The regulation of muscular strength, J. Assoc. Phys. Ment. Rehabil. **11:**41-47, 1957.

12. Sherrington, C.: The integrative action of the nervous system, New Haven, Conn., 1961, Yale University Press.

RECOMMENDED READINGS

Adams, W. C., and McCristal, K. J.: Foundations of physical activity, Champaign, Ill., 1968, Stipes Publishing Co.

The Alliance: Physical activity programs and practices for the exceptional individual, third national conference, Long Beach, Calif., 1974-79, The Office of the Los Angeles County Superintendent of Schools, Division of Special Education.

American National Red Cross: Swimming for the handicapped: instructors manual, Washington, D.C., 1975, American National Red Cross.

Arnheim, D. D.: Area I physical activity: general stretching. In Larson, L. A., editor: Encyclopedia of sport sciences and medicine, New York, 1971, Macmillan Publishing Co., Inc.

Barney, S., Hirst, C., and Jensen, R.: Conditioning exercises: exercises to improve body form and function, St. Louis, 1972, The C. V. Mosby Co.

Barrett, M., et al.: Foundations for movement, Dubuque, Iowa, 1968, William C. Brown Co., Publishers.

Berger, R. A.: Optimum repetitions for the development of strength, Res. Q., **33:**334, 1962.

Billig, H. E., Jr., and Lowendahl, E.: Mobilization of the human body, Stanford, Calif., 1949, Stanford University Press.

Carr, D. B., et al.: Sequenced instructional programs in physical education for the handicapped, Los Angeles City Schools Special Education Branch, Physical Education Project, P.L. 88-164, Title III, December 1970.

Christina, R.: The relationship of kinesthesis to physical education, Phys. Educ. **24:**167-168, 1967.

Cooper, K. H.: Aerobics, New York, 1972, Bantam Books, Inc.

Cooper, K. H., and Cooper, M.: Aerobics for women, New York, 1973, Bantam Books, Inc.

Cratty, B. J.: Movement behavior and motor learning, ed. 3, Philadelphia, 1973, Lea & Febiger.

Daniels, L., and Worthingham, C.: Therapeutic exercise, Philadelphia, 1977, W. B. Saunders Co.

Davis, E. C., Logan, G., and McKinney, W.: Biophysical values of muscular activity, Dubuque, Iowa, 1965, William C. Brown Co., Publishers.

Digennaro, J.: Individualized exercise and optimal physical fitness, Philadelphia, 1974, Lea & Febiger.

Doolittle, L., and Paschal, J.: The effect of a rope jumping program upon cardiovascular efficiency, Calif. Assoc. Health Phys. Educ. Rec. J. **30:**11, 1968.

Drury, B. J.: Posture and figure control through physical education, Palo Alto, Calif., 1966, National Press Books.

Fait, H. F.: Special physical education, Philadelphia, 1972, W. B. Saunders Co.

Falls, H. B., Wallis, E. L., and Logan, G. A.: Foundations of conditioning, New York, 1970, Academic Press, Inc.

Glass, J.: Exploring movement, Freeport, N.Y., 1966, Educational Activities, Inc.

Guide for programs in physical education and recreation for the mentally retarded, Washington, D.C., 1968, American Alliance for Health, Physical Education, and Recreation.

Guidelines for adapted physical education, Harrisburg, Pa., 1966, Department of Public Instruction, Commonwealth of Pennsylvania.

Hackett, L. C.: Water learning, Palo Alto, Calif., 1970, Peek Publications.

Hackett, L. C., and Jenson, R. G.: A guide to movement explorations, Palo Alto, Calif., 1967, Peek Publications.

Hayden, F. J.: Physical fitness for the retarded, Toronto, 1964, Metropolitan Toronto Association for Retarded Children.

Huber, J. H., and Vercollone, J.: Using aquatic mats with exceptional children, J. Phys. Educ. Rec. **47:**44, 1976.

Jokl, E.: Nutrition, exercise, and body composition, Springfield, Ill., 1964, Charles C Thomas, Publisher.

Kendall, F. P.: A criticism of current tests and exercises for physical fitness, Phys. Ther. **45:**187-197, 1965.

Keogh, J.: Motor performance of elementary school children, Los Angeles, 1965, Department of Physical Education, University of California.

Kraus, H., and Raaf, W.: Hypokinetic disease, Springfield, Ill., 1961, Charles C Thomas, Publisher.

Krusen, F. H., editor: Handbook of physical medicine and rehabilitation, Philadelphia, 1971, W. B. Saunders Co.

Larson, L. A.: Fitness, health, and work capacity, New York, 1974, Macmillan Publishing Co., Inc.

Licht, S.: An exploration and analytical survey of therapeutic exercise, Am. J. Phys. Med. **46:**1, 1967.

Licht, S., and Johnson, E. W.: Therapeutic exercise, Baltimore, 1965, Waverly Press, Inc.

Lilly, L. J.: An overview of body mechanics, Palo Alto, Calif., 1967, Peek Publications.

Logan, G., and Dunkelberg, J.: Adaptations of muscular activity, Belmont, Calif., 1964, Wadsworth Publishing Co., Inc.

Lowman, C. L.: Analysis of exercises commonly misused, Phys. Educ. **24:**115-116, 1967.

Lowman, C. L.: Technique of underwater gymnastics, Los Angeles, 1937, American Publications, Inc.

Mathews, D. K., Kruse, R., and Shaw, V.: The science of physical education for handicapped children, New York, 1962, Harper & Row, Publishers.

Metheny, E.: Body dynamics, New York, 1952, McGraw-Hill Book Co.

Moffroid, M. T., and Whipple, R. H.: Specificity of speed of exercise, Phys. Ther. **50:**1692-1699, 1970.

Mott, J. A.: Conditioning and basic movement concepts, Dubuque, Iowa, 1968, William C. Brown Co., Publishers.

Mueller, G. W., and Christaldi, J.: A practical program of remedial physical education, Philadelphia, 1966, Lea & Febiger.

Myers, C. R., Golding, L. A., and Sinning, W. E.: The Y's way to physical fitness, Emmaus, Pa., 1973, Rodale Press.

Oermann, K. C., Young, C. H., and Mitchell, J. G.: Conditioning exercises, games, tests, Annapolis, Md., 1960, U.S. Naval Institute.

Olson, E. C.: Conditioning, Columbus, Ohio, 1968, Charles E. Merrill Publishing Co.

O'Shea, J. P.: Scientific principles and methods of strength fitness, Reading, Mass., 1969, Addison-Wesley Publishing Co., Inc.

Perceptual-motor foundations: a multidisciplinary concern, Proceedings of the perceptual-motor symposium sponsored by the Physical Education Division, American Association for Health, Physical Education, and Recreation, Washington, D.C., 1969, American Association for Health, Physical Education, and Recreation.

Physical fitness in business and industry, Washington, D.C., 1972, President's Council on Physical Fitness and Sports.

Rathbone, J., and Hunt, V.: Corrective physical education, Philadelphia, 1965, W. B. Saunders Co.

Royal Canadian Air Force: Royal Canadian Air Force exercise plans for physical fitness, New York, No date, Essandess Special Editions.

Ruff, W. R.: Physical conditioning through weight training, Palo Alto, Calif., 1966, National Press Books.

Rusk, H. A.: Rehabilitation medicine, ed. 4, St. Louis, 1977, The C. V. Mosby Co.

Shepard, R. J.: Endurance fitness, Toronto, 1969, University of Toronto Press.

Sigerseth, P. O.: Physical activity: general flexibility. In Larson, L.A., editor: Encyclopedia of sport sciences and medicine, New York, 1971, Macmillan Publishing Co., Inc.

Vitale, F.: Individual fitness programs, Englewood Cliffs, N.J., 1973, Prentice-Hall, Inc.

6

Tension control

Tension is described by Cratty[6] as being overt muscular contraction caused by an emotional state or increased muscular effort. Nervous tension results from anxiety and from the hectic pace of our society. The anxious person is one who tends to worry and has an unusual amount of undefined fear. A continued state of nervous tension may be manifested in pathological systemic conditions. Prolonged anxiety and emotional stress may also lead to psychosomatic disorders.

Selye[20] suggested the existence of a general adaptation syndrome (GAS) that occurs in animals and humans when they are subjected to continual emotional stress. The GAS is composed of three consecutive stages: the *alarm reaction,* which represents normal bodily changes caused by emotion; the *resistance to stress,* or one's adjustment to the alarm reaction, which requires considerable energy resources; and the *exhaustion stage,* in which the energy storehouse is used up. The exhaustion stage may lead to the death of single cells, organs, organ systems, or the entire organism. The pathological conditions of hypertension, rheumatism, arthritis, ulcers, allergies, and other conditions have been described by some authorities as possibly caused by stress. The overanxious person has a high level of cerebral and emotional activity, coupled with nervous muscular tension that may eventually lead the individual to the exhaustion stage and perhaps to psychosomatic disorders. It is commonly accepted in medicine that chronic stress may lead to one or more disease states.[20]

It is desirable for all persons to be able to consciously control their tension levels. It is particularly important for persons having high degrees of tension attributable to some emotional or physical problem to be able to attain a relaxed state at will. Pain and nervous distress are accentuated and compounded by disorders of the mind and body. Characteristically, persons with cardiovascular, respiratory, or rheumatic (as well as other) conditions need to develop the ability to reduce their tension levels.

Of extreme importance to all physical educators is the ability to instruct their students in the skill of recognizing abnormal tensions and reducing them. It is even more important for adapted physical educators, who deal directly with individuals with special problems, to be able to recognize overt signs of abnormal muscular tension levels and to teach ways of overcoming them.

RELAXANTS

Relaxation is freedom from nervous tension and anxiety. All persons seek relaxation at some time or another; however, practices leading to relief of tension differ from one culture to another. Many different techniques for achieving relaxation are currently in vogue in the United States. Most of these practices yield an immediate release from tension, but some result in long-range deleterious effects on the mind and body.

Pills, powders, and drinks

The American public annually spends millions of dollars, both legally and illegally, on medicinal agents and alcoholic beverages for the express purpose of reducing an uncomfortable sense of tension or attaining a state of euphoria. Drug abuse is an ever pressing problem in the world today.[9] Individuals seeking relief from painful anxieties and feelings of inadequacy attempt escape through drugs that alter neural activity. Common categories of those agents used for relaxation and alteration of the personality are psychotomimetic drugs, narcotics, analgesics, sedatives, ataractics or tranquilizers, and depressives.

Psychotomimetic drugs. Psychotomimetic or hallucinogenic agents such as LSD (lysergic acid diethylamide) and mescaline are often used by individuals who are dissatisfied with their lives and are seeking the peace of mind and understanding that comes with an expanded consciousness. The psychotomimetic used in very small doses produces a toxic psychosis that may cause perceptual distortions of any one or all of the senses. Users of such hallucinogens may end up with a "bad trip" resulting in altered behavior, which is manifested in irrationality and uncommon fears.

Narcotics. Derivatives of opium, especially morphine, are used medically for their sedative and analgesic actions. Unfortunately, they are also sought for their euphorigenic properties, particularly found in heroin. Addicts of opiates and opiatelike narcotics are attempting to relieve emotional pain that is found in daily anxieties and hostilities that are difficult to cope with.[9]

Marijuana, unlike the opiates, is not considered physiologically addicting. Its sole source is the plant *Cannabis sativa*. When smoked, the marijuana leaf may produce euphoria, sedation, and hallucinations in the user. The user may display an altered consciousness, expressing feelings of lightness, gaiety, and detachment from reality.

Analgesics. Salicylates are used in a number of compounds that may be applied to the body externally or internally. Acetylsalicylic acid (aspirin) represents the most common compound. The salicylate has the ability to reduce inflammation and pain. As a pain reliever, it has a definite effect on the musculoskeletal system. Although it does not produce sedation or euphoria, as do the opiates, there is recent indication that aspirin has some tranquilizing qualities. It might be speculated that aspirin's great use as a tension reducer is attributable not to its tranquilizing effects, but mainly to its ability to relieve muscular discomfort that is below the pain threshold level.[5]

Sedatives. Barbiturates are considered hypnotic and sedative drugs and are widely used by persons for sleep-inducing or (in smaller dosages) calming effects. The physiological effects of barbiturates are not well understood; however, there are some indications that a general depression of the central nervous system takes place. Barbiturates are highly habit-forming and are addicting to the user. The chronic user of barbiturates is in a constant state of severe depression, which manifests itself in numerous personality changes.

Tranquilizers. Tranquilizers, or ataractics, have become increasingly prominent in medicine and in the patent drug industry. Used for tension and anxiety, tranquilizers affect the sympathetic nervous system by suppressing synaptic stimuli. The main use of ataractics in medicine has been in the areas of behavioral disorders and mental disease. The hyperirritable patient who becomes tranquilized is more amenable to psychotherapy. For much of the general public, tranquilizers have increasingly become a crutch for coping with daily stress.

Depressives. Ethyl alcohol has hypnotic qualities and has been used systemically for centuries as a generalized depressant. It is believed to block the synaptic connections of nerve impulses in the central nervous system, producing varying degrees of depression. Alcohol is an anesthetic to the higher faculties, and thus it brings about a state of temporary relaxation. Depression of the higher brain centers results in diminished control of emotional behavior and decreased movement control.

Rituals, systems, and methods

Most people practice various methods of achieving relaxation in daily life. Some methods may be very beneficial to health, whereas others, as mentioned before, may be deleterious to health. Some methods may be momentary, whereas others are more lasting and involve an established routine or ritual. In Western civilization, many such techniques are used, for example, imagery, physical therapy, psychology and religion, and exercise.

Imagery. Imagery involves word symbolization or auditory stimulation to evoke mental pictures that are both pleasing and relaxing; for example, while in a comfortable position, a person can imagine that he or she is either floating on a cloud or becoming increasingly heavy while gradually sinking deeper and deeper. Listening to soothing music of a slow tempo may result in a state of calm; viewing a beautiful landscape painting may conjure the feeling of quiet and peace.

Physical therapy. To achieve a relaxed state, Americans use many methods that come under the classification of physical therapy. Some common methods are the use of the sauna or steam bath, hydromassage, hot water soaks, and massage.[22] For example, the Finnish sauna bath has been used for centuries as a means to decongest engorged muscles after exercise and to increase relaxation in tense musculature. The European practice of repeatedly heating the body to temperatures of 185° F for 15 minutes and following this with a cool shower is fast becoming a popular technique in America. It invokes a euphoric feeling of physical well-being and relaxation. Many resort hotels and spas are now offering sauna baths and hydromassage in small warm-water pools, followed by an envigorating dip in a large cool swimming pool. Hydromassage is a popular form of relaxing the body. The water is agitated around the body by means of a machine that forces jets of water from various openings in the pool. The pressures applied to the body by the water soothe nerve endings, providing the recipient with a sense of reduced muscular tension.

Since recorded history, some form of manual massage has been used as a means of bringing about a physiological response. Defined as the systematic manipulation of the soft tissues of the body, massage may be applied in numerous ways: through the use of mechanical vibrators, rollers, or agitated water or, most commonly, through the laying on of hands. Many experts indicate that hands, when controlled by a knowledgeable operator, offer the most efficient way to apply massage. Through physiological, mechanical, and psychological effects, massage can produce relaxation. The most frequently used technique is effleurage, which allows the hands to glide lightly over the body in a slow rhythmical pattern, passively reducing muscular tension.

Psychology and religion. The tenets of psychology and religion often try to aid persons who are seeking peace within themselves. Millions of books are sold with such themes as achieving self-renewal, overcoming personal conflicts, or attaining peace in a tension-filled world.

Recently, some Americans have become interested in following some of the Eastern religions and philosophies, the foundations of which are set in inner contemplation and meditation. There are various forms of meditation, most of which begin by having the subject assume a comfortable posture and then focus on some external or internal object. Transcendental meditation employs a mantra—a specific single sound or short phrase that is repeated over and over. Focusing on an object or making a continuous sound helps the meditator avoid distracting thoughts that creep into his or her consciousness. Scientific research has determined that meditation can significantly reduce mental anxiety and muscular tension.[15] A recent meditation approach that blends both Eastern and Western concepts is titled *the relaxation response*.[4] This method uses the three basic elements found in most meditation and conscious relaxation techniques: (1) proper posture, (2) dwelling on an object or sound, and (3) the assumption of a passive attitude. In the relaxation response, the participant sits quietly in a comfortable chair with the eyes closed; progressively relaxes the muscles, starting with the feet and moving up the body; and then breathes through the nose, saying *one* to himself or herself on each inhalation and expiration for 10 to 20 minutes.

One of the most significant biomedical advances in recent times has been the development of biofeedback methods. Through training, individuals can increase their alpha brain waves, which predominate in the mentally relaxed state.[14] Using machines that monitor the brain waves and are designed to make a sound when alpha waves are present, the subject learns to control anxiety and bring about mental and physical relaxation at will.[14]

For many persons, hypnosis is a means of reducing anxieties and muscular tension psychotherapeutically. Hypnosis has been defined as "an artificially induced passive state in which there is increased amenability and responsiveness to suggestions and commands, provided that these do not conflict seriously with the subject's own conscious or unconscious wishes." Under hypnosis, various suggestions about relaxation can be made to the subject, dealing with such things as reducing worry, anxiety, or fear; decreasing pain; and relaxing muscles.[16,17]

Exercise. Most persons would agree that the body senses a reduction in tension after any physically fatiguing activity.[13] Electromyographic studies show that neuromuscular tension levels decrease significantly with vigorous exercise, particularly in persons having high tension levels; however, effects are usually transitory.[7]

Other forms of exercise that result in a relaxed state are specifically rhythmical motion, muscle stretching, and the physical exercise system of hatha-yoga, known as āsana. Music and rhythm are used extensively for the purpose of initiating coordinated movement and relaxation. Synchronization of specific movement patterns, as expressed through kinesthesia, is the basis for skilled activity. Rathbone[18] indicates that rhythmical exercise relieves the feeling of fatigue and residual tension. Activities that have as their basis a continuous or even sequence of movement (such as walking, dancing, swimming, or bicycle riding) result in reduced tension. Muscle stretching, which is designed to increase joint flexibility, also tends to reduce tension within the musculotendinous unit. It is logical therefore to presume that an articulation that is unencumbered by tight restricting tissue will also be one that is capable of relaxation. Stretching the body helps overcome the discomfort of stiffness and allows the various body segments to relax. Research indicates that a steady progressive stretch tends to decrease the myostatic reflex and reduce muscle tension, whereas the ballistic or jerky stretch increases the tension state. Many of the āsanas of hatha-yoga tend to improve joint range of motion. Each yoga posture is executed slowly and deliberately. It is considered by devotees that relaxation occurs as the mind and body become harmonious.

CONSCIOUS CONTROL OF MUSCULAR TENSION

The most easily learned beneficial means of reducing nervous tension is through conscious control.[8] Physiological benefits such as reduced oxygen consumption, respiratory rate, heart rate, and muscle tension result from willed relaxation.

Two excellent techniques for consciously reducing tension are progressive relaxation and autogenic training. Edmund Jacobson, a physiologist-physician, is known as the father of progressive relaxation.[10-12] His technique emphasizes relaxation of voluntary skeletal muscles. During progressive relaxation training an individual becomes aware of muscular tension and learns to consciously release that tension in specific muscle groups. Autogenic training in relaxation was developed by H. H. Schultz, a German neurologist.[19] This technique is designed to reduce exteroceptive and proprioceptive stimulation through mental activity described as *passive concentration*. Using this method an individual brings to mind mental images that promote a relaxed state.

Jacobson's system starts with muscles of the left upper extremity and moves to the right upper extremity, followed by the left lower extremity, right lower extremity, abdominal muscles, respiratory muscles, back, pectoral region, shoulder muscles, and facial muscles. Persons are encouraged to gradually stiffen each body part and then to slowly release that same tension.[10]

Autogenic training begins with phrases that suggest heaviness of the whole body and then the individual parts, followed by phrases that suggest warmth or regularity to the body, heart, respiratory system, and abdominal area. A third set of phrases promotes images of colors and relaxing in warm, soft, pleasant surroundings.[19]

These techniques, used individually and in combination, reduce nervous tension and tactile defensive responses in children.[1]

MUSCLE TENSION REDUCTION

To the physiologist, relaxation indicates a complete absence of neuromuscular activity (zero).[10] The relaxed body part does not resist stretch but rather reflects the lengthened state of muscle fibers. An overt sign of relaxation is a limp and completely motionless body part. Through relaxation of overly tense muscles, a number of positive effects can occur. Some of these effects may be seen in respiration, circulation, and neuromuscular coordination.

Respiration. The reduction of tension in the thorax and muscles of respiration allows for a greater capacity of inspiration and expiration. With this increased capacity, there is a more efficient exchange of oxygen and carbon dioxide within the body. For persons with breathing disorders, relaxation of the thoracic mechanism allows for a greater respiratory potential.

Circulation. Relaxation of tense skeletal muscles allows the blood to circulate unimpeded by constricted blood vessels to all the bodily tissues. A person with cardiovascular disease is greatly aided when the ability to reduce muscular tension at will is achieved. Blood pressure may be reduced by diminishing outside resistance, which subsequently decreases the strain on heart and blood vessels.

Neuromuscular coordination. In order for the body to move uninhibited, there must be a smooth synchronization of muscles. Differential relaxation or controlled tension attributable to the reciprocal action of agonist and antagonist muscles provides for coordinated movement without undue fatigue. Persons who, as a result of neuromuscular or cerebral problems, express poor coordination must learn to relax tense muscles differentially in order for their purposeful movement to be smooth, accurate, and enduring.

IMPLICATIONS FOR PHYSICAL EDUCATION

Learning to relax is a motor skill and must be considered an important part of the total program of physical education. As a skill, relaxation must be taught and practiced for competency. Too often, teachers of physical education are concerned with gross movement activities alone. To lie down when tired or to practice relaxation when tense or overanxious is considered a waste of time by many teachers. This narrow point of view eliminates consideration of a very important aspect of the field of physical education. Relaxation is of special impor-

tance to many atypical as well as typical students.

A number of positive benefits can be accrued by disabled children who have conscious control of their tension levels. Needed energies can be conserved and better control of emotions can result (fears and anxieties become less intense). Sleep comes easier, the acquisition and conduction of motor skills are enhanced, pain and physical discomfort become less intense, and the ability to learn may be improved. Relaxation therefore becomes a vital tool in the total machinery of the educational process.

Teaching a system of relaxation

The adapted physical education instructor can teach a variety of relaxation techniques depending on time and available conditions. As has been described earlier in this discussion, imagery and tension recognition provide a convenient means of learning to relax. Both may be combined and used with success in the typical 30-minute physical education period.

Identifying abnormal tension areas in the body requires the performance of a series of muscle contractions and relaxations. In this modified system of progressive relaxation, muscle contractions should be performed gradually and slowly for 30 seconds and then a "letting go" of the tension should be made for 30 seconds in an attempt to obtain a "negative" state. The student is continually reminded to tense only those muscles the instructor indicates. An attempt is made by the pupil to keep all other body areas relaxed while contracting a single part. Special consideration is given to those areas of the body that are difficult to relax, for example, the low back, the abdominal, the shoulder, the neck, and the eye regions. After the guided session, the student makes a record of those areas that were difficult to relax. Eventually, with diligent practice, the student will have to tense and relax only those areas that are difficult to relax. In doing so, the student can achieve at will a general decrease of muscular tonus throughout the entire body.

Preliminary requirements

In order for the student to develop a keen perception of tension and learn to relax, the instructor should make provisions for a number of environmental and learning factors that may strongly affect the ability to reduce body tension.

Room. The room in which relaxation exercises are conducted should have a comfortable temperature (between 72° and 76° F); it should be well ventilated with no chilling drafts. The light may be dimmed or turned off and signs may be posted outside to prevent interruption of the relaxation lesson.

Dress. The student should wear comfortable, warm, loose-fitting apparel and no shoes.

Equipment. In actuality, very little equipment is needed to teach relaxation. Ideally, five small pillows or rolled-up towels and a firm mat are useful; however, relaxation can be accomplished on any comfortable surface without the use of props. A pencil and paper should be available and in close proximity to all students so that they can record personal reactions after the session.

Positioning. Although a person can learn to relax while standing or sitting, the ideal position for tension recognition is lying supine on a firm mat with each body curve comfortably supported by a pillow or towel (Fig. 6-1). Contour support is afforded the curves of the cervical and lumbar vertebrae; each forearm is supported, resulting in a slight bend to each elbow; and the knees, like the elbows, are maintained in a slightly flexed position with thighs externally rotated. By affording minimal support to the body curves and limbs, free muscle contraction can take place while the individual is in a comfortable, relaxed position. If,

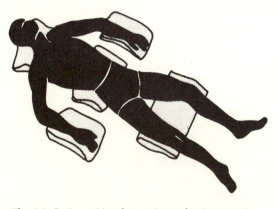

Fig. 6-1. Basic position for tension reduction exercises.

however, equipment is not available for joint support, a flat mat surface will suffice.

Sound. A number of techniques utilizing sound may be used by the teacher to aid the student in acquiring the right frame of mind for relaxing. Soft music playing in the background may be beneficial. If music is not available, the monotone pattern of a metronome clicking at 48 or fewer beats per minute may be helpful. Most important, however, whether there is sound equipment or not, is the voice of the instructor, which should be quiet, slow, rhythmical, and distinct.

Breathing. During the relaxation session, the student is instructed to take slow, deep inhalations through the nose and make long, slow exhalations through the mouth. Gradually, through breath control, the student consciously tries to let go of all the bodily tensions. As relaxation occurs, breathing becomes increasingly slow and shallow.

Using imagery. The tension recognition technique involves two distinct phases: a *contraction phase,* whereby the subject contracts a particular muscle or group of muscles to sense tension, and a *letting go phase,* whereby the subject seeks a complete lack of tension or negativeness. To aid the pupil in the second phase, the teacher encourages the use of imagery. The student is told to imagine very relaxing things. Imagery-inducing statements such as "your body is heavy against the floor," "your body is gradually getting warmer," "imagine your heart beating regularly and calmly like a clock ticking," and "listen to the sound of your breathing" may help a student relax. Children at the elementary school level have keen imaginations and respond readily to such suggestions as that they imagine their bodies as snowmen on a hot day or as butter in a hot pan.

Sleep. The pupil should be instructed that developing awareness of tense body areas and the ability to relax consciously without falling asleep is the main purpose of the exercise session. However, if sleep does occur during the session, it should be considered a positive reaction.

Procedure

There are a number of ways the instructor can proceed. The teacher can instruct the pupils by having them start with contracting their facial muscles and then moving downward to finish in the lower limbs or, conversely, by having them move from foot to head. If less time is available, using large muscle groups and progressing to the smaller muscles of the body is another alternative. Whatever the technique used, the goals are the same and the teacher will soon develop a style that seems to work best.

Because of the limited amount of time available in the physical education period, many sessions may be required before adequate desired results are reached. A home program should be encouraged for those persons who find it difficult to let go of tension.

Directions to the student

For expediency in the physical education setting, each muscular contraction phase and each relaxation phase is conducted for approximately 30 seconds, providing a total of 1 minute for each step. During the introductory session, the muscle contraction should be intense enough to cause a degree of fatigue. For each subsequent session, the tension becomes less and less, requiring a greater perceptual sensitivity. The following is a sample of a relaxation session given to a group of students in a typical school setting.

Step 1. Lie still for a minute and stare at an object on the ceiling. Do the eyes feel as though they are getting heavy? As this occurs, gradually let them close. Take five deep breaths, inhaling and exhaling slowly. Think of all the joints of the body as being very relaxed.

Step 2. Curl the toes downward and point both feet downward toward the end of the mat (Fig. 6-2). Feel the tension in the bottoms of the feet and behind the legs. Keep the mouth relaxed and continue to breathe deeply and slowly. Remember, while tensing one area of the body, all other parts should be relaxed. Now, release the muscle contractions slowly, trying to let go to a complete relaxed state. Feel the body getting extremely heavy and sinking into the mat.

Step 3. Curl the toes and both feet backward toward the head (Fig. 6-3). Sense the tenseness on the tops of the feet and legs. Remember not to reinforce the movement by tensing other parts of the body. Breathe easily and relax. Let go of the muscle contraction, allowing the feet and ankles to go limp slowly.

Step 4. Leaving the legs in their original position, with the knees slightly bent, press down against the mat with the heels, attempting to curl the legs backward (Fig. 6-4). Feel the tension in the back of the thighs and buttocks. Remember, while holding this contraction, all other parts of the body should be at ease. Relax, slowly feeling the discomfort of tension completely leave the body.

Step 5. Remain in the same position as in step 4 and straighten the legs to full extension (Fig. 6-5). Feel the tightness in the tops of the thighs. Now, let go. Breathing should come easily and in a relaxed manner and a profound sense of heaviness should be present throughout the body.

Step 6. With the legs and thighs in the original resting position, draw the thighs upward to a bent (flexed) position, with the heels raised off the mat

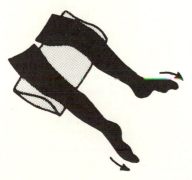

Fig. 6-2. Step 2.

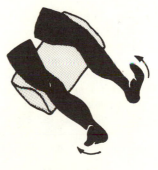

Fig. 6-3. Step 3.

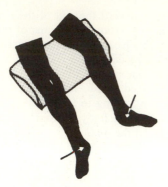

Fig. 6-4. Step 4.

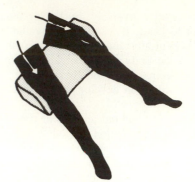

Fig. 6-5. Step 5.

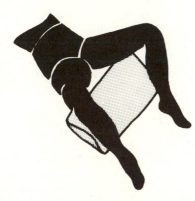

Fig. 6-6. Step 6.

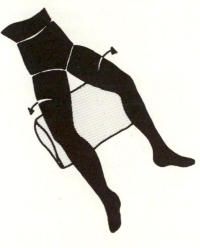

Fig. 6-7. Step 7.

about 3 inches (Fig. 6-6). The tension felt should be primarily in the bend of the hip. Try to keep all other muscle groups relaxed. Return slowly to the starting position and then let go to negative again.

Step 7. Forcibly rotate the thighs outward (Fig. 6-7). Feel the muscle tension in the outer hip region. Do not let tension creep into other parts of the body. Now, slowly relax the hip rotators. Go limp.

Step 8. Rotate the thighs inward (Fig. 6-8). Feel the muscle tension deep in the inner thighs. Relax

slowly, let go of all tension, and let the thighs again rotate outward. Sense the body sinking deeper into the mat.

Step 9. Squeeze the buttocks (gluteal muscles) together tightly and tilt the hips backward (Fig. 6-9). The only muscular tension that should be felt is in the buttocks and low back region. Again, be acutely aware of other tensions that may be occurring in the body. Now, let go of the contraction and try to sense the joints becoming extremely loose.

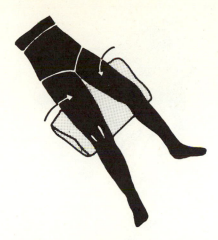

Fig. 6-8. Step 8.

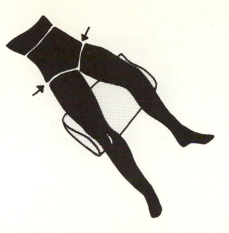

Fig. 6-9. Step 9.

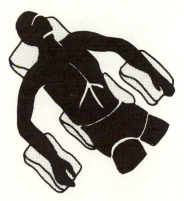

Fig. 6-10. Step 10.

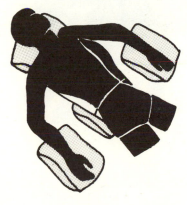

Fig. 6-11. Step 11.

Step 10. Tighten the abdominal muscles by pressing downward on the rib cage while rolling the hips backward; at the same time, flatten the low back (Fig. 6-10). The tension felt is both in the abdominal muscles and in the low back region. Inhale slowly and let the back settle into the mat.

Step 11. Inhale and exhale slowly and as deeply as possible three times (Fig. 6-11). A general tension should be felt throughout the rib cage. After the last forced inspiration and expiration, return to normal quiet breathing and sense the difference in tension levels.

Step 12. Accentuating the curve of the neck (cervical spine), press the head back and lift the upper back off the mat (Fig. 6-12). The tension felt should be in the back of the neck and upper back. Settle slowly back to the mat.

Step 13. Next, pinch the shoulders back,

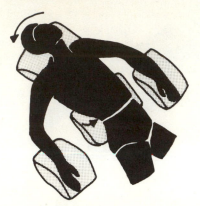

Fig. 6-12. Step 12.

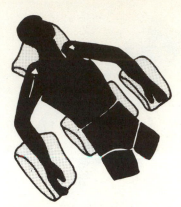

Fig. 6-13. Step 14.

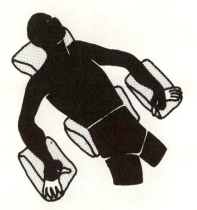

Fig. 6-14. Step 15.

Fig. 6-15. Step 17.

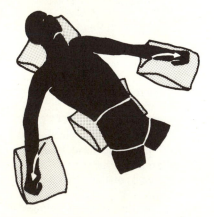

Fig. 6-16. Step 18.

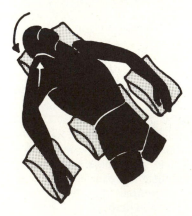

Fig. 6-17. Step 19.

squeezing the two shoulder blades (scapula bones) together. Tension is felt in the back of the shoulders. Release the contraction slowly and fall easily back to the mat. Be aware of any residual tension that might remain after returning to the mat.

Step 14. Leaving the arms in the resting position, lift and roll shoulders inward so that tension is felt in the front of the chest (Fig. 6-13). Do not reinforce this by contracting other muscles. Now, allow the shoulders to drop back to the mat in the resting position. Feel the tension leave the chest.

Step 15. Spread and grip the fingers of both hands. Do this three times (Fig. 6-14). The tension felt is in the hands and forearms. As the fingers are gripped and spread, be sure not to lift the elbows off the mat. After the third series, let hands and forearms fall limply back to their supports.

Step 16. Make a tight fist with both hands and slowly curl the wrists backward, forward, and to both sides. Tension should primarily be felt at the fist, wrist, and forearm. After these movements, allow fingers and thumbs to open gradually.

Step 17. Make a tight fist with both hands and slowly bend (flex) the forearms at the elbows against the upper arms, at the same time lifting the arms at the shoulders (Fig. 6-15). Tension is felt in the front part of the forearms, in the biceps regions, and in the front part of the shoulders. After the flexion of the shoulders, the arms should be slowly uncurled and returned to the resting position; relax each segment separately until the arms become limp, motionless, and negative.

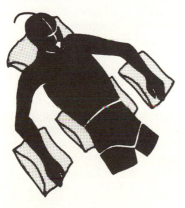

Fig. 6-18. Step 21.

Step 18. Make a tight fist with both hands, stiffen the arms, and press hard against the mat (Fig. 6-16). Tension should be felt in the forearms and the back of the upper arms and shoulders. Hold the pressure against the mat for 30 seconds and then release slowly.

Step 19. Shrug the right shoulder; then bend the head sideward (laterally flex neck), touching the ear to the elevated shoulder (Fig. 6-17). The only tension that should be felt is in the upper right shoulder and the right side of the neck. Release the contraction, slowly returning the neck and shoulder to the resting positions.

Step 20. As in step 19, shrug the left shoulder; then laterally flex the neck, touching the ear to the elevated shoulder. The only tension that should be felt is in the upper left shoulder and the lateral muscles of the neck. Release the contraction, slowly returning the neck and shoulder to the resting position.

Step 21. Bend the head forward, touching the chin to the chest (Fig. 6-18). Tension is felt in the front of the neck. Relax and slowly return the head to the resting position. Continue to concentrate on the body as being extremely heavy and at a zero state.

Step 22. Lift eyebrows upward; wrinkle the forehead. Feel the tension in the forehead region. Let the face go blank.

Step 23. Close the eyelids tightly and wrinkle the nose. Tension is felt in the nose and eyes. Let the face relax slowly. Concentrate on the tension leaving the face.

Step 24. Open the mouth widely as if to yawn. Feel the tension in the jaw. Now, let the mouth close slowly and lightly.

Step 25. Bite down hard and then show the teeth in a forced smile. Tension should be felt in the jaw and lips. Slowly allow the face to return to a blank expression. Be sure not to tense other parts of the body when contracting the facial muscles.

Step 26. Pucker the lips hard as if to whistle. Sense tension at the edge of the mouth. Let the tension melt away.

Step 27. Push the tongue hard against the roof of the mouth. Let go. Push the tongue against the roof of the mouth again as hard as possible. Relax. Push the tongue against the upper teeth. Relax. Sense the contraction of the tongue muscles. As you do this exercise, try not to use any other body parts. Relax.

Step 28. Lie very still for a short while and try to be conscious of those body areas that were difficult to relax. Move slowly and take any position desired. Relax and rest.

Step 29. Try to hold the color of black or white in the mind's eye. Once you see one color, do not let any other color or picture slip into your mind.

Step 30. At the end of relaxation tell the students to roll to one side and sit up slowly.

Teacher evaluation

Although the most accurate indication of abnormal tension is by electromyographic tests, subjective evaluation still has its place for the physical education instructor. Tension is easily observable through mannerisms such as extraneous movements or muscle twitches (eye twitches, finger movements, stiffness, changes of body position, playing with hands, and vocal sounds of all kinds). The instructor should test muscle resistance by lifting the students' arms or legs after the relaxation session. Limbs that have a residual tension do not feel limp or lifeless; they tend to feel stiff and unyielding. The instructor tells the students that they will be tested for relaxation at the end of the session. The following four factors may be made apparent by the tests: (1) whether the student assists the movement, (2) whether the student resists the movement, (3) whether the student engages in positioning body parts, or (4) whether the student ideally displays a complete lack of tension.*

Student evaluation

After the exercise session, the students are asked to answer questions about their personal reactions, writing their answers on a sheet of paper by their side. Some suggested questions include the following:

1. What was your general reaction to the session—good, bad, or indifferent?
2. Were you comfortable for the whole time? If not, what disturbed you?

3. Did you sense the tensions and relaxations at all times? If not, why not?
4. Were there areas of the body that you just could not continually relax? What were they?

Questions such as these help the student identify reactions to the relaxation period. It may require a number of sessions for the student to identify tense body regions accurately. While learning to relax individual parts, the student will gradually be able to relax larger and larger segments and eventually the whole body at will.

RELAXING THE PHYSICALLY IMMATURE

Conscious control of muscular tension is usually very difficult for physically immature persons. A program of relaxation training must be commensurate with the subjects' developmental and maturational levels. Before a training program can be effectively instituted, the subjects must understand what tension and relaxation are and how they are contrasted. The concept of relaxation can be taught by having the students pretend their arms are like rubber bands, that they are melting like snowmen on a very hot day, or that they are rag dolls that cannot stand up. Another good technique to develop the concept of tightness and looseness is to have the participants stiffen whole bodies for about 30 seconds and then gradually let go of the tension by pretending to be a pat of butter melting in a very hot pan (Fig. 6-19). Following this activity, the instructor can introduce questions such as "How does it feel to be relaxed?" or "Doesn't it feel better to be relaxed than stiff and tense?" Once the subjects perceive the difference between tensing and releasing tension, the instructor can begin to develop skill programs that gradually take the students from a total body program to a segmental relaxation program.[2]

DIFFERENTIAL RELAXATION

Decreasing and increasing muscular tension levels at will requires varying degrees of coordination (Fig. 6-20). All skilled movement requires differential relaxation. A technique that has been found beneficial in training individuals to selectively control specific muscles is known as the *muscle tension recognition and release method*.[2,3] This technique starts with the subject tensing and letting go of the entire body and proceeds to *bilateral body*

---

*See also Crowe, W. C., Arnheim, D. D., and Auxter, D.: Laboratory manual in adapted physical education and recreation, St. Louis, 1977, The C. V. Mosby Co.

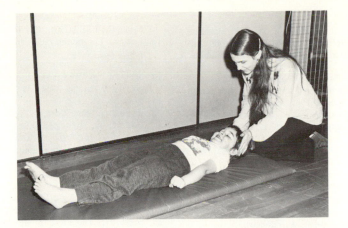

Fig. 6-19. Stiffening the entire body to learn the difference between muscle tension and relaxation. (Courtesy of California State University, Audio Visual Center, Long Beach, Calif.)

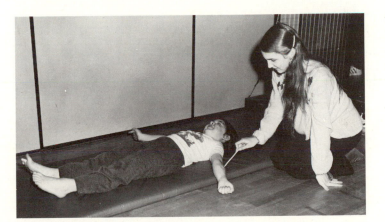

Fig. 6-20. Learning to differentiate specific body areas by tensing and relaxing on command. (Courtesy of California State University, Audio Visual Center, Long Beach, Calif.)

control in which the subject learns control of both upper limbs and then of both lower limbs. Following successful demonstration of bilateral limb control, the subject advances to *unilateral body control,* whereby muscular tension is increased on one side of the body and completely released on the other, for example, tensing the right arm and leg and relaxing the left arm and leg. From unilateral control, the subject progresses to *cross lateral body control,* which involves tensing the opposite arm and leg. The last stage of differential relaxation training is the isolation and relaxation of specific body parts at will. In general, differential relaxation training is a useful tool for developing total body control, increasing body awareness, and reducing anxiety. However, this technique cannot force maturation and should be limited to the particular developmental level of the individual.

REFERENCES

1. Anneberg, L.: A study of the effect of different relaxation techniques on tactile deficient and tactile defensive children, Unpublished masters thesis, University of Kansas, 1977.
2. Arnheim, D. D., and Pestolesi, R. A.: Developing motor behavior in children: a balanced approach to elementary physical education, St. Louis, 1973, The C. V. Mosby Co.
3. Arnheim, D. D., and Sinclair, W. A.: The clumsy child: a program of motor therapy, ed. 2, St. Louis, 1979, The C. V. Mosby Co.
4. Benson, H.: The relaxation response, New York, 1975, William Morrow & Co., Inc.
5. Collier, H. O. J.: Aspirin, Sci. Am. **209:**96-108, 1963.
6. Cratty, B. J.: Movement behavior and motor learning, Philadelphia, 1973, Lea & Febiger.
7. deVries, H. A.: Physiology of exercise, ed. 2, Dubuque, Iowa, 1974, William C. Brown Co., Publishers.
8. Frederick, A. B.: Tension control, J. Health Phys. Ed. Rec. **38:**42-44, 78-80, 1967.
9. Goth, A.: Medical pharmacology: principles and concepts, ed. 9, St. Louis, 1978, The C. V. Mosby Co.
10. Jacobson, E. O.: Progressive relaxation, Chicago, 1938, The University of Chicago Press.
11. Jacobson, E. O.: Self-operation control, Philadelphia, 1964, J. B. Lippincott Co.
12. Jacobson, E. O.: Modern treatment of tense patients, Springfield, Ill., 1970, Charles C Thomas, Publisher.
13. Larson, D., editor: Encyclopedia of sports science and medicine, New York, 1971, Macmillan Publishing Co., Inc.
14. Melzack, R.: The promise of biofeedback: don't hold the party yet, Psychol. Today **9:**18-22, 80-81, 1975.
15. Naranjo, C., and Ornstein, R. E.: On the psychology of meditation, New York, 1971, The Viking Press, Inc.
16. Powers, M.: Advanced techniques of hypnosis, ed. 4, Hollywood, Calif., 1956, Wilshire Book Co.
17. Powers, M.: A practical guide to self-hypnosis, Hollywood, Calif., 1963, Wilshire Book Co.
18. Rathbone, J. L.: Relaxation, Philadelphia, 1969, Lea & Febiger.
19. Schultz, H. H., and Luthe, W.: Autogenic training, New York, 1959, Grune & Stratton, Inc.
20. Selye, H.: The stress of life, New York, 1956, McGraw-Hill Book Co.
21. Selye, H.: Stress without distress, Philadelphia, 1974, J. B. Lippincott Co.
22. Tappan, F. M.: Massage techniques, New York, 1961, Macmillan Publishing Co., Inc.

7

Underdevelopment and low physical vitality

One of the objectives of physical educators is to develop in their students the physical characteristics necessary to perform the activities of daily living without undue fatigue. Furthermore, the outcome of the development of these physical characteristics is to be able to perform motor skills competently.

The problem of the physical and motor underdevelopment and low vitality of the handicapped is a major concern of physical education. Chronically ill persons with debilitating conditions are particularly prone to poor physical vitality and development. Persons with cardiorespiratory conditions such as chronic bronchitis and various heart defects (Chapter 12) are particularly prone to poor physical fitness and are a special challenge to the physical education instructor. Handicapped children as well as normal children often lack prerequisite physical and motor abilities to successfully participate in sport skills and the activities of daily living.

MOVEMENT EFFICIENCY

It is important for handicapped children to move as efficiently as possible. Inherent in movement efficiency is *motor fitness,* which can be defined as the ability to effectively perform movement activities that require strength, flexibility, and endurance. All human movement requires relative levels of muscular strength, joint flexibility, and stamina as well as the ability to use these motor components in activities requiring balance and coordination.[1,23] *Motor fitness* refers to tasks that require neuromuscular coordination for task performance and involve coordination of many large muscles. Fundamental movement patterns such as running and jumping are included in this group. Physical fitness, on the other hand, involves less skilled performance than does motor fitness in that, by and large, refined neuromotor integration is not required to successfully perform fitness tasks. The components of physical fitness are generally described as strength, flexibility, and endurance.

PHYSICAL AND MOTOR FITNESS

Motor fitness is an area of physical education designated in the regulations of P.L. 94-142[43] that is to be developed for handicapped persons.

Whereas strength, flexibility, and endurance are prerequisites to movement, the integration of these prerequisites into qualitative movement involves motor fitness. Thus, motor fitness refers to performance of motor skills.

Physical fitness deals with the primary prerequisites for efficient movement so that there can be adaptation to muscular demands. It also refers to the acquisition of muscular strength and endurance and cardiovascular endurance to be employed for a given task. For the purpose of this discussion, flexibility will also be included as a prerequisite physical fitness component. Muscular strength, flexibility, and endurance can be further analyzed into areas relevant to specific movements that involve specific muscular responses. Subsumed under physical fitness is the development of the posturing mechanism. Poor posture involves the lack of physical fitness of specific muscle groups. The development of appropriate posture is discussed in Chapter 9. The more general aspects of physical fitness as it relates to muscular strength and endurance and cardiovascular fitness are discussed in this chapter.

Physical fitness and motor fitness are important aspects of the total physical education program for handicapped children. This has been verified by incorporating the development of physical and motor fitness in the legal definition of physical education. Therefore, it is important that attention be given to procedures for conducting instruction of physical and motor fitness activities that conform with the regulations of P.L. 94-142.[47]

Gilhool and Stutman[21] indicate that the first step in converting statutes into practice is detailed study of the plain language of the law and the regulations. However, intensive study of the plain language of the law regarding the nature of implementation of physical and motor fitness programming raises some interesting questions. An attempt will be made to identify questions raised by such study and appropriate procedures that may assist in answering the questions. Table 7-1 indicates the regulations from P.L. 94-142 that apply to the conduct of physical and motor fitness programs and that raise questions.

The developmental process has been described in detail in Chapter 2. However, in review, it means progression of the individual on a performance continuum. It involves a process that affects the individual as a result of participation in qualitative experiences that extend the present level of educational performance. The qualitative experience can be equated with the short-term instructional objective.

Physical fitness activities are designed to develop strength and flexibility in specific muscle groups. On the other hand, motor fitness activities assist the child with movement to cope dynamically with the changing demands of the environment.

Table 7-1. Regulations from P.L. 94-142 that apply to physical and motor fitness

Regulations from P.L. 94-142	Questions raised
Physical Education means the development of physical and motor fitness. . . .	What is development? What are physical and motor fitness activities? What is physical and motor fitness?
There must be full preevaluation to determine the educational needs.	What is an educational need? How is an educational need determined? What evaluation instruments shall be used to determine the educational needs? When has there been *full* evaluation?
Special Education [special physical education in this case] must . . . meet the unique needs of such child [physical and motor fitness needs].	What is a unique need? How are unique needs in the areas of physical and motor fitness determined? What are the procedures for meeting the unique physical and motor fitness needs of handicapped children?

Full evaluation of physical and motor fitness

The full evaluation of a handicapped child's physical and motor fitness requires comprehensive assessment in ability areas identified through research.[20] For instance, muscular strength can be broken down into muscular strength of the knee extensors, hip extensors, elbow flexors, arm flexors, and abdominal muscles. A severe loss of strength in any one of these muscle groups may seriously affect the attainment of specific sport skills. Thus, a full evaluation of physical education needs would entail knowledge of the child's ability in many areas of strength. The same analysis could be applied to flexibility. For every joint and action of the body there are normative levels of performance. Full evaluation would take into consideration all aspects of total physical fitness. For instance, from an evaluation of posture (see Fig. 9-36, pp. 254 to 255), specific physical activities can be identified to meet postural needs. However, a postural evaluation is only one type of physical fitness evaluation.

The procedures for determining educational needs have been described in Chapter 4. In review, an educational need is determined by identifying a discrepancy between a child's performance on a physical or motor fitness task and normative expectations for that task. For example, if the normative expectancy of a 6-year-old child's broad jump performance is 60 inches, but the child can jump only 45 inches (the performance capability of a normal 4-year-old child), then there is a need for the development of broad-jumping ability. Thus, full evaluation to determine the unique needs of the child is based on the discrepancy between actual performance and normative performance. The charts on expected normative performance in Chapter 2 should assist in identifying normal expectancies of children for these tasks.

Physical and motor fitness assessment instruments

Physical and motor fitness test instruments must be selected that can provide comprehensive information about the abilities and educational needs of handicapped children. Some of the specific tests batteries accepted in the field of physical education are the AAHPER Physical Fitness Test,[44] the Kraus-Weber Test, the Physical Fitness Index[14] and the Test of Physical and Motor Ability Structure.[20] Studies on the motor abilities of handicapped persons identify domains for measurement by selection of specific tests. Factor studies on the motor abilities of the mentally retarded have been conducted by Rarick and Dobbins[41] and by Rarick and McQuillian.[42] Other test batteries adapted to handicapped populations are those of Johnson and Londeree[27] and the Special Fitness Test for the Mentally Retarded.[44] Thus, it is suggested that test items selected for preevaluation of handicapped children be domain referenced so that there is opportunity to associate educational programming with the test. Full evaluation can best be achieved through comprehensive representation of the identified domains for physical and motor fitness.

MEETING UNIQUE NEEDS

Full evaluation of physical and motor fitness enables specific programming for the child.[47] However, it becomes apparent that to acquire a full evaluation of a handicapped child, it is not feasible to test for all of the specific tasks represented by a subarea of physical and motor fitness. Stated another way, if an individual exhibited no gross observable deficiencies in strength or flexibility, it would not be feasible to test each action at each joint for flexibility or each muscle of each muscle group for strength and endurance. Therefore, it is necessary to acquire an evaluation by identifying classes of related behaviors. For example, to evaluate the behavior of jumping, it would be desirable to sample one form of many jumping behaviors, such as the two-footed standing broad jump. One test—the two-footed standing broad jump—would be used to infer abilities in related activities such as jumping over a hurdle, jumping backward, jumping sideways, jumping over a hurdle backward, running and jumping for height, and running and jumping for distance. Thus, from the results of a single test, measuring ability in one task, one would be able to infer the child's ability in several related tasks. This procedure of selecting tests through which inferences of ability can be made to other similar and related tasks is called *domain reference testing*.[18] Such testing is desirable for securing a full evaluation of the educational perfor-

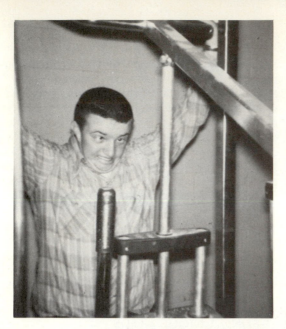

Fig. 7-1. Unique needs are met through the appropriate selection of activity that requires the performer's best efforts. (Courtesy of Julian Stein, American Alliance for Health, Physical Education, Recreation, and Dance and Denton State School, Denton, Tex.)

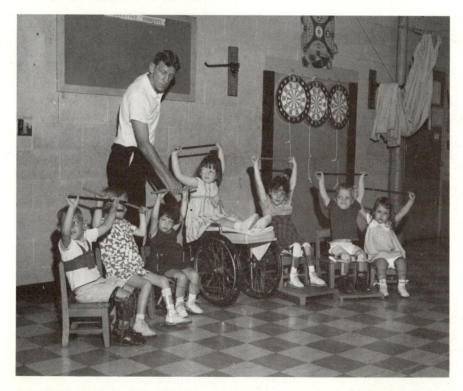

Fig. 7-2. Movement of the arms backward may develop extent flexibility. (Courtesy of Julian Stein, American Alliance for Health, Physical Education, Recreation, and Dance and University Hospital School, University of Iowa, Iowa City.)

mance in physical and motor fitness and in all other areas mandated for instruction of handicapped children. Factor analysis research employs procedures that specifically identify subabilities of physical and motor fitness to enhance domain-referenced testing for the purpose of acquiring full preevaluation data.

Unique needs in physical and motor fitness

A short-term instructional objective of an activity that represents a needed domain from preevaluation data is called a unique need. Short-term instructional objectives are tasks that extend present levels of educational performance. However, the instructional objective must be in needed physical and motor fitness subdomains. For instance, if preevaluation data indicate that a 6-year-old child's present level of educational performance for a broad jump is 45 inches and the normative expectancy is 60 inches, the instructional objective

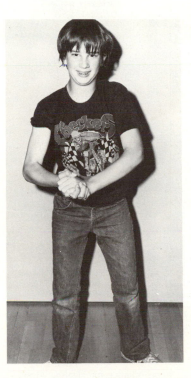

Fig. 7-3. A display of static muscle exertion. (Courtesy of California State University, Audio Visual Center, Long Beach, Calif.)

should be 46 inches. An instructional objective less than 45 inches is inappropriate, because that level of performance has already been met. On the other hand, an objective much greater than the present level of performance would likewise fail to meet the present educational needs of the child. Thus, educational needs are met through selection of specific tasks for which there is application of detailed and specific measurement to enhance the learning and development processes. Furthermore, the tasks that children perform must fall within the domains expressed in the preevaluation. Thus, in the case at hand, the comparison of the child's performance against a standard is discrepant to such an extent that programming in the specific domain is desirable.

Procedures for determining unique needs

Litigation in federal courts indicates that another aspect of a unique need is a functional deficit in skills required for self-sufficiency in community living.[2a] Thus, in a practical sense, prerequisite demands for physical and motor fitness should be studied in relationship to motor skills required in recreation and community living in the environments where handicapped persons are most likely to live.

The ultimate purpose of preevaluation in the areas of physical and motor fitness is to determine which activities will meet the unique needs of the handicapped child. The delivery of the instructional process that achieves this end is called special education. The procedures to be employed for determining the unique needs of the handicapped child in the areas of physical and motor fitness are as follows:

1. Identify motor skills to be taught in physical education that can be expressed as self-sufficient recreational skills and activities of daily living in the community.
2. Select physical and motor fitness areas associated with the skills needed for self-sufficiency.
3. Identify prerequisite levels of physical and motor fitness necessary for independent recreation and activities for daily living in the community.
4. Test for present levels of educational performance in physical and motor fitness domains.

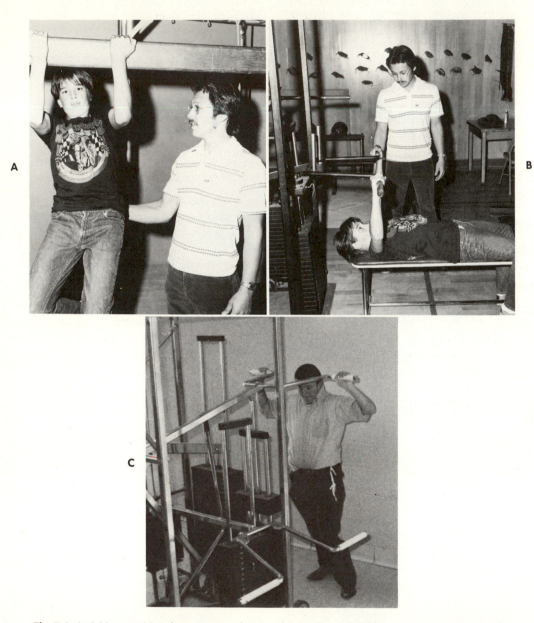

Fig. 7-4. Activities requiring dynamic strength. (**A** and **B** Courtesy of California State University, Audio Visual Center, Long Beach, Calif. **C** Courtesy of Julian Stein, American Alliance for Health, Physical Education, Recreation, and Dance, and Denton State School, Denton, Tex.)

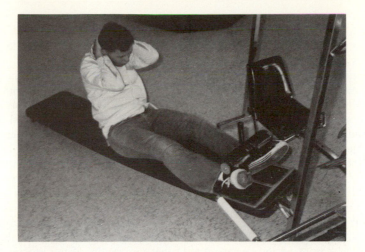

Fig. 7-5. The surface upon which the sit up is performed can be raised to make the task more difficult, thus enabling the construction of a development sequence. (Courtesy of Julian Stein, American Alliance for Health, Physical Education, Recreation, and Dance and Denton State School, Denton, Tex.)

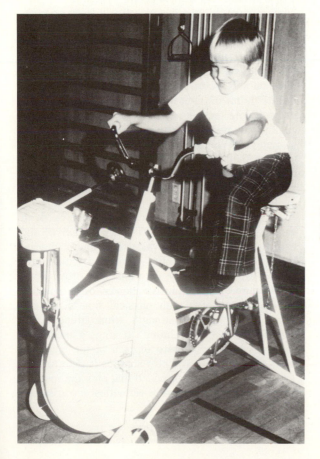

Fig. 7-6. Building stamina by bicycling. (Courtesy of California State University, Audio Visual Center, Long Beach, Calif.)

5. Compare the child's performance with normative community standards to determine whether there is sufficient discrepancy to indicate an educational need.
6. If it is determined that there is a need in an identified domain, then ascertain present levels of educational performance on tasks related to the domain and postulate short-term instructional objectives.

Operational definitions of the physical components, adapted from Fleishman,[20] are as follows:

1. *Extent flexibility:* Ability to stretch muscles as far as possible (Fig. 7-2)
   EXAMPLE: Toe touch activities
2. *Static strength:* Maximum force that a subject can exert for a brief period, where the force is exerted continuously to this maximum (Fig. 7-3)
   EXAMPLE: Pulling against dynamometers
3. *Dynamic strength:* Ability to exert muscular force repeatedly and move one's own approximate body weight (Fig. 7-4)
   EXAMPLES: Chinning, dips on parallel bars, push-up activities (activities 18, 25, 26 to 32, and 35 to 38 in Chapter 5)
4. *Trunk strength:* Dynamic strength specific to the trunk muscles, particularly the abdominals (Fig. 7-5)
   EXAMPLES: Sit-ups, knee-chest curls
5. *Stamina:* Capacity to continue maximum effort requiring prolonged muscular exertion over time
   EXAMPLES: Distance running, rope jumping, bench stepping, bicycling (Fig. 7-6)

The following are descriptions of components that are included in the motor fitness areas:

1. *Dynamic flexibility:* Ability to make rapid flexing or extension movements in which the resiliency of the muscles in recovery from distortion is critical
   EXAMPLES: Activities 10, 39, and 40 in Chapter 5
2. *Explosive strength:* Ability to expend a maximum of energy in one or a series of explosive acts (Fig. 7-7)
   EXAMPLES: Broad jump, high jump, shot put, 50-yard dash, and shuttle run (AAHPER test) (Fig. 7-8)
3. *Gross body coordination:* Ability to coordinate the simultaneous actions of different parts of the body while making gross body movements
   EXAMPLE: Rope jumping
4. *Gross body equilibrium:* Ability to maintain equilibrium despite forces that disturb balance when an individual must depend on vestibular and kinesthetic cues (Fig. 7-9)
   EXAMPLES: Walking a balance beam or jumping on a trampoline

When programs for the physically subfit are implemented, it is desirable to be more comprehensive with regard to programming for general physical and motor fitness components. Therefore, programs for the subfit should be comprehensive so that the results of the program can be generalized to many physical and motor aspects of life.

Physical and motor fitness abilities are the prerequisites to learning and efficient execution of sport skills. Therefore, physical and motor fitness programming should be comprehensive so that handicapped children can effectively learn and perform the sport skills of the physical education curriculum.

The Individual Education Program of P.L. 94-142 requires the fulfillment of development of physical and motor fitness of handicapped children. Furthermore, implicit in the act is a systematic way of achieving these goals. To achieve the outcomes of physical and motor fitness the question to be answered is "What are the physical and motor fitness abilities that can be developed in an individual?" Once this question is answered, a concrete plan for interrelating program objectives, diagnosis, and remediation can be made.

To meet the unique physical and motor needs of handicapped children it is necessary to analyze and isolate subabilities of physical and motor fitness. In this discussion, abilities associated with motor fitness are gross body coordination, gross body equilibrium, and explosive power or strength.[20] Abilities associated with physical fitness are dynamic strength, static strength, trunk strength, extent flexibility, etc. Through testing, a profile of strengths and weaknesses in each of the analyzed areas of physical and motor abilities is determined. Thus, information is provided that aids the instructor in selecting appropriate activities according to a specific pupil's need.

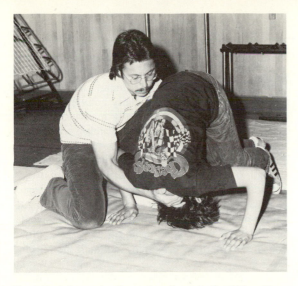

Fig. 7-7. A forward roll requires dynamic flexibility. (Courtesy of California State University, Audio Visual Center, Long Beach, Calif.)

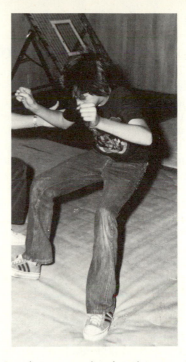

Fig. 7-8. Completing a standing broad jump, which illustrates the use of explosive strength. (Courtesy of California State University, Audio Visual Center, Long Beach, Calif.)

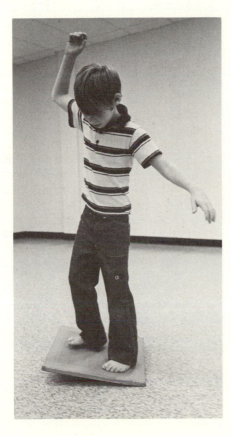

Fig. 7-9. The balance board helps the student develop gross body equilibrium. (Courtesy of the Special Education Early Childhood Intervention Program, University of Kansas, Lawrence.)

TAXONOMY OF PHYSICAL AND MOTOR FITNESS

A taxonomy is a classification system that specifically identifies discrete abilities. The establishment of a taxonomy is the first step in developing an approach to meet the unique measured needs of children. A taxonomy, in this case, is a means of categorizing diverse physical actions in such a way that useful relationships among activities are established. It simplifies and identifies the way in which individuals possess traits in common and yet differ in characteristics. It is extremely useful in describing performance on a wide variety of tasks.

The development of a taxonomy makes it possible to formulate goals, select tests relevant to those goals, and then more precisely specify activity objectives for individuals according to target deficiencies. Thus, if the instructor makes use of a taxonomy, the advantages are as follows: a profile of abilities may be generated and appropriate activities may be selected according to each child's needs. Thus, each child, regardless of developmental status and disability, works toward the acquisition of skills commensurate with his or her abilities.

Before a taxonomy can be justified, there must be evidence that supports discrete identifiable physical and motor properties that exist within each physical and motor ability. Factor analysis studies tend to describe the ways in which individuals may be different. This statistical technique assists in the classification of motor tasks into ability categories and thus enables the construction of a taxonomy. Such components are discussed in the following pages.

STRENGTH

Strength is that factor of physical fitness that allows a person to overcome a resistance through muscular exertion. Three discrete strength subabilities identified by Fleishman[20] are *explosive strength*, *static strength*, and *dynamic strength*. Explosive strength is apparent in those activities requiring movement, speed, and sudden changes in direction, for example, in running through an obstacle course or in throwing an object for distance. Static or isometric strength involves a brief maximum muscular contraction that requires little muscle shortening. Dynamic strength, on the other hand, involves repeated isotonic muscular contractions.

Normal muscle capacity is maintained at a level that is in keeping with our daily activities. Consequently, children who habitually maintain minimal levels of physical activity may develop subaverage strength or continue in a condition of low vitality. However, through proper training, the general strength of the body may be increased. This is usually done by providing a training stimulus greater than the normal daily stress requirement of a particular muscle or group of muscles. The traditional method of strength training is through the application of the overload principle, in which the training

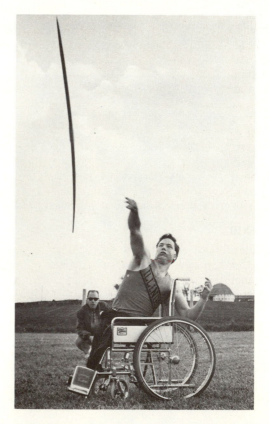

Fig. 7-10. Throwing the javelin requires explosive strength of the arms. (Courtesy of Julian Stein, American Alliance for Health, Physical Education, Recreation, and Dance and Rehabilitation Education Center, University of Illinois, Champaign-Urbana, Ill.)

stimulus exceeds the student's present level of performance. For best results, training should be pushed to the point of fatigue. This enhances the total effect of training more effectively than if training is interrupted prior to the fatigue point.[25] A general axiom in strength training that generally yields good results for increasing muscular strength would be: "Greater work effort rather than long duration of effort." To make optimal gains in strength training, it has been recommended that the training stimulus be increased at least every 14 days, for the overload effect is not as great unless resistance is increased periodically. In the case of weaker children, the training effects will be great at first; however, with the acquisition of greater strength, slower progress will be made.[25]

Some muscle groups are more susceptible to strength training than are others. Muscle groups that are used most strenuously in day-to-day activity are those that respond less readily to strength training. Among them are the muscles of the forearm and the arm, whereas the gastrocnemius, gluteal, and hip extensor muscles respond more favorably to stimulus training.[25] In accord with this concept is the fact that atrophied muscles respond five or six times more favorably to strength training than do well-trained groups of muscles. Stated in another way, the trainability of muscle groups shows a direct relationship to their use in the activities of daily living (Chapter 5).[25]

FLEXIBILITY

Flexibility is the range and degree of motion through which one extremity can move in relation to another. It is generally agreed that varying degrees of flexibility are required for efficiency of joint movement and motor performance. Although the optimal amount of flexibility for successful performance is not clearly understood, there seems to be a consensus that each activity has it own desirable amount of flexibility.[14] When considering just how much flexibility is needed by the individual, all eventualities should be taken into consideration. A highly elastic and mobile body should allow for sudden uncommon or unexpected movements.

There is no single factor that determines the differences in the flexibility of one individual as compared with another. Variance in flexibility can be attributable to heredity, a difference in joint struc-

ture, the extent of elasticity in connective tissue that is found throughout the body, the extent of reciprocal coordination and muscular tension, and muscle viscosity. Thus, there is no single factor that accounts for the ability of a joint to move through a given range.

Although it is generally thought that its elasticity changes as the body grows older, studies indicate that flexibility varies more with individual movement habits and growth patterns than with age.[3] It can be concluded therefore that in order to maintain or increase body mobility and joint range of movement, an individual must engage in a great variety of gross and fine motor activities that involve a full range of movement of the joints employed.

Two common types of exercise for increasing flexibility are the ballistic and static, or gradual, stretching techniques. In the ballistic technique, a rebounding movement is initiated that is controlled and slowly employs the principle of reciprocal muscle action. Consequently, moving muscles pull the body part into a stretch position while the opposing set of muscles relaxes. To avoid the possibility of injury to the musculotendinous unit, stretching by the ballistic method is not carried to the point of discomfort. The student is cautioned against engaging in lunging and uncontrolled movements. Static (or gradual) stretching, on the other hand, discourages the bobbing action of the ballistic technique by maintaining the stretch position for a period of 30 seconds or longer. The participant is instructed to stretch a little beyond the point of discomfort. Logan and Egstrom[32] studied the effects of static and ballistic stretching on the sacrofemoral angle and concluded that both types of exercise were equally effective. However, in a comparison of ballistic and static stretching, de Vries[17] indicates that static stretching tends to decrease the chances of muscle strains in preactivity warm-up (Chapter 5).

MUSCULAR ENDURANCE

Muscular endurance and cardiovascular endurance refer to a person's ability to engage in continuous activity without performance decrement. Although both forms of endurance possess this property, there are differences: muscular endurance involves repeated contractions of muscles, whereas cardiovascular endurance is an individual's capacity to use oxygen during physical activity.[7,8]

Well-constructed programs of physical activity can be of significant value to children who are lacking in muscular endurance or cardiovascular fitness. There is evidence that systematic muscular exercise leads to an increase in height and weight as well as to an increase in the function of the vital organs. Another value of physical exercise programs in assisting children who are physically unfit is producing organic changes in the lungs and circulatory system and improving their function in normal living.

It is the hope of the physical educator that favorable attitudes toward physical exercise can be instilled in all students. It is commonly believed that exercise is one of the factors deterring the onset of hypokinetic disease, primarily of the cardiovascular system. Exercise reduces hypertension (which is often caused by anxiety and emotional stress), serves as an outlet for nervous tension (Chapter 6), and helps maintain the elasticity of the blood vessels. However, there is no royal road to fitness, for it requires time and energy. In the development of muscular endurance and cardiovascular fitness, each bout of exercise must be a little stronger than the previous one; in this way, each bout will lead to progressive efficiency. (See the discussions of cardiovascular fitness in Chapters 5 and 12.)

POSTURAL FITNESS

As will be discussed in detail in Chapter 9, good body alignment is essential for efficient movement. Faulty posture and poor body mechanics produce an imbalance in muscle strength and extensibility that results in the expenditure of more energy than is necessary in the performance of a motor activity. Moreover, faulty posture either causes or results from distortions in body awareness and an inaccurate sense of body position.

COORDINATED MOVEMENT

Motor fitness is essential for coordinated movement to take place. In order for a person to achieve success in a great variety of physical activities, there must be present an effective interweaving of all the various factors of motor fitness. Awkward movement behavior implies asynchronous and inefficient muscle action.[2]

APPRAISING MOTOR FITNESS

It is of the utmost importance that great care be taken in the selection of tests that evaluate the status of an individual student with respect to subdevelopment in physical and motor areas. The purpose of a test may be to screen or diagnose physical and motor deficiencies. In setting up programs of developmental activities, it is important to ensure that evaluative tests be of a diagnostic nature. A diagnostic test enables the physical educator to assess the student's present level of educational performance for a task that represents an ability. From these data, programs can be set up to measure the student's progress from that point in programming. Such a procedure, in many instances, provides motivation for continuing activities of the program.

Criteria for the selection of tests are as follows:
1. The test should relate to fundamental abilities that can be improved through the program.
2. The test must relate to a task that is a goal of the Individual Education Program, where there has been common agreement between the school and the parents as to the utility of the goal once achieved.
3. Screening batteries should be carefully evaluated so that no two tests measure the same abilities. The test should cover as many different areas of motor and physical development as possible.
4. Tests that should be selected are those that have the best scientific foundation. Some of the information that should be known about the test includes its reliability, the consistency with which the same results are acquired, its validity (does the test measure what it claims to measure?), the norms that make it possible to compare the test results with a comparable random sampling of population, and the feasibility of its administration (the amount of time and equipment required and the degree of difficulty in administering the test).

Selected tests for classifying, grading, and diagnosing physical and motor deficiencies are discussed specifically in Chapters 2, 5, 7, 9, 11, and 12 and in the laboratory manual for this text.

PROGRAMMING FOR MOTOR FITNESS

Besides the developmental exercises found in Chapter 5, which are designed for specific body areas and conditions, the adaptive physical educator can employ the circuit training concept to increase a student's level of physical development and vitality.

It is well established that a progressive resistive exercise program is the best method for the development of muscular strength and that an interval training program of running, swimming, rope skipping, and bicycle riding is best for the development of circulorespiratory endurance. Therefore, the conditioning system that best meets the needs of both strength and circulorespiratory endurance is the circuit training method.[8] Circuit training has the potential to fulfill specific diagnosed areas of deficiencies among students through the selection of carefully arranged exercises. Each numbered exercise in a circuit is called a station. Therefore, there can be many stations throughout a particular gymnasium with persons of varying deficiencies routed to the stations that have exercises prescribed to meet each person's particular deficiency. The circuit training system is extremely adaptable to a great variety of situations and has the potential to meet individual differences that are present within a particular class. The advantages of a circuit training system in developing subaverage physical and motor factors are the following: (1) it can cope with most diagnosed deficiencies, (2) it has the potential of applying the progressive overload principle, and (3) it enables a large number of performers to train at the same time and yet meets the individual needs of each performer.

Circuit training usually involves the introduction of a time element into training, which often forces the participant to perform at submaximal levels. However, this need not be entirely the case. Each performer can be assigned a specific circuit for a prescribed number of repetitions at each station. If a person wishes to develop both cardiovascular and strength variables, the load may be of a submaximal nature so that the person may continuously engage in exercise while moving from station to station. However, if the strength component is a more desirable outcome, then fewer repetitions with a large dosage should be achieved before the person moves to the next station. After one circuit lap has been completed, it is at the discretion of the instructor to move the student through a second or third lap, depending on the total dosage desired for a given student. The advantages of the circuit system are as follows:

1. It is adaptable to a number of varying situations.
2. It can be used by 1 or 100 persons and fits almost any time requirements.
3. Progression is assured.
4. A person always works at his or her present capacity and then progresses beyond that.
5. It provides a series of progressive goals, which is a powerful motivating force.
6. It may use variables such as load, repetition, and time and consequently it may develop motor and physical developmental characteristics that have been identified by diagnostic testing.
7. It has the possibility of providing a vigorous bout of exercise in a relatively short period of time.
8. Any number of stations can be constructed to meet any identifiable need.
9. The student knows what must be done because of the construction of an individualized program.

Regardless of the system of training used in the developmental program, it should always be kept in mind that the primary goal of the system is to meet the individually diagnosed needs of each child in the program through planned progressive exercise. If this principle is applied, chances are that the program will be beneficial to the physical and motor development of the child.

Fig. 7-11 shows the implementation of a circuit program. This circuit program consists of 10 different exercises at separate stations, each performed according to a prescribed number of repetitions and load. It must be remembered that there are as many stations possible as there are exercises or areas of subdevelopment. The illustration shows five different levels at each station, permitting four steps of progression. Individuals subjectively select a starting level, and when a criterion of 10 repetitions is reached they move to the next level. Progression depends on the ability to meet a set number of repetitions, which will enable the individuals to move on to the next progressive level. At each station, it is desirable to place on the wall a card naming the item and showing the five levels of performance. The load and number of repeti-

Name of exercise	Developmental levels*				
	I	II	III	IV	V
	Wt.	Wt.	Wt.	Wt.	Wt.
Two arm curl	40	50	55	60	65
Military press	50	60	65	70	75
Deep knee bends	70	80	85	90	95
Dead lift (straight leg)	70	80	85	90	95
French curl (or dip) with dumbbell	10	15	20	25	30
Situps (time)	--	--	--	--	--
Bench step-ups (time)	--	--	--	--	--
Bench press	55	60	65	75	85
Lateral raises (dumbbell)	5	10	15	20	25
Pushups (time)	--	--	--	--	--

*When 10 repetitions are reached, advance to the next developmental level.

Fig. 7-11. A suggested circuit training program.

tions should be initially selected to meet the capabilities of the average students in the class; however, from this point weights are adjusted to determine students' present levels of educational performance so that short-term instructional objectives can be determined. Also, it must be remembered that it is not necessary for all students to participate at each of these 10 stations. Therefore, students may be routed to four, five, or six stations according to their needs as compared with normative performance. Any station may be devised that meets a physical or motor need of children, and a progressive program may be established.

SELECTED FITNESS PROBLEMS

As mentioned earlier in this chapter, the problem of underdevelopment and low physical vitality is closely associated with a great number of organic, mental, and emotional problems discussed throughout this book. However, three major problem areas transcend most, namely, malnutrition, anemia, and aging.

Malnutrition

The term *malnutrition* means poor nutrition, whether there is an excess or a lack of nutrients to the body. In either instance, the individual who is malnourished has relatively low physical vitality, may be underdeveloped, and has other serious disadvantages.[5]

Underweight

It is important that the cause of physical underdevelopment be identified. One of the causes for physical underdevelopment may be a lack of physical activity, which, consequently, does not provide opportunity for the body to develop to its physical potential. However, there are some children who are physically underdeveloped partially because of undernutrition. When a person's body weight is more than 10% below the ideal weight indicated by standard age and weight tables, this may indicate that undernutrition is a cause. Tension, anxiety, depression, and other emotional factors may restrict a person's appetite, causing insufficient caloric intake and weight loss. Impairment to development of the body may also ensue. In culturally deprived areas, diets in some instances may be deficient in proper nutrition as a result of insufficient food, idiosyncrasy, and lack of appetite because of some organic problem. Proper nutrition and exercise go hand in hand in growing children. One without the other may cause lack of optimal physical development. The role of the physical educator in dealing with the underweight person is to help establish sound living habits with particular emphasis paid to proper diet, rest, and relaxation. The student should be encouraged to keep a 5-day food intake diary, after which, with the help of the teacher, a daily average of calories consumed is computed. After determining the average number of calories taken in, the student is encouraged to increase the daily intake by eating extra meals that are both nutritious and high in calories. *

Overweight

Many persons in the United States are overweight. Obesity, particularly in adults, is considered one of the great current medical problems because of its relation to cardiovascular and other diseases. The frequency of overweight among male patients, as reported by Master, Jaffe, and Chesky,[34] was nearly 40% in patients with angina pectoris, coronary insufficiency, and hypertension and nearly 50% in those with coronary occlusions as compared with approximately 20% in the populations used as controls.

Overweight may be defined as any excess of 10% or more above the ideal weight for a person and obesity is any excess of 20% or more above the ideal weight. Obesity constitutes pathological overweight that requires some means of correction. There are several factors that must be considered in determining whether a person is overweight. Among these are sex, weight, height, age, general body build, bone size, muscular development, and accumulations of subcutaneous fat.

In the past, there has not been sufficient attention given to the diagnosis of the large number of overweight children in our modern society. Research on the incidence of overweight children in our schools has indicated estimates of 10% or more.[36] The incidence therefore is of such significance that attention to prevention and remediation should be provided by public school doctors, nurses, and health and physical educators in our schools.

Overweight persons have a greater tendency than normal or underweight individuals to contract diseases of the heart, circulatory system, kidneys, and pancreas. They also have a predisposition to be afflicted with structural foot conditions and joint pathology because of their increased weight and a lack of motor skill to accommodate the excess weight.

The basic reason for overweight is that the body's food and caloric consumption is more than the physical activity or energy expended to utilize them. Consequently, the excess energy food is stored in the body as fat, leading to overweight. In many instances, overeating is a matter of habit. Thus, the body is continually in the process of acquiring more calories than are needed to maintain a normal body weight.

Overweight and obesity have many causes. Among them are (1) caloric imbalance from eating incorrectly in relationship to energy expended in the form of activity; (2) dysfunction of the endocrine glands, particularly the pituitary and the thyroid, which regulate fat distribution in the body; and (3) emotional disturbance.

There is impressive evidence that obesity in adults has its origin in childhood habits. There seems to be a substantial number of overweight adults whose difficulty in controlling their appetite stems from childhood.[40] The social environment may have some influence on obesity. Gurney[23] found that 73% of the children he investigated were obese when both parents were overweight, 41% when only one parent was obese, and 10% when both parents were of average weight. In the preschool years, thinness rather than obesity is the general developmental characteristic of children. However, during the early school years and up to early adolescence, children seem susceptible to excess fat deposition.

A belief prevalent among some authorities is that a great portion of obesity is caused by emotions. They theorize that children at the age of 7 years

---

*See also Crowe, W. C., Arnheim, D. D., and Auxter, D.: Laboratory manual in adapted physical education and recreation, St. Louis, 1977, The C. V. Mosby Co.

are particularly susceptible to obesity from overeating in order to compensate for being unhappy and lonely. Evidently, eating may give comfort to children. This particular period is significant because it is when children are transferring close emotional ties from the family to peer relationships. In the event that children do not successfully establish close friendships with other children, they feel alone. Therefore, a compensatory mechanism of adjustment is eating, which gives comfort. Eating may also be used as a comfort when children have trouble at home or at school.

Adverse effects of obesity. Obese children, in many instances, exhibit characteristics that are of an immature nature socially and emotionally. It is not uncommon for obese children to dislike the games played by their peers, for obesity handicaps them in being adept at the games in which their peers are adequate. These children are often clumsy and slow, objects of many stereotyped jokes, and incapable of holding a secure social position among other children. Consequently, these children may become oversensitive and unable to defend themselves and thus may withdraw from healthy play and exercise. This withdrawal from activity decreases the energy expenditure needed to maintain the balance that combats the obesity. Therefore, in many instances, obesity leads to sedentary habits. It is often difficult to encourage these children to participate in forms of exercise that permit great expenditure of energy.

Obesity may be an important factor as children form ideas about themselves as persons and about how they think they appear to others. The ideas that they have about themselves will be influenced by their own discoveries, by what others say about them, and by the attitudes shown toward them. If the children find that their appearance elicits hostility, disrespect, or negative attention from parents and peers, these feelings may affect their self-concept. Traits described by their parents and peers may affect their inner feelings and may be manifested in their behavior, for children often assess their worth in terms of their relationships with peers, parents, and other authority figures.

When children pass from the child-centered atmosphere of the home into the competitive activities of the early school years, social stresses are encountered. They must demonstrate physical abilities, courage, manipulative skill, and social adeptness in direct comparison with other children of their age. The penalties for failure are humiliation, ridicule, and rejection from the group. Obesity places a tremendous social and emotional handicap on children. Therefore, educators should be concerned with and give these children all possible assistance and guidance in alleviating or adjusting to obesity.

Evaluating obesity. There are many ways that overweight or obesity can be determined; some of these are highly technical methods requiring sophisticated equipment, whereas others are relatively simple, but less valid. One of the least recommended means of measuring fatness is comparison of data about the individual with normative age, sex, and height/weight tables. These tables do not normally allow for the person who may have a preponderance of muscle tissue in place of fat or for those with wide frames and/or heavy skeletal structures. The most accurate method of determining fatness that can easily be used by the adaptive physical educator is the direct application of an-

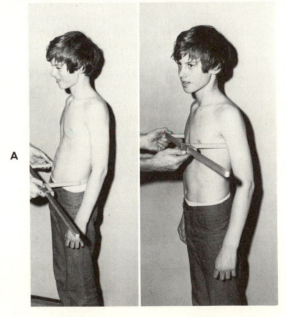

Fig. 7-12. Determining lateral diameter of the pelvis, **A,** and chest, **B.** (Courtesy of California State University, Audio Visual Center, Long Beach, Calif.)

thropometric measurement such as the Pryor width-weight technique and skin fold measurement.[40]

The Pryor method predicts body weight based on an individual's skeletal structure. By ascertaining the lateral diameter of the chest at the nipple line and the width of the pelvis at the iliac crest (Fig. 7-12) and then comparing these measurements with the height and age of the individual, a predicted weight is determined.[39] Fig. 7-13 shows the Pryor method in predicting weight for boys 2 to 6 years of age.

Skin fold measurement provides both a simple and accurate method of assessing quantitatively the fat content of the human body.[47] The skin fold cal-

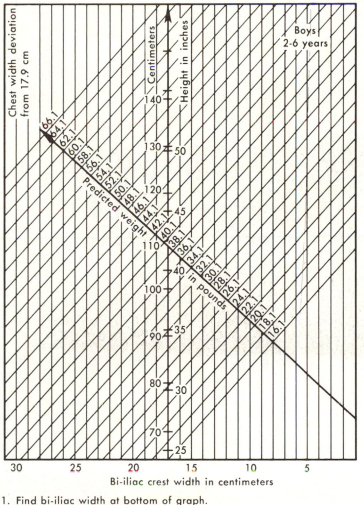

1. Find bi-iliac width at bottom of graph.
2. Follow the vertical channel indicated, up to standing height.
3. Take nearest slant axis to predicted weight.
4. Correct for chest width if necessary. (Go up 1 unit or down 1 unit for each centimeter that the chest measurement exceeds or falls short of the mean at the top of the graph.)

Fig. 7-13. Predicting weight for boys 2 to 6 years of age through the use of the Pryor method.

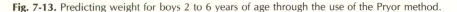

iper is applied to locations on the body where a fold of skin and subcutaneous fat can be lifted between the thumb and the forefinger so that it is held free of the muscular and bony structure. The skin fold caliper has become an evaluation tool for universal comparability of fat fold measurements. The accepted national recommendation is to have a caliper designed so as to exert a pressure of 10 gm/mm^2 on the caliper face. The contact surface area to be measured should be in the neighborhood of 20 to 40 mm.^{2} The skin fold measurement to be obtained should be picked up in standard fashion. The recommended method is to pinch a full fold of skin and subcutaneous tissue between the thumb and forefinger, at a distance of about 1 cm from the site on which the caliper is to be placed, and then to pull the fold away from the underlying muscle.[47] The calipers are then applied to the fold about 1 cm below the fingers so that the pressure on the fold at the point measured is exerted by the faces of the calipers and not by the fingers. The handle of the caliper is then released and a recording is made to the nearest 0.5 mm. When skin folds are thick, the recording should be made 2 or 3 seconds after the caliper pressure is applied.

Although the skin fold at the triceps site has been thought by many to adequately represent total body fat, it is advisable, for the greatest accuracy, to take measurements at several additional body sites (Table 7-2). Durnin and Rahaman,[19] for example, used four sites for their study of body fat content of 13- to 34-year-old persons: the biceps, the triceps, the subscapular, and the suprailiac areas (Table 7-3). Their method of taking skin fold measurements was as follows:

1. All subjects were seated.
2. Only measurements of the right side were taken.
3. The *biceps* were measured over the midpoint of the muscle (Fig. 7-14) while the forearm was resting supinated on the subject's thigh.
4. The *triceps* were measured at a point half the distance between the olecranon and acromion process while the arm was hanging vertically (Fig. 2-7, *A*).
5. The *subscapular* region was measured just below the tip and to the lateral side of the inferior angle of the scapula (Fig. 2-7, *B*).
6. The *suprailiac* region was measured just above the iliac crest at the midaxillary line (Fig. 2-7, *C*).

Table 7-2. Obesity standards for white Americans*†

Age (years)	Skin fold measurements (mm)	
	Men	Women
5	12	14
6	12	15
7	13	16
8	14	17
9	15	18
10	16	20
11	17	21
12	18	22
13	18	23
14	17	23
15	16	24
16	15	25
17	14	26
18	15	27
19	15	27
20	16	28
21	17	28
22	18	28
23	18	28
24	19	28
25	20	29
26	20	29
27	21	29
28	22	29
29	23	29
30-50	23	30

*Minimum triceps skin fold thickness in millimeters indicating obesity. Figures represent the logarithmic means of the frequency distributions plus one standard deviation.
†Adapted from Seltzer, C. C., and Mayer, J.: Postgrad. Med. **38:**101-107, 1965.

Durnin and Rahaman studied thin, intermediate, and obese adolescent boys and girls from the ages of 13 to 16 years and young adult men and women from the ages of 21 to 34 years. They also approximated the percentages of the subjects' body fat based on the four skin fold sites (Table 7-4).

Implications for physical education. Since overweight children often cannot perform the activities of the physical education program efficiently, it is not uncommon for them to dislike many of these activities. Often, as a result of their inability to participate in the program, they are the objects

Table 7-3. Measurements required to determine total skin fold thickness at four skin fold sites (biceps, triceps, subscapular, and suprailiac)*

Body build	Skin fold measurement (mm)			
	Men	**Women**	**Boys**	**Girls**
Thin				
Mean	24.0	31.2	22.4	33.3
Standard deviation	7.1	6.3	5.3	9.5
Intermediate				
Mean	34.7	39.9	29.7	36.2
Standard deviation	15.7	10.0	7.6	8.8
Plump and obese				
Mean	57.2	66.0	43.2	49.0
Standard deviation	21.4	22.7	13.2	13.6

*Adapted from Durnin, J. V. G. A., and Rahaman, M. M.: Br. J. Nutr. **21:**681-689, 1967.

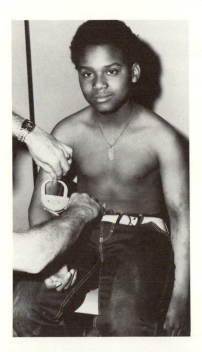

Fig. 7-14. Biceps skin fold measurement.

Table 7-4. Percentages of fat corresponding to the total of skin fold measurements at four sites (biceps, triceps, subscapular, and suprailiac)*

Total skin fold measurement (mm)	Body fat (%)			
	Men	**Women**	**Boys**	**Girls**
15	5.5	—	9.0	12.5
20	9.0	15.5	12.5	16.0
25	11.5	18.5	15.5	19.0
30	13.5	21.0	17.5	21.5
35	15.5	23.0	19.5	23.5
40	17.0	24.5	21.5	25.0
45	18.5	26.0	23.0	27.0
50	20.0	27.5	24.0	28.5
55	21.0	29.0	25.5	29.5
60	22.0	30.0	26.5	30.5
65	23.0	31.0	27.5	32.0
70	24.0	32.5	28.5	33.0
75	25.0	33.5	—	—
80	26.0	34.0	—	—
85	26.5	35.0	—	—
90	27.5	36.0	—	—
95	28.0	36.5	—	—

*From Durnin, J. V. G. A., and Rahaman, M. M.: Br. J. Nutr. **21:**681-689, 1967.

of practical jokes and disparaging remarks made by other children. In such an environment, obese and overweight boys and girls become unhappy and ashamed and often withdraw from the activity to circumvent emotional involvement with the group.[33] The physical educator should attempt to create an environment that will enable the obese child to have successful experiences in the class, thus minimizing situations that could degrade the child's position as a person of positive worth. The physical educator is also challenged with regard to developing attitudes on the part of the nonhandicapped majority. Consequently, proposing the acceptance of children with differences to the normal group is an important and worthwhile goal of the physical educator.

There can be no one program for the remediation of children who are overweight. It is necessary that the true cause of the problem be found. When the cause of overweight or obesity is known, there are several avenues available for treatment; they are as follows:

1. Control of the diet by reduction of caloric intake
2. Medical treatment in the case of a glandular dysfunction
3. Counseling when emotional causes are at the root of the problem
4. Counseling on the consequences of obesity to the total personality
5. A program of exercise within the capacity of the child to increase energy expenditure in order to balance the caloric intake
6. Disruption of sedentary ways of living

It is sound reasoning in combating obesity and overweight to attempt to change living patterns in terms of physical activity and diet rather than to go into crash programs for fast reduction of weight. The habits of everyday living are of longer range than the crash programs and more value will be accrued by this type of living in the long run.

Obese and overweight students should be guided into activities that can be safely performed and successfully achieved. This will tend to encourage them to participate in more vigorous activities.[9,36] Some of the activities that can be used to combat obesity are general conditioning exercises, jogging, dancing, rhythms, swimming, and sports and games. Much can be done for these children with personal guidance, encouragement, and selection of the proper developmental experiences for individual children.

Weekly weigh-ins in which a certain number of pounds is scheduled to be lost in a given week provide program incentives. Sustained reduction over a period of time may afford opportunities for establishing permanent patterns for exercise and eating. The value of the weigh-in is that it projects a precise goal for the student to achieve each week. Furthermore, the exercise program in which the student engages should be progressive. Exercises based on calculated energy expenditures are initiated with slight progression ensured in the program with each successive day of attendance. Suggested activities are walking, jogging, bicycle riding, rope jumping, swimming, stair and hill climbing, and stepping up on and down from a bench. The main purpose of these exercise programs is to sustain moderate activity over a period of time in order to expend calories. If the student can be induced to engage in more than one exercise bout a day, this is of greater value.

Anemia

Anemia is a condition of the blood in which there is a deficiency of hemoglobin, which delivers oxygen to body tissues. This deficiency of hemoglobin may be a result of the quantity contained in the red corpuscles of the blood or a reduction in the number of red corpuscles themselves.

The physical education teacher should be aware of the characteristics that anemic persons display. In many instances, anemic persons appear to be pale because their blood is not as red as that of typical persons. Persons with anemia tire easily because of impaired oxidation in the muscles, and they also may become short of breath. Consequently, in many instances, the rate of breathing is increased. As a rule, children with anemia fatigue more easily than do typical children, are often unable to make gains in physical strength, and are impaired in learning motor skills.

Some of the symptoms that may give rise to suspecting anemia are an increased rate of breathing, a bluish tinge of the lips and nails (because the blood's color is not as red), headache, nausea, faintness, weakness, fatigue, and a lack of strength.

Causes

There are many diverse reasons for the occurrence of anemia. The following are some of the main ones: (1) great loss of blood; (2) decreased blood production within the system; (3) diseases such as malaria, septic infections, and cirrhosis of the liver; (4) poisons such as lead, insecticides, and arsenobenzene; and (5) chronic dysentery, intestinal parasites, and diseases associated with endocrine deficiency and vitamin deficiencies. Anemia is symptomatic of a disturbance that in many cases can be remedied. Inasmuch as there are several varieties of anemia, the method of treatment is dependent on the type of anemia present.

Types

There are several forms of anemia. *Chlorosis* is a form of anemia that is characterized by a reduced amount of hemoglobin in the corpuscles and usually occurs in young women at about the time of puberty. Anemia can be caused by excessive hemorrhage, in which case the specific gravity of the blood is reduced because there is a greater proportion of fluid in comparison with corpuscles in the blood. Occurring less often than chlorosis, *pernicious anemia* is characterized by a decrease in the number of red corpuscles. It can cause changes in the nervous system, along with loss of sensation in the hands and feet. In *aplastic anemia,* the red bone marrow that forms blood cells is replaced by fatty marrow. This form of anemia can be caused by radiation, radioactive isotopes, and atomic fallout. Certain antibiotics may also be causative factors. *Iron deficiency anemia* is a form of anemia that afflicts millions of American women. It is caused by insufficient iron to replace that which is lost during each mentrual period. One prevalent type of anemia among blacks is *sickle cell anemia.* This type afflicts 8% of all blacks in the United States. Jones, Shainberg, and Byer[28] indicate that 50% of the blacks afflicted with this disease die before they reach the age of 20 years.

Treatment

The various forms of anemia require different treatments. Chlorosis may be remedied or cured by increasing the amount of iron-bearing foods in the diet. However, pernicious anemia requires the intramuscular injection of liver extracts. Aplastic anemia may be corrected by transplanting bone marrow from healthy subjects and by utilizing the male hormone testosterone, which is known to stimulate the production of cells by the bone marrow if enough red marrow is present for the hormone to act on. In the case of iron deficiency anemia, treatment consists of improving the iron content of the diet or taking diet supplements that contain iron. Vitamin B_{12}, which is important for bone marrow actvity, is also an important ingredient in treating pernicious anemia. The gastric juice appears to be missing the substance, produced in the lining of the stomach, that promotes the absorption in the intestine of vitamin B_{12}, which is stored in the liver and released as required for the formation of red blood cells in the bone marrow.[45]

Implications for physical education

The final decision regarding the nature of physical education activities for a child with anemia should be made by medical personnel. A well-conceived and supervised physical education program can be of great value to the child who has anemia. Exercise stimulates the production of red blood cells through the increased demand for oxygen. However, to be beneficial, an activity must be planned qualitatively with regard to the specific anemic condition. It is not uncommon for children who have anemia to be retarded in the development of physical strength and endurance. Identification of the anemic condition and its cure often may result in significant gains in physical fitness and muscular endurance. The alert physical educator conceivably will be able to assist in the identification of anemia and thus to refer the student to medical authorities who may, in turn, alleviate the condition. Anemia that is undiagnosed may have social implications because of the possibility of curtailment in motor skill and physical development and may set the child apart from peers in social experiences.

Aging

The science that studies aging is called *gerontology,* whereas the field of *geriatrics* is concerned more specifically with diseases and management of old age.[1]

Aging is relative. Chronological age, the age in years, is a poor indicator of the stage of a person's

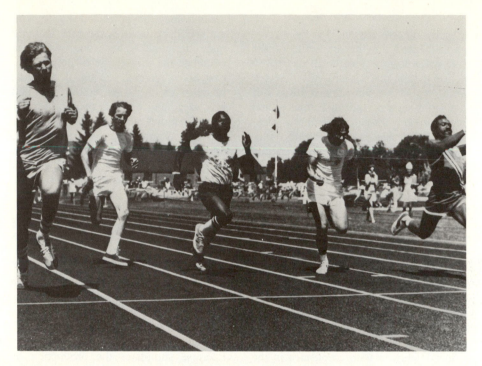

Fig. 7-15. Mentally retarded adults have an opportunity to participate in athletic competition in the Special Olympics. (Courtesy of the Joseph P. Kennedy Foundation, Special Olympics, Washington, D.C.)

total development. Aging per se does not progress or decline at an even rate. There is great variability in anatomical, physiological, and psychological aging. Consequently, a person may have a chronological age of 50 years, the heart and arteries of a person aged 30 years, and a mental vitality of a person aged 25 years.

Therefore, aging must be considered a dynamic biological process of growth and development and not merely degeneration or organic regression.[15] Physiological aging, in general, produces a loss of the essential functioning and the gradual degeneration of organs. The collagenous substances within the connective tissues of the body, such as those found in tendons and ligaments, become hardened and inelastic. Organs that undergo aging lose their ability for normal nutrient and metabolic transfer between the cellular structures and blood. Microscopic degeneration resulting in cellular death spreads and progresses to organs and subsequently to an entire organ system. Senescence occurs when the death rate of cells is greater than the rate of their respective reproduction.

Problems in aging

The cardiovascular system (CVS) is vital to the normal functioning of the entire body. Aging affects the CVS efficiency and subsequently results in alterations in the rate and efficiency of oxygen nutrient utilization. With age, connective tissue and fat content increases within inner surface membranes and cavities of the heart. The senile heart moves from an oblique to a more upright position. Valves become inelastic, resulting in a tendency toward dilation and muscular incompetency in the heart, with subsequent arrhythmia. Coronary arteries supplying the heart become thickened at their innermost lining (intima). Blood vessels, particularly arteries, display age by their inelasticity and thinning muscular walls. Stretched arteries become more twisted in their course. Degeneration and the collection of fat deposits further weaken artery walls. After structural arterial change comes a functional rise in systolic blood pressure and a lowering of diastolic pressure. The aging person's lungs gradually become inelastic, smaller, and, in general, less viable. Chest excursion may be hampered by the rigidity of the thorax as a result of the calcification of cartilaginous tissue. An inability to inhale or expand the chest fully produces lowered vital capacity and a decreased breathing capacity.

With senescence comes a number of musculoskeletal changes, primarily degeneration and atrophy of muscle fibers and resultant strength loss, cartilage calcification, and softening of bony structures through absorption of mineral matter (osteoporosis). Joint changes also occur, resulting in articular degeneration and eventually arthritis. Disuse is the reason given for accentuated osteoporosis and muscular atrophy. Evidence indicates that strength diminishes very slowly during the mature adult period and increases its rate of decline after the fifth decade.

Gross brain size diminishes with age; microscopic studies show degeneration of the nerve ganglion cells as well as the highly specialized supporting elements of the nervous system. Anderson and Langton[1] indicate that with brain atrophy and cellular degeneration there occur increased cerebrospinal fluid, thickened dura mater, and a decrease of general blood circulation with a resultant decrease in metabolism. Such alterations are manifested in slower learning and motor response, inability to visually accommodate near points (presbyopia), and a decrease in auditory acuity.

Organs of internal secretion, such as thyroid, pituitary, and adrenal glands, start a definite regression as aging progresses. Bodily functions controlled by the endocrine glands, such as basal metabolism rate (BMR) and resistance to infection, decline with age. Also, the reproductive organs decline rapidly and cease to function at about 50 years of age for the female and 65 years of age for the male. Increasing age brings with it a decrease in androgenic hormones and increases in the speed of atrophy of muscular tissue and internal organs.

Wolff[50] summarized the basic findings of scientific investigation on the changes produced in aging:

1. An increase in connective tissues
2. A gradual loss of connective tissue elasticity
3. A disappearance of nervous system cells
4. A reduction of normal cells
5. An increase in the amount of fat
6. A decrease in the ability to use oxygen
7. A decrease in blood volume while resting
8. A decrease in vital lung capacity
9. A decrease in muscle strength
10. A decrease in the amount of hormones and endocrine excretion

All adults are affected to some degree by pathological aging. A number of factors cause an individual's aging process to be either atypically slow or prematurely fast, namely, heredity, general adaptation to stress, and particular style of living. An individual's constitutional inheritance affects the aging process because it passes on deficiencies or the predisposition for certain diseases. Heredity also helps determine an individual's ability to adapt to life's stresses. Selye's[43] general adaptation syndrome (GAS) indicates that each individual is born with a given store of genetic energy that must be considered in the process of adaptation. Worry, fatigue, and constant muscular tension, together with improper physical activity, may constitute a life-style that would tend to exhaust genetic energies and result in premature aging.

As a person grows older, there is increased susceptibility to the condition of tissue deterioration. In general, the most common degenerative diseases are considered to be those of the heart, arteries, and kidneys. Anderson and Langton[1] describe arteriosclerosis, hypertension, nephritis, and heart disease as a degenerative quartet. Arteriosclerosis, cancer, arthritis, rheumatic disorders, nervous diseases, and mental breakdowns are considered the most prevalent aging disorders.

Many authorities have attributed premature aging and degenerative diseases, primarily in the area of the cardiovascular system,[9,22] to American living practices. A cause has not been singled out, but rather there appears to be a multitude of causes. The main ones might be listed as hypoactivity, overweight, excessive cigarette smoking, and worry.[34]

Over 100,000 Americans die each year from some major disease of the heart and/or blood vessels, not to mention those who are permanently disabled by such disease. This number accounts for about one half of the deaths that occur annually in the United States. Besides cardiovascular disease, the adult population suffers from untold orthopedic, emotional, and metabolic disorders that may be attributed directly or indirectly to contemporary life-styles.

Exercise and aging

To prevent involution, atrophy, and ultimate cellular and organ deaths, tissue stimulation must occur. Mateeff[35] states that "exercise is that vital factor that alone is capable not only of stopping the processes of involution and atrophy but also of reversing them, which promotes and brings into play the processes of self-repair and self-renovation at the molecular level in organisms of the aging." Planned progressive exercise can produce such positive gains as increased strength and skeletal muscle hypertrophy, hypertrophy of the heart with the resultant training effect of decreased heart rate, increased ability to expend energy, more efficient use of oxygen, a greater vital capacity, and improved body suppleness from increased joint mobility.[37] Bortz[6] indicated that physical activity helps delay the diminution of sex hormone excretion. Activity therefore can maintain the anabolic protein-building qualities of the sex glands and concomitant muscle strength. Many physically active

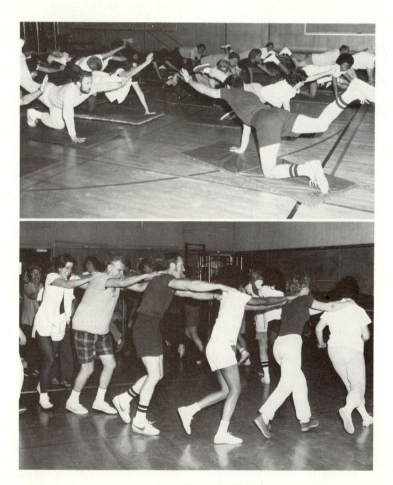

Fig. 7-16. An adult exercise program. (Courtesy of the Faculty Fitness Club, California State University, Long Beach, Calif.)

older persons express a higher level of vitality, ability to sleep, mental capacity, and desire for socialization than do their sedentary counterparts.

To offset many of the problems of premature aging, preventive conditioning programs have been emerging in the United States, primarily in YMCA's, colleges, universities, municipal recreation departments, and private organizations. However, the government, insurance companies, and industries have been slow to respond to this need because of a lack of concrete evidence that preventive measures can be applied to the subfit adult. In these supervised programs, adults can remedy or offset the debilitating influences of inactivity. (Fig. 7-16).

As discussed previously, aging progresses at varying speeds in different persons and in different organs within the same person. However, the organ system that should be of the greatest concern to the average American today is the cardiovascular system. It is reported that degeneration occurs in this system after 20 years of age. Stein indicates that the total peripheral vascular resistance increases 1.7%/year, heart work output decreases 0.6%/year, and resting cardiac output and maximum work rate decrease about 1%/year.[46]

However, Hutinger[26] indicates that physical activity is a key for delaying the aging process. Indeed, he reports that men in their sixties and seventies possess the capability of achieving percentages of improvement in the functional use of the heart and lungs and have a physical work capacity comparable to that of young men.[16] The decline in physical work capacity is normally from 9% to 15% during the ages from 45 to 55 years. However, Kasch[29] indicates that through a program of endurance with running and swimming at an average 86% intensity of maximum oxygen uptake, the normal decline in work capacity was forestalled. Thus, the use of systematic exercise as an intervention technique to retard the onset of aging of the cardiovascular system appears to have merit.

Although there is evidence of diminished functioning as a result of the aging process, there is also evidence that elderly handicapped persons can still develop function. This is made particulaly evident by a case reported by Gold (see Chapter 3). A mentally retarded person with an I.Q. of 19 was trained to complete a 14-part bicycle brake assembly in 20 trials. This person was also physically handicapped and legally blind. In that same study a 72-year-old mentally retarded woman with an I.Q. of 47, also legally blind, learned this same assembly task, although the rate of acquisition was approximately five times that of the previously mentioned subject. This task required a minimum of physical and motor fitness; nevertheless, when behavioral technology is applied to the acquisition of skills and ability by aged handicapped persons, positive developmental benefits result. It is conceivable that prerequisite physical and motor fitness abilities may be developed in some aged handicapped persons as well. If increased functioning of an aged person can be attained in tasks, perhaps the increase of skill attainment in these tasks represents physical and motor fitness components.

There is speculation as to just how much development can be achieved in motor and physical fitness in aged persons. The full expected benefits from physical education programs that are systematically implemented by trained personnel are as yet unknown. However, aged persons, whether handicapped or not, should receive systematic instructional programs consisting of positive developmental objectives in areas of physical and motor fitness.

It has been pointed out that the fit, as compared with the unfit, individual has the ability to deliver oxygen to the body as it is required. On the other hand, an unfit person experiences a greater energy demand than physical capacity to deliver it.

Research studies and clinical observations point to the fact that regular physical activities may contribute to fitness by preventing obesity and by decreasing the possibility of premature coronary heart disease. Exercise for the mature adult increases the individual's potential for withstanding the stresses of life.[30,34] Most authorities agree that the cardiovascular benefits from exercise are as follows:

1. Improved oxygen economy of the heart
2. More effective parasympathetic and sympathoinhibitory counterbalances
3. Slower heart rate at rest and less acceleration during effort
4. Faster heart deceleration after exercise
5. Reduction of peripheral blood vessel resistance
6. Increased residual blood volume of the heart

7. Improved coronary blood flow as a result of increased collateral capillarization of heart muscle
8. Prolongation of coagulation time and a lowering of the serum cholesterol level

Although there are positive signs that exercise may be beneficial to the cardiovascular system, proof must come through further research. Studies have attempted to obtain definitive information from programs designed to *intervene actively* in living patterns of subjects who are postcoronary patients or who are considered high-risk subjects, as determined by an electrocardiograph stress test. Such tests are administered by a cardiologist who determines whether there are ischemic heart changes after exercise. Test results serve as a useful index for the amount of exercise in which an individual can safely engage.[3,24]

Implications for physical education

With an increased awareness of the deleterious effect of inactivity on the sedentary adult population, physical education has emerged with new importance. Through the efforts of many disciplines, the public is beginning to realize that proper exercise can be a deterrent to many characteristics of premature physiological aging as well as to their concomitant diseases.

Research and studies have resulted in new concepts about the type of physical fitness activities best suited for adults. Continuity of well-planned activities can serve as a preventive conditioner. Isotonic exercise is preferable to isometric exercise, particularly for persons with a history of cardiovascular disease. Isometric exercise may result in irregular heartbeats, premature ventricular contractions, and abnormally fast heartbeats in heart disease patients.

A multidisciplinary approach has resulted from medicine's concern for premature cardiovascular disease and the positive effects of proper exercise. The physician, physical educator, applied physiologist, and many other professional persons are lending their skills to help solve the problem of adult physical fitness. With the implementation of many medically oriented adult physical education programs, there is an increased need for trained adapted physical education teachers who understand the problems and needs of the adult popula-

tion. Establishing individualized physical education programs for adults is one of the greatest challenges of our times.

REFERENCES

1. Anderson, C. L., and Langton, K.: Health principles and practice, ed. 6, St. Louis, 1970, The C. V. Mosby Co.
2. Arnheim, D. D., and Pestolesi, R. A.: Developing motor behavior in children: a balanced approach to elementary physical education, St. Louis, 1973, The C. V. Mosby Co.
2a. Armstrong vs. Kline, In the United States District Court of Appeals, Civil Action 78-132, 78-133, 78-172 (Third Circuit Court), 1980.
3. Astrand, I.: Clinical and physiological studies of manual workers 50-64 years old at rest and during work, Acta Med. Scand. **162:** 155, 1958.
4. Billing, H. E., and Lowendahl, E.: Mobilization of the human body, Stanford, Calif., 1949, Stanford University Press.
5. Bogert, L. J., et al.: Nutrition and physical fitness, ed. 9, Philadelphia, 1973, W. B. Saunders Co.
6. Bortz, E. L.: Creative aging, New York, 1963, Macmillan Publishing Co., Inc.
7. Clarke, H. H.: Circulatory-respiratory endurance improvement, Phys. Fitness Res. Digest Ser. 4, No. 3, Washington, D.C., 1973, President's Council on Physical Fitness and Sports.
8. Clarke, H. H.: Development of muscular strength and endurance, Phys. Fitness Res. Digest Ser. 4, No. 1, Washington, D.C., 1973, President's Council on Physical Fitness and Sports.
9. Clarke, H. H: Exercise and fat reduction, Phys. Fitness Res. Digest Ser. 5, No. 2, Washington, D.C., 1975, President's Council on Physical Fitness and Sports.
10. Clarke, H. H.: Joint and body range of movement, Phys. Fitness Res. Digest Ser. 5, No. 4, Washington, D.C., 1975, President's Council on Physical Fitness and Sports.
11. Clarke, H. H.: Physical fitness testing in schools, Phys. Fitness Res. Digest, Ser. 5, No. 1, Washington, D.C., 1975, President's Council on Physical Fitness and Sports.
12. Clarke, H. H.: Strength development and motor-sports improvement, Phys. Fitness Res. Digest Ser. 4, No. 4, Washington, D.C., 1974, President's Council on Physical Fitness and Sports.
13. Clarke, H. H.: Towards a better understanding of muscular strength, Phys. Fitness Res. Digest Ser. 4, No. 1, Washington, D.C., 1973, President's Council on Physical Fitness and Sports.
14. Clarke, H. H., and Carter, G. H.: Oregon simplification of the strength and physical fitness indices, Res. Q. **30:**3-10, 1959.
15. Course syllabus: principles and practice of geriatric rehabilitation, New York, 1960, New York College, Metropolitan Medical Center, Physical Medicine and Rehabilitation Department.
16. de Vries, H. A.: Exercise intensity threshold for improvement of cardiovascular respiratory function in older men, Geriatrics **25:**94-101, April 1971.
17. deVries, H. A.: Warm-up effects of relaxation and stretch-

ing techniques upon gross motor performance, Unpublished doctoral dissertation, University of Southern California, 1961.

18. Donlon, T.: Referencing test scores: introductory concepts. In Hively, W., and Reynolds, M. C., editors: Domain referenced testing in special education, Arlington, Va., 1975, Council for Exceptional Children.

19. Durnin, J. V. G. A., and Rahaman, M. M.: The assessment of fat in the human body from measurements of skin fold thickness, Br. J. Nutr. **21**:681-689, 1967.

20. Fleishman, E. A.: The structure and measurement of physical fitness, Englewood Cliffs, N.J., 1963, Prentice-Hall, Inc.

21. Gilhool, T., and Stutman, N.: Integration of severely handicapped students: toward criteria for implementing and enforcing the integration imperative of P.L. 94-142 and Section 504, Philadelphia, 1977, Public Interest Law Center of Philadelphia.

22. Guild, W. R.: How to keep fit and enjoy it, New York, 1967, Cornerstone Library, Inc.

23. Gurney, R.: Hereditary factors in obesity, Arch. Intern. Med. **57**:557-561, 1956.

24. Haskell, W. L., and Fox, S. M.: The possible place of stress testing to discover and physical activity to prevent coronary heart disease, South. Med. J. Assoc. **59**:642-647, 1966.

25. Hettinger, T.: Physiology of strength, Springfield, Ill., 1961, Charles C Thomas, Publisher.

26. Hutinger, P. A.: A key for delaying the aging process, Swimmer Magazine, February/March 1979, pp. 36-41.

27. Johnson, L., and Londeree, B.: Motor fitness testing manual for the moderately mentally retarded, Washington, D.C., 1976, American Alliance for Health, Physical Education, and Recreation.

28. Jones, K., Shainberg, L., and Byer, C.: Principles of health science, New York, 1975, Harper & Row, Publishers.

29. Kasch, F.: Physiological variables during 10 years of endurance exercise, Med. Sci. Sports Spring **8**:5-8, 1976.

30. Kraus, H., and Hifschland, R. P.: Minimum muscular fitness in school children, Res. Q. **25**:178-188, 1954.

31. Kraus, H., and Raab, W.: Hypokinetic disease, Springfield, Ill., 1961, Charles C Thomas, Publisher.

32. Logan, G. A., and Egstrom, G.: Effects of slow and fast stretch on the sacrofemoral angle, Paper presented to AAHPER Southern District Convention, Albuquerque, N.M., April, 1955.

33. Lourie, R. S.: A pediatric-psychiatric viewpoint on obesity, Pediatrics **20**:552-556, 1957.

34. Master, A. M., Jaffe, H. L., and Chesky, K.: Relationship of obesity to coronary disease and hypertension, J.A.M.A. **153**:1449-1501, 1953.

35. Mateeff, D.: Problems of the fight for longevity, Quest, 1964.

36. Mayer, G.: Obesity in school children, Nutr. Rev. **15**:233, 1957.

37. Mayer, J.: Middle-aged man must exercise, Postgrad. Med. J. **40**:127-132, 1966.

38. Morgan, R. E., and Adamson, G. T.: Circuit training, London, 1961, G. Bell & Sons, Ltd.

39. Pryor, H. B.: Charts of normal body measurements and revised width-weight tables in graphic form, J. Pediatr. **68**:615-631, 1966.

40. Pryor, H. B.: Width-weight tables, ed. 2, Stanford, Calif., 1936, Stanford University Press.

41. Rarick, G. L., and Dobbins, D. A.: Basic components in the motor performance of educable mentally retarded children: implications for curriculum development, Berkeley, Calif., 1972, University of California.

42. Rarick, G. L., and McQuillian, J. P.: The factor structure of motor abilities of trainable mentally retarded children: implications for curriculum development, Project No. H23-2544, for the Department of Health, Education, and Welfare, Bureau of Education for the Handicapped, Berkeley, Calif., 1977, University of California.

43. Selye, H.: The stress of life, New York, 1956, McGraw-Hill Book Co.

44. Special fitness test manual for mildly mentally retarded persons, Washington, D.C., 1976, American Alliance for Health, Physical Education, and Recreation.

45. Stecher, P. G., et al.: The Merck index, ed. 8, Rahway, N.J., 1968, Merck & Co., Inc.

46. Stein, J.: Adaptation of the internal system to general exercises and calisthenics, Phys. Educ. **17**:1-6, 1960.

47. U.S. Public Health Service: Obesity and health, Washington, D.C., 1966, U.S. Government Printing Office.

48. Vodala, T. M.: Individualized physical education program for the handicapped child, Englewood Cliffs, N.J., 1973, Prentice-Hall, Inc.

49. Wilkes, E. T.: A survey of three hundred obese girls, Arch. Pediatr. **77**:441-452, 1960.

50. Wolff, K.: The biological, sociological, and psychological aspects of aging, Springfield, Ill., 1959, Charles C Thomas, Publisher.

51. Youth fitness test manual, Washington, D.C., 1965, American Alliance for Health, Physical Education, and Recreation.

RECOMMENDED READINGS

Behnke, A. R., and Wimore, J. H.: Evaluations and regulations of body build and composition, Englewood Cliffs, N.J., 1974, Prentice-Hall, Inc.

Bowerman, W. J., and Harris, W. E.: Jogging: a physical fitness program for all ages, New York, 1967, Grosset & Dunlap, Inc.

Clarke, H. H.: Muscular strength and endurance in man, Englewood Cliffs, N.J., 1966, Prentice-Hall, Inc.

Cooper, K. H.: Aerobics, New York, 1970, Bantam Books, Inc.

Guthrie, H. A.: Introductory nutrition, ed. 4, St. Louis, 1979, The C. V. Mosby Co.

The healthy life: special report, New York, 1966, Time-Life Books.

Williams, S. R.: Nutrition and diet therapy, ed. 3, St. Louis, 1977, The C. V. Mosby Co.

8

Modifying sports and games

No program of adapted physical education should be considered complete unless it includes provision for modifying sports and games.

There are two broad aspects of the physical education program. One is the portion of the program in which the student engages in activity for the purpose of individual development of skills and abilities. The other involves the expression of these skills in the playing of games. There may be development of individual skills in playing games, but because of the lack of control of specific conditions this development evolves, for the most part, by chance. The primary value of playing the game is to learn rules and strategies and derive benefit from the social interaction with teammates. This chapter will address the problem of adapting sports and games for the purpose of including handicapped children in games with their peers in an integrated setting, the regular class.

SECTION 504 AND MODIFICATION OF SPORTS AND GAMES

Chapter 1 discussed in detail the need for accommodating individual differences in the least restrictive environment. Section 504 of the Rehabilitation Act of 1973[16] states clearly that "no handicapped person shall be excluded from participation," in this context from participation in sports and games with the nonhandicapped. Furthermore, it also indicates that handicapped persons shall not be denied benefits of programs, in this case benefits of participation in sports and games. Thus, methods must be developed that will help the handicapped to participate to the greatest extent possible in games and sports activities with the nonhandicapped. P.L. 94-142[17] indicates that physical education should *develop* physical and motor fitness, fundamental motor patterns and skills, team sports skills, and lifetime sports skills. Although developmental activities are essential for conducting physical education programs for the handicapped, accommodations must be made for them to participate in sports and games. There are many reasons that it is desirable to include a program of modified sports and games for these students. Some of the reasons for including adapted sports activities in the program are the following:

1. Handicapped students need activities that have carryover value. They may continue exercise programs in the future, but they also need training in sports and games that will be useful to them in later life.
2. Modified sports have therapeutic value if they are carefully structured for the students.
3. Modified sports and games should help handicapped persons learn to handle their bodies under a variety of circumstances.
4. There are recreational values in games and sports activities for students who are facing the dual problem of getting a good education and overcoming some type of handicap; some

of their special needs can best be met through recreational kinds of activities.

5. A certain amount of emotional release takes place in play activities and this is important to students with disabilities.
6. The modified sports program, whether it is given every other day or several weeks out of the semester, tends to relieve the boredom of a straight exercise program. No matter how carefully a special exercise program is planned, it is difficult to maintain a high level of interest if the students participate in this kind of activity on a daily basis.

Many handicapped students will be mainstreamed and attend regular physical education classes. Some of these students will not need modification of sports and games to participate. However, for some activities in regular class some handicapped students will need such modification. Sometimes students in regular physical education

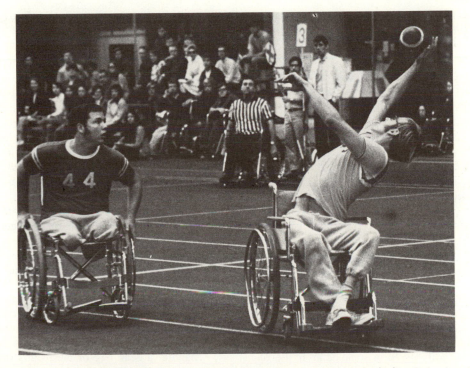

Fig. 8-1. An individual in a wheelchair stretches to catch a long pass. (Courtesy of Julian Stein, American Alliance for Health, Physical Education, Recreation, and Dance and Rehabilitation Education Center, University of Illinois, Champaign-Urbana, Ill.)

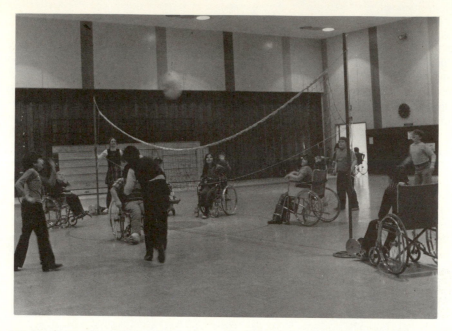

Fig. 8-2. Handicapped persons participating in a volleyball game in which the area has been reduced. (Provided through Unit on Programs for the Handicapped, American Alliance for Health, Physical Education, Recreation, and Dance.)

classes who sustain injuries or come back from illnesses need special exercises or special activity programs. When cooperation exists between the medical service and the teachers of the adapted and the regular physical education classes, these students are assigned to the adapted class for their physical education so that they can profit from the special attention provided there.

When one hears the term *adapted games and sports,* two kinds of activities might very well come to mind: (1) there are certain kinds of physical education activities that lend themselves especially well to activity programs for students who have some kind of a physical handicap and (2) almost any activity that can be engaged in by students in a regular physical education class in public or private schools can be modified to the special needs of students. In its broadest sense, the adapted sports and games program should include both categories. Each is discussed in some detail in the following sections of this chapter.

Practically all games and sports in which students regularly participate in physical education classes can, with minor modifications, be made

safe and interesting for the handicapped. In general, the rules, techniques, and equipment of a game or activity should be changed as little as possible when modifying for handicapped students. One should, however, retain as many of the elements of the regular game or activity as possible. Some of the ways that regular physical education and sports activities can be modified are the following:

1. The size of the playing area can be made smaller, reducing the amount of activity proportionately.
2. Often, larger balls or larger pieces of equipment can be introduced to make the game easier or to slow down the tempo.
3. For other types of games and sports, a smaller, lighter ball or striking implement may be necessary (plastic or styrofoam balls and plastic bats) or an object that is easier to handle (a bean bag or Nerf ball) can be substituted.
4. More players can be added to a team, reducing the amount of activity and the responsibility of individuals in a game.

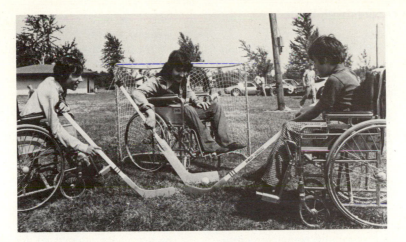

Fig. 8-3. Equipment and facilities can be altered to accommodate handicapped persons. (Provided through Unit on Programs for the Handicapped, American Alliance for Health, Physical Education, Recreation, and Dance.)

5. Minor rule changes can be made in the contest or game while as many of the basic rules as possible are retained.
6. The amount of time allowed for play can be reduced by providing shorter quarters, or the total time for a game can be reduced.
7. An attempt can be made to avoid *headlining* by any one player. In games such as softball, soccer, and football, players can be required to rotate positions frequently so that all the participants will have an opportunity to perform various kinds of activities and play various positions (as long as a particular position or activity would not be contraindicated for any one of the participants).
8. The number of points required to win a contest can be reduced.
9. Free substitutions can be made, allowing the students alternately to participate and then rest while the contest continues.

These modifications can be made in a game or contest whether the students participate in handicapped-only or regular physical education classes.

If the handicapped child participates in a handicapped-only class, it is possible to provide activities similar to those of regular physical education classes by using many of the sports fundamentals that are involved and by practicing them in drill types of activities. An example would be playing such basketball games as "twenty-one," "two on two," and "around the world" or taking free throws as lead-up activities to the sport. Punting, passing, running pass patterns, and place kicking may be done in preparation for participation in football. Pitching, batting, throwing, catching, fielding, and games such as "over the line" can be played as lead-up activities for softball. Serving, stroking, volleying, and the like can be practiced as lead-up activities for tennis. In all cases, these activities serve as modifications of a sport or game, provide interesting activities for the student, and ensure similar kinds of drills to those being engaged in by the regular physical education student. They also help handicapped students become more skillful in various activities, so that when they return to a regular class or are able to participate in the whole game or sport, they are able to do so with a reasonable degree of success.

TYPES OF ADAPTATIONS FOR THE LEARNER

There are three broad groups of handicapped children who require modified games and sports: (1) children who are orthopedically handicapped and have impaired movement, (2) those who have sensory problems and cannot interpret events in the environment, and (3) those who are capable of limited activity but possess movement capability. Each of these requires different techniques of adapting the classroom environment.

Adaptations for children with limited movement

There are several options to accommodate individual problems for children with limited movement. First, games may be selected that circumvent the inability to move. This enables handicapped children to participate in a normal environment with their peers. However, it is obvious that such activity will comprise but a small part of the games and sports of the total physical education program. Second, in team sports it is not uncommon for specific positions of a sport to require different degrees of movement. Thus, those children who are limited in movement capability assume those positions that require less movement. Third, the rules of the game can be modified, enabling equitable competition between the handicapped and the nonhandicapped. Fourth, aids can be introduced that accommodate the inability so that adjustments can be made to the game. Any one or a combination of these principles of adaptation may be employed to enable handicapped children to participate in regular classes.

Adaptations for children with sensory problems

Children who are blind and deaf have different problems from those who are limited in movement. Their basic problem is that of receiving appropriate information from the environment in which they must perform a physical task. Blind or visually limited children have difficulty interpreting information required for participation in games involving projectiles and rapidly changing conditions requiring visual assessment. On the other hand, the deaf are usually impaired in such activities as rhythm and in receiving instruction and information that rely on the auditory mechanism. In both cases, adaptations can be made to include these children in activities utilizing the functional senses. Blind persons require adaptive environments when kinesthesia and audition are used for communication. Deaf persons must have amplification of auditory signals. Detailed suggestions for adapting games for children with sensory problems can be found in Chapter 14.

Adaptations for children with limited activity

Children who have heart conditions, asthma, or other disabilities that contraindicate intense and/or prolonged activity may need adaptation of the amount and intensity of the activity. There are at least three procedures for these types of adaptation: first, games can be selected that do not require considerable activity; second, rest periods can be introduced at intervals commensurate with the children's functional capabilities; third, the children can be assigned to positions that require lesser degrees of physical involvement. Any one or a combination of the adaptive techniques may enable handicapped children to participate in regular physical education classes.

PROCEDURE FOR ADAPTING SPORTS AND GAMES

Teachers who attempt to include handicapped children in games and sports in the regular physical education class must be able to apply principles of adapting the sports and games to each child. It is beyond the scope of this book to compile adaptations of games for a wide range of handicapping conditions. Therefore, it is desirable for physical education teachers of the handicapped to apply principles of adapting sports activity. Below is a suggested procedure for adapting a sport or game to a handicapped child:

1. Select and analyze the sport or game to be played.
2. Identify the problems the individual child will have in participating in the sport or game.
3. Make the adaptations to the sport or game.
4. Select principles of adaptation that may apply to the specific situation.

PRINCIPLES FOR ADAPTING SPORTS AND GAMES

There are at least two interrelated considerations that physical education teachers must make to effectively modify games and sports activities to accomodate handicapped children. First, the nature of the handicaps should be considered. Children who have sensory impairments and those who have limited mobility or are prescribed to limited activity possess different needs of modification. Second, the nature of the physical education activity is an important consideration. Specific tasks are more easily adapted to particular types of handicaps. Third, specific principles of adaptation should be applied in modifying games and sports. The next

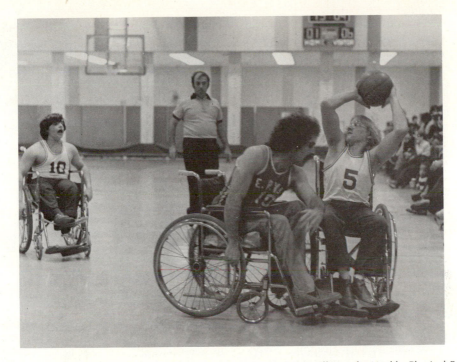

Fig. 8-4. Wheelchair basketball. (Courtesy of Julian Stein, American Alliance for Health, Physical Education, Recreation, and Dance and Human Resources Center, Albertson, N.Y.)

Table 8-1. Modifications for handicapping conditions

Handicap	Activity	Modification
Blind	Archery	Pegs in the ground for stance
Blind	Class management	Environment that is ordered and consistent
Blind	Running	Ropes for guidance
Blind	Swimming	Ropes that designate the swimming lane
Blind	Class management	Reference points that indicate the location of the child in the play area
Blind	Softball	Concrete or sand for base paths
Blind	Softball	Concrete bases slightly raised above base path
Blind	Softball	Different texture of ground or floor when near a surface that could result in a serious collision
Blind	Track	Sand, different texture of surface at finish line, and ropes for guidance
Mentally retarded	Class management	Pictures or stick symbols to communicate rather than written or spoken words
Learning disabled	Class management	Environment free from distractions
Learning disabled	Body management	Footprints and handprints to assist direction of body parts
Physically handicapped	Mobility	Handrails
Blind	Class management	Auditory cues to identify obstacles in the environment
Blind	Class management	Tactile markings on the floor
Blind	Class management	Rings or ropes that hang from the ceiling to indicate student's location
Blind	Class management	Boundaries of different texture
All handicapped	Swimming	Swimming pool with nonslip bottom

portion of the chapter indicates the principles that assist in the accommodation of a wide variety of handicapping conditions in a considerable number of sport skills and games. Some suggested principles are as follows:

1. Design the instructional environment to accommodate the individual.
2. Introduce special devices, aids, and equipment to assist the individual.
3. Utilize special instructional techniques to accommodate the individual.
4. Introduce precautionary safety measures to meet the individual's needs.
5. Provide special feedback for tasks to facilitate learning.
6. Employ nonhandicapped peers to assist with instruction.
7. Train the individual for mobility and understanding the environment.

The instructional environment

The physical education facility can be designed to accommodate persons with handicapping conditions. Such adaptations of the environment might be handrails to enable physically handicapped persons to move safely and support themselves, or visual and auditory cues, for children with sensory impairment to provide information for appropriate physical activity. Altering the design of the instructional environment is particularly useful for adapting sports and games for children with sensory impairment and those with deficient mobility. Examples of applying this principle to specific types of handicapping conditions and specific activities are listed in Table 8-1.

Special devices, aids, and equipment

Special devices, aids, and equipment are used by handicapped children to respond successfully in physical activity. With blind persons, audible balls are used in games involving projectiles. Introduction of this special equipment enables the blind and partially sighted to participate in such games as soccer, basketball, and softball. Physically handicapped children use crutches for locomotion in game activity. Equipment designed specifically for them may also enable participation in many activities (Fig. 8-5). Some examples of special equipment and devices are listed in Table 8-2.

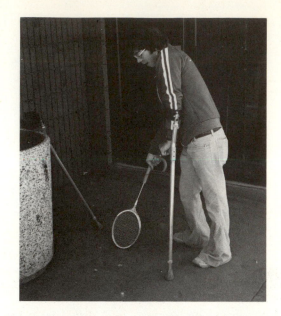

Fig. 8-5. Modification of equipment and the playing environment enables physically handicapped person to participate in racquet sports. (Courtesy of Julian Stein, American Alliance for Health, Physical Education, Recreation, and Dance and Alameda Unified School District, Hayward, Calif.)

Special instructional techniques

Special instructional techniques enable the physical education teacher to communicate activities to handicapped children. Some of the techniques that can be used are controlling the attention of the learner, precise verbal instructions, and appropriate selection of the sensory avenue for communication. Children with sensory disorders must receive instructional communication through the remaining effective avenues. Thus, instruction must be adapted by utilizing the appropriate sensory avenue. Furthermore, children who are incapable of understanding complex verbal instructions and explanations need concise and sometimes multisensory techniques of instruction. Examples of special instructional techniques for handicapped children are listed in Table 8-3.

Special task feedback

Handicapped children need to know the effects of their performance on tasks of physical activity. However, in the case of children with sensory im-

Table 8-2. Special devices, aids, and equipment for handicapping conditions

Handicap	Activity	Device, aid, or equipment
Orthopedically handicapped	Bowling	Lighter ball
Orthopedically handicapped	Softball	Whiffle ball bat
Learning disabled	Ball catching	Balloon or large ball
All handicapped	Swimming	Flotation to increase buoyancy
All handicapped	Gymnastics	Safety belt
All handicapped	Gymnastics	Soft mat to protect the performers

Table 8-3. Instructional techniques for handicapping conditions

Handicap	Instructional technique
Blind	Give clear auditory signals with a whistle or megaphone.
Blind	Instruct through manual guidance.
Blind	Use braille to teach cognitive materials before class.
Blind	Encourage tactual exploration of objects to determine texture, size, and shape.
Mentally retarded	Instruct simply and concisely.
Mentally retarded	Model what is to be done with a simultaneous verbal description and visual model of the behavior.
Blind	Address the child by name.

pairment, some activities provide little knowledge as to the quality of performance. For example, blind children do not have the opportunity to receive visual feedback on tasks that require the use of a projectile. Therefore, buzzers or bells may be inserted in a basket to inform a blind person when a basket has been made. In addition, as has already been mentioned, gravel may be placed around stakes for horseshoes to inform as to the accuracy of a toss. On the other hand, deaf persons must be able to receive visual feedback. Therefore, electrical lighting devices can be incorporated into the task equipment.

It is not possible to magnify the feedback for certain types of motor tasks for specific types of learners. Therefore, it is suggested that peers be trained to provide feedback for one another. Feedback is particularly important when the physical education teacher is working with short-term instructional objectives. An essential component of the objective is the criterion (see Chapter 4), which indicates whether the task has been completed to mastery. Thus, attention to modification of the feedback properties of tasks increases the quality of programming for handicapped children.

Peer assistance

Nonhandicapped peers can assist the handicapped child with instruction in mainstream situations. The nature of this assistance will depend on the nature of the task and the handicapping condi-

tion. For instance, if a child is blind, peer assistance may be required for movement in the play area or for feedback regarding performance. On the other hand, if a child is mentally retarded, peer assistance may involve the instruction of correct techniques and feedback on the task response. If the child is deaf, peer assistance may involve communicating instructional content. However, when nonhandicapped peers take part in the instructional process with handicapped children, it is necessary that such management does not deter the learning of the nonhandicapped. Thus, peer assistance to the handicapped involves a small part of the class period and minimally disrupts the performance of the nonhandicapped.

Mobility and orientation training

Mobility and orientation training is an adaptive technique that applies particularly to children with limited vision. Orientation training refers to teaching the structure of the environment, whereas mobility training involves teaching how to move in the structured environment. It is suggested that a program of mobility and orientation training be provided to blind children so that they may learn about play areas where physical activity occurs. Such a program expands the capability of participation in physical education, increases confidence to move with greater authority, provides greater safety to the blind while they are participating. Thus, programs of mobility and orientation train-

Table 8-4. Safety measures for handicapping conditions

Principle	Handicap	Safety measure
Protection of vulnerable parts of the anatomy	Blind	Protect eyes
	Orthopedically handicapped	Protect physically disabled part
	All handicaps	Protect all body parts, spotting in gymnastics
Protection of aids	Partially sighted	Protect eyeglasses
	Hard of hearing	Protect hearing aid
Safe equipment	Blind	Use a sponge ball for softball, volleyball, and many projectile activities
Structure of safe environment	Blind	Check play areas for obstacles and holes in the ground
	Blind	Carry out activity away from walls
Activity according to ability	Blind	Avoid activities that require children to pass each other at high speeds
	All handicapped	Close supervision of all potentially dangerous activity
	Heart condition	Schedule frequent rest periods

ing are valuable ways to modify participation in sports and games for blind children.

Safety measures

Handicapped persons often have limited capability to cope with events while participating in activities that may endanger their safety. Precautions that can be taken to reduce the chance of injury are the following:

1. Protection of specific vulnerable parts of the anatomy.
2. Structure of activities commensurate with the child's abilities.
3. Protection of vital areas of disability through the use of aids such as orthopedic braces, prostheses, crutches, and canes.
4. Selection of safe equipment.
5. Structure of a safe environment.

Examples of applying these principles to specific handicapping conditions are listed in Table 8-4.

Physical education instructors of the handicapped must constantly be aware of any situations in the adapted activity program that would be hazardous to students in their classes. They must also be alert to any situations that would tend to aggravate the condition of any of the students. For these reasons, each activity must be assigned to a student on an individual basis, predicated whenever possible on the student's interest, but, more important, based on the good judgement of the physical education teacher and on the recommendations of the physician. All students in the program must be cautioned to watch for certain signs indicating that they or their classmates are involved in inappropriate activity. Students should be instructed to stop an activity and report to the instructor if any of the following conditions are noted: (1) pain in any part of the body, (2) dyspnea (shortness of breath), (3) abnormal amount of flushing about the face, (4) feeling of general systemic fatigue, or (5) cyanosis (blueness of the lips).

If students are observed to have these conditions or if they report them to the instructor, their activity program must immediately be reevaluated and modification of their activity programs may be necessary.

SELECTED ADAPTED GAMES

A large selection of interesting games geared to the interest and ability levels of various age and disability groups can be found in a number of standard sources in the library. These will often be listed under the categories of games or recreational activities recommended for the elementary, the junior and senior high school, or the college age level; according to the type of activity involved, for example, *quiet games, low organization games,* and *active games;* or according to the type of activity area needed, for example, table games, indoor games, and outdoor games. Some authors have even organized their adapted sports and games according to disabilities so that the teacher

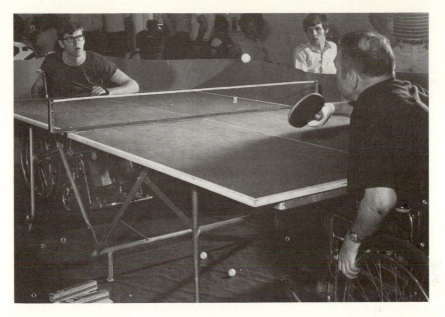

Fig. 8-6. The environment for table tennis is modified so that the balls that go off the table remain close enough to be retrieved by the students. (Courtesy of Julian Stein, American Alliance for Health, Physical Education, Recreation, and Dance and Rehabilitation Education Center, University of Illinois, Champaign-Urbana, Ill.)

can find recommended activities under such headings as cardiac conditions, asthma, or cerebral palsy. Many of these games can be used as described, but others will have to be modified for use in the adapted program. Careful study of these references and a little ingenuity on the part of teachers will enable them to select a number of these games for inclusion in the program (Table 8-5).

Adapted games and sports are generally offered in one of several activity areas in the physical education plant: the adapted physical education room, the gymnasium, the blacktop area, the fields, the pool, or the dance studio.

Indoor games

Contests and relays can be organized to include some of the actual exercises and activities in which the students participate during their regular developmental exercise programs. A typical lesson might consist of the following activities: a short formal warm-up for all students led by the instructor, followed by 15 minutes of special and group exercises done by individuals and small groups of students in the class, and then a 10-minute game and activity period under the general direction of the teacher.

A few examples of the kinds of activities that might be given in this type of a situation follow. A posture relay might be conducted with squads chosen by the instructor according to their special abilities or limitations. The students would run a traditional type of relay but would be walking with headboards or books balanced on their heads, thus working for good balance and good body mechanics as they participate in the relay. A game of swat tag with students deployed in a circular formation could be used in a similar way. This is a very popular kind of activity. A pigeon-toe walk relay might involve short distances but require that the student throw the foot into an overcorrected position while involved in this lap of the relay. There might be relays for students to pick up marbles with the toes and drop them into a box, using an activity similar to an exercise that they might have in the exercise program for their feet. Over-the-head and under-the-leg passing relays are popular,

Text continued on p. 208.

Table 8-5. Suggested activities, games, and sports for adapted physical education classes

	Hindman[9]		Chapman[3]
	Book I	Book II	
INDOOR GAMES			
Quiet games			
Card games			212-213
Concentration (2 players)	140		
Authors (4-8 players)	141		
Go fish (3-6 players)	142		
Wild eights (crazy eights) (2-4 players)	143		
Card cutting			221
Paper and pencil games			
Ticktacktoe (2 players)	147		
Battleship (2 players)	149		206-208
Table games			
Pyramid (2 players)	151		
Checkers (2 players)			
Dominoes (2 players)	92, 212		
Chess (2 players)			
Crokinole (carom) (2-4 players)	195		
Shuffleboard (table or floor) (2-4 players)	210-212		
Croquet (2-4 players)			
Active games			
Races and relays			
Head-balance race (or relay)	165		
Ping-Pong race (or relay)	166		
Paper clip relay (5-8 players on team)	174		
Arch pass relay (4-8 players on team)	178		
Car (pencil) relay (4-8 players on team)	180		
Hand clasp relay (4-8 players on team)	181		
Folding chair relay (4-8 players on team)	183		
Through-the-hoop relay (4-8 players on team)	184		
Sitting through-the-hoop relay (4-8 players on team)	184		
Rubber band relay (4-8 players on team)	185		
Over-and-under relay (8-20 players)			248-249
Throwing objects			
Balloon throw (shot put) (any number)	186		
Balloon hammer throw (any number)	186		
Playing card throw (any number)	186		220
Soda straw throw (javelin) (any number)	187		
Ball blow (asthma) (any number)	188		
Indoor lawn bowling (2-6 players)	193		
Indoor quoits (2-4 players)	194		
Bean bag board (2-4 players)	200		219, 238
Magic-square toss (2-4 players)	202		
Ball-board (2 players)	204		
Ring toss (2-4 players)			250

Eisenberg[6]	Pomeroy[13]	Fait[7]	Arnheim and Pestolesi[2]	Van Hagen, Dexter, Williams[18]	Anderson, Elliot, LaBerge[1]	ERCA[5]
363						
443						
432-434 439-440				465 908-909 583-585		
		235-241	229-241	427-432		GR 1-23
				491-492		
379			239			
				593	183	GR 26
421-422 387-388 387-388 387-388 387-388		235-241				GTC 1-24
423 426-429 426-427	316 309	237		536-538 536-538 536-538		
422-423	316					GTC 5

Continued.

Table 8-5. Suggested activities, games, and sports for adapted physical education classes—cont'd

	Hindman[9]		Chapman[3]
	Book I	Book II	
INDOOR GAMES—cont'd			
Games for adapted room			
Elementary school			
Tag with variations (5-20 players)		10-27	
Posture tag (5-20 players)		24	
Pom-pom pullaway with variations (10-20 players)		39-44	
Snatch-the-handkerchief with variations (10-20 players)		56-58	245
Hopscotch and variations (5-20 players)			
Swat tag with variations (15-30 players)		65, 81	39
Circle rush (10-25 players)		89	
Circle squat with variations (10-25 players)		175	
Simon says with variations (10-25 players)		177	251-252
Follow the leader (2-25 players)			246
Statues (10-20 players)			
Secondary school and college			
Rec-room shuffleboard (2 players)	210-212		
Table shuffleboard (2 players)	212		
Tenpins (bowling) with variations (2 players)		184	
Medicine ball (2-20 players)			262
Stall bar activities			265-266
Steal the bacon (15-30 players)			252-253
Swat tag with variations (15-30 players)		65, 81	239
Follow the leader with variations (2-20 players)			246
Wastebasket basketball (4-20 players)			
OUTDOOR GAMES AND SPORTS			
Games of low organization			
Dodge ball with variations (15-30 players)		112-119	244-245
Around the world (2-8 players)		224	
Twenty-one with variations (2-8 players)		224-229	268-269
Punt drive (association football) (4-20 players)		246-247	
Tetherball (2 players)		268-270	253-254
Parachute play			
Games and sports			
Field hockey with variations (12-22 players)		403-408	
Football variations		367-368, 397-400	275
Basketball variations (2-10 players)		362-365	257-258, 291-292
Table tennis with variations (2-4 players)		280-282	267-268
Bowling			272
Shuffleboard with variations (2-4 players)		216-220	262-263
Golf with variations			259-260
Archery (archery golf)		202	
Goal hi			258-259
Volleyball and Newcomb with variations (4-20 players)		250, 254-260	269-270
Softball with variations (4-20 players)		311-329	273-274

Eisenberg[6]	Pomeroy[13]	Fait[7]	Arnheim and Pestolesi[2]	Van Hagen, Dexter, Williams[18]	Anderson, Elliot, LaBerge[1]	ERCA[5]
463-469		229-241	224-227 227-239	410	238	GFC 1-15 GFC 14
475						
466		239				GL 11
467						GPG 3, 4 GCF 40
336		238	239 226	486-487	153	
341				411		
	308	239	233	421		
439-440				908-909		
439				908		
449		242	234	641		GCF 42
467						
373						
480		234	231-243			GTC 17-21
		243-244	244	409, 683-684	189	GB 7
			255		283	GB 9
			255	799-800	283	
			257	671-672	256	
444	320		245	588, 917	197	GPG 12
		244-246	200-201			
		298-301	257-260	752-774 659-661, 745-751, 756-761, 792-799	243-265	GT 1-6
		290-293	247-256	661-668, 678-679 720-749	274-300	GB 1-13 GR 29-31
343	321	281-286		789-791		
	311	265-266		634, 889	208-211	
439	317	286-288		892-894		
	313	268-276				
	310	262-265				
				649-652		
	323	301-303	248, 254-255	801-811	311-332	GV 1-9
	321	294-298	248-249, 260-263	566-581	353, 369, 190	GBA 1-21

Continued.

Table 8-5. Suggested activities, games, and sports for adapted physical education classes—cont'd

	Hindman[9]		Chapman[3]
	Book I	**Book II**	
Outdoor games and sports—cont'd			
Games and sports—cont'd			
Paddle tennis		278-280	
Tennis with variations (2-4 players)		261-262, 270-278	275
Croquet (roquet) (2-6 players)		199-201	240-242
Horseshoe pitching (2-4 players)		203	261-262
Quoits (2-4 players)		206	
Lawn bowling with variations (2-4 persons)		207-213	256
Handball with variations (2-4 players)		283-288, 295	
Deck tennis (quoitennis) (2-8 players)		252-253	256-257
Badminton (2-4 players)		262-266	254, 255
Aerial darts (2-4 players)		266-268	
Soccer with variations (2-24 players)			273
Kickball with variations (2-24 players)			247-248
Pateca (2-4 players)			
Track and field			
Aquatic games and activities			
Water games			
Swimming			274
Baseball type (4-20 players)		322-323	
Basketball type (4-20 players)		370	270
Water polo (4-20 players)			275-276
Outdoor education			
Boating and canoeing			
Fishing			
Camping, hiking, and nature study			
Rhythm and dance			88-116
Square dance			106-116
Social dance			98-102
Folk dance			104-106
Fundamental rhythms			
Creative rhythms			
Running and jogging			

Eisenberg[6]	Pomeroy[13]	Fait[7]	Arnheim and Pestolesi[2]	Van Hagen, Dexter, Williams[18]	Anderson, Elliot, LaBerge[1]	ERCA[5]
		275-278		669-670 411, 653, 853-854	200	GPG 8, 11
	312 316			764-768		
485			257	549-552, 561 868-870	208-211 198-199 321, 332	
	310	278-281		561, 855-860		
	323	241	250, 255	773-788	222-250	GS 1-7, GR 32
486-487			249		212-218	
		270-272	257	484-485	339-347	GTF 1-10
489-493 84, 490	317-320			152-153		
	310 312			875-876		
		329-337				
236 494-540		257-259 259 256-257 254-256	218-223 208-218 205-206 206-208	191-197 204 211, 214 207-210, 931	440-446 412-438 377-384 385-398	RF 1-18 RSD 1-24 RFD 1-44 RF 19-25
			257	172-175		PFA 10, 11 PFC 3-5

as is passing a volleyball, basketball, or medicine ball back over and through a squad line. Another activity that has proved quite successful is participation in an obstacle course. Students move through each obstacle, performing an exercise or stunt or demonstrating a skill as required (Fig. 8-2). Many games that can be played in a small space and indoors can be selected from one of the standard game books. Such selections should be appropriate for the age levels, the interest levels, and the capacities of the students. Lists of such games and activities are included in Table 8-5.

Games

Some games require more space than do other games. Such games may require the use of multipurpose rooms, outside blacktop areas, swimming pools, dance studios, or athletic fields. Whenever possible, it is desirable to have handicapped students participate in a variety of activities outdoors (Fig. 8-3). Games of low organization lend themselves to this kind of activity and prove to be very popular with the students in the adapted class. Many of these games require no special type of floor or deck space and involve the use of equipment that is readily available from the regular physical education program. Lead-up activities for football, basketball, speedball, volleyball, soccer, softball, hockey, and the like can also be offered.

Special areas for modified sports

It is also possible for special adapted sports areas to be constructed to provide the kinds of activities that would lend themselves particularly well to students with severe handicaps. Special areas for adapted sports are described in Chapter 20. These special areas allow for participation in a variety of activities all concentrated in one area so that they can be supervised by one adapted physical education instructor. Paddle tennis, modified volleyball, croquet, shuffleboard, horseshoes, deck tennis, and table tennis provide interest and activity for handicapped students.

MODIFYING SPORTS AND GAMES FOR SELECTED DISABILITIES

Since most physical, mental, and emotional handicaps are quite individual in terms of what the person can and cannot do, only selected examples of how a variety of activities can be modified will be offered in this chapter. Complete texts have been written on this subject and these and other references are recommended for further study in Table 8-5 (Fig. 8-7).

Aquatics

1. Provide a device (metronome, music, etc.) that emits a sound or signal so that blind or visually handicapped persons retain their orientation while in the pool.
2. Teach persons with one arm to swim the side stroke with the remaining arm on the lower side of the body to allow them to retain balance and breathe without difficulty.
3. Teach students with partial loss of locomotion to move in the swimming pool, where body weight is minimal and muscle reeducation and body locomotion can take place during a carefully graded exercise and/or activity program.

Team sports

1. *Volleyball.* A volleyball game is modified for a senior high school class by changing it as follows. Nine players are permitted on each team, a serve can be helped over the net by a teammate for selected players, and two players are permitted to catch and then throw the ball in place of a proper pass. All other rules and techniques are the same as for a regular game.
2. *Softball.* A junior high school class of girls are playing "over the line," an adaptation of softball. The rules are modified as follows. A runner is provided for one of the girls, the line over which the ball must be hit is moved closer to the batter for three of the girls, and seven players are permitted on each team.

Dual sports

1. *Badminton.* Four students in wheelchairs and four students with mild cardiac disorders are scheduled for a game of badminton with four players on each side. Those in wheelchairs play up front; each is backed up by a cardiac teammate. Players do not rotate and each side is permitted two side outs before relinquishing the serve. The serve is alternated between the person playing short and the person playing deep. Only the serving team scores.

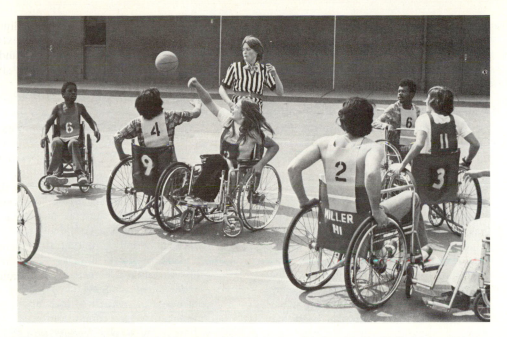

Fig. 8-7. Wheelchair basketball. (Courtesy of Lyonel Avance, Los Angeles City Unified School District, Special Education Division, Los Angeles, Calif.)

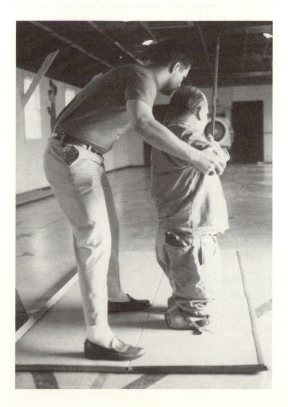

Fig. 8-8. Students who understand the fundamentals of archery can assist their handicapped peers with the mechanics of shooting in archery. (Courtesy of Julian Stein, American Alliance for Health, Physical Education, Recreation, and Dance and Coldwater State School and Hospital, Coldwater, Mich.)

2. *Table tennis.* A game of table tennis is modified so that a boy with crutches can compete with a boy with one arm. The only changes necessary are that the boy with crutches plays only one side of his half of the table. The amputee serves by balancing the ball on his paddle, throwing it up in the air, and striking it for the serve. If the ability level is still different, a handicap can be applied to the score until competition is equalized.

Individual sports

1. *Archery.* Archery can be modified in many ways to meet the special needs of boys and girls in adapted physical education classes. Blind students need a raised pointer along the ground or floor to direct them toward the target. They also need a rack to guide them in the placement of their front and back hands (to aid in giving direction and also to show how far to pull). Students with loss of strength in one hand may need to have the bow strapped to that hand. The arrow can then be properly drawn and released with the other hand. Students with leg involvement can have other students retrieve their arrows and they can shoot from crutches or wheelchairs.

2. *Bowling.* Most children and adults can be taught to bowl, regardless of their physical handicaps. Bowling can be set up in the gymnasium, on the green, or at regulation bowling alleys. Adaptations for a wheelchair bowler might consist of utilizing a smaller or lighter ball or, in cases of bilateral hand and arm weakness, a ball with a handle that snaps back or holding a special chute in the patient's lap, from which the ball is rolled to hit the pins. Wheelchair bowlers and those with problems of ambulation can use a preliminary arm swing rather than the traditional walking approach to increase the momentum and accuracy of their delivery.

Dancing and rhythms

Participation in rhythmic activities provides an important recreational outlet for many disabled persons and often provides therapeutic values as well. Many students with neuromuscular problems, including some types of cerebral palsy, can benefit from rhythmic exercises and may also profit from various types of dancing. Increased relaxation, coordination, and timing are often experienced during rhythmic activities performed to the tempo of a metronome, record, or tape or to sound patterns provided by other students using drums, tambourines, and rhythm sticks (see Fig. 20-19). Some adaptations may be necessary to protect individuals as they participate in various types of rhythmic activities. These adaptations include the following:

1. Many activities are extremely vigorous and stimulating and should be contraindicated for the severely handicapped. Time limits and scheduled rest periods should be provided.

2. Certain students, such as the mentally retarded, may need a considerable amount of individual attention during rhythmic activities, and progress may be very slow until fundamentals are learned.

3. Placement of students should be carefully considered in relation to their ability to hear the music, see the demonstration, and imitate a skill or move about easily in a dance pattern (either square or modern).

4. Psychological and emotional needs of the students may be better satisfied in rhythmic types of activities than in many other adapted activities. The proper type and amount of activity must be carefully selected by a competent and understanding teacher.

SELECTED ADAPTED SPORTS

Many handicapped students can participate in selected sports offered in the regular physical education program. However, if handicapped children are assigned to handicapped-only classes, teachers should organize sports activities that are similar to those of the regular physical education classes. These sports activities should be offered in the appropriate activity area, using equipment as similar as possible to that being used by the regular classes and with only minor adaptations in the rules of the contest when necessary.

Swimming activities and therapeutic exercises in the pool

Handicapped students can profit from a swimming program specifically designed to meet their needs. Although swimming facilities are usually heavily scheduled, it is often possible for the teacher of handicapped persons to offer a unit on swimming either between regular classes or by using the shallow end of the pool or a smaller teaching pool if one is available. It is important to remember that each handicapped student must be considered individually in relation to a program of swimming activities. Teaching some of the students regular swimming strokes and aquatic games and activities might very well aggravate conditions that already exist. Thus, already strong muscles would be overstrengthened at the expense of weak ones. It is therefore necessary that some students either be taught adaptations of the regular swimming strokes or activities or be provided with therapeutic exercise programs designed to help them strengthen their weak areas.[11]

Adapting sports and games for use in the pool

Adapting therapeutic exercises for use in a pool is covered in Chapter 5. Adapting sports and games and choosing perceptual-motor activities for use in an aquatics program are presented in the following sections of this chapter.

Shallow-water activities

Water volleyball. Water volleyball is an excellent activity because of its recreational, fitness, and teamwork values. Modification of rules and techniques should be based on the abilities of the players involved and might include any of the following:

1. Allow for an assist on the serve (or a substitute server).
2. Reduce the size of the playing area and increase the number of players (since it is very difficult to move from place to place and cover more than a minimal area).
3. Allow more flexibility in passing techniques (four or more passes allowed on a side and standard bump pass not required).
4. For the severely handicapped, use a lighter ball.
5. Allow players to use flotation devices, if necessary. (If inner tubes are used, the valve stems should be removed or taped down to prevent injury to players.)

Water polo. Water polo allows walking, running, swimming, and passing to advance the ball toward the opponents' goal. The ball is not out of bounds until it actually passes across the edge of the pool, that is, the ball can strike the pool edge

and rebound into the pool and it is still in play. Other modifications of rules and techniques may include any of the following:

1. Use a larger, lighter ball.
2. Allow those who need them to use flotation devices; the ball may then be carried in the tube for a maximum of five arm strokes.
3. Allow no player contact.
4. Allow no more than five walking or running steps to be taken before the ball is passed or shot.
5. Increase the number of players and reduce the size of the playing area.
6. On the pool deck, use regular playground benches turned on their sides, with the legs turned toward the pool, as goals.

Water basketball. Water basketball allows for walking, running, swimming, and passing to advance the ball toward the opponents' basket. The ball is not out of bounds until it passes completely across the pool edge. Other modifications of rules and techniques may include any of the following:

1. Use a smaller, lighter ball.
2. Allow those who need them to use flotation devices; the ball may then be carried in the tube for a maximum of five arm strokes.
3. Allow no player contact.
4. Allow no more than five walking or running steps to be taken before the ball is passed or shot.
5. Increase the number of players and reduce the size of the playing area, if necessary.
6. Offensive players cannot shoot from closer than 8 feet from the basket.
7. Mount regular basketball backboards and baskets on frames that sit on the pool deck at either end of the playing area. The baskets should be placed so that they are 12 to 18 inches above the water's surface. Another adaptation is to place tires on the side of the pool or inner tubes in the pool to serve as baskets.

Deep-water activities

All the games described in the previous section can be played in deep water, but some further modifications may be necessary.

Water volleyball. A possible modification of rules for deep-water volleyball may be as follows:

1. Serves may be made from a sitting position

on the side or an overhand pass type serve, which may be assisted over the net, may be allowed.

2. A small court size or a large number of players is necessary, since players can only cover an area a little less than their reach in each direction.

3. All types of passes are permitted and the number of passes and repeat hits should be increased (this improves the game and allows for rallies to take place).

4. All or some of the players may use flotation devices, life jackets, inner tubes, etc.

5. A lighter ball may be used.

6. The net should be suspended with its top about 3 feet above the water surface; a paddle tennis or badminton net may be used in place of the regulation volleyball net.

Water polo. Possible modifications of rules for water polo in deep water may be as follows:

1. All or some of the players may use flotation devices.

2. Players using tubes for flotation may carry the ball in their tubes for not over five arm strokes before they must pass the ball or shoot.

3. Players with life jackets and those swimming freely may not use more than five arm strokes before they must pass the ball or shoot.

4. No player contact should be allowed; that is, the ball only should be played.

5. The size of the playing area may need to be reduced or the number of players increased according to the abilities of the contestants.

Water basketball. Suggested modifications for deep-water basketball will be the same as those for water polo in deep water.

Perceptual-motor activities in the pool

A variety of perceptual-motor activities can be included in aquatic programs. Activities can be planned so that the participants will be able to keep their heads above the water at all times; underwater activities can be planned in which participants look at or retrieve objects that are either at the bottom of or are suspended in the water. In addition to the

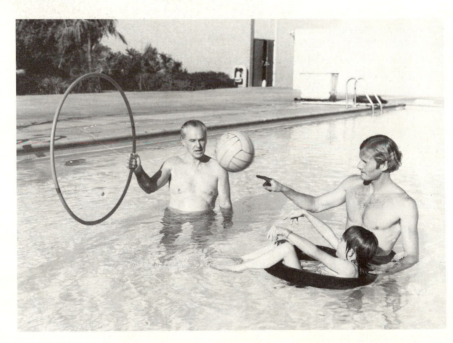

Fig. 8-9. College instructor and teacher-in-training provide aquatic skills instruction. (Courtesy of California State University, Audio Visual Center, Long Beach, Calif.)

motor activity involved, considerable learning can take place if the objects in the pool are of different shapes and colors, if they have numbers or letters printed on them, and if the clinician or teacher includes conceptual development as a part of each appropriate activity. Some of the different types of equipment that can be used in the aquatic program are described in the following sections.

1. Balls of different sizes and weights can be thrown, pushed, sunk, or used to support the student. They can be employed in a variety of games and activities (Fig. 8-9).

2. Hoops, like hula hoops (of various colors and sizes), normally float on the surface and can be used as targets in throwing activities; the student can be positioned inside or outside of them. The hoops can be weighted on one side so as to float vertically, thereby serving as a tunnel through which to dive and swim, or they can be weighted so as to sink to the bottom to be stood in, to be walked around, to serve as a target, or to be dived for and brought to the surface.

3. Floating plaques of various sizes, shapes, and colors can be used with the previously described equipment either as targets or to be thrown into a target. Students can be asked to identify plaques of different sizes, shapes, or colors or with given numbers or letters on them; to arrange several of them in various patterns; or to pass them to another person in a specified order. Plaques can also be weighted so as to float suspended in the water or so as to sink to the bottom of the pool.

4. Face masks, snorkels, fins, and swim gloves may also be used where appropriate to assist vision in the water, to aid persons with breathing problems, or to facilitate movement through the water.

5. Flotation devices such as life jackets, inner tubes (automobile, motorcycle, bicycle, etc.), styrofoam blocks, kickboards, and the like can also be used either to support an individual or one of the limbs or for many of the activities previously described. A flotation device may provide for many new and different types of experiences for persons with a variety of disabling conditions and often will serve as a vehicle to help these per-

sons overcome fears and apprehensions associated with learning to swim. Such items as life jackets and inner tubes may facilitate participation in a variety of aquatic activities and sports.

Excellent materials and activities involving therapeutic exercises, water games, and activities in the pool are offered by Lowman,[11] Daniels and Davies,[4] Fait,[7] Mathews, Kruse and Shaw,[12] and the American National Red Cross.[15]

Rope skipping

Rope skipping is an excellent activity to include in physical education programs for the handicapped. It involves exercise for a large number of the muscles of the body; it is helpful in the development of balance and coordination; and it is an excellent activity for the development of muscular endurance and cardiovascular efficiency. Since many handicapped students spend much of their time in sedentary activities, endurance activities such as rope skipping, jogging, and swimming should be a part of their total physical education experience.

Manufactured ropes with handles, some with special swivel action that facilitates turning the rope rapidly, can be purchased, or ropes can be cut from lengths of $1/4$- or $3/8$-inch diameter clothesline or nylon rope. The latter ropes are quite satisfactory and several different lengths can be cut to accommodate the various lengths needed by the students in the class. Longer lengths of rope can be used in cases in which two persons turn one or two ropes for another person to jump (Fig. 8-10). The more advanced jumper can even jump a single short rope while jumping the long rope turned by others.

Students of all ages may have some trouble in learning to skip rope. It requires patience and practice to become proficient. It is such an interesting, challenging activity that time limitations may have to be placed on certain students so that they do not overdo. Students who are under par or who experience cardiovascular insufficiency may need to have a modified program of rope skipping set up especially to meet their needs and limitations. Using heavier, slower turning ropes, with definite allotted time periods (interspersed with required rest periods), these students may be allowed to partici-

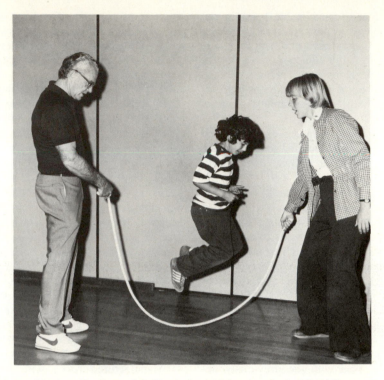

Fig. 8-10. Rope skipping. (Courtesy of California State University, Audio Visual Center, Long Beach, Calif.)

pate in rope skipping without overexertion on the approval of their physicians.

A student can learn the basic footwork involved in skipping rope simply by jumping in place on both feet at the same time; on one foot at a time, using the same foot; and on one foot at a time, alternating the feet. The hand, wrist, and arm motion can be practiced by taking both handles of the rope in one hand. Rotating the hand and wrist with the hand held down by the side of the hip, the center of the rope can be swung in a large arc in a plane parallel to the direction the student is facing. This should be practiced with each hand separately if the student is having trouble with the hand and wrist motion.

The student is then ready to put these two drills together and learn various patterns of jumping with a rope. Probably the easiest pattern to learn is to execute one single jump with each turn of the rope so that as the rope nears the feet, the student jumps just enough to clear it and to allow it to continue its swing over the head. The rope can either be turned to the front or to the rear and both types of rope skipping should be learned. The following are other types of rope jumping:

1. Jumping two times to each turn of the rope (This can be done on one or both feet.)
2. Alternating feet with each turn of the rope as in running in place
3. Jumping with one foot in front of the other so that the student "rocks" over the rope first with one foot and then with the other (either foot can be put forward in this drill)
4. Spinning the rope twice for each jump
5. Crossing the hands in front of the body as the rope swings over the head so that the jump is made with each hand placed by the opposite hip and then uncrossing the hands prior to the next jump
6. Jumping on both feet with one ankle crossed over the other
7. Jumping forward and back or side to side over a line drawn on the floor

All these styles of jumping can be executed

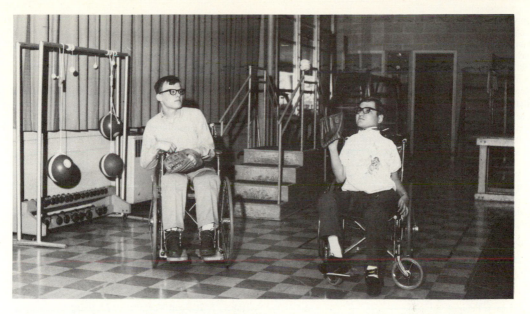

Fig. 8-11. Sports activities for children in wheelchairs. (Courtesy of Julian Stein, American Alliance for Health, Physical Education, Recreation, and Dance.)

while the rope is swung either forward or backward and all should be practiced both ways until perfected.

After these patterns have been learned, they can be worked into numerous combinations to challenge those of all ability levels in the program.[2,5,8]

SUGGESTED ACTIVITIES, GAMES, AND SPORTS FOR ADAPTED PHYSICAL EDUCATION CLASSES

The activities, games, and sports listed and classified in Table 8-5 are described in detail in standard texts on recreation, games, and stunts; in specific texts for some of the better-known sports and games; or in special sources on recreation for the handicapped. Two or three references are given for each activity presented in the chart in order to facilitate finding descriptions of the activities. Additional information about sports and games can be found in Stafford,[14] Hunt,[10] Pomeroy,[13] and Fait.[7]

Many of the games and sports listed can be used with handicapped children without modification. In many cases, modified forms of the activity are suggested in the text. Any game can be modified as much as desired by applying the techniques suggested earlier in this chapter (Fig. 8-11).

The full reference for each book cited in Table 8-5 appears in the reference list at the end of the chapter. Additional information on adapting activities is given in Chapters 12, 14, and 16.

REFERENCES

1. Anderson, M. H., Elliot, M. E., and LaBerge, J.: Play with a purpose, New York, 1966, Harper & Row, Publishers.
2. Arnheim, D. D., and Pestolesi, R.A.: Developing motor behavior in children: a balanced approach to elementary physical education, St. Louis, 1973, The C. V. Mosby Co.
3. Chapman, F. M.: Recreation activities for the handicapped, New York, 1960, The Ronald Press Co.
4. Daniels, A. S., and Davies, E. A.: Adapted physical education, ed. 3, New York, 1975, Harper & Row, Publishers.
5. Educational Research Council of America: Physical education program guide, Columbus, Ohio, 1969, Charles E. Merrill Publishing Co.
6. Eisenberg, H., and Eisenberg, L.: Omnibus of fun, New York, 1956, Association Press.
7. Fait, H. F.: Special physical education, Philadelphia, 1972, W. B. Saunders Co.
8. Fitness for children through hopscotch, rope skipping, peg board, Sacramento, Calif., 1957, California State Department of Education.
9. Hindman, D. A.: Complete book of games and stunts, Englewood Cliffs, N.J., 1959, Prentice-Hall, Inc.
10. Hunt, V. V.: Recreation for the handicapped, Englewood Cliffs, N.J., 1955, Prentice-Hall, Inc.

11. Lowman, C. L.: Technique of underwater gymnastics, Los Angeles, 1937, American Publications, Inc.
12. Mathews, D. K., Kruse, R., and Shaw, V.: The science of physical education for handicapped children, New York, 1962, Harper & Row, Publishers.
13. Pomeroy, J.: Recreation for the physically handicapped, New York, 1964, Macmillan Publishing Co., Inc.
14. Stafford, G. T.: Sports for the handicapped, Englewood Cliffs, N.J., 1950, Prentice-Hall, Inc.
15. Swimming for the handicapped: instructor's manual, Washington, D.C., 1960, American National Red Cross.
16. U.S. Department of Health, Education, and Welfare, Federal Register (May 4) 1977, pp. 22676-22702.
17. U.S. Department of Health, Education, and Welfare, Federal Register (August 23) 1977, pp. 42474-42518.
18. Van Hagen, W., Dexter, G., and Williams, J. F.: Physical education in the elementary school, Sacramento, Calif., 1941, California State Department of Education.

RECOMMENDED READINGS

Abernathy, K., et al.: Jumping up and down, San Rafael, Calif., 1970, Academic Therapy Publications.
Adams, W. C., Daniel, A., and Rullman, L.: Games, sports, and exercises for the physically handicapped, Philadelphia, 1972, Lea & Febiger.
Boehm, D. A.: The family game book, New York, 1967, Doubleday and Co., Inc.
Bond, G.: An adapted surfing device, Unpublished master's thesis, California State University, Long Beach, 1974.
Borst, E., and Mitchell, E.: Social games for recreation, New York, 1959, The Ronald Press Co.
Bowerman, W. J., and Harris, W. E.: Jogging, New York, 1967, Grosset & Dunlap, Inc.
Brownell, C. L., and Moore, R. B.: Recreational sports, Mankato, Minn., 1969, Creative Educational Society, Inc.
Carr, D. B., et al.: Sequenced instructional programs in physical education for the handicapped, P.L. 88-164, Title III, December 1970, Los Angeles, 1970, Los Angeles City Schools Special Education Branch, Physical Education Project.
Chaney, C., and Kephart, N. C.: Motoric aids to perceptual training, Columbus, Ohio, 1968, Charles E. Merrill Publishing Co.
Clark, D. E.: Physical education: a program of activities, St. Louis, 1969, The C. V. Mosby Co.
Counselman, J. E.: The science of swimming, Englewood Cliffs, N.J., 1969, Prentice-Hall, Inc.
Cowart, J., and Dressel, M.: Sport adaptions for a student without fingers, J. Phys. Educ. Rec. **47:**46, 1976.
Cratty, B. J.: Development games for physically handicapped children, Palo Alto, Calif., 1969, Peek Publications.
Cratty, B. J.: Movement behavior and motor learning, ed. 3, Philadelphia, 1973, Lea & Febiger.
Cratty, B. J., and Breen, J. E.: Educational games for physically handicapped children, Denver, 1972, Love Publishing Co.
Crowe, W. C., Arnheim, D. D., and Auxter, D.: Laboratory manual in adapted physical education and recreation, St. Louis, 1977, The C. V. Mosby Co.
Dauer, V. P.: Dynamic physical education for elementary school children, Minneapolis, 1972, Burgess Publishing Co.

Designs for dance, Washington, D.C., 1968, American Association for Health, Physical Education, and Recreation.
Donnelly, R., et al.: Active games and contests, New York, 1958, The Ronald Press Co.
Drowatzky, J. N.: Physical education for the mentally retarded, Philadelphia, 1971, Lea & Febiger.
Fredrick, A. B.: 212 ideas for making low-cost physical education equipment, Englewood Cliffs, N.J., 1963, Prentice-Hall, Inc.
Graham, D., and Ingersol, J. B.: Helping adolescents get moving: the reality therapy approach, J. Phys. Educ. Rec. **46:**32-33, 1975.
Guide for programs in physical education and recreation for the mentally retarded, Washington, D.C., 1968, American Association for Health, Physical Education, and Recreation.
Hackett, L. C.: Movement exploration and games for the mentally retarded, Palo Alto, Calif., 1970, Peek Publications.
Harris, J. A.: Fun O' File, Minneapolis, 1970, Burgess publishing Co.
Hayes, S.: The use of rhythmical activities in adapted physical education, Unpublished master's thesis, University of California at Los Angeles, Los Angeles, 1957.
How we do it book, ed. 3, Washington, D.C., 1964, American Association for Health, Physical Education, and Recreation.
Huber, J. H., and Vercollone, J.: Using aquatic mats with exceptional children, J. Phys. Educ. Rec. **47:**44, 1976.
Klafs, C.: Rhythmic activities for handicapped children, Unpublished doctoral dissertation, University of Southern California, Los Angeles, 1957.
Kratz, L. E.: Movement without sight, Palo Alto, Calif., 1973, Peek Publications.
Kraus, R.: Recreation leader's handbook, New York, 1955, McGraw-Hill Book Co.
Latchaw, M.: A pocket guide for games and rhythms for the elementary school, Englewood Cliffs, N.J., 1958, Prentice-Hall Inc.
Lawrence, C. C., and Hackett, L. C.: Water learning, Palo Alto, Calif., 1975, Peek Publications.
Merrill, T.: Activities for the aged and infirm: a handbook for the untrained worker, Springfield, Ill., 1967, Charles C Thomas, Publisher.
Moran, J. M., and Kalakian, L. H.: Movement experiences for the mentally retarded or emotionally disturbed child, Minneapolis, 1974, Burgess Publishing Co.
Mulac, M. E.: Games and stunts for school, camp, and playground, New York, 1969, Harper & Row, Publishers.
Physical activities for the mentally retarded (ideas for instruction), Washington, D.C., 1968, American Association for Health, Physical Education, and Recreation.
Physical activity programs and practices for the exceptional individual, third national conference, Long Beach, Calif., 1974, The Alliance for Health, Physical Education, and Recreation.
Physical activity programs and practices for the exceptional individual, fourth national conference, Los Angeles, 1975, The Alliance for Health, Physical Education, and Recreation.
Pomeroy, J.: ''Recreation unlimited'': an approach to community recreation for the handicapped, J. Phys. Educ. Rec. **46:**301, 1975.
Practical guide for teaching the mentally retarded to swim,

Washington, D.C., 1969, American Association for Health, Physical Education, and Recreation.

Schmais, C.: What is dance therapy? J. Phys. Educ. Rec. **47:**36, 1976.

Shivers, J. S., and Fait, H. F.: Therapeutic and adapted recreational services, Philadelphia, 1975, Lea & Febiger.

Smith, H.: Water games, New York, 1967, The Ronald Press Co.

Stein, J. U.: Special olympics instructional manual, Washington, D.C., 1972, American Association for Health, Physical Education, and Recreation and the Joseph P. Kennedy, Jr. Foundation.

Stoner, W. T.: Trampoline lesson plans for teaching trampoline, Whittier, Calif., 1973, Remedial Physical Education, Lowell Joint School Districts.

Williams, A. M.: Recreation in senior years, New York, 1962, Associated Press.

Witengier, M.: An adaptive playground for physically handicapped children, Phys. Ther. **50:**821-826, 1970.

PART THREE

Programming for specific problems

An understanding of specific types of disabilities found in adapted physical education classes at the elementary, secondary, and college levels of instruction should prepare the teacher of persons with these disabilities to be better able to apply assessment procedures, to set reasonable performance objectives, and to plan appropriate exercise and activity programs for these students.

9

Posture and body mechanics

An individual's posture, in a large measure, determines the impression that he or she makes on other persons. Good posture gives the impression of enthusiasm, initiative, and self-confidence, whereas poor posture often gives the impression of dejection, lack of confidence, and fatigue. We know that faulty posture does not necessarily indicate illness; however, we also know that good posture and body mechanics help the internal organs assume a position in the body that is favorable to their proper function and that allows the body to function most efficiently. Good posture should not be confused with the ability to assume static positions in which the body is held straight and stiff and during which good alignment is achieved at the sacrifice of the ability to move and to function

properly. Possibly, *good body mechanics* would be a better term to use in describing the proper alignment and use of the body during both static and active postures.

The term *body mechanics* is sometimes defined as the static and the functional relationships between the parts that make up the body and the body as a whole. Regardless of what we call it, there is general agreement that the human body operates best when its parts are in good alignment and are maintained thus while sitting, standing, walking, or participating in a variety of occupational and recreational types of activities. It is important to remember that there is no such thing as a normal posture for an individual. Certain anatomical, ethnological, and mechanical principles have been developed over the years that aid physicians, therapists, and physical educators in the identification of faulty body mechanics both in static and in moving postures. Proper body mechanics and posture help individuals keep their bodies in proper balance with as small an expenditure of energy as possible and with the minimum amount of strain.[6,10,11]

The center of gravity of the human body is located at a point where the pull of gravity on one side is equal to the pull of gravity on the other side. This center of gravity (higher in men than in women) falls in front of the sacrum at a point ranging from approximately 54% to 56% of the individual's height when standing. The center of gravity is changed any time the body or its segments change position.

In the upright standing position, the human body is relatively unstable. Its base of support, the feet, is small; its center of gravity is high; and it consists of a number of bony segments superimposed on one another, bound together by muscles and ligaments at a large number of movable joints. Any time the body assumes a static or dynamic posture, these muscles and ligaments must act on the bony levers of the body to offset the continuous downward pull of gravity.

Whenever the center of gravity of the body falls within its base of support, a state of balance exists. The closer the center of gravity is to the center of the base of support, the better will be the balance or equilibrium. This has important implications for the individual both in terms of good posture and as it relates to good balance for all types of body movement. The body is kept well balanced for activities in which stability is important, whereas it may be purposely thrown out of equilibrium when movement is desired, speed is to be increased, or force is to be exerted on another object.[1,13,14]

As the human being matures, balance for both static and dynamic positions becomes more automatic. An individual develops a feel for a correct position in space so that little or no conscious effort is needed to regulate it and attention can be devoted to other factors involved in movement patterns. This feeling for basic postural positions as well as for dynamic movement is controlled by certain sensory organs located throughout the body. The eyes furnish visual cues relative to body position. The semicircular canals of the inner ear furnish information on body equilibrium. Receptors in the tendons, joints, and muscles also contribute to the individual's ability to feel the body's position in space. The loss or malfunction of any of these sense organs requires that major adjustments be made by the individual to compensate for its loss. Such adjustments are part of the functions performed by the physician-physical educator-therapist team.[1,5]

Therefore, it is important for physicians, teachers, and parents to include, as part of the training of children and youth, the proper use of the body and, whenever necessary, programs for the correction of defects in posture and body mechanics. There are many causes of poor posture and poor body mechanics. Included among these are such factors as environmental influences, psychological conditions, pathological conditions, growth handicaps, congenital defects, and nutritional problems. Any one of these may have an adverse effect on the posture of the growing child, the adolescent, or

the adult. Posture of the young child is discussed on pp. 37 to 38.

Environmental factors that may cause poor posture include such things as improper shoes, narrow or short socks, clothing that does not fit the growing youngster properly, and overfatigue and overwork, especially with the growing child and adolescent. Also of concern are improper seating, including chairs, tables, and desks and other insufficient objects of furniture, including short or sagging beds and poor mattresses. Some types of toys that cause asymmetrical development may have an adverse effect on the posture of the child. Examples are scooters, skateboards, skating on one skate—in fact, the unilateral use of any type of toy. Psychological problems that may lead to postural deviations include such things as egotism, shyness, modesty, hypersensitiveness, and depression. Pathological conditions, too, often lead to both functional and structural postural deviations. Some of these are faulty vision and hearing; various cardiovascular conditions; tuberculosis; arthritis; and neuromuscular conditions resulting in atrophy, dystrophy, and spasticity. Growth handicaps include some of the following types of conditions: weaknesses in the skeletal structure and in the muscular system, growth divergencies of various sorts, fatigue, and glandular malfunctions. Congenital defects include amputations, joint and bone deformities, spina bifida, clubfoot, and the like (Chapters 10 and 11). Nutritional problems include underweight, overweight, and poor nourishment.

GOOD POSTURE AND BODY MECHANICS

Before we identify some of the deviations in posture and the methods used to determine the presence and severity of these conditions, it might be beneficial to look rather carefully into the matter of what constitutes good posture and good body mechanics in various body positions.

Good posture might be defined as a position (or positions) that enables the body to function to the best advantage with regard to work, health, and appearance.[12]

Standing posture

In the standing position, the body should be held erect and well balanced but not in a stiff or posed manner. The feet should be approximately parallel and a comfortable distance apart. The weight of the body should be equally distributed over the feet and borne on the heel, along the lateral side of the bottom of the foot, and across the total ball of the foot with the assistance of the five toes. The legs should be straight but not stiff. The pelvis should be balanced over the top of the legs with the lower abdomen kept flat and with a normal amount of anteroposterior curvature in the lower back. The upper back should also have a normal amount of anteroposterior curvature; the shoulders should be

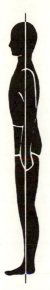

Good total alignment

Segments balanced over one another

Comfortable, alert position

A Excellent

Slight malalignment

Segments not balanced directly over one another

Note head forward, upper body flexed, knees slightly flexed

B Good

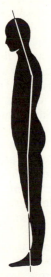

Poor total body alignment

Segments poorly balanced over base of support

Note forward head, exaggerated spinal curves, faulty leg alignment

C Fair

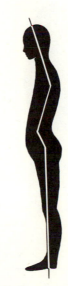

Very poor total body alignment

Body segments show total imbalance

Exaggerated curves are shown throughout body

D Poor

Fig. 9-1. Four-figure system for rough assessment of posture (used to identify students in need of a more discriminating type of posture examination).

held level and comfortably balanced with the head high, chin in, and the lobe of the ear directly over the center of the tip of the shoulder. The chest should be held high but not stiff. The shoulder blades should be flat against the back of the rib cage; the arms should hang comfortably at the

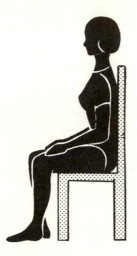

Fig. 9-2. Good sitting posture.

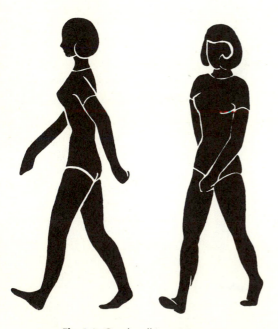

Fig. 9-3. Good walking posture.

sides. Looking at the individual from the front or rear view, the pelvis should be level, the shoulders level, the spine straight, and the head erect above the shoulders.

A side view of the person would show the following segments balanced and superimposed directly above one another: a point $1\frac{1}{2}$ inches anterior to the external malleolus, a point just posterior to the patella, the center of the hip, the center of the shoulder, and the lobe of the ear (Fig. 9-1). This test for body alignment, called the plumb line or gravity line test for standing posture, is described in a later section of this chapter.

Sitting posture

The position of the body while sitting is similar to the position of the body while standing; that is, the head is held erect, the chin is kept in, normal anteroposterior curves are maintained in the upper and lower back, and the abdomen is flat. The hips should be pushed firmly against the back of the chair. The thighs should rest on the chair and help support and balance the body. The feet should be flat on the floor or the legs comfortably crossed at the ankles. The shoulders should be relaxed and level with the chest kept comfortably high (Fig. 9-2).

Correct posture in walking

The basic position of the body in walking is similar to that of the standing posture, but all parts of the body are also involved in moving through space. The toes face straight ahead or toe out very slightly as the leg swings straight forward; the heel strikes the ground first, with the weight being transferred along the lateral side of the bottom of the foot. The weight is then shifted to the forward part of the foot and balanced across the entire ball of the foot. The step is completed with a strong push from all the toes. The upper body should be held erect with the arms swinging comfortably in opposition to the movement of the legs. The head is held erect with the chin tucked in a comfortable position. The chest is held high, the shoulder blades are flat against the rib cage, and the shoulders are held even in height (Fig. 9-3).

Persons with deviations in their sitting, standing, or moving posture and body mechanics should receive special attention so that prevention or correction of these problems becomes a part of their Individual Education Programs. Suggestions for corrective and preventive measures, for measurement, and for program adaptations are presented in this chapter as a part of the discussion of each deviation. Specific program information designed to meet the requirements of the Individual Education Program developed as a part of P.L. 94-142 is given in the last section of this chapter. Chapters 5 and 10 present detailed information on specific posture and body mechanics problems together with programs of exercises and activities for these conditions.

The spinal column

Viewed from the front or rear, the spinal column should be straight. However, when the spine is viewed from the side, or lateral view, curves normally exist in various vertebral segments. The cervical spine is slightly hyperextended, stretching from the base of the skull to about the top of the thoracic vertebrae. The dorsal or thoracic spine is flexed throughout the length of the thoracic verte-

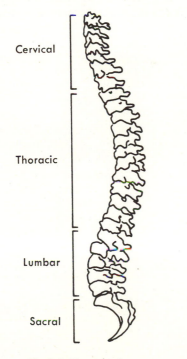

Fig. 9-4. Normal spine.

brae. The lumbar curve is hyperextended throughout the length of the lumbar vertebrae and the sacral curve is flexed and extends throughout the sacral and coccygeal vertebrae. These curves are present in the spinal column to help the individual maintain balance and to absorb shock and they should be considered normal unless they are exaggerated (Fig. 9-4).

POOR POSTURE ALIGNMENT PATTERNS

Postural deviations are ordinarily noted during examination of the individual from the lateral, anterior, and posterior views. In conducting a posture examination, it is considered best to perform the examination from the base of support upward. Thus, if deviations are noted at one level, they can be checked to see if compensatory deviations have occurred in areas above that particular level.

As each condition in this section is described, causes of the deviation are listed and suggestions for prevention and correction are given. These, together with the exercise programs outlined in Chapter 5, which suggest specific muscle realignment and development exercises for each condition, should provide adequate information for teachers and therapists to plan Individual Educational Programs for participants (handicapped or nonhandicapped) in their programs.

Postural deviations
Foot and ankle

Postural deviations of the foot and ankle can be observed while the student is standing in the upright position or participating in activities that involve walking or running. The evaluation of the foot should be made by observing it from the anterior, lateral, and posterior views and should involve both a walking and a static examination of the feet. The number of persons with deviations of the foot is large at all age levels and the number of persons who suffer with painful feet increases with increasing age. Muscles and joints of the foot and ankle become weakened from age and misuse. Pain associated with faulty mechanics in the use of the feet also begins to show up with increased age. The good mechanical use of the feet throughout life plus other factors such as good basic health, the maintenance of a satisfactory level of physical fitness, proper choice of shoes and socks, and proper attention to any injury or accident to the foot should serve as preventive measures to the onset of weak ankles and feet in later life.

The foot consists of seven irregularly shaped tarsal bones bound together by strong ligaments to make up the posterior half of the foot. These bones articulate anteriorly with five metatarsal bones, long and narrow in shape, which, in turn, are joined distally with the 14 phalanges that make up the toes (Fig. 9-5). The tarsal bones articulate with the distal end of the tibia through the talus bone to form the ankle joint. When the individual is standing in the upright position, the body weight is transferred from the tibia, through the talus, into the calcaneus and the navicular bones. The body weight is transferred anteriorly in the foot through the three cuneiform bones and the cuboid bone, located just anterior and lateral to the navicular (scaphoid), then, through these bones to the metatarsals, and, finally, to the phalanges. The total body weight is borne on the heel and the forepart of the foot with the anterior weight fairly well distributed across the heads of the five metatarsal bones. The first metatarsal bone and the two sesamoid bones located just under its distal head assume a slightly greater portion of the total weight on the anterior part of the foot. The bottom surfaces of the toes should also rest on the floor and should be active in helping support the foot both in the standing position and while walking.

The foot consists of a longitudinal arch that extends from the anterior portion of the calcaneus bone to the heads of the five metatarsal bones. The medial side of the longitudinal arch is usually considerably higher than the lateral side, which, as a general rule, makes contact throughout its length with the surface on which it is resting (Fig. 9-6, *A* to *C*). This is particularly true when the body weight is being supported on the foot. The longitudinal arch is sometimes described as two arches, a medial and a lateral arch, extending from the anterior aspects of the heel to the heads of the metatarsal bones. However, it is currently most frequently described as one long arch that is dome shaped and higher on the medial side than on the lateral side. On the forepart of the foot, in the region of the metatarsal bones, a second arch can be distinguished that runs across the forepart or ball of the foot. This arch, called the transverse or metatarsal arch, is slightly dome shaped, being

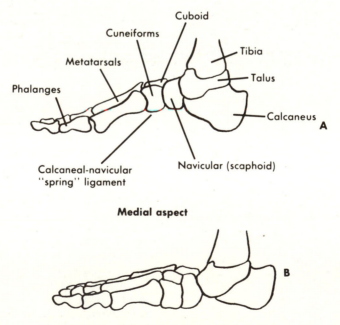

Fig. 9-5. Bones of the foot. **A,** Normal foot. **B,** Flatfoot.

higher at the proximal ends of the metatarsal bones than at the distal ends. It often is considered a continuation of the dome-shaped long arch described previously, and thus we have just one dome-shaped arch of the foot (Fig. 9-6, *D* and *E*).

Although these arches are described and named differently in the literature and there appears to be a difference of opinion in relation to the importance of their height, there is substantial agreement about the need for correct structure and placement of the bones, the importance of the strong ligamentous bands that help hold the bones in place to form the arches of the foot, and the need for good muscular balance between antagonistic muscles that support the foot. All these factors have an important effect on the position of the foot under both weight-bearing and non—weight-bearing conditions. A foot is considered strong and functional when the following conditions are present:

1. The foot is pain free.
2. The bones are properly placed and bound together by strong ligamentous bands (especially the calcaneonavicular ligament and the long plantar ligament).
3. The feet have adequate muscle strength (especially the posterior tibial muscle and the long flexor muscles of the toes) to support the longitudinal arch of the foot.
4. The bones have strong ligamentous and fascial bindings and well-developed small intrinsic muscles of the foot are present to maintain proper strength of the arch in the metatarsal region (Chapters 5 and 10).

In addition to considering the structure of the foot and ankle, it is also necessary to consider other factors such as the range of movement in the foot and ankle; the support of the body by the foot and ankle; and the effect that various positions of the foot, ankle, knee, and hip have on the mechanics of the foot itself. A consideration of the various movements possible in the foot and ankle, together with a description of the terminology used to describe these movements, should help clarify the discussion of those deviations of the foot and ankle

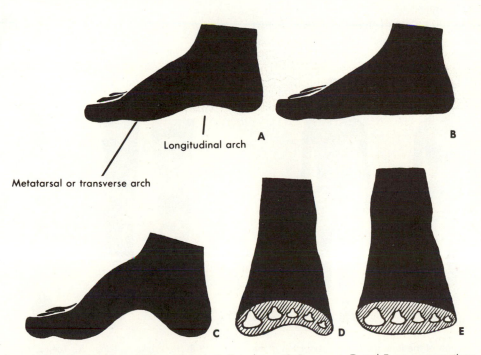

Longitudinal arch

Metatarsal or transverse arch

Fig. 9-6. Arches of the foot. **A,** Normal foot. **B,** Pes planus. **C,** Pes cavus. **D** and **E** are cross-sections of the arch. **D,** Normal metatarsal arch. **E,** Flat metatarsal arch.

that are presented in more detail in later portions of this chapter. The ankle joint is a hinge joint, and therefore only dorsiflexion and plantar flexion are possible. The numerous articulations between the individual tarsal bones and between the tarsal and metatarsal bones allow for inversion and eversion of the foot and for abduction and adduction of the foot.

Movements of the foot are as follows:

Dorsiflexion: Movement of the top of the foot in the direction of the knee

Plantar flexion: Movement of the foot in the opposite direction, in the direction of the sole of the foot

Inversion: Tipping the medial edge of the foot upward or *varus* (walking on the outer border of the foot)

Eversion: Tipping the lateral edge of the foot upward or *valgus* (walking on the inner border of the foot)

Adduction: Turning the whole forepart of the foot in a medial direction

Abduction: Turning the forepart of the foot in a lateral direction

Pronation: Combination of tipping the outer border of the foot up and toeing out (eversion with abduction)

Supination: Combination of tipping the inner edge of the foot upward while toeing in (inversion with adduction)

It should also be remembered that it is possible to turn the foot into toed-in and toed-out positions by rotating the lower leg when the knee is bent and by rotating the whole leg at the hip when the knee is straight. Thus, when an individual toes in or toes out while walking or standing, the examiner must determine whether this is the result of a foot deviation or a rotation of the leg (Fig. 9-7). Many foot and ankle deviations are closely linked to alignment problems occurring in the leg above the region of the ankle.

Pes planus. Pes planus, or flatfoot, refers to a lowering of the medial border of the longitudinal arch of the foot. The height of this side of the longitudinal arch may range anywhere from the extremely high arch known as *pes cavus*, to the so-

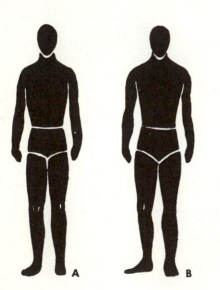

Fig. 9-7. Abduction of the foot and leg. **A,** Abduction of the foot. **B,** Toeing out of the foot resulting from outward rotation of the hip joint. Note difference in position of patella.

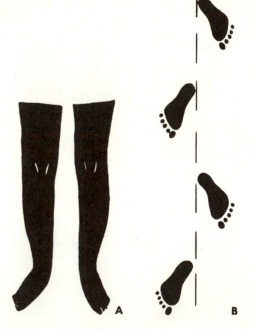

Fig. 9-8. Improper walking. **A,** Toeing out and walking across medial border of the foot. **B,** Footprints show outward rotation or splayfoot position while walking.

called normal arch, and down to a position in which the medial border lies flat against the surface on which the individual is standing. When this side of the foot is completely flat, the medial border of the foot may even assume a rather convex appearance to the observer (Fig. 9-6, *A* to *C*). Pes planus may be the result of faulty bony framework, faulty ligamentous pull across the articulations of the foot, an imbalance in the pull of the muscles responsible for helping to hold the longitudinal arch in its proper position, or racial differences. The specific cause may often be linked to improper alignment of the foot and leg and to faulty mechanics in the use of the foot and ankle.

When the foot is held in a toed-out or abducted position while standing and walking, there is a tendency to throw a disproportionate amount of body weight onto the medial side of the foot, thus causing stress on the medial side of this arch. Over a period of time, this stress may cause both a gradual stretching of the muscles, tendons, and ligaments on the medial aspect of the foot and a tightening of like structures on the lateral side. When the individual walks with the foot in the abducted or toed-out position, these same factors are again accentuated and, in addition, there is a tendency for the individual to rotate the leg medially in order to have it swing in alignment with the forward direction of the step. When the leg is swung straight in line with the direction being traveled and with the foot toed out, the individual will walk across the medial side of the foot with each step (Fig. 9-8). This not only weakens the foot but also predisposes the individual to a condition called tibial torsion. Since the individual is walking with the leg in basically correct alignment, but with the foot abducted and/or toed out, malalignment results. Thus, when the foot and leg alignment are examined, it will be found that when the legs and kneecaps face straight forward, the feet are in the abducted position; when the feet are aligned in a position parallel to one another, the kneecaps are facing in a slightly medial direction (tibial torsion). This may produce strain and possibly cause a lowering of the medial side of the longitudinal arch.

Correction of pes planus must involve a reversal of the factors and conditions just described. The total leg from the hip through the foot must be properly realigned so that the weight is balanced over the hip, the knee, the ankle, and the foot itself. The antagonistic muscles involved must be reoriented so that those that have become stretched (tibial muscles) are developed and tightened and those that have become short and tight (peroneal muscles) are stretched; thus, the foot is allowed to assume its proper position. The muscles on the lateral side of the foot must be stretched (peroneal group). The gastrocnemius and soleus muscles, which sometimes become shortened in the case of flatfoot, exert an upward pull on the back of the calcaneus bone, thus adding to the flattening of the arch. These muscles must also be stretched whenever tightness is indicated. The major muscle group that must be shortened and strengthened is the posterior tibial muscle, which is extremely important in terms of supporting the longitudinal arch, along with help from the long and short flexor muscles of the toes. The individual must also be given foot and leg alignment exercise in front of a mirror in order to observe the correct mechanical position of the foot while exercising, standing, walking, and actively using the feet. (See Chapter 5 for special exercises.)

Such activities as walking in soft dirt, on grass, or in sand with the foot held in the proper position can do much to help strengthen the foot and realign it with the ankle and hip. Emphasis here should be on walking straight over the length of the foot, placing the heel down first, with the weight being transferred along the outer border of the foot and with an even and equal push-off from the forepart of the foot and the five toes. In actual practice, the great toe should be the last toe to leave the surface on the push-off.

Pes cavus. Pes cavus is a condition of the foot in which the longitudinal arch is abnormally high. This condition is not found as frequently in the general population as is pes planus. If the condition is extreme, the student is usually under the special care of an orthopedic physician. Special exercises are not usually given for the high arch unless the person has considerable associated pain, requiring special corrective procedures recommended by the physician (Fig. 9-6, *C*).

Pronation of the foot. Since the ankle joint is a hinge joint allowing only plantar flexion and dorsiflexion, pronation of the ankle—as it is sometimes called—is actually a condition of pronation

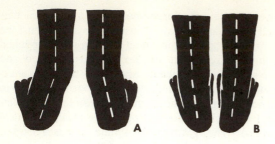

Fig. 9-9. Faulty foot and ankle positions. **A,** Foot and ankle pronation. **B,** Supinated foot.

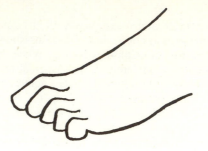

Fig. 9-10. Hammer toes.

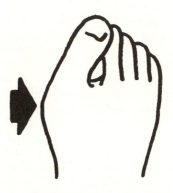

Fig. 9-11. Hallux valgus.

of the foot. As described previously, this is a combination of abduction of the foot itself and eversion. Since pronation involves eversion, the medial border of the foot is lowered as it is in the flat longitudinal arch. When this condition occurs, the forward part of the foot is also abducted, a condition caused by a shifting of the calcaneus bone downward and inward. This also changes the relationship of the talus to the other tarsal bones so that the tarsal-metatarsal and the metatarsal-phalangeal articulations must adapt, thus causing the abduction of the forepart of the foot[9] (Fig. 9-9). The reverse of this condition, one that involves inversion and adduction of the forepart of the foot, is called supination of the foot.

Viewed from the front of the individual being examined, the pronated foot is characterized by the turning of the forepart of the foot outward, by the lowering of the medial side of the longitudinal arch, by the prominence of the scaphoid or navicular bone, and by the prominence of the internal malleolus of the ankle. From the posterior view, the same conditions of the forepart of the foot are present, the internal malleolus will be prominent, and the Achilles tendon bows inward or medially (Helbing's sign). Correction of pronation of the foot is similar to that described for pes planus or flatfoot. Special exercises are described in Chapter 5.

Proper foot and leg alignment. Proper foot and leg alignment has been mentioned previously in rather general terms. More specifically, when properly aligned, the leg should be straight and the foot should be facing straight forward or in a slightly toes-out position. A plumb line held so that it hangs in line with the anterior inferior spine of the

ilium passes through the center of the patella, the center of the ankle, and the second toe of the foot. When viewed from the rear, the gravity line should pass through the center of the knee, the leg, and the calcaneus bone. The Achilles tendon must appear straight with no curvature.

Metatarsalgia. Two types of metatarsalgia may be recognized in a thorough foot examination. The first is a general condition, involving the transverse (metatarsal) arch, in which considerable pain is caused by the pressure of the heads of the metatarsal bones on the plantar nerves. The second type, Morton's toe, is more specific and is discussed in a later portion of this chapter.

Metatarsalgia in general may be caused by undue pressure being exerted on the plantar surface of the foot by the heads of the metatarsal bones. This pressure ultimately causes inflammation and therefore results in pain and discomfort. Its causes relate to such factors as wearing shoes or socks that are too short or too tight, wearing high-heeled shoes for long periods of time, and participating in various types of occupational or athletic endeavors that place great stress on the ball of the foot. The mechanism of injury may result in a stretching of the ligaments that bind the metatarsophalangeal joints together and therefore pressure is exerted on the nerves in this area. Correction involves the removal of the cause, if this is possible, and the assignment of special exercises to increase flexibility of the forepart of the foot. Exercises are then assigned to strengthen and shorten the muscles on the plantar surface, which may aid in maintaining a normal position in the metatarsal region. The physician may prescribe special shoes or suggest that an arch support or metatarsal bar be worn to support the metatarsal region of the foot to help reduce pain (Fig. 9-6, *D* and *E*).

Morton's toe. Morton's toe, often called *true metatarsalgia,* is more specific than the general breakdown of the metatarsal arch described previously. The onset of true metatarsalgia is often abrupt and the pain associated with it may be more intense than that found in general metatarsal weakness. In true metatarsalgia, the fourth metatarsal head is severely depressed, sometimes resulting in a partial dislocation of the fourth metatarsophalangeal joint. The abnormal pressure on the plantar nerve often produces a neuritis in the area, which, in turn, causes intense pain and disability. Treatment consists first of the removal of the cause of the condition. The orthopedic physician will advise which procedure will follow this. A second type of Morton's toe is characterized by the presence of a second metatarsal bone that is longer than the first metatarsal bone.

Hammer toe. In hammer toe, the proximal phalanx of the toe is hyperextended, the second is flexed, and the distal phalanx is either flexed or extended. This condition will often result from congenital causes or from having worn socks or shoes that are too short or too tight over a prolonged period of time (Fig. 9-10). Tests must be made to see whether the condition has become structural. If the condition is functional in nature and the affected joints can be stretched and loosened, corrective measures may be taken to reorient the antagonistic muscle pull involved in this deviation. The first step, however, must be the removal of the cause and, in severe cases, an orthopedic physician should be consulted relative to special

bracing, splinting, or surgery for correction of this condition.

Hallux valgus. A faulty metatarsal bone or shoes or socks that are too short, too narrow, or too pointed can cause a deviation of the toe known as hallux valgus. In this condition, the great toe is deflected toward the other four toes at the metatarsophalangeal joint (Fig. 9-11). The exposed medial side of the metatarsophalangeal joint is thus subject to undue pressure and irritation from the shoes and the result is often a bunion in this region of the foot. As irritation continues, the body's natural defense is to deposit calcium over the metatarsophalangeal joint and under the bunion. This increases the size of the joint and also the amount of pressure that occurs in this area of the foot. Correction of this condition must first involve consultation with a physician and usually requires the removal of the calcium deposit and the bunion. Further corrective measures would be to prescribe proper socks and shoes to allow sufficient room for the great toe to be held in the normal straight position. As an added precaution, both the standing and walking positions of the foot should be analyzed to determine whether the foot is being used in proper alignment. If the foot is not properly aligned and is toeing out excessively, remedial measures should be taken to correct this alignment in order to prevent a further aggravation of hallux valgus.

Lateral posture examination

Deviations in the foot and ankle were discussed in detail in an earlier section of this chapter.

The knee. The instructor's eyes, in examining the student from the side, move upward from the foot and ankle through the knee. Common deviations that may be noted in the position of the knee consist of either a hyperextended knee *(genu recurvatum)* or a hyperflexed knee. The normal position of the knee should be straight but not stiff. It is possible to correct both forward and backward knee by realigning the pull of the muscles that control its flexion and extension and by reorienting the student to the proper position of the leg (see Chapter 5). Bent knee and "back" knee, respectively, often will be associated with flat lower back and lordosis of the lumbar spine (Fig. 9-12).

The pelvis. The normal pelvis is inclined forward and downward at approximately a 60-degree

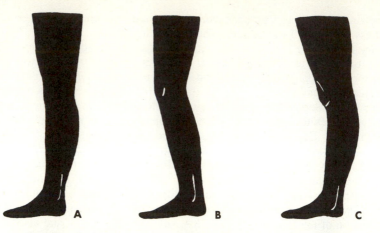

Fig. 9-12. The knee. **A,** Normal. **B,** Bent (flexed). **C,** Hyperextended.

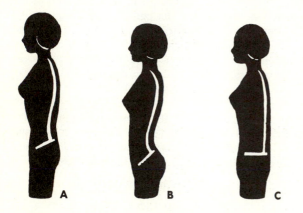

Fig. 9-13. Pelvic positions. **A,** Normal. **B,** Forward (downward) pelvic tilt. **C,** Backward (upward) pelvic tilt. Note position of spine as pelvic position changes.

angle when a line is drawn from the lumbosacral junction to the symphysis pubis. Any variation in this angle, with the pelvis tipping (tilt) downward and forward, would usually result in a greater curve of the lumbar spine; by the same token, a variation in the angle, with the pelvis tipping upward and backward, would tend to produce a flatness in the lumbar area. Since the sacroiliac joint is basically an immovable joint and only a minimum amount of motion takes place at the lumbosacral joint, pelvic inclination and lumbar spinal curves are closely linked (Fig. 9-13). Since exaggerated spinal curves may limit normal motion in

the low back, both lordosis and flat low back require special attention.

Lordosis. Lordosis is an exaggeration of the normal hyperextension in the lumbar spine. It is usually associated with tight musculature in the lower erector spinae or sacrospinalis muscle group, tightness in the iliopsoas and rectus femoris muscle groups, and either weak or stretched abdominal muscles. Correction of this condition would therefore necessitate stretching and loosening the lower erector spinae, the iliopsoas, and the rectus femoris muscles, together with assigning exercises designed to shorten and tighten the abdominal muscle group. It may also be important to develop muscular control of the gluteal and hamstring groups, which can exert a downward pull on the back of the pelvis. The development of the gluteal and hamstring groups can help the individual assume a correct position while stretching, while exercising, and even while in the static standing position, but these muscles must be relaxed when the individual wishes to walk, move, or run. It is then necessary for the abdominal muscles to hold the front of the pelvis up and to maintain the desired curvature in the lower back. A condition called *ptosis* (visceroptosis) is often associated with a forward pelvic tilt and lordosis. This condition is characterized by a sagging of the lower abdominal muscles and a protrusion of the lower abdominal area. It can also be corrected by shortening, tightening, and strengthening the abdominal muscle groups (Figs. 9-13, *B,* and 9-14, *A*).

Flat lower back. A flat lower back condition can develop when the pelvic girdle is inclined upward at the front, thereby decreasing the normal curvature of the lumbar spine. Often associated with this condition are tight hamstring and gluteus maximus muscles with weakened and stretched iliopsoas and rectus femoris muscles, coupled with weakness in the lumbar section of the erector spinae muscle group. A flat back can be corrected by stretching and increasing the flexibility of the hamstring and gluteal muscles and by developing, shortening, and tightening the iliopsoas, the rectus femoris, and the erector spinae groups (Fig. 9-14, *B*).

In the correction of both lordosis and flat low back, the individual student must learn to reorient the standing position by learning to feel what it is like to stand with the body in the correctly aligned position. It is helpful for the student to practice this corrected position while standing sideways to a regular or three-way mirror and observing the body in the correct mechanical position. A gravity line painted on the mirror or a plumb line hung down the length of the mirror will assist the student in realigning the body (Figs. 9-13 and 9-14).

Kyphosis. Kyphosis is an abnormal amount of flexion in the dorsal or thoracic spine. An extreme amount of kyphosis is called *humpback*. This condition ordinarily involves a weakening and stretching of the erector spinae and other extensor muscle groups in the dorsal or thoracic regions, along with a shortening and tightening of the antagonist (pectoral) muscles on the anterior side of the chest and shoulder girdle (Fig. 9-15, *A*). Its correction is effected largely by stretching the anterior muscles of the chest and shoulders (Fig. 20-9) so that the spinal extensor and shoulder girdle adductor muscle groups can be developed, strengthened, and shortened in order to pull the spine back into a more desired position. Often associated with kyphosis, but not necessarily found with it, are forward or round shoulders, flat chest, and winged scapula.

Forward or round shoulders. Forward or round shoulders is a condition involving an abnormal position of the shoulder girdle. This condition usually exists when the anterior muscles of the

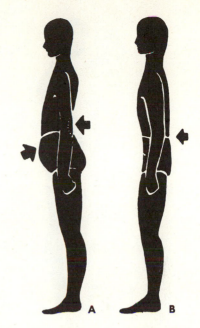

Fig. 9-14. A, Ptosis and lordosis. **B,** Flat back.

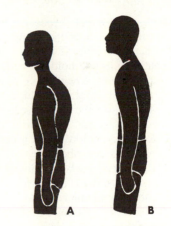

Fig. 9-15. A, Kyphosis. **B,** Forward or round shoulders.

shoulder girdle (pectoral muscles) become shortened and tightened and the retractors or adductors of the shoulder girdle (rhomboids and trapezius muscles) become loose, weak, and stretched. It is often associated with a flat chest and kyphosis. The basic correction of this condition is to stretch and loosen the anterior muscles of the chest and shoulder girdle and to develop, strengthen, and shorten

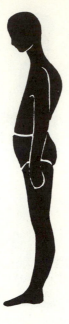

Fig. 9-16. Fatigue slump with kypholordosis.

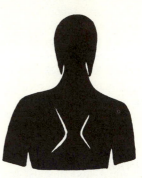

Fig. 9-17. Winged scapula.

the adductor muscles of the shoulder girdle (Fig. 9-15, *B*).

The student with either kyphosis or forward shoulders should also practice standing and sitting in good alignment in front of a mirror to get the feeling of what it is like to hold the body comfortably in proper balance. When the correct position becomes easy and natural, the student will no longer have to rely on the mirror and the visual cues associated with its use.

Kypholordosis. Kypholordosis is a combination of the two deviations described previously: that of kyphosis in the upper back and lordosis in the lower portion of the spine (Fig. 9-16). Often, one of these deviations is a compensation for the other and involves the body's attempt to keep itself in balance. Correction of kypholordosis consists of the same basic principles that are involved in correcting the individual conditions described previously; however, time can often be saved in the exercise program by assigning certain exercises that would be beneficial for the correction of both conditions. The exercise assignment sheet in Chapter 5 lists exercises that can be assigned to aid in the correction of all these conditions.

Flat upper back. A flat upper back would be the opposite of a kyphotic spine and would involve a decrease or absence of the normal anteroposterior spinal curve in the dorsal or thoracic region. Exercises and activities that would be beneficial for this condition include stretching the posterior muscles of the upper back to allow their antagonists on the anterior side of the body to be developed and shortened (Chapter 5).

Winged scapula. Winged scapula is a condition that involves the abduction or protraction of the shoulder blades (the medial border of the affected scapula being a greater distance from the spinal column than normal). A projection of the medial border of the scapula posteriorly and a protrusion of the inferior angle are other concomitants of this condition (Figs. 9-17 and 20-25). It is a very common condition among young children, who exhibit it especially when their arms are raised forward to the shoulder level. This results from lack of shoulder girdle strength; ordinarily, the condition will be outgrown as the child begins to participate in hanging and climbing activities for the development of the muscles of the shoulder girdle. In the adolescent and the young adult, the condition is one that involves unequal pull on the antagonist muscles of the shoulder girdle; corrective measures may be necessary to correct it. In general, the procedure to follow would be to stretch and loosen the anterior

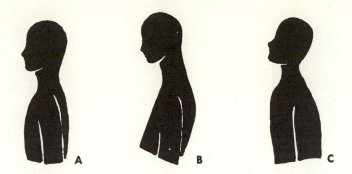

Fig. 9-18. Forward head and cervical lordosis. **A,** Normal head position. **B,** Forward head. **C,** Cervical lordosis.

muscles of the shoulder girdle and to develop the retractors or adductors of the scapula, involving both the trapezius and the rhomboid muscles. Developmental exercises for the serratus anterior muscle also are necessary, since it has a major responsibility for keeping the scapula in the correct position flat against the rib cage.

Forward head. Forward head is one of the most common postural deviations. It often accompanies kyphosis, forward shoulders, and lordosis. Two factors are involved in analyzing the causes of and in correcting forward head. The extensors of the head and neck are often stretched and weakened because of the habitual malposition of the head in the forward position. Correcting this condition involves bringing the head into proper alignment, with the chin tucked so that the lower jaw is basically in line with the ground and so that the chin is not tipped up when the head is drawn back. This involves reorientation of the head and neck so that the individual knows what it feels like to hold the head in the correct position. The antagonist muscles involved must be reeducated to hold the head in a position so that the lobe of the ear approximates a position in line with the center of the shoulder (Fig. 9-18, *A* and *B*).

Cervical lordosis. Cervical lordosis may result from an attempt to compensate for other spinal curves occurring at a lower level in the spinal column or from incorrect procedures in attempting to correct a forward head. The spinal extensors are often tight and contracted so that the head is tilted well back and the chin is tipped upward (Fig. 9-18, *C*). As in the case of forward head, a reedu-

cation of the antagonistic muscles and the proprioceptive centers involved is necessary so that the lower jaw is held in line with the ground. In the correction of cervical lordosis and forward head, the student must learn to assume the proper position and must exercise in front of a mirror in order to recognize the correct position (Fig. 9-18, *A*). Special exercises for the correction of cervical lordosis and forward head are found in Chapter 5.

Posterior overhang (round swayback). In posterior over-hang, the upper body sways backward from the hips so that the center of the shoulder falls in back of the gravity line of the body. To compensate for this position, the hips and thighs may move forward of the gravity line, the head may tilt forward, and the chest may be flat. Correction of a posterior overhang involves a reorientation of the total body so that its several parts are returned to a position of alignment. The student is instructed to work in front of a mirror and align the body with a gravity marker on the mirror. Alternatively, the instructor may check and correct the student's posture. The exercise program includes a reeducation of the antagonistic muscles so as to enable the student to return the body to a position of balance. Those muscle groups needing special attention are the abdominal muscles, the antagonist muscle groups responsible for anteroposterior alignment of the tilt of the pelvis, the adductor muscles of the shoulder girdle, and the extensor muscles of the upper spine. The student must stand tall, with chin tucked and abdomen flat, to correct this condition (Fig. 9-19).

Fatigue slump. Fatigue slump is a term used to

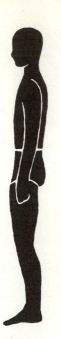

Fig. 9-19. Posterior overhang.

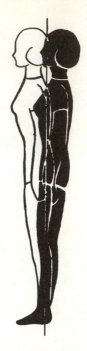

Fig. 9-20. Forward and backward leans.

describe a rather complete breakdown in the alignment of the total body. Children, from the upper elementary school grades through the first year or two of high school, are especially susceptible to this condition (both physically and emotionally). These early adolescent years are times of physical, emotional, and mental stress that may often result in a general "sagging" of the whole body. The student will often have all of the following postural deviations: back knees, forward pelvic tilt, lordosis, kyphosis, forward shoulders, and forward head. The student may also have some lateral deviations such as a low shoulder and a head tilt.

Since part of the cause of fatigue slump may be linked to a period of rapid growth of bone, joint, and muscle, symmetrical development may not occur. Corrective measures for fatigue slump must include a consideration of both physical and emotional factors. Students must be motivated to want to work toward the correction of their posture. Motivation for boys should include such factors as strength and motor proficiency, whereas girls may be more interested in body poise and esthetics. This may be a very individual matter at this age level; motivation must be based on individual

needs and interests. The actual physical correction of the fatigue slump is a twofold matter involving the realignment of antagonistic muscle groups throughout the body and the development of a feeling for sitting, standing, and moving with the body properly aligned. Realignment techniques previously described and exercises given in Chapter 5, especially those that develop the antigravity (extensor) muscles of the body and stretch their antagonists, should be assigned. The student should also work on body alignment (sitting, standing, and moving) in front of a mirror or a competent observer so that he or she can develop a feeling for the newly acquired correct posture. Correction of total body malalignment is difficult and requires a vigorous exercise regime, coupled with sufficient self-discipline to overcome whatever emotional and mental factors are contributing to the problem (Fig. 9-16).

Body leans. When viewed from the side, the total body may lean a considerable distance either forward or backward of the line of gravity. When the total body, from foot to head, is in good alignment, but leans forward or backward from the ankle so that the lobe of the ear is positioned either

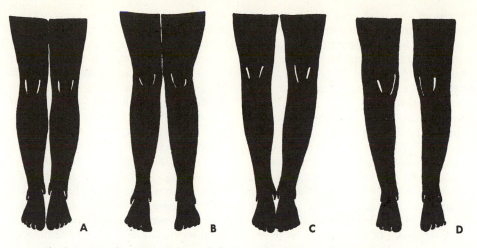

Fig. 9-21. Leg alignment. **A,** Normal. **B,** Knock-knees. **C,** Bowleg. **D,** Tibial torsion.

anterior or posterior to the gravity line, the condition is considered to be a total body lean (Fig. 9-20). If body leans are not corrected, as the individual attempts to compensate for the lean and bring the body back to a balanced standing position, the body often will be transferred into one or more of the postural conditions discussed previously. Correction of the forward or backward lean of the total body is largely a matter of reorientation of the proprioceptive centers of the body to enable the individual to feel when the body is in correct alignment in the standing position. Checking the body against a gravity line or a plumb line hung vertically down the face of the three-way mirror is an excellent way for the student to check the forward or backward deviation and to recognize the feel of standing with the body in the correct position. Symmetrical exercises can then be assigned so that the student can develop the flexibility and strength necessary to hold the body in correct alignment.

Anterior and posterior posture examinations

Deviations of the foot and ankle that would be noted in examining a student from the anterior or posterior view were discussed in an earlier section of this chapter.

The knee. Three conditions involving the knee and the upper and lower leg may be noted when a student is examined from the anterior or posterior view. Bowlegs and knock-knees are recognized from either of these two views, whereas tibial tor-

sion is more easily identified when the student is examined from the anterior view.

Bowlegs (genu varum). Bowlegs can be identified by examining a student with a plumb line, by comparing alignment of the leg with one of the vertical lines of the posture screen, or by having the student stand with the internal malleoli touching and the legs held comfortably straight. In the latter test, if a space exists between the knees when the malleoli are touching, the individual may be considered to have bowlegs. Unless this is either a functional condition in the young child (which may be outgrown) or a condition related to hyperextending the knees and rotating the thighs in order to separate the knees, corrective measures ordinarily must be prescribed by an orthopedic physician. Hyperextended and rotated knees causing a bowleg can be corrected by having the student assume the correct standing position and by developing proper balance in the pull of the antagonistic muscles of the hip and leg[2] (Fig. 9-21, *C*).

Knock-knees (genu valgum). Knock-knees can be identified as described in the section on bowlegs; however, in this case, when the inner borders (medial femoral condyles) of the knees are brought together, a space exists between the internal malleoli. Knock-knees may be related to pronation of the ankle and weakness in the longitudinal arch. Correction involves realignment of the antagonist muscles of the leg and foot, which control proper alignment. This usually involves developing the outward rotators of the thigh and shortening and tightening the structures that traverse the medial side of the leg at the knee; those on the lateral side should be stretched. Correction of this condition will also involve realignment of the foot, the ankle, and the hip (Fig. 9-21, *B*). Knock-knees also may be related to tibial torsion.

Tibial torsion. Tibial torsion, or twisting of the tibia, is identified by examining the student from the anterior view. When the feet are pointed straight ahead, the individual with tibial torsion will have one or both of the kneecaps facing in a medial direction, or when the kneecaps are facing straight forward, the feet are rotated in a toed-out position (Fig. 9-21, *D*). Correction of this condition involves realignment of the total leg, with emphasis being placed on the regions of the ankle, knee, and hip. The outward rotators of the hip and the thigh must be developed, whereas muscles on the medial and lateral side of the foot and ankle must be properly stretched and strengthened to obtain proper alignment. Special exercises for these problems of leg alignment are described in Chapter 5.

Lateral pelvic tilt. A lateral pelvic tilt, in which one side of the pelvis is higher or lower than the other side, can be observed during both the anterior and the posterior posture examinations. These conditions can be evaluated by marking either the anterior superior iliac spines or the posterior superior iliac spines of the ilium and then observing their relative height through the grids of a posture screen. The examiner can also evaluate the height of the pelvis by placing his or her fingers on the uppermost portion of the crest of the ilium and by observing the relative height of the two sides of the pelvis (Fig. 9-22). A lateral pelvic tilt may result from such things as unilateral ankle pronation, knock-knees, bowlegs, a shorter long bone in either the lower or upper portion of one leg, structural anomalies of the knee and hip joint and deviations in the pelvic girdle, or a scoliotic spine, all of which are discussed in Chapters 10 and 11. Before an exercise program for a lateral pelvic tilt is initiated, its cause must be determined by a physician, who may then suggest either symmetrical or asymmetrical exercises to realign the pelvic level. The position of the pelvic girdle as viewed from the anterior or posterior view has very definite implications for the position of the spinal column as

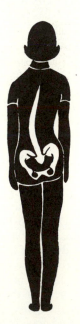

Fig. 9-22. Lateral pelvic tilt.

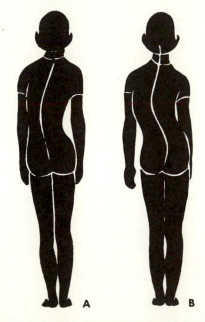

Fig. 9-23. Scoliosis. **A,** Total left C curve. **B,** Regular S curve.

it extends upward from the sacrum. A lateral tilt of the pelvis will be reflected in the spinal column above it, since the sacroiliac and the lumbosacral joints are semi-immovable. The resulting lateral spinal curvatures are discussed in the next section of this chapter. Lateral tilt of the pelvis may also be related to a twisting of the pelvic girdle itself. This is a complicated orthopedic problem involving, in addition to the pelvis, resultant manifestations in both hip joints, the legs, and the vertebral column. Such cases should be referred to the orthopedic physician for treatment and for advice relative to a special exercise program.

Scoliosis. Scoliosis is a rotolateral curvature of the spine. When viewed from the front or from the rear, a scoliotic spine has a curvature to one side; in advanced stages, it may curve both to the left and to the right. Scoliosis curves are ordinarily described in relation to their position as the individual is being viewed from the rear. A curvature is described as a simple C curve to the left or right. In a more advanced stage, compensation above or below the original curve may occur and the resulting curvature is described as a regular S curve or a reverse S curve. Examples of scoliotic curves are shown in Fig. 9-23.

Initially, a lateral deviation of the spine may involve only a simple C curve to the left or right in any segment of the spine, depending on the cause of the problem, the resulting change in soft tissues, and the pull of the antagonist muscles. These curves are often functional in nature and thus are correctable through properly assigned stretching and developmental exercises under the guidance of a physician. Untreated spines will often become progressively worse, involving permanent structural changes.

Scoliosis is often caused by asymmetry of the body. Lateral pelvic tilt, low shoulder, asymmetrical development of the rib cage, or lateral deviation of the linea alba may be involved in a "cause" or "effect" relationship with a rotolateral curve of the spine. Evidence of this would be found in one or more of the following bodily changes:

1. When the thoracic vertebral column is displaced laterally, the rotation of the vertebral bodies is in the direction of the convexity of the curve.
2. Lateral bending of the spine is accompanied by a depression and protrusion of the intervertebral discs on the concave side, with a greater separation between the sides of the vertebrae on the convex side of the lateral curve.
3. There is an imbalance in the stability and pull of the ligaments and muscles responsible for holding the vertebral column in its normal position. Muscles and ligaments on the concave side become tight and contracted, whereas those on the convex side become stretched and weakened. Muscle atrophy may occur.
4. Changes in the rib cage involve a flattening and depression of the posterior aspects of the ribs on the concave side, with a posterior bulging of the ribs on the side of the convex spinal curve. The opposite is true of the anterior aspect of the chest. There the ribs on the concave side are prominent, whereas they are flattened or depressed on the convex side.

The treatment of scoliosis is rather specific, depending on the cause of the condition and the resulting changes in the spinal column. Students with scoliosis must be referred to an orthopedist for examination and recommendations relative to stretching and developmental exercises. These may be either symmetrical or asymmetrical in nature. Some orthopedic physicians believe that the treatment of scoliosis should be very specific and will indicate the types of asymmetrical exercises that should be engaged in by the student. Others subscribe to the theory that the cause of scoliosis should be eliminated if possible, but that only symmetrical types of exercise should be assigned for this condition. Both types of exercise for scoliosis are presented in Chapter 5.

Since scoliosis of the spine is a very complicated and difficult type of condition to diagnose and treat, it is necessary for the adapted teacher or therapist to rely on the advice of the physician relative to the types of activities and exercises that should be prescribed for the student. Since lateral spinal curves are accompanied by a certain amount of rotation of the spine, a great deal of skill is required to diagnose and treat the condition correctly. Recommendations relative to types of games, sports, and activities should therefore be indicated by the examining physician. Although scoliosis is usually

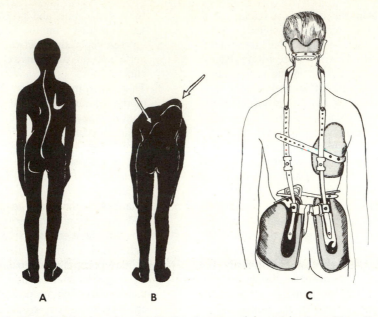

Fig. 9-24. Scoliosis. **A,** Rotolateral curve. **B,** Rotation viewed from Adam's position. **C,** Milwaukee brace.

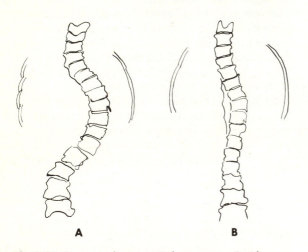

Fig. 9-25. Severe scoliosis. **A,** Before surgery. **B,** After surgery and corrective procedures.

recognized when the student is examined from the posterior view, the student with scoliosis often will also exhibit certain characteristics of asymmetry when checked from the anterior view. These include asymmetry of the rib cage and a lateral deviation of the linea alba.

Scoliosis in young girls. During the last several years, the importance of identifying and treating scoliosis in young girls between the ages of 9 and 13 or 14 years has been stressed by orthopedic physicians. Early detection by physical education teachers, therapists, and nurses and immediate referral to a physician who *specializes* in scoliosis treatment may prevent permanent deformity in many of these young persons.

Treatment may consist of utilization of casts or braces (Fig. 9-24) combined with a special exercise program assigned by the physician. Exercise programs without the cast or brace are not usually recommended. Cases that are not discovered early may require surgery with spinal fusion or the insertion of rods along the vertebral column to straighten the severely curved spine (Fig. 9-25).

Physicians at the Los Angeles Orthopedic Hospital and the Orange County Orthopedic Hospital in California have successfully treated large numbers of young girls and have spearheaded campaigns to provide for early diagnosis of this serious problem.

Treatment of patients with severe scoliosis (Chapter 5 includes specific exercises for scoliosis) may include any or all of the following:

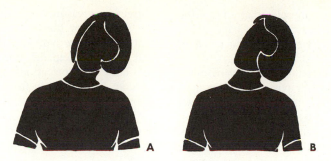

Fig. 9-26. Faulty head positions. **A,** Head tilt. **B,** Head twist.

1. Removal of the cause, if possible.
2. Assignment of symmetrical exercises, especially for the abdomen, back, and hip regions.
3. Promoting mobilization of tightness in soft tissue in the trunk, shoulder girdle, and hip region.
4. Giving asymmetrical exercises to tighten muscles on the convex side of the curves on the recommendation of an orthopedic physician.
5. Recommendation of traction of the spine by the physician.
6. Assignment of exercises to increase the strength and the anteroposterior balance and alignment of the spine.
7. Specific prescription of any derotation exercises by the physician.

Physical educators who specialize in adapted physical education and specialists in therapeutic recreation should inform those teaching regular physical education, the school nurse, and other health-related personnel of the importance of screening young persons for scoliosis and other body mechanics problems early. The students can then be involved in preventive programs under the guidance of a physician who specializes in the diagnosis and care of scoliosis and other serious orthopedic problems.

Shoulder height. It is rather common for an indvidual to have one shoulder higher or lower than the other. This condition usually results from asymmetrical muscle or bony development of the shoulder girdle or lateral curvature in the spinal column. Correction of an abnormal curve in the spine may result in the shoulders returning to a level position, although corrective exercises may be required in the process. When the cause is muscular in origin, correction is a relatively simple matter of developing the strength of the weaker or lower side and stretching the contracted side. This also involves a reorientation of the student's feeling for the correct shoulder and body alignment. Exercise for a low or high shoulder should be done in front of a regular or three-way mirror to enable the student to learn to feel the position of the body when it is being held in proper alignment. (See Chapter 5 for special exercises.)·

Head tilt or twist. When viewed from the anterior or posterior view, the head may be either tilted directly to the side or tilted to the side with a concomitant twisting of the head and neck (Fig. 9-26). In either case, it is necessary to reorient the student to the proper position of the head. Very often, deviations in the position of the head and neck are compensatory for other postural deviations located below this area. The correction of these conditions should accompany the reorientation and correction of the position of the head itself.

The correction of the head position will involve reeducating the antagonist muscles responsible for holding the head in a position of balance, plus reorienting the student in terms of holding the head in the correct position. This will involve the appropriate proprioceptive centers and balance organs. The exercise program for correction of the condition should be rather specific in terms of those muscle groups that are stretched and developed. Moreover, the exercise program should be practiced with the individual standing in front of a mirror so that he or she can visualize the correct position and develop the feeling of holding the head in correct alignment. Selected exercises used in stretching and developing muscles that control the position of the head are presented in Chapter 5. A discussion of torticollis (wryneck) is included in Chapter 10.

Body tilt. Another deviation that may be noted in the anterior and posterior posture examinations is a problem of body alignment in which the total body is tilted to the left or right of the gravity or plumb line (Fig. 9-27). Standing with the body tilted to the side causes increased strain on the bones, joints, and muscles and may result in compensation being made to bring the body back into a position of balance over its base of support. Often, this compensation results in the hips and shoulders being thrown out of alignment, leading to the development of a lateral curvature in the spine. Correction of this condition involves an analysis of the causative factors of the tilt, such as unilateral flatfoot, pronated ankle, knock-knee, or short leg. On the other hand, standing out of balanced alignment may be habitual with the student. Before correction of the lateral body tilt can be accomplished, unilateral deviations must be corrected. Specific suggestions for the correction of a weak foot, ankle, or knee are contained in another section of this chapter. Together with these specific

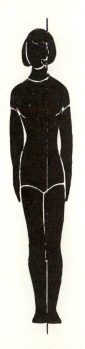

Fig. 9-27. Body tilt.

corrective measures, exercises should be given to the student for body tilt. Exercises and activities that involve the symmetrical use of the total body and that will help the student learn to stand with the body in correct alignment and balance are needed. Exercising in front of the mirror will give the student a visual concept of the feeling of standing with the body in a balanced position, which should help to effect a correction of a lateral tilt of the body. (Special exercises are described in Chapter 5.)

TESTS AND MEASUREMENTS FOR POSTURE AND BODY ALIGNMENT

Tests and measurements can be used in adapted physical education to evaluate improvement, to aid in instruction, to determine whether body parts are properly aligned, and to motivate students to work toward correction of body malalignment. Some of the tests and measurements traditionally used in adapted physical education programs are not high in validity and reliability but may still be of some use in identifying deviations, in helping the instructor explain malalignments to students, and in motivating students to work toward self-improvement. If any or all of these values are obtained from testing the students, it should be a worthwhile part of the total program. Assessment procedures such as those presented in the next several pages must be used to meet the requirements of P.L. 94-142. The data thus obtained are used to formulate specific performance objectives for each person and to aid in the development of Individual Education Programs. (Also see previous discussions in this chapter of each deviation, suggested exercise programs in Chapter 5, and activities in Chapter 8 for ideas on program planning.)

Tests and measurements can be made more useful if instructors carefully observe the following matters in their testing procedures:

1. Obtain the best testing equipment possible.
2. Keep all equipment in correct working condition.
3. Use correct testing procedures.
4. Use the same piece of testing equipment on successive tests, if possible.
5. Have the same person administer each successive test.
6. Test under similar conditions, for example,

before a workout each time, at the same time each day, or at the same time in each period.

7. Record all information accurately and indicate the date that the test was given.

8. Determine accurately the location of landmarks used in measurement.

9. Attempt to standardize all procedures and provide a written description of these procedures so that they can be followed on each occasion by any teacher or tester.

Tests for the foot
Podiascope

Description. The podiascope is a device used to observe the plantar surface of the foot under weight-bearing conditions. It consists of a wooden box (usually made of ³/₄-inch thick plywood) approximately 14 inches square with the top surface of ³/₄-inch thick plate glass. The front side is left open. Inside the box, under the glass and facing toward the open side, is an adjustable mirror slanting downward at approximately a 45-degree angle. The mirror is mounted on a piece of wood and made adjustable so that its back edge can be moved up and down to facilitate viewing the bottom of the foot from various angles in front of the podiascope or when it is placed in front of a wall mirror so that the student can view the feet (Fig. 9-28).

Instructions for use. The podiascope is placed on a bench or table. The glass top is thoroughly cleaned and the student stands on the glass facing toward the open side. The instructor, seated so as to be able comfortably to look into the mirror, can then observe the reflection of the bottoms of the student's feet. After approximately 1 minute of standing on the glass, the weight-bearing surfaces of the feet begin to show up as pale white areas, whereas the non–weight-bearing areas are pink in color. The examiner will then be able to observe the following:

1. The shape of the longitudinal arch
2. The height of the longitudinal arch
3. The areas of stress on the bottom of the foot (indicated by darker colorations and caluses that occur from abnormal pressures during weight bearing)

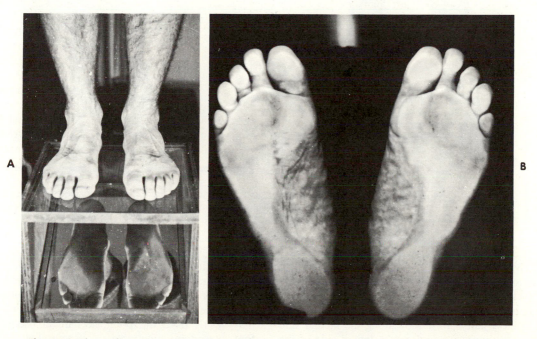

Fig. 9-28. The podiascope examination. **A,** Subject standing on podiascope. **B,** Photograph of feet through podiascope.

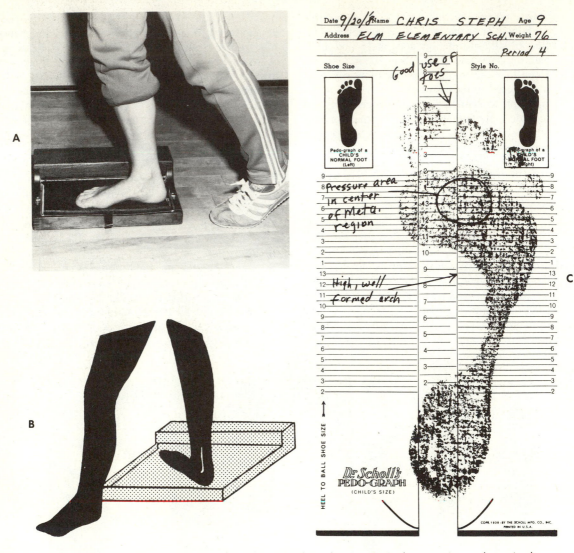

Fig. 9-29. Footprint examinations. **A,** Making a pedograph print. **B,** Student stepping on large-sized pedograph. Note badly abducted foot position. **C,** Pedograph print with markings used to show findings from the podiascope examination. (**A,** Courtesy of California State University, Audio Visual Center, Long Beach, Calif.)

4. Whether the toes are bearing their share of the weight, whether they are straight, and whether the second toe projects forward a greater distance than does the great toe.
5. Heavy callus formation along the medial side of the great toe and on the lateral side of the heel, indicating abnormal use of the foot

6. Callus formation in the metatarsal arch region

These calluses may reflect pressure of one metatarsal bone or may be large, reflecting pressure across the total transverse arch. Pressure or stress may result from the poor mechanical use of the foot caused by functional or structural deviations or from activities that produce heavy friction to the foot, such as dancing, cross-country running, and basketball.

Uses and limitations. The podiascope can be used to examine the longitudinal and transverse arches of the foot while weight bearing and to check for areas of stress and strain on the foot. By placing the podiascope in front of a regular or three-way mirror, the student can observe the foot problems that have been discovered and described by the instructor. A permanent record can be made of the podiascope findings by photographing the bottom of the foot through the glass. If photography is not used, a permanent record of the examination can be recorded on a pedograph print by the instructor (Fig. 9-29).

Pedograph

Description. A pedograph is an ink print that is made of the bottom of the foot under weight-bearing conditions. This print is made by placing either a special or a blank piece of paper directly beneath a rubber sheet, the underside of which has been inked. The student is then instructed either to step on the rubber sheet with full weight or to take a walking step across the pedograph so that a permanent print of the foot under weight-bearing conditions is recorded. The William M. Scholl Company (Chicago, Ill.) commercially produces a pedograph machine for use by the general public. A device of this type is satisfactory for school use; however, similar equipment can be constructed by the adapted physical education teacher or the maintenance or industrial arts department of the school.

Instructions for use. The footprint machine is placed on the floor directly in front of the student, with the paper placed under the rubber sheet. The student is then instructed to step on the print with the full body weight being borne as in normal use. The print of the foot can be taken as the individual steps directly on and off the rubber sheet or it can be taken as the individual takes a normal walking step across it. The latter would indicate the pattern of weight bearing during normal walking; however, to permit the individual freedom in the placement of the foot, the pedograph must be larger than the Scholl pedograph. To accommodate the foot in whatever position is usual for the student, a 14- by 16-inch space is needed.

Uses and limitations. Although the pedograph

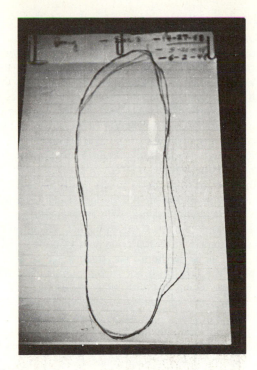

Fig. 9-30. Foot tracing. Note improvement shown in successive examinations (lines on medial side of foot move progressively toward the midline of the foot) as leg, foot, and ankle are realigned. (See Fig. 20-8.)

does not indicate deviations as clearly as does the podiascope, it will furnish a permanent print for study and for comparison during later examinations. If a pedograph print is made prior to the time the podiascope examination is performed, information that is obtained from the podiascope examination can be recorded by the instructor on the pedograph print. This can be done by writing explanatory notes on the pedograph or by circling areas of special significance on the print, for example, abnormal patterns of weight bearing, prominent calluses, and poor alignment of the toes and feet (Fig. 9-29, *C*).

The pedograph print can also be used to record the results of a foot tracing made to show the amount of medial displacement of and pronation in the foot and ankle. The procedure for making a foot tracing is described in detail in this chapter in the section discussing the ankle (Fig. 9-30).

Height of the longitudinal arch test

Description. The height of the longitudinal arch of the foot seems to be of interest to some doctors, therapists, and physical educators, especially if the measurement of its height is one that compares the arch under weight-bearing and non–weight-bearing conditions. The functional flatfoot may be a painful flatfoot and the height of the arch, in this case, will often show considerable difference when weight-bearing and non–weight-bearing measurements are compared.

Instructions for use. The test involves measurements made of the height of the scaphoid bone. The instructor first marks, with either a skin pencil or a ballpoint pen, the farthest medial projection of the scaphoid or navicular bone with a dot or a short line parallel to the floor. The student is then asked to place the foot on a flat surface without bearing weight on it and the instructor measures the distance from the supporting surface to the mark on the scaphoid bone. The student then places weight on the foot and the height of the mark is again measured. The difference in the height of the mark is compared with the scale found in Fig. 9-37.

Uses and limitations. The height of the long arch test can be used with students who have functional flatfoot and for those with ankle pronation. It is a relatively easy test to administer; however, difficulty may be encountered in finding the medialmost projection of the bone on some subjects.

It should be remembered that there is no direct relationship between the height of the arch and the strength of the foot. Many persons with very low arches, or even with flatfeet, are free of pain and also highly successful in terms of athletics and other physical endeavors. However, measurement of the height of the arch and examination of the foot for proper mechanics can provide information that is useful to the instructor in the assignment of special exercises to strengthen the foot, for recommendations relative to good mechanics in the use of the foot, and for other matters such as recommending proper footwear and special care of the feet.

Tests for the ankle

The ankle joint is a hinge joint, capable of only two fundamental motions: dorsiflexion and plantar flexion. However, because of its close connection with the bones of the foot and because it is superimposed directly above the foot bones, certain foot deviations are also reflected in the position of the ankle. Therefore, it is necessary in doing a complete foot examination not only to examine the foot, but also to examine the structures located above it, including the ankle, the knee, and the hip.

Foot and ankle tracings

Description. Lowman, Colestock, and Cooper[10] described a technique of making a tracing around a person's foot with a pencil that is held perpendicular to the surface on which the person is standing. The pencil thus reflects indentations and prominences around the edge of the foot as the tracing is made. The tracing will also show other projections above the region of the sole of the foot such as the medial aspect of the scaphoid bone, the position of the medial malleolus, and the position of the lateral malleolus. Young[11] devised a small block arrangement with a pencil inserted so that the block slides in a position perpendicular to the sheet on which the tracing is made and the mark made by the pencil reflects more accurately the foot and ankle position described previously (Fig. 9-30).

Instructions for use. The student assumes a normal standing position, with the feet about 6 inches apart, either on pedograph prints previously made of the feet or, if preferred, on two blank pieces of paper. The instructor then traces an outline around the foot, making sure that the front edge of the tracer is kept in firm contact with the foot and that the pencil is recording properly on the paper. The lower surface of the tracer is kept flat on the paper as it slides around the edge of the foot. To standardize procedures, the same tracer, with a different colored pencil in the tracer, should be used each time an individual is retested. Thus, the second tracing can be made on the same paper and directly compared with the first. When this is done, it is important to compare the complete tracing of the foot on each of the examinations so that if, during a second examination, the total foot is shifted to the medial or lateral side of the position taken during the first tracing, the individual reading the tracing will not suspect that improvement or change has taken place. When the foot is placed in the same position each time and the medial side of the tracing moves toward the center of the foot on successive tests, that is, less prominence of the scaphoid bone and internal malleolus, improvement in pronation and alignment is indicated (Fig. 9-30).

Uses and limitations. Foot tracings can be used to show the deviations in the foot and ankle position that have been observed by the instructor during the posture and foot examinations. Of particular importance are such factors as abduction of the forepart of the foot, medial protrusion of the scaphoid bone, and medial displacement of the internal malleolus, all of which will show up rather clearly in the tracing. Seeing this illustration of the deviation, and then observing how changes can take place when the muscles are reeducated so that the inside of the foot and arch are realigned should serve as motivation for students to work toward improvement of pronation of the feet and ankles and abduction of the feet. Special exercises for realigning the foot and the ankle are presented in Chapter 5.

Achilles tendon test

Description. The Achilles tendon test is usually conducted as part of a total posture examination; however, it must also be a standard procedure for all foot examinations. This test is made from the rear of the student and involves viewing the alignment of the heel cord of the individual while he or she is standing in a normal position. It can be made by viewing the student while he or she stands behind the posture screen, by using a plumb line for comparison, or by simply viewing the heel cord and estimating the degree of straightness or the amount of inward curve that is present in the Achilles tendon.

Instructions for use. The individual to be tested stands with the back turned toward the instructor, who stands 5 to 10 feet behind the student. The instructor then uses the vertical lines of the posture screen, a plumb line, or judgment to determine whether the heel cord is straight. The Achilles tendon of a properly aligned foot and ankle will not curve inward or outward. However, an individual who has pronation of the ankles will often reflect a bowing inward of the heel cord (Helbing's sign); conversely, a person with supinated feet will display outward bowing. When ankle pronation is present, the inner malleolus will be more prominent and the scaphoid bone will protrude in a medial direction. The forepart of the foot may also be turned out and the medial side of the foot may be depressed (Fig. 9-9).

Tests for knock-knees and bowlegs

Description. Tests for knock-knees and bowlegs are used to determine whether the individual's legs are straight or are either knock-kneed or bowlegged and the approximate extent of either of the latter conditions.

Instructions for use. The individual is asked to assume a normal standing position while the general leg alignment is observed from the front and rear. The student then is requested to slide the legs together until either the inner sides of the condyles of the knees or the medial malleoli touch. If the inner sides of the knees come together first and the ankle bones are still separated, a knock-knee condition exists. The extent of this deviation can be determined by measuring the distance between the internal malleoli. If, on the other hand, the internal malleoli touch and the medial condyles of the knees are separated, a bowleg condition exists. This condition can be measured by determining the distance between the inner sides of the knees. Inside calipers can be used to measure the amount of deviation or, if this equipment is not available, the instructor can measure the approximate distance with a tape measure or with small pieces of wood that have been cut for this purpose in various predetermined widths ranging from $1/2$ to 3 inches.

Uses and limitations. The amount of knock-knee or bowleg can also be estimated while the individual stands behind a posture screen by observing the leg alignment in relation to the vertical lines of the grid. If heavy fat pads exist on the medial side of the leg just above the knee, it may be difficult to obtain an accurate measurement with either of these two tests. Consequently, the individual is instructed to bring the inner sides of the condyles of the knees together firmly on the knock-knee test. When a measurement of the distance between the inner sides of the knees is made, it should be made with enough pressure to eliminate the effect of the musculature and the fatty pads that may be present in this region. Tests for alignment of the total leg are described in the following section.

Tests for leg alignment

Description. The alignment of the leg can be evaluated from the anterior, lateral, or posterior view. Each of these positions will give the examiner an opportunity to look for certain basic factors related to good segmental balance and alignment in the foot, ankle, knee, and hip.

Instructions for use. These examinations can be made with the individual standing behind a posture screen, using the vertical lines of the screen or a plumb line as a reference. When the examination is made from the anterior view, the student is instructed to stand in a normal posture facing the examiner. After they have been located for the student by the instructor, the anterosuperior spines of the ilium are marked with a skin pencil or the student is instructed to hold the index finger on these points. The instructor then moves to a position 5 to 10 feet away from the student and holds the gravity line out at full arm's length in order to sight through it, observing certain pertinent landmarks on the student. When the gravity line falls just medial to the anterosuperior spine of the ilium, it should pass down the leg through the center of the knee, the center of the ankle joint, and then through a point between the first and second toes of the foot (Fig. 9-31, *B*). Any deviation from these positions could indicate a knock-knee (genu valgum) or bowleg (genu varum), respectively, depending on whether the plumb line fell lateral to or medial to the correct position at the center of the knee. A pronated or supinated ankle or an abducted or adducted foot would likewise be identified according to its relationship to the plumb line.

After examining the student and evaluating the normal standing position, the instructor can have the student make whatever corrections are necessary to bring the foot, ankle, knee, and hip into proper alignment. The correctly aligned position is then practiced while standing, walking, and running.

When the gravity line examination is made to determine anteroposterior deviations in leg alignment, the student is viewed through the posture screen or evaluated with the plumb line from a position directly to the side. The student is asked to assume a normal standing position and certain landmarks are checked by the instructor against the gravity line. This runs through the center of the hip (approximately through the center of the greater trochanter of the femur bone), just posterior to the kneecap, and about 1 to 1 1/2 inches anterior to the outer ankle bone (external malleolus) or approximately in line with the center of the scaphoid (navicular) bone (Fig. 9-31, *A*). Any deviation from this alignment indicates either that the individual has a forward or backward lean of the total body or a deviation in the region of the knee in which there is either abnormal hyperextension (genu recurvatum) or hyperflexion (bent knee). These conditions can be described to the student and efforts can be made to realign the body in correct balance. The student should then exercise the appropriate muscles and practice this new position until it becomes natural to stand with the legs in proper alignment (Fig. 9-12).

Uses and limitations. These tests are usually given in connection with, or in addition to, the

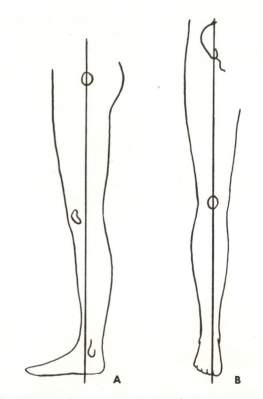

Fig. 9-31. Leg alignment tests. **A,** Lateral view examination. **B,** Anterior view examination.

general posture examination. They should supplement the general examination and should call particular attention to problems that exist specifically in the leg and foot. Measurements on this test are not precise and will be dependent on the subjective judgment of the instructor. However, the plumb line or the posture screen serves as a good point of reference from which to make fairly accurate judgments. Exercise programs for the various conditions that might be discovered in these examinations are described in Chapter 5.

Tests of the pelvic girdle
Anteroposterior deviations

Description. Tests for an increased pelvic angle, sometimes called a forward (downward) pelvic tilt, and for an upward (backward) tilt of the pelvis are made while the person is examined from the lateral view. Several tests are available for use by the instructor. The first test compares the position of the anterosuperior spine of the ilium with the symphysis pubis. In correct pelvic alignment, these two landmarks fall on the same vertical line. If the anterosuperior spine of the ilium falls in a plane

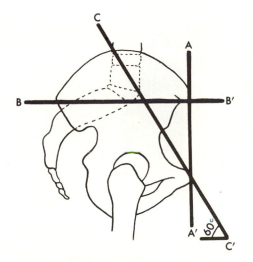

Fig. 9-32. Anteroposterior pelvic tilt examinations. *A-A',* Anterosuperior spine and symphysis pubis in vertical alignment; *B-B',* Anterosuperior spine and posterosuperior spine in horizontal alignment; *C-C',* Line connecting lumbosacral joint with symphysis pubis forms a 50- to 60-degree angle with a horizontal line.

anterior to the line of the symphysis pubis, the student has a condition described as a *forward* (anterior) or *downward* pelvic tilt, whereas the reverse would be described as a *backward* (posterior) or *upward* pelvic tilt.

A second test involves a comparison of the position of the anterosuperior spine of the ilium with the posterosuperior spine of the ilium. In this case, the two landmarks fall on the same horizontal line. If the anterosuperior spine of the ilium falls in a plane that is lower than the posterosuperior spine, the individual has an *increased forward* (anterior) or *downward* pelvic tilt. If the reverse is true, the individual has a *decreased backward* (posterior) or *upward* pelvic tilt.

The third test is called the pelvic angle test. This consists of locating the lumbosacral joint and the symphysis pubis and drawing an imaginary line connecting these two segments. The angle that results when this line joins a horizontal plane of the body can be compared by the instructor with the so-called normal angle of 50 to 60 degrees of pelvic inclination[13] (Fig. 9-32).

Uses and limitations. Any one of these tests can be used to help determine the amount of pelvic inclination. A completely objective evaluation of pelvic inclination is difficult to make for several reasons. The individual may be very heavy, with large fat pads anteriorly and posteriorly that make it difficult to make any evaluation of either the pelvic position or the pelvic angle. The individual may be wearing bulky clothes that cover the region of the pelvis and low back and therefore make visual inspection difficult. The individual may also have a very large buttock region or a large anterior overhang of the lower abdominal region, which makes a subjective evaluation very difficult to make. Usually one set of the measurements described previously can be obtained while the individual is examined and they will allow the instructor to make a more accurate evaluation. The relationship between the tilt of the pelvis, the alignment of the upper leg and knee, and the lower portion of the spine has been discussed in an earlier portion of this chapter. It is important to check the amount of pelvic inclination of any student with bent or back knee or with lordosis or flat lower back. For a more objective evaluation of pelvic tilt, an x-ray examination is necessary.

Lateral deviations

Description. Lateral tilt of the pelvis can be evaluated from either the anterior view or the posterior view. Usually the examination is made from both views in order to verify that a lateral tilt exists and to look for torques in the pelvis. These tests are usually made by evaluating the individual with the horizontal lines of the posture screen.

Instructions for use. For the anterior examination, the anterosuperior spines of the ilium are either marked with a skin pencil or located by the instructor and the student is instructed to place one index finger on each spine. The student then stands behind the posture screen with the feet placed an equal distance to either side of the center (gravity) line of the screen. The instructor then steps back 10 to 12 feet from the screen, directly at its center, and sights through the screen to determine whether the anterosuperior spines fall on the same horizontal line. The posterior examination is conducted in the same manner, with the posterosuperior spines of the ilium being marked and the individual checked from the posterior view. The amount of deviation in the height of the spines can then be estimated and recorded on the student's posture examination form (Fig. 9-38, *C*).

If the instructor so desires, a measuring tape can be used to check the distance from the floor to the anterosuperior spine of the ilium on each side in order to determine whether the leg lengths are identical. Individual segments of the leg can also be measured in an attempt to determine where any deviation in length exists, for example, measuring the distance from the internal malleolus to the patella or to the anterosuperior spine on each side. Another technique that can be used to determine how much difference there is in the height of the sides of the pelvis involves the use of leg length blocks. These blocks are approximately 12 inches long and 3 inches wide and vary in thickness from $1/8$ to $1 1/2$ inches at $1/4$-inch intervals. Any one or combination of these blocks can be placed underneath the foot of the leg on the low side of the pelvis until the pelvis is level, as viewed through the grids of the posture screen. If the student stands on this board with the back to the posture screen,

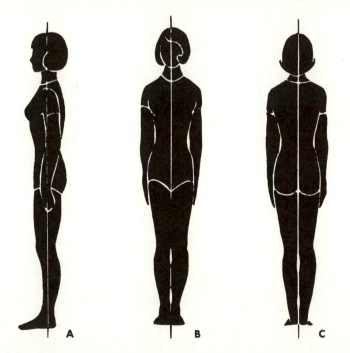

Fig. 9-33. Plumb line tests. **A,** Lateral examination. **B,** Anterior examination. **C,** Posterior examination.

any resulting improvement in the lateral alignment of the spine can be observed. If the student wears a lift in the shoe but does not have one for the gym shoes, these same blocks can be placed under the foot while he or she is exercising in the adapted physical education room. Students with marked deviations in the height of the pelvis or with pain associated with pelvic tilt should be referred to an orthopedist for a more extensive examination, for recommendations relative to the need for a lift in the shoe, and for advice on special exercises and activities.

Other tests of the pelvic girdle

Jorris[7] devised an instrument, called the *tilt-o-meter*, with which anteroposterior and lateral pelvic tilts can be measured. Where it is possible to locate the same landmarks as were described previously, it is possible to use the Jorris tilt-o-meter to obtain an evaluation of the amount of tilt of the pelvis.

Total body examinations
Plumb line tests

Description. A plumb line can be held by the instructor or can be hung so that it falls between the person being examined and the instructor. It is used as a vertical line or reference to check both the anteroposterior and the lateral body alignment of the student. Certain surface landmarks on the body that align with a gravity line of the human body have been located by kinesiologists and engineers. These surface landmarks can be used as points of reference in conducting examinations designed to see how well the body is balanced and how well its segments are aligned in the upright position.

Lateral view. From the lateral view (anteroposterior deviations), starting at the base of support and working up the body, the gravity line should fall at a point about 1 to 1½ inches anterior to the external malleolus, just posterior to the patella, through the center of the hip at the approximate center of the greater trochanter of the femur, through the center of the shoulder (acromial process), and through the lobe of the ear.

Anterior view. From the anterior view (lateral deviations), the gravity line should fall an equal distance between the internal malleoli and between the knees; should pass through the center of the symphysis pubis, the center of the umbilicus, the center of the linea alba, the center of the chin, and the center of the nose; and should bisect the center of the upper portion of the head.

Posterior view. The landmarks to be checked in the posterior examination (lateral deviations) would include the following: the same points as those checked in the anterior examination in the region of the ankle and the knee, the cleft of the buttocks, the center of the spinous processes of the spinal column, and the center of the head. The plumb line does not provide as many points of ref-

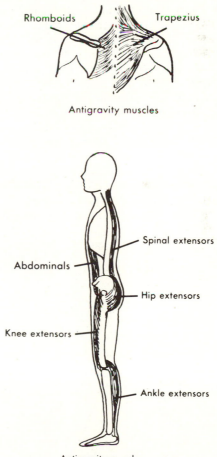

Fig. 9-34. Antigravity muscles involved in maintaining erect posture.

erence as does the posture screen, since only one vertical line is available to be used as a reference for all anteroposterior and lateral postural deviations (Fig. 9-33). The posture grid provides both vertical and horizontal lines to be used as reference points for evaluating all segments of the body in relation to their contribution to a well-balanced, comfortable standing position, which is maintained by proper use of the antigravity muscle groups of the body (Fig. 9-34).

Posture screen

Description. A posture screen consists of a rectangular frame, mounted on legs so that it stands upright and laced with string so that a 2-inch-square grid pattern (4- and 6-inch squares are recommended by some) crosses the frame. The vertical lines are parallel to a center (gravity) line and the horizontal lines are exactly at right angles to the gravity line. The center line is usually of a color different from that of the other strings. This makes it easy to identify and to use in comparison with the landmarks described previously. It is possible to have a conformator built into the side of the posture screen, thus allowing the teacher with limited budget and space to have two pieces of apparatus in one. The conformator will be described later under the discussion of anteroposterior curvature of the spine (Figs. 9-40 and 20-26).

Instructions for use. The student should wear as little clothing as possible during the posture examination. Tight-fitting trunks for boys and girls,

with a halter-type top for girls, are suggested. Neither shoes nor socks should be worn. It is almost impossible to administer an accurate examination if such landmarks as the ankle bones, kneecaps, spines of the pelvis, spinous processes of the vertebrae, medial borders of the scapula, and linea alba cannot be observed.

The posture screen should be checked for proper alignment with a plumb line to be sure that the gravity line is actually true and that the screen is also plumb when viewed from the side. It is then necessary to locate a point, about 18 inches from the posture screen, where the student will be centered properly behind the gravity line. This point is determined by having the instructor move to a position 10 to 15 feet away from the posture screen and standing in alignment with the center string while holding a plumb line out in front. Sighting through the plumb line and the center line of the screen, a point can be marked on the floor 18 inches behind the screen. This point will be in alignment with the instructor and the center line itself. Thus, when the student stands behind the screen with the exterior malleoli 1½ inches behind this point, it is possible to evaluate the posture from the anterior, posterior, and lateral views in relation to the center line of the screen (Fig. 9-35).

A posture screen may be used to give quick superficial screening examinations to identify students in need of special posture correction programs or it may be used to give a very thorough examination to those students who have been

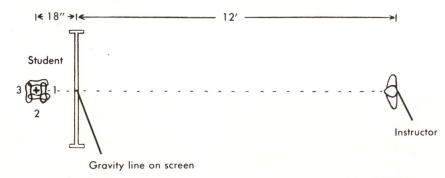

Fig. 9-35. Alignment of posture screen as viewed from above. *1,* Anterior, *2,* lateral, and *3,* posterior examinations.

screened previously and have been identified as being in need of special programs for the correction of their posture and body alignment.

A posture examination is much more meaningful to the student and far more useful to the teacher if the findings are carefully recorded by the examiner (especially during review of the material obtained in the examination prior to setting up an exercise or activity program or when doing a reevaluation of the pupil several months after the original examination). The examination record must provide space for the instructor to record the findings of the examination quickly and accurately. Provisions should be made for recording the severity of each of the conditions identified in the examination. The findings of successive examinations can also be recorded on the same form. An example showing a three-way figure with the proper labels and with numbers to indicate the severity of the conditions discovered is shown in Fig. 9-36, *B*. With this kind of prepared examination form, the instructor can very quickly identify deviations observed through the posture grid and can record them on the card by drawing a diagonal line through the number that indicates the severity of the condition: first degree, slight; second degree, moderate; and third degree, severe (Fig. 9-37). No other writing is necessary unless the instructor identifies something that does not appear on the chart or wishes to record special information to be used at a later time. Successive examinations can be made on the same posture form by using different colored pencils to indicate second, third, or fourth examinations. In this way, improvement can be shown through the use of the cumulative record.

Anterior view. The student is instructed to stand directly behind the posture screen with the internal malleoli of the ankles placed 1½ inches posterior to and an *equal* distance from the + mark on the floor (see Fig. 9-35). This will place the student in the proper position so that the surface landmarks of the body will fall in correct alignment in relation to the center (gravity) line of the screen. The student is then instructed to stand as he or she would normally. The instructor should take a position about 10 to 15 feet back from the posture screen and in direct line with the center line. The posture examination record can be mounted on a clipboard held by the examiner or a lectern can be used to hold the forms so as to facilitate recording the findings. Since the feet serve as the base of support, it is important to examine the student from the base of support upward in checking for proper body alignment. Specific examinations for the foot, ankle, knee, and leg have been covered in preceding sections of the chapter; they will be reviewed very briefly in this section, largely in terms of their influence on posture and the alignment of the rest of the body.

The feet should be checked to see if they are pointed straight forward or toeing in or out. The longitudinal arch should be higher on its medial than on its lateral side. The inner and outer malleoli should be about equal in prominence and the scaphoid bone should not project unduly medially. The ankles and knees should be straight, with the kneecaps facing directly forward when the feet are held in the straight forward position. The height of the kneecaps and the anterosuperior spines of the ilium should be even. The gravity line passes midway between the ankle bones, between the knees, and then falls directly through the umbilicus, the linea alba, the center of the chin, and the center of the nose. As the instructor's eyes move up the body from the region of the pelvis to the shoulders, the symmetry of the sides of the body must be checked. Any abnormal curvature or creasing on one side of the trunk (not found on the other side) should lead to a more careful examination to determine whether a lateral sway or tilt of the body or a lateral curvature of the spine exists. Lateral spine curvature must be checked if any deviations in the position of the umbilicus or of the linea alba exist or if there are any apparent differences in the depth of the sides of the chest.

With boys, the nipple levels are compared, and with both boys and girls the heights of the creases made where the arms join the body should be checked to be sure that the two creases on either side are symmetrical. It is also necessary to check to see if one arm hangs closer to the trunk than the other (Fig. 9-38, *B*). The shoulder height must be checked to see if the shoulders are level. If the pelvis is found to have a lateral pelvic tilt or if a high or low shoulder is noted, the student is then checked for a lateral curvature of the spine. Al-

California State University, Long Beach
PHYSICAL EDUCATION DEPARTMENT
Adapted physical education appraisal

Name _____ Age _____ Date _____
      Last   First   Middle

Year in school _____

Physical disability (Be exact, give dates.) (This information is obtained from the student or parent.)

_____
_____
_____

Other disabilities and injuries discovered (Be exact, give dates.) _____

_____
_____
_____

Results of physical examination (This information is obtained from the physician.)

Classification   A   B   C   1   2   3   4   5   6   7   8   9   0

_____
_____

Recommendation of physician _____

_____
_____

Assignment in adapted physical education class   Temporary   Permanent   Strict   Mild

Nutritional status information _____

Examination number	1	2	1	2

Pryor index   Behnke index _____

   Age (years, months) _____   Weight (normal) _____

   Height (inches) _____   Weight (actual) _____

   Pelvis width (cm) _____   Weight (variation) _____

   Chest width (cm) _____

   Weight (normal) _____   Other tests _____

   Weight (actual) _____   _____

   Weight (variation) _____

Skin fold measurements (mm) _____

   Triceps _____ = % _____   Biceps _____ = % _____

   Scapular _____ = % _____   Suprailiac _____ = % _____

Body type (Sheldon) _____

   Endomorph   Mesomorph   Ectomorph

   1 2 3 4 5 6 7   1 2 3 4 5 6 7   1 2 3 4 5 6 7

Follow-up examinations

Examination	Dates checked	Examination	Dates checked
Blood pressure		Anthropometric measurements (Specify.)	
Heart		1. Girth	
Cardiogram		2.	
Others		3.	
X-ray films		4.	
Photography		Nutrition	
Posture		Diet analysis	
Divergency		Basal metabolism	
Foot		Other tests	
Tracings			
Pedograph			
Podiascope			
Joint measurements			

Code used on this appraisal sheet

Severity of condition	Record of examinations
Calipers	
Goniometer	1 degree = Noticeable to First examination—Black pencil
Tracings	slight Second examination—Blue pencil
Spine	2 degree = Moderate Third examination—Red pencil
Tracings	3 degree = Severe Fourth examination—Green pencil
Conformator	

A

Fig. 9-36. Adapted physical education appraisal. **A,** Front. **B,** Back. See text for explanation of appraisal of scoliosis conditions marked with an asterisk.

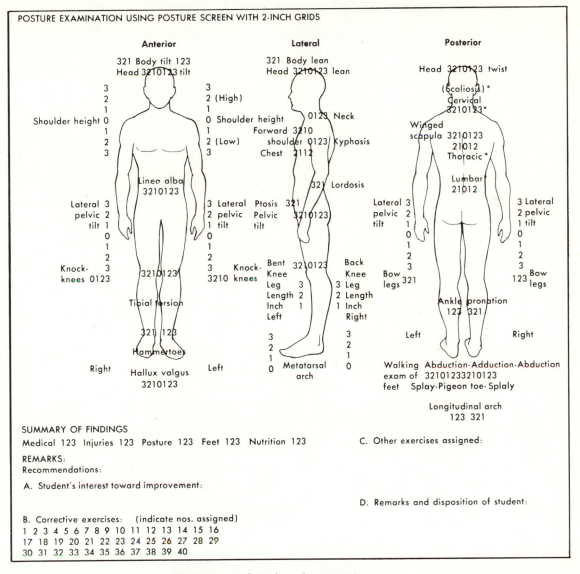

POSTURE EXAMINATION USING POSTURE SCREEN WITH 2-INCH GRIDS

Anterior

321 Body tilt 123
Head 3210123 tilt

3
2
1
Shoulder height 0
1
2
3

Lineo alba
3210123

Lateral 3
pelvic 2
tilt 1
0
1
2
Knock- 3
knees 0123

3210123

Tibial torsion

321 123

Hammertoes

Right   Hallux valgus   Left
3210123

Lateral

321 Body lean
Head 3210123 lean

3
2 (High)
1
0 Shoulder height
1
2 (Low)
3

0123 Neck
Forward 3210
shoulder 0123 Kyphosis
Chest 2112

321 Lordosis

3 Lateral Ptosis 321
2 pelvic Pelvic
1 tilt 3210123
0
1
2
3 Knock-
3210 knees

Bent 3210123   Back
Knee   Knee
Leg   3   3 Leg
Length 2   2 Length
Inch   1   1 Inch
Left   Right

3   3
2   2
1   1
0 Metatarsal 0
   arch

Posterior

Head 3210123 twist

(Scoliosis) *
Cervical
3210123 *

Winged
scapula 3210123
21012
Thoracic *

Lumbar
21012

Lateral 3   3 Lateral
pelvic 2   2 pelvic
tilt 1   1 tilt
0   0
1   1
2   2
3   3
Bow   Bow
legs 321   123 legs

Ankle pronation
123 321

Left   Right

Walking Abduction-Adduction-Abduction
exam of 32101233210123
feet   Splay-Pigeon toe-Splaly

Longitudinal arch
123 321

B

SUMMARY OF FINDINGS
Medical 123 Injuries 123 Posture 123 Feet 123 Nutrition 123   C. Other exercises assigned:

REMARKS:
Recommendations:

A. Student's interest toward improvement:

                                                                D. Remarks and disposition of student:

B. Corrective exercises: (indicate nos. assigned)
1 2 3 4 5 6 7 8 9 10 11 12 13 14 15 16
17 18 19 20 21 22 23 24 25 26 27 28 29
30 31 32 33 34 35 36 37 38 39 40

Fig. 9-36, cont'd. For legend see opposite page.

DEGREE OF DEVIATION CHART
Individual posture examination using a posture screen with 2-inch grids

Anterior view		Lateral view		Posterior view	
Condition	**Degree of severity**	**Condition**	**Degree of severity**	**Condition**	**Degree of severity**
Body tilt	1 inch = 1 degree	Body lean	1 inch = 1 degree	Head twist	Subjective evaluation
Head tilt	½ inch = 1 degree	Head lean	½ inch = 1 degree	Scoliosis (see cervical, thoracic, lumbar)	½ inch = 1 degree at each spinal level
Shoulder height	½ inch = 1 degree	Forward shoulders	Subjective evaluation (check tip of shoulder with gravity line)	Winged scapula	Subjective evaluation and measure distance between scapulae
Linea alba	½ inch = 1 degree	Kyphosis	Subjective evaluation and /or conformator	Lateral pelvic tilt (compare postero superior spines of ilium)	¼ inch = 1 degree
Lateral pelvic tilt (anterior, superior spines of ilium)	½ inch = 1 degree	Chest	Subjective evaluation	Bowlegs (measure at the knees)	½ inch = 1 degree
Knock-knees (measure at the ankles)	½ inch = 1 degree	Lordosis	Subjective evaluation and /or conformator	Ankle and foot pronation	Subjective evaluation, Helbing's sign, and foot tracer
Tibial torsion	Subjective evaluation	Ptosis	Subjective evaluation	Abduction (splay foot) or adduction (pigeon toe)	Subjective evaluation and foot tracer
Hammer toes	Subjective evaluation	Pelvic tilt	Mark anterior and posterior spines of ilium and compare height	Longitudinal arch	Height of scaphoid bone ¼ inch = 1 degree
Hallux valgus	Subjective evaluation	Bent and back knee	Subjective evaluation re: gravity line		
Leg length	Measure legs or use leg length boards and posture screen	Metatarsal arch	Subjective evaluation or pedograph print and podiascope		

Fig. 9-37. Individual posture examination degree of deviation chart. These figures were developed over a 10-year period for use with college students at the University of California at Los Angeles and California State University at Long Beach.

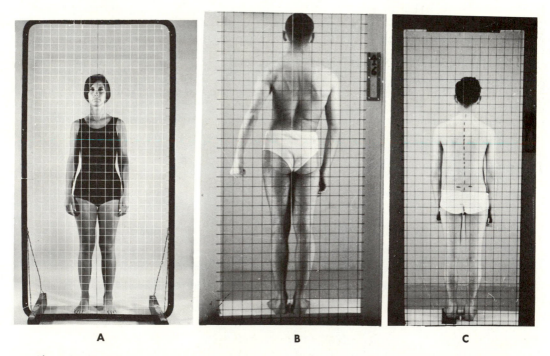

A B C

Fig. 9-38. Posture examinations with a posture screen. **A,** Anterior view examination. **B,** Structural scoliosis. **C,** Functional scoliosis. Note spinal alignment when a leg lift board is placed under the left foot.

though lateral curvatures will not occur with all the previously noted conditions, these types of conditions may serve as possible indicators of such a problem. The examiner next checks the head position to be sure that it is held in alignment with the gravity line and to determine if there is any twisting of the head and neck. Finally, the total body should be viewed in terms of whether it is being held in good alignment and balance and to see if any lateral tilts of the total body exist (Fig. 9-38).

Posterior view. The student is instructed to assume the same position in relation to the posture screen as in the anterior examination, except that the back is now turned to the screen, that is, with the inner ankle bones over the marker on the floor. The posterior examination should give the instructor an opportunity to double-check many of the conditions noted from the anterior view and will also allow the instructor to make an evaluation of certain other conditions that cannot be checked during the anterior view examination. Foot alignment can again be checked, with special emphasis this time being placed on whether the forepart of the foot is abducted, the top part of the calcaneous bone is rotated medialward, the heel cords are bowed in, and the inner and outer malleoli are of approximately equal prominence. It should also be checked to see if the inner sides of the malleoli and the inner sides of the femoral condyles are about the same distance apart and if the legs are in good, straight alignment. Previous judgments about bowlegs and knock-knees can be double-checked in the posterior view. The level of the hips can also be checked.

The gravity line passes directly up through the cleft of the buttocks and through the center of the spinous processes of each of the vertebrae, bisecting the head through its center. The posterior examination is the best for scoliosis (rotolateral curvature). If a lateral curvature exists, further examinations should be made to see if there is any rotation or torque in the pelvic girdle. The degree of lateral deviation and the amount of rotation that has taken place in the spinal column should also be checked. All the areas where lateral deviation of the spine could be present are indicated on the posture card, along with a place to indicate the degree of severity. The examination of the spinal column can be made more meaningful, if scoliosis is suspected, by marking the posterior surfaces of the spinous processes of the vertebrae with a skin pencil so that the curves can be observed more accurately (Figs. 9-38, *B* and *C*). The sides of the trunk are also checked as they were in the anterior view for any abnormal unilateral curvatures and for any creases or bulges on one side only, which would indicate the presence of a tilt or of a lateral spinal curve.

From the posterior view, the shoulder blades, or scapulae, are viewed to determine whether they are flat against the rib cage, whether the medial borders have been pulled laterally in abduction, and whether the medial border and the inferior angle of the scapula project outward from the back of the rib cage. This latter condition is known as a *winged scapula.* The distance between the medial borders of the scapulae can be measured with a tape measure and this distance can be compared with measurements taken after corrective exercises have been assigned to pull the scapulae together and flatten them against the rib cage. The head position must also be checked from the posterior view to verify the findings of the anterior examination relative to the presence of a head tilt or head twist.

If differences between the anterior and the posterior examinations occur, they may be a result of the fact that the student is sighting on the gravity line in the anterior view and is standing in a stiff or posed position. If this visual cue is used by the student, it should be removed. One way to do this is to have the individual close the eyes at the conclusion of the posterior examination; keep the feet in exactly the same position; bend over at the waist; and freely swing the arms, shoulders, and upper body back and forth from side to side. Then have the student stand up again, keeping the eyes closed; double-check the posture from the posterior view. This should help to identify the natural standing body alignment (one that *feels* comfortable to the student) and should rule out the factors of posing and using the eyes for correct alignment.

Lateral view. For the lateral or side view, the student stands with the left side to the screen (the side facing the screen is the one shown on the posture examination form). One foot is placed on either side of the + drawn on the floor, with the inner malleolus about $1\frac{1}{2}$ inches behind its center. Deviations in alignment and posture can readily be observed through the screen. Abnormalities in flexion and extension of the toes may be easier to see from the side than they were from the front. The lateral examination is used to verify conditions noted in other phases of the examination. The whole conformation of the foot should also be checked for such things as redness, swelling, heavy calluses, undue rotation, or pressure on the various areas of the feet and ankles.

The center line of the screen should pass about 1 inch anterior to the external malleolus, just behind the patella at the knee, and through the center of the hip at about the center of the greater trochanter of the femur bone. If the student has back knee, the gravity line will fall too far forward in relation to the patella; if the student has bent knee, it will fall too far back (toward the center of the knee).

If the student has a total forward or backward lean of the body, alignment is basically correct at all joints, except the ankle, where he or she is leaning too far forward or backward. In this case, the examiner will find that the reference points become progressively farther out of alignment with each segment from the foot to the head. If the alignment is correct at the ankle and at the shoulder, but the center of the hip is too far forward, the individual will have a total body sway, whereas if the hips are too far back, the individual will have a distorted position of the low back and buttocks. If the alignment is correct at the ankle, knee, and hip, but the shoulder and the head are positioned too far posteriorly, the student will have what is called a posterior overhang. It is quite easy to identify these various conditions when the body landmarks are viewed in relation to the gravity line of the posture screen (Fig. 9-39). The amount of deviation is ascertained by judging the distance the affected body parts are out of alignment in relation to the grids of the posture screen. Corrective procedures for leans and sways are presented in Chapter 5.

Forward or backward pelvic tilt can be quickly checked in the examination through the posture screen by marking either the anterior and posterior superior iliac spines and checking them against the horizontal lines of the screen or by marking the anterior spine of the ilium and the symphysis pubis and checking this alignment against one of the vertical lines. It is usually easier to evaluate these landmarks if the student places a finger on each of them so that they can be seen more easily by the examiner.

The vertebral spine should then be checked throughout its length for what would be termed its normal curvatures. In the region of the lower back, the two conditions that are noted are (1) excessive hyperextension in the lumbar spine, a condition called *lordosis,* and (2) too little curve in the lumbar spine, known as *flat low back.* When the lumbar spine goes into a flexion curve, it is called *lumbar kyphosis.* This is not observed frequently, however. Usually associated with these lower back conditions are a pelvic tilt forward (with lordosis) and a pelvic tilt backward (with a flat low back). Often associated with these conditions, especially with lordosis, is abdominal *ptosis.* Ptosis refers to a relaxation of the lower abdominal muscles with a sagging of the abdomen forward, often accompanied by misplacement of the pelvic organs. The degree of severity of this deviation must be judged subjectively (Fig. 9-14).

In the region of the chest and shoulders, the nor-

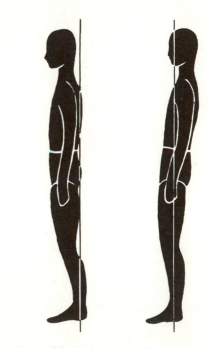

Fig. 9-39. Total body forward and backward leans (plumb line test).

mal curvature of the spine is one of mild flexion. The abnormal condition that would be looked for in the thoracic spine is an excessive amount of flexion in this region, which, in its severest form, is called *humpback*. Any abnormal increase in flexion is known as *kyphosis*. Kyphosis is often associated with a flattening of the chest and rib cage and, frequently, with deviations in the alignment of the shoulder girdle, called *forward shoulders* and *winged scapula*. Although these four conditions are often found in the same individual, they do not necessarily occur together. The winged scapula, mentioned in the posterior examination, should be checked again from the lateral position

to see whether the inner border projects to the rear and whether the inferior angle projects outward from the rib cage. The degree of deviation in forward (round) shoulders is judged subjectively and is related to how far forward of the gravity line the center of the shoulder falls.

In the region of the neck, the most common condition found is a forward position of the cervical vertebrae accompanying a forward head. An abnormal amount of hyperextension in the cervical or neck vertebrae exists when the individual has attempted to correct a faulty head position by bringing the head back and the chin up. All the antero-posterior curves of the spine (discussed previously)

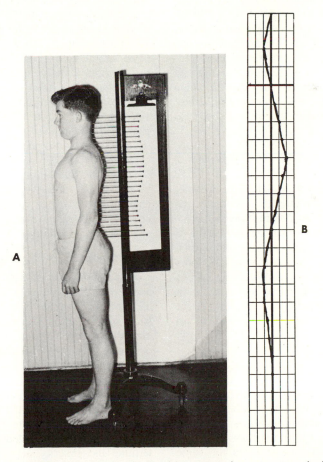

Fig. 9-40. A, Conformator examination for charting life-size spinal curves on attached sheet of paper. **B,** Conformator examination charted to scale on the posture examination card or graph paper by viewing conformator through the grids of a posture screen. (See Fig. 20-26.)

can be judged subjectively as to the degree of severity or can be measured more objectively through the use of a conformator (Fig. 9-40).

If the instructor believes that students are posing for the examination, the technique described at the last part of the posterior examination can be used to disorient them.

In all the examinations described previously, the instructor must be alert to the possibility that one postural deviation often leads to, causes, or is the result of another. It is a pattern of the human body to attempt to keep itself in some semblance of a state of balance (homeostasis). Therefore, when one segment or various segments of the body become malaligned, it is customary (sooner or later) for the body to attempt to compensate for this by throwing other segments out of alignment, thus obtaining a balanced position. An example of this would be the individual with lordosis who compensates with kyphosis and forward head. The individual with a simple C scoliosis curve in the spine may compensate for this with a complex S curve (an effort to return the spine, and thus the body, to a state of balance).

Tests for functional-structural conditions
Description

Several tests may be used to determine whether spinal curvatures are functional (involving the muscles and soft tissue) or structural (involving the bones). Postural deviations that are the result of muscle and soft tissue imbalance are considered functional and will often disappear when the force of gravity is removed. Structural posture deviations have gone beyond the soft tissue stage, with involvement of the supportive bones and connective tissue, and are not eliminated by the removal of gravitational influences.

Instructions for use

Prone lying test. The prone lying test is designed to check anteroposterior or lateral curves of the spine. Functional curves will disappear or will be decreased when the student assumes the prone position on a bench, a table, or the floor.

Hanging test. The hanging test has the same uses as the prone lying test. The individual hangs by the hands from a horizontal support. Functional curves disappear or are decreased in this position (Fig. 9-41, *B*).

Adam's test. The Adam's test is used to determine whether a lateral deviation of the spine (scoliosis) is functional or structural. The student assumes a normal standing position, then gradually bends the head forward, continuing with the trunk until the hands approximate the toes. The instructor stands a short distance behind the student and observes the student's spine and the sides of the back as the student *slowly* bends forward. If the spine straightens and if the sides of the back are symmetrical in shape and height, the scoliosis is considered functional (Fig. 9-41, *C*). Corrective procedures should be started under the direction of a physician.

If the spine does not straighten and if one side of the back (especially in the thoracic region) is more prominent (sticks up higher) than the other as the student bends forward, the scoliosis is judged to be structural (Fig. 9-41, *D*). In structural cases, the rotation of the vertebrae accompanying the lateral bend of the spine causes the attached ribs to assume a greater posterior prominence on the convex side of the curve. This curve does not disappear in the Adam's test after bony changes occur in the spinal column. Structural cases must be cared for by an orthopedist.

Uses and limitations. The Adam's test is used by physicians, therapists, and physical educators to analyze lateral spinal curves. It provides an evaluation of scoliosis, which can be verified by x-ray examination, if desired.

Photography

Photography can be used in many aspects of the adapted physical education program, especially in all types of posture examinations. It can be used successfully in photographing the individual behind the posture screen. This has some advantages over other kinds of examinations, since it provides a permanent record of how the student actually looked at the time of the examination. It also serves as a motivating device, since the student can then see deviations and the instructor can point out what can be done to correct them. The posture picture also may be evaluated by the instructor to determine the severity of various conditions, especially when a posture screen is used, since deviations can then be evaluated in relation to the grids of the screen. In doing posture photography through a posture screen, it is necessary to stan-

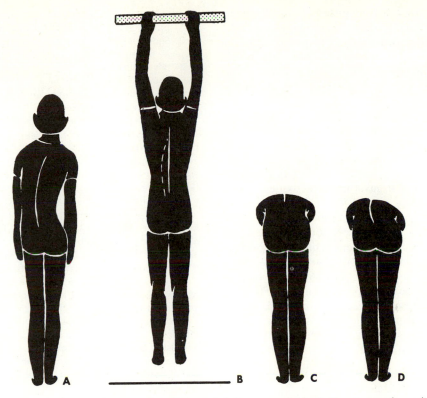

Fig. 9-41. Test for functional-structural scoliosis. **A,** Left C curve scoliosis. **B,** Hanging test for scoliosis. Note straight line indicates spinal position during hanging test. **C,** Adam's test showing functional scoliosis. **D,** Adam's test showing structural scoliosis.

dardize procedures completely so that photographs can be taken quickly and accurately when the need arises. This can be done by determining the proper distance, the proper settings for the camera, and the proper lighting to be used. It is also important to provide a proper backdrop behind the subject so that a clear, well-defined picture is obtained each time a student is photographed (Figs. 9-38 and 20-26). The use of videotape is also an excellent way to record and study posture. The teacher and student can immediately evaluate the static and moving posture pictures thus recorded.

Moving posture examinations

Description. Many persons have been critical of static posture evaluations, indicating the following:

1. Students are likely to pose in this type of examination.
2. When a plumb line or posture screen is used,

the student may use it to obtain visual cues to correct faulty posture.
3. The posture examination does not indicate the student's habitual standing posture.
4. No attention is given to posture and alignment as they would relate to students' movements in activities.

For these reasons, it is wise to include, as a part of the total posture examination, certain phases in which the students are actually in motion and during which they may or may not know that they are being examined. This may be accomplished in several different ways. One is to deploy the class for exercises, observing them as they perform during the exercise program and when they remain in a standing or sitting position between exercises. To enable the examining teacher to identify those students with major deviations and to record this properly on the student's examination form, students must either be organized in a fashion in which the instructor knows all the students by name or by a number or students may be removed from the group as posture deviations are noted. Their names should then be taken so that the posture deviations noted are recorded for the proper students.

Another technique that can be used to evaluate posture and body mechanics during movement is to have the students gather in a large circle around the teacher, or with the teacher standing at the periphery of the circle, and then have the students walk, run, or do various kinds of activities as they move continuously around the circle. The teacher or therapist identifies those children who are in special need of posture correction and removes them from the circle. Their names are then recorded, along with the appropriate information regarding their posture deviations. As a part of each of these two types of examinations, especially if they are given in lieu of any type of static examination, the students should also assume a normal standing position with the teacher evaluating posture from the front, lateral, and rear views.[4,10]

INDIVIDUAL EDUCATION PROGRAMS FOR POSTURE PROBLEMS

Persons with severe posture and body mechanics problems should have proper assessment, and the Individual Education Programs should then provide for activities and special exercises to balance antagonistic muscles and to help with the development of specific and total body proprioception to provide the maximum degree of correction possible. Two examples of such programs follow.*

Case 1. An 8-year-old child has badly pronated and abducted feet and ankles. Helbing's sign is observed, showing marked inward curvature in the Achilles tendons of both feet. Test information is gathered as follows. A foot and ankle tracing is made of each foot with the foot tracer as described in a previous section of this chapter. This will be compared with later tracings to indicate improvement (Fig. 9-30). Using a goniometer the number of degrees of abduction (toeing out) of each foot is measured and recorded.

Performance objectives for this child might include the following:

---

*See also examples in Crowe, W. C. Arnheim, D. D., and Auxter, D.: Laboratory manual in adapted physical education and recreation, St. Louis, 1977, The C. V. Mosby Co.

1. Show an improvement of $1/2$ inch in foot and ankle pronation as measured with a foot tracer.
2. Show an improvement of 10 degrees of foot adduction as measured with a goniometer by the instructor or physical therapist.

Muscle strength tests also can be used as criteria of progress. Evaluation tests will be administered by the instructor or physical therapist.

Exercises and activities recommended include the following: exercises (see Chapter 5) for *warm up* and for *stretch* of the heel cord and the lateral muscles of the lower leg (No. 10, bicycle, and No. 12, foot circling) and specially assigned work on the heel cord stretch and supinator boards (Fig. 20-14); and developmental exercises to strengthen the medial side of the foot and ankle and to help to turn the foot into the normal straight position (No. 15, knee rotator, and No. 14, foot curling). The person should also practice walking with the medial edge of each foot parallel to the edge of a line 2 inches wide painted on the floor and work on correct standing positions in front of a mirror. Good standing and walking mechanics and concentration on the feeling of the *corrected* positions of the foot, ankle, and leg must be stressed at all times.

Motivation techniques might include "before and after" still or moving picture photography, assessment of progress using the two assessment tests on a monthly basis, and keeping a record card of repetitions, resistance used, and distance traveled during exercise and activities (see Fig. 5-47).

Case 2. Persons with severe third degree postural or functional kyphosis of the thoracic spine. Assessment procedures include x-ray examination by an orthopedic physician, conformator test by the adapted physical education teacher, and muscle testing by the teacher or physical therapist. Under the guidance of an orthopedic physician or a physiatrist, if needed, a program of flexibility exercises for the anterior chest (pectoralis minor and pectoralis major) and strengthening and shortening exercises of the extensors of the back (sacrospinalis) and the abductors of the shoulder girdle (rhomboideus major, rhomboideus minor, and trapezius) are recommended.

Performance objectives might include the following:

1. Stop the progress of the kyphosis and show an improvement of 5 degrees by the end of the eighth month as measured by the physician with x-ray films.
2. Show an improvement of $1/4$ inch in the dorsal curve as measured by a second test with conformator at the end of the eighth month.
3. Show an improvement of 5 pounds in scapular adduction (rhomboideus major, rhomboideus minor, and trapezius) and 7 pounds in extension of the thoracic spine (sacrospinalis) as measured by a cable tensiometer at the end of the seventh month.

Exercises and activities include the following: for general *warm up* of the upper trunk—No. 1, supine stretch and No. 39, jumping jack with variations; to *stretch* the anterior chest and shoulder girdle—passive stretching in the hook lying position, arms in inverted T position with a rolled-up towel between the scapulae (Fig. 20-9), and No. 4, neck, back, and shoulder tightener; to *strengthen* and *shorten* the spinal extensors and the shoulder girdle abductors—No. 6, neck flattener at mirror, and No. 29, chin lift. Other activities to be recommended include swimming the elementary backstroke concentrating on fully extending the thoracic spine; relaxing in the supine position on a mat or the floor with arms extended overhead and with the back of the hands and elbows resting on the floor; and practicing standing tall and straight in front of a mirror, then walking around the room and return to check the moving and static posture in the mirror. (See Chapters 5 and 7.)

Individual Exercise Programs can be written in a similar way to accommodate all of the different conditions discussed in this chapter, using the assessment tools described. Additional exercises and activities are discussed in Chapters 5, 6, and 10.

REFERENCES

1. Adams, W. C., et al.: Foundations of physical activity, Champaign, Ill., 1972, Stipes Publishing Co.
2. Barham, J. N., and Wooten, E. P.: Structural kinesiology, New York, 1973, Macmillan Publishing Co., Inc.
3. Clarke, H. H.: Application of measurement to health and physical education, Englewood Cliffs, N.J., 1967, Prentice-Hall, Inc.
4. Corrective physical education, Los Angeles, 1958, Los Angeles City Schools.
5. deVries, H. A.: Physiology of exercise for physical education and athletics, Dubuque, Iowa, 1973, William C. Brown Co., Publishers.
6. Hansson, K. G.: Body mechanics and posture, J.A.M.A. **128:**947-953, 1945.
7. Jorris, T. R.: The relationship between abdominal muscle shortening and anterior-posterior pelvic tilt, Unpublished doctoral dissertation, University of California at Los Angeles, Los Angeles, 1960.
8. Kelly, E. D.: Adapted and corrective physical education, New York, 1965, The Ronald Press Co.
9. Logan, G., and Dunkelberg, J.: Adaptations of muscular activity, Belmont, Calif., 1964, Wadsworth Publishing Co., Inc.
10. Lowman, C. L., Colestock, C., and Cooper, H.: Corrective physical education for groups, Cranberry, N.J., 1928, A. S. Barnes & Co., Inc.
11. Lowman, C. L., and Young, C. H.: Posture fitness significance and variances, Philadelphia, 1960, Lea & Febiger.
12. Morrison, W. R., and Chenoweth, L. B.: Normal and elementary physical diagnosis, Philadelphia, 1955, Lea & Febiger.
13. Rasch, P. J., and Burke, R. K.: Kinesiology and applied anatomy, Philadelphia, 1975, Lea & Febiger.
14. Wells, K. F., and Luttgens, K.: Kinesiology: scientific basis of motion, Philadelphia, 1976, W. B. Saunders Co.

RECOMMENDED READINGS

Barrett, M., et al.: Foundations for movement, Dubuque, Iowa, 1968, William C. Brown Co., Publishers.
Billig, H. E., Jr., and Lowendahl, E.: Mobilization of the human body, Stanford, Calif., 1949, Stanford University Press.
Broer, M. R.: An introduction to kinesiology, Englewood Cliffs, N.J., 1968, Prentice-Hall, Inc.
Crowe, W. C.: The use of audio-visual materials in developmental (corrective) physical education. Unpublished master's thesis, University of California at Los Angeles, Los Angeles, 1950.
Crowe, W. C., Arnheim, D. D., and Auxter, D.: Laboratory manual in adapted physical education and recreation, St. Louis, 1977, The C. V. Mosby Co.
Davis, E. C., Logan, G., and McKinney, W.: Biophysical values of muscular activity, Dubuque, Iowa, 1965, William C. Brown Co., Publishers.
Drury, B. J.: Posture and figure control through physical education, Palo Alto, Calif., 1966, National Press Books.
Kendall, H. O., and Kendall, F. P.: Developing and maintaining good posture, Phys. Ther. **48:**319-336, 1968.
Krusen, F. H., editor: Handbook of physical medicine and rehabilitation, Philadelphia, 1971, W. B. Saunders Co.
Lilly, L. J.: An overview of body mechanics, Palo Alto, Calif., 1967, Peek Publications.
Metheny, E.: Body dynamics, New York, 1952, McGraw-Hill Book Co.
Mueller, G. W., and Christaldi, J.: A practical program of remedial physical education, Philadelphia, 1966, Lea & Febiger.
Rusk, H. A.: Rehabilitation medicine, ed. 4, St. Louis, 1977, The C. V. Mosby Co.
Williams, M., and Lissner, H. R.: Biomechanics of human motion, Philadelphia, 1977, W. B. Saunders Co.
Williams, M., and Worthingham, C.: Therapeutic exercises for body alignment and function, Philadelphia, 1957, W. B. Saunders Co.

10

Musculoskeletal disorders

Acute

The National Safety Council in their 1974 report, which surveyed the number of accidents occurring during the years 1971 through 1973, indicated that there were annually over 62 million accidents causing activity restriction. Of that number, there were over 14 million disabilities so serious as to result in confinement in bed.[1] A significant number of accidents also occurs as the result of sports activities. The young person is subject to many physical hazards that may be attributed to living an active life. There are hundreds of thousands of sports injuries sustained each year, with well over 41,000 serious enough to require hospitalization.[7]

By their very nature, many sports and recreation activities invite injury. The "all out" exertion required, the numerous situations requiring body contact, and the play that involves the striking and throwing of missiles establish hazards that are either directly or indirectly responsible for the many and varied injuries suffered by those engaged in sports.[2] The highest incidence of sports injuries is in the category of sprains and strains, with the greatest number occurring to the lower limbs.

Often, the physical educator or the recreational therapist is called on to assist individuals, both young and old, who have an acute musculoskeletal condition. It is not uncommon that the adapted physical educator or therapist must help in managing a physical education class or must establish a reconditioning program for a person after a recreation or sports injury has been incurred.

Handicapped persons are especially vulnerable to acute injuries that often complicate their lifestyles and further limit their opportunities to be involved in the activities of daily living and in exercise and recreation programs important for their total fitness. Proper rehabilitation programs are, therefore, necessary for such persons. Proper evaluation techniques must be utilized and long-term goals and performance objectives must be included in their Individual Education Programs. Pre- and postevaluation techniques and suggested exercise and activity programs are presented throughout this chapter for each acute condition. Selected examples of Individual Education Programs for acute musculoskeletal conditions are also included.

The acute traumatic injury is characterized as being *sharp* and *intense,* having *rapid onset,* and usually being of *short duration*. Trauma to the musculoskeletal system causes tissue to be either compressed or elongated. Classification of injuries falls into two broad categories: exposed and unexposed. Exposed injuries are wounds that expose external tissue, whereas unexposed injuries are those that occur to underlying tissue.[7]

The reaction of the body to those traumatic forces that tear, crush, overstretch, or shear tissue produces the classic inflammatory quintet: *local heat, swelling, redness, pain,* and *loss of function*. Immediately after injury, there occurs first, constriction of blood vessels and, then, capillary dilation. After capillary dilation, an osmotic fluid imbalance causes blood and exudation of serum to extravasate into the surrounding tissue areas. Pain is produced by swelling and resultant pressure on sensory nerves as well as hormones that destroy tissue. Associated with inflammation is the removal of debris by phagocytosis and repair. Contained within the serum exudate are the ingredients for repair that, eventually, form a granulation tissue scar.[2]

UNEXPOSED INJURIES

In general, unexposed or internal injuries affecting the musculoskeletal system fall into two categories: trauma by compression and trauma by stretching.

Trauma by tissue compression

Injuries to the body that occur by compression of tissue are (1) contusions resulting from sudden and direct blows to the body or other forces that compress and crush tissue and (2) the chronic pressure conditions produced by a constant abnormal external force on the body.

An acute injury to the body can produce varying degrees of muscle spasm and vascular hemorrhage with associated pain. Repeated contusions to a single area under constant abnormal pressure can cause chronic inflammatory conditions. However, chronic compression problems are most apparent with persons who have worn poorly fitting shoes over a long period of time. Shoes that are too long, too short, too narrow, or too pointed cause toes to become deformed (Chapter 9).

Trauma by tissue stretching

Those injuries that occur primarily by the mechanism of stretch are described as strains, sprains, dislocations, and fractures.

Strains

A strain is described as a pulled muscle, with trauma being attributed to an excessive stretch or forcible muscular contraction. The extent of injury is characterized as *first, second,* or *third degree* and, additionally, as *slight, moderate,* or *severe*. The pathological condition ranges from little or no hemorrhage and low-grade inflammation to the severe rupture of the musculotendinous unit or complete evulsion of a tendon from its bony attachment.

Sprains

Direct or indirect trauma to a joint, affecting its stabilizing connective tissue, results in a sprain. An articulation forced beyond its anatomical limitations can result in pathology in ligamentous, capsular, and synovial membranous tissue as well as tendons crossing or contiguous to the joint. As in strains, sprain severity is depicted by first, second, and third degrees and ranges from a very minor tearing to complete separation of supporting structures. The recipient of a sprain may have symptoms ranging from minimal discomfort to severe joint tenderness, loss of function, and swelling.

Dislocations

The traumatic displacement of a bone from its usual position within a joint is generally termed a dislocation. More specifically, a complete articular disunion is called a *luxation,* whereas a partial separation is considered a *subluxation*. Many severe sprains have, in reality, been dislocations that have spontaneously reduced themselves into proper alignment. The pathological condition that occurs as a result of a dislocation is extensive, with stretching and tearing of articular tissue as well as those tendons associated with movement of the part. Besides affecting the structure of stabilization, avulsion chip fractures may occur from the force of trauma. Once an articulation has been disrupted by such force as to cause severe sprain, subluxation, or luxation, recurrence is very possible. A chronic recurring dislocation often requires surgical intervention to reestablish stabilization.

Fractures

Fractures represent interruptions in the continuity of a bone and are classified as either closed or open. A closed fracture is one in which there is no external wound; conversely, an open fracture displays external tissue damage. Although fractures are commonly caused by shearing forces, they can occur as a result of direct external forces that crush the bone.

After a fracture, there is damage to the periosteum and adjacent soft tissue structures, primarily blood vessels, nerves, connective tissue, and muscles. There is hemorrhaging and noticeable inflammation. The repair and healing of the bone ends involve a number of processes, namely, formation of a granulation tissue mass, fibrous connective tissue junction, or hard callus and the final development of new rigid bone.

BASIC CONCEPTS IN PHYSICAL RECONDITIONING

The major concern of the adapted physical educator with individuals who have experienced serious acute traumatic impairments is one of reconditioning. The term *reconditioning* implies that through an exercise program, an individual will be returned to the same degree of conditioning as before the injury. In cooperation with the physician, the teacher establishes an individually designed exercise program for the student.

Prolonged bed rest or inactivity after trauma to the musculoskeletal system results in delayed recovery. Physicians and reconditioning specialists generally agree that an exercise program is needed for all muscular and skeletal involvements, whether preoperative preparation, postoperative recovery, or general rehabilitation of acute conditions. It is important that the affected person engage in a general physical fitness program as well as rehabilitation of the injured part.

A relatively healthy individual who has incurred an acute musculoskeletal impairment should *avoid inactivity* as a means to restoration. Lack of activity results in muscular atrophy and the loss of joint flexibility and general coordination. Prolonged bed rest may lead to a generalized debilitation that may extend the recuperation period. Authorities generally agree that a carefully guided program of activity encourages healing and shortens the time of recovery, particularly in cases of acute musculoskeletal conditions.

The traumatic conditions discussed in this chapter are commonly found to occur to active persons, those involved in accidents, the weak, and the infirm. Each condition is described in terms of its *anatomical implications, mechanism of injury,* and *pathological condition,* and a *rationale for reconditioning* is presented. There is no intent here to give a complete discussion of all traumas, but to discuss those injuries that have a high incidence among the school-aged and early adult populations.

THE FOOT, ANKLE, AND LEG

The 26 bones composing the skeleton of the foot are primarily structured for strong, flexible, coordinated movement. Architecturally, the foot forms an anterior metatarsal arch, an outer longitudinal arch, and the high inner longitudinal arch on its medial aspect. The main function of the arch is to absorb the shock of weight bearing and to allow space for plantar muscles, nerves, and blood vessels. Body weight is conducted to the foot via the leg bone of the tibia through the supporting bone, the talus. A mortise is formed by the malleoli of the fibula and the tibia and, with the aid of collateral ligaments, it stabilizes the talus. Below the talus is the calcaneus. The foot makes surface contact with the calcaneus and the metatarsal heads. An intricate system of plantar muscles and elastic and inelastic connective tissue serves to uphold the shape and arches of the foot. Additional support is afforded by a suspension of muscles stemming from the leg and ending within the longitudinal arch. Dorsiflexion, together with plantar ankle flexion, is permitted at the talotibial articulation, whereas inversion and eversion of the foot take place at the talocalcaneal and intertarsal joints.

Structurally, the ankle joint is relatively strong as a result of its bony and ligamentous arrange-

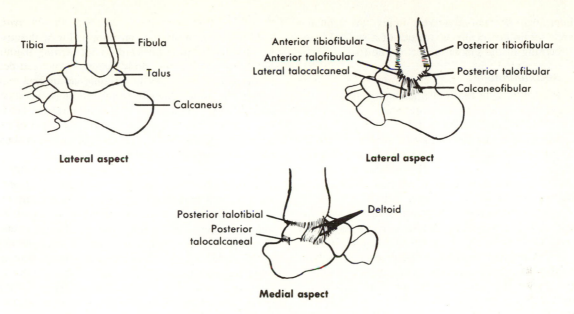

Fig. 10-1. Bones and ligaments of the ankle.

ments. Because of the direction of weight bearing, the medial collateral, as compared with the lateral collateral, ligament offers the greatest ankle stability. Bony strength is added to the medial collateral ligament by the arrangement of the talus over the calcaneus. Laterally, the ankle is architecturally weaker and more subject to sprains than on the medial side (Fig. 10-1).

The leg is composed of the tibia and fibula and the soft tissues surrounding them. Three fascial chambers contain the muscles, blood vessels, and nerves. The anterior compartment contains those constituents that control the action of dorsiflexion, namely, the tibialis anterior, the extensor hallucis longus, the extensor digitorum longus, the anterior vessels, and the anterior tibial nerves; a lateral compartment houses the muscles of the peroneus longus and the peroneus brevis; and a posterior compartment confines the motor mechanisms of plantar flexion and inversion, primarily the soleus, posterior tibialis, long flexors of the toes, and gastrocnemius muscles. The main weight-bearing bone of the leg is the tibia. It is triangularly formed at its upper two thirds and changes to a more oval shape in the lower one third. The fibula's primary function is serving as a point for muscle attachment. Connecting the fibula and tibia is the strong tissue sheet of the interosseous membrane.

Foot injuries

The foot is extremely vulnerable to trauma. Serious injury may occur as a result of the following:
1. An individual's falling from a height and landing on the feet
2. Objects falling on the foot
3. Striking toes against an immovable object
4. Twisting and wrenching forces

Fractures to the phalanges are most common consequent to a stubbing action; to the talus and calcaneus consequent to falling; and to the metatarsals consequent to objects falling on them, although fractures at the base of the fifth metatarsal are associated with severely sprained ankle and violent foot inversion. Spontaneous fractures can arise from prolonged use of feet, as occurs in walking or running. Tendon and connective tissue injuries have the highest incidence in the plantar and lateral aspects of the foot. However, sprains and strains may occur at almost any site. The sprained foot commonly affects ligaments that stabilize the intertarsal or tarsometatarsal joints. A traumatic arch sprain can occur as a result of a sudden overstretching of the plantar aspect of the foot.

Reconditioning

Reconditioning the foot after injury involves the prevention of edema and fluid stasis; immobilization, when applicable; mobilization; and graded exercises. The tendency toward swelling after injury requires the physical therapy of immediate elevation, pressure, and cold application. Uncontrolled edema may result in eventual fibrosis and chronic irritation.

Physical restoration is implemented during the convalescent period by active movements of the toes within the margins of pain and safety (Fig. 10-2). The physical educator must give consideration to the main foot functions and redevelopment of the injured muscles (see Chapter 5 and Figs. 5-13 and 5-14).

Ankle injuries

Most ankle injuries occur as a result of the foot being forcibly turned inward or outward on the leg while supporting the body weight. The primary cause of ankle injuries is stepping on uneven surfaces. The highest incidence of trauma to the ankle occurs when the foot is violently inverted; however, the most serious pathological condition results from eversion, which affects the main supporting tissues of the ankle and longitudinal arch. The scope of ankle injuries ranges from the mild stretching of stabilizing ligamentous tissue to fractures of both malleoli, or even ankle dislocation.

An ankle sprain results in stretched or torn ligamentous fibers and muscle tendons. The inversion sprain affects the anterior tibiofibular ligament, the anterior talofibular ligament, the calcaneofibular ligament, and the posterior talofibular ligament in varying degrees, not to mention the straining of the peroneal tendons (Fig. 10-3, *A*). Eversion sprains

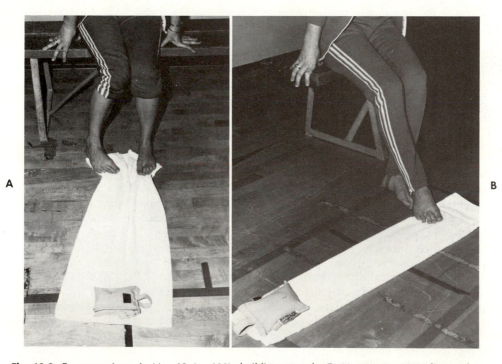

Fig. 10-2. Foot exercises. **A,** No. 13 (p. 129), building mounds. **B,** No. 14 (p. 129), foot curling. (Courtesy of California State University, Audio Visual Center, Long Beach, Calif.)

primarily affect the medial collateral deltoid ligament, with an associated pathological condition in the plantar ligaments and tendons. Severe abnormal twisting of the foot, inwardly or outwardly, can result in fractures of the lateral or medial malleolus such as are incurred in skiing injuries.

Serious ankle damage is manifested in loss of movement and inability to bear weight. Marked swelling, pain, and discoloration (ecchymosis) often are displayed. Severe ankle joint derangement often requires immobilization by cast or strapping and the prevention of weight bearing for a varied length of time.

Reconditioning

Care of severe acute ankle affections demands control of edema by means of cold pressure, elevation, support by adhesive strapping, or casting. Weight bearing may be restricted and crutches may be required or a plaster walking case may be applied for immobilization in the care of fractures or severe sprains.

The primary objective of ankle reconditioning is to restore normal joint function. Movement at the tibiofibular-talar articulation approximates 20 degrees of dorsiflexion and 45 to 60 degrees of plantar flexion. Normal movement may be encouraged immediately after injury, once fracture has been ruled out. Early exercise often aids in venous and lymphatic drainage. When initial soreness decreases, the physician may allow the patient to engage in modified activity and limited weight bearing.

The saying "Once a sprain, always a sprain" points up the fact that stretched or torn ligaments do not repair themselves. Exercise cannot be expected to restore injured ligaments nor can it be expected to fully strengthen strained tendons crossing the ankle joint. Therefore, full ankle stability after severe derangement is doubtful and should not be expected.

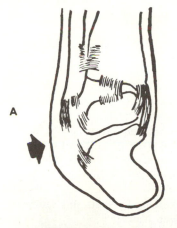

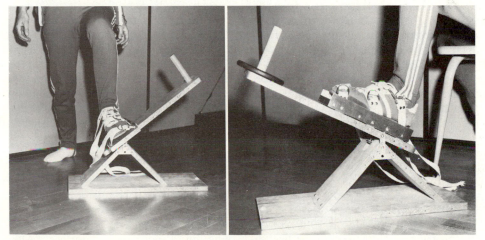

Fig. 10-3. A, Lateral ankle sprain. **B,** Ankle exercise machine; foot eversion. **C,** Foot dorsiflexion. (**B** and **C** Courtesy of California State University, Audio Visual Center, Long Beach, Calif.)

With the permission of the physician, the student may begin a graded program of inversion, eversion, plantar flexion and dorsiflexion, and exercises against resistance. To provide normal mechanical continuity between ankle and foot, an exercise program should also include toe and arch routines. A number of choices of ankle resistance devices are available to the individual with a sprained ankle. Specialized resistance machines, weighted iron boots, sandbags, and manual resistance may afford an overload program to the injured ankle (Fig. 10-3 and Chapter 5).

The criterion for resumption of normal activity should be whether the student can pass a variety of ankle stress tests, such as the following:

1. Walking without a limp
2. Balancing on the ball of the foot of the affected limb without pain
3. Jumping up and down with ease while bearing full weight on the affected ankle
4. Running at full speed in a zigzag pattern

The Individual Education Program for a handicapped person with a second degree (moderate) inversion range of motion, pain, swelling, and loss of strength may be done by a physical therapist, by the examining physician (who should in each instance rule out bone fracture by means of an x-ray examination) or examinations might reveal a loss of 10 degrees of dorsiflexion and 15 degrees of plantar flexion of the ankle, swelling on the lateral side of the ankle and foot, pain resulting from all ankle joint actions, and inability to fully bear weight on the affected foot. Muscle tests given when pain has subsided result in a rating of "good-fair" using standard muscle-testing procedures.[5]

Muscle testing. The long-range goal would be to help the young person to return to a normal gait in walking on flat surfaces and to resume participation in all previous activities. Objectives might include the following:

1. The student will regain 10 degrees of dorsiflexion and 15 degrees of plantar flexion in the affected foot and ankle, as measured with a standard goniometer, by the end of the sixth week.
2. The student will be able to do 10 toe raises on the affected foot by the end of the twelfth week.
3. The ankle everters (peroneus longus and per-

oneus brevis) will test "normal" on the standard muscle test by the end of the twelfth week.
4. The student will be able to execute each of the four stress tests (described in the preceding paragraph of this discussion) by the sixteenth week.

Suggested exercises and activities might include the following:

1. For increased range of motion in the foot and ankle:
   a. Exercise No. 12, foot circling (Fig. 5-15).
   b. Flutter kick drill sitting at edge of pool, progressing to kick bracketed at side of pool, to flutter kick with use of kickboard.
2. For increased strength of foot and ankle muscles:
   a. Use of ankle exercisor for development of plantar and dorsal flexors, everters, and inverters (Fig. 10-3). Use progressive resistance technique, starting with one-fourth the maximum number of repetitions (see p. 112, DeLorme's technique).
   b. Exercise No. 30, toe lifts (Fig. 5-33).
3. For further preparation to perform stress tests:
   a. Walking forward and backward in chest-deep water.
   b. Walking on flat surfaces, concentrating on good foot and leg mechanics.
   c. Slow jogging on soft, flat surfaces.
   d. Rope skipping (Fig. 5-43 and pp. 137-138).

The subject should advance through the suggested progressions with the instructor's approval predicated on absence of pain during and following an activity and on increased flexibility and strength as measured periodically by the instructor and as described in the previous paragraph.

Shin splints

Shin splints is a condition associated with pain in the area of the anterior or posterior aspect of the tibia. It most often occurs to athletes or active individuals who engage in repetitive walking or running on a nonresisting surface. Although shin splints may occur suddenly and transitorily, it may also appear gradually and become a chronic disability. Many factors have been attributed to causing shin splints; the primary causes are the following:

1. Running or walking on nonresistant and uneven surfaces
2. Poor running or walking form
3. Running on the balls of the feet too early in the training program
4. Postural and structural foot anomalies[10]

Most authorities agree that shin splints is a chronic inflammation of the muscles and connecting tissue in the shin region, primarily resulting from irritation to the calf muscles and plantar flexors; however, it occasionally occurs from irritation to the dorsiflexors of the ankle and the peroneals located on the anterior and lateral sides of the leg.

Nontraumatic problems of the shin region, such as stress fractures, anterior tibial syndrome, and leg overuse, may, in their early stages, closely resemble shin splints. The stress fracture occurs spontaneously in the tibia or fibula from overuse, whereby the synergistic muscle coordination is overcome by fatigue. Acute anterior tibial compartment syndrome is considered a very serious condition leading to ischemic necrosis from hemorrhage within the fascial boundaries.

Reconditioning

Physical therapy of shin splints requires heat, rest, supportive strapping, and static stretching in positions of plantar and dorsiflexion (Fig. 10-4). deVries[6] determined that muscle spasm is an important cause of the shin splint symptoms and could be relieved by a daily routine of static stretching of both the anterior and posterior aspects of the lower leg.

THE KNEE AND THIGH

The knee has an extremely high incidence of injury among active young persons, particularly those engaged in football and skiing. As an articulation, the knee is considered to be an unstable ginglymus, or hinge type, joint. Having an extremely shallow bony structure, the knee's functional stability is based mainly on the support of its muscles and ligamentous arrangement. Structurally, the knee joint is the largest and one of the most complicated joints in the body. It is formed by the lateral and medial femoral condyles, the tibia, and the patella. Two semioval cartilages (menisci) serve to deepen the shallow depression of the tibia. Ligamentous stability is afforded the knee,

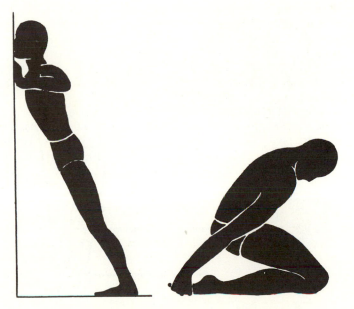

Fig. 10-4. Stretching for shin splints.

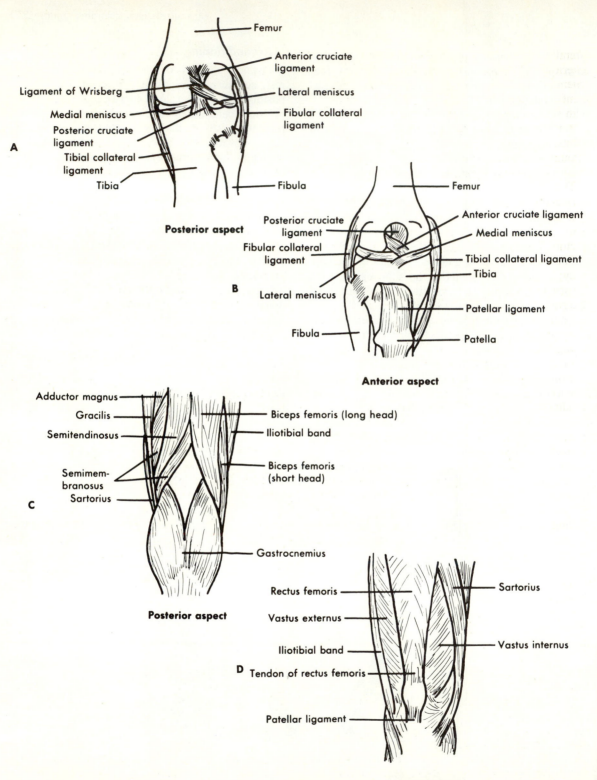

Fig. 10-5. Knee anatomy.

laterally and medially, by collateral ligaments and, anteriorly and posteriorly, by internal cruciate ligaments (Fig. 10-5, *A* and *B*). The primary movements of the knee consist of flexion and extension, with some secondary internal and external rotation. Although the ligaments prevent abnormal movements, the primary knee joint stability is acquired through the gastrocnemius, the hamstring, and the quadriceps muscles (Fig. 10-5, *C* and *D*).

The thigh consists of the femur and associated musculature, blood vessels, and nerves. There are four groups of thigh muscles, based on their primary action: flexors, extensors, abductors, and adductors.

The patella is the largest sesamoid bone in the body; it lies within the quadriceps muscle tendon. Its primary function is to provide protection to the anterior aspect of the knee joint and to increase the mechanical advantage during extension. The two most prevalent injuries of the patella in the active young person are dislocation and fracture.

Acute patellar dislocations may result from a direct blow or sudden twist when the knee is flexed. Dislocations of this type happen most often to individuals who have poor quadriceps tone or a shallow patellar groove. *Genu valgum*, or knock-knee, is also a contributing factor, along with the increased tibial femoral angle that is common in the physically mature female. O'Donoghue[9] described the mature female as being more prone to patellar dislocations because of her broader pelvis, resulting in an increased angle at the patella, therefore pulling laterally on full knee extension. Treatment of the dislocated patella often requires corrective surgery and immobilization. Activity is then increased through a graded quadriceps exercise program.

Fractures of the patella are not as prevalent as dislocations. They result from a direct blow or from a sudden severe pull that fragments some portion of the patella. Because of the possibility of developing a roughened articular surface, surgery may be required to remove a portion of, or the entire, patella.

Repeated trauma to the kneecap can lead to the condition known as chondromalacia, which is a softening of the articular surface. Chondromalacia eventually develops into degenerative changes and a state of chronic inflammation. Other articular surfaces that commonly develop chondromalacia in the

rapidly growing adolescent are the knee and hip (Chapter 11).

Knee sprains

Because of the structural shallowness of the knee joint, it is very vulnerable to abduction, adduction, and torsion injuries. Violent activity, as in football or skiing, places great stress on the knee joint. Injury often follows when the foot is planted firmly and the knee is either struck from the outside inward or rotated on its long axis.

The *medial collateral ligament* has the highest incidence of sprain. Medial collateral knee sprain occurs often when the knee receives a direct blow, which causes the foot to evert and the knee to be forced inward in an unlocked position. Although not usually as serious as the medial, the lateral collateral knee sprain results from a forced adduction of the leg and an internally rotated knee. In both instances, there is an instability of the affected side besies a tendency toward effusion, hemarthrosis (blood in the joint), and pain.

The *anterior cruciate ligament* can be abnormally stretched or torn by a violent internal rotation of the femur while the foot is planted with the thigh adducted and the knee flexed or by hyperextension while the leg is internally rotated on the femur at the knees. Conversely, the posterior cruciate ligament can be injured when the femur is externally rotated and the foot is fixed with the knee in a flexed and adducted position. A fall on a flexed knee can also result in a posterior cruciate sprain. Anterior cruciate injury results in forward displacement of the tiba in relationship to the femur, whereas the posterior cruciate sprain results in backward displacement and instability. In each case of injury, there is usually swelling and effusion of blood into the joint.

The mechanism *hyperextension knee sprain* can result from a direct force to the planted foot, causing the knee to move backward abnormally. Depending on the severity of trauma, the hyperextension injury can result in sprain to the medial collateral and anterior cruciate ligaments, besides straining tissue in the popliteal region.

Reconditioning

Very often, the physical educator will be charged with helping a student who is about to have, or who is recovering from, knee surgery.

There has been a recent trend toward early knee surgery when symptoms reveal definite joint derangement, especially in the "unhappy triad," indicating trauma to the medial collateral ligament, medial meniscus, and anterior cruciate ligament.

Profound atrophy and weakness are common to the quadriceps extensor mechanism after knee injury or surgery. Weak quadriceps muscles, in general, mean a defective and unstable knee joint. Physical restoration of the knee requires a concentrated exercise regimen for strength and flexibility of the gastrocnemius and both the quadriceps and hamstring muscle groups. Eliminating the hamstring and gastrocnemius muscles from the reconditioning program results in failure to provide a balance of knee strength and leaves the student vulnerable to additional trauma.[9]

A graduated exercise program of reconditioning will, in most instances, consist of the following seven procedures:

1. Quad setting
2. Straight leg raises with hip flexion
3. Straight leg raises with hip extension
4. Toe raises
5. Leg swings
6. Hamstring conditioning
7. Progressive resistance exercises

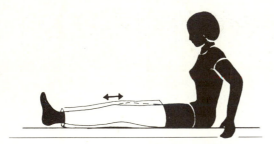

Fig. 10-6. Quad setting.

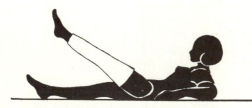

Fig. 10-7. Straight leg raises with hip flexion.

Quad setting (Fig. 10-6), or muscle tensing, is a procedure in which the student performs an isometric or static contraction of the quadriceps muscles for a period of between 6 and 10 seconds, without knee movement and until some fatigue is sensed. Many physical educators and therapists start this exercise immediately after injury to prevent muscle wasting or after knee surgery in an attempt to restore normal muscle strength as soon as possible.

Straight leg raises with hip flexion (Fig. 10-7) are executed against gravity, first in a sitting position, which emphasizes the three single-joint muscles of the quadriceps group at the knee, and then, gradually, in the supine position, which brings into action all four muscles. The effectiveness of the exercise is increased by the individual leaning back on the hands to a final position of long lying. The second and third exercise positions increase the stress placed on the rectus femoris muscle. The student attempts to maintain the knee in a locked position while raising the leg about 6 inches above the level of the hip. When 15 to 20 repetitions can be accomplished for two or three bouts during the day without undue discomfort, the physician may allow graduation to leg swings. Gradual resistance can also be applied to the straight leg raising exercise by progressively adding sandbags to the extended leg.

Straight leg raises with hip extension (Fig. 10-8) should be executed to exercise the gluteus maximus and hamstring muscles. The student takes a prone position and lifts the affected leg approximately 6 inches above the hip level. Like the straight leg raise with hip flexion, this exercise is conducted 15 to 20 times, with two to three bouts daily. Sandbag weights can also be applied for progressive resistance exercise (Fig. 10-9).

Because the gastrocnemius (Fig. 10-10) assists in flexion at the knee as well as in plantar flexion

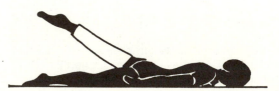

Fig. 10-8. Straight leg raises with hip extension.

at the ankle and because it provides posterior stability, it should be included in the reconditioning exercise regimen. Exercise of the gastrocnemius can best be accomplished by the progression of toe pointing without weight bearing, weight bearing and *toe raises,* and weight bearing plus resistance, for example, carrying a weight in the hands or on the shoulder and initiating toe raising (see Fig. 5-33). From 15 to 20 repetitions should be initiated in each set of exercises. A full stretch of the Achilles tendon should be attempted after each toe raise, which is accomplished by standing with the ball of the foot on a raised block 1 to $1\frac{1}{2}$ inches thick.

Leg swings (Fig. 10-11) may be incorporated with the straight leg raises or may be reserved as a progressive movement, depending on the extent of knee damage and the physician's recommendations. The patient executes them by sitting on a table or bench and freely swinging the lower leg in flexion and extension and gradually increasing the arc of the swing. The primary purpose of leg swings is to aid in muscle redevelopment, restore joint flexibility, and increase normal circulation for the resolution of effusion or joint swelling. Resumption of normal knee movement should be encouraged as soon as possible without hindering the healing process.

Hamstring strength is essentially for the posterior support of the knee. Too often, this muscle group is neglected in the total knee reconditioning program. Lying in the prone position, the student

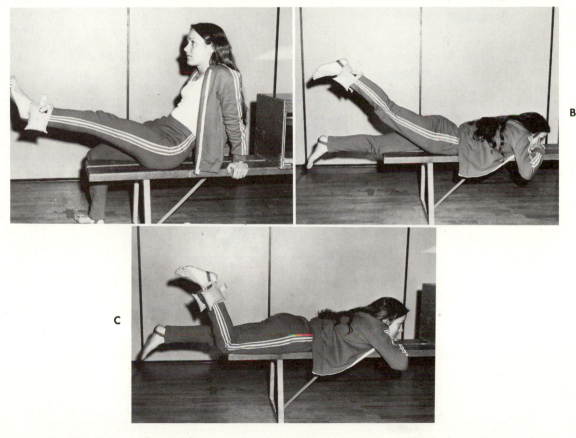

Fig. 10-9. Using sandbag weights in a progressive resistance exercise program for the knee. (Courtesy of California State University, Audio Visual Center, Long Beach, Calif.)

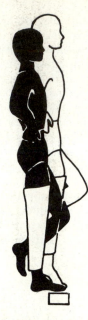

Fig. 10-10. Toe raises.

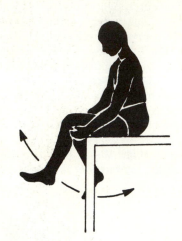

Fig. 10-11. Leg swings.

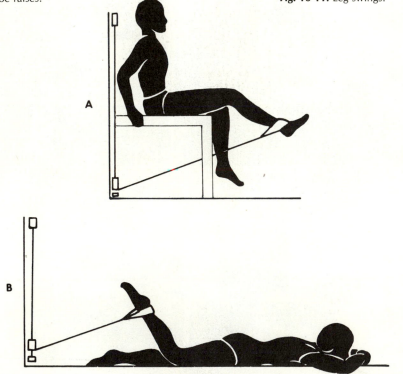

Fig. 10-12. A, Knee extension against resistance. **B,** Knee flexion against resistance.

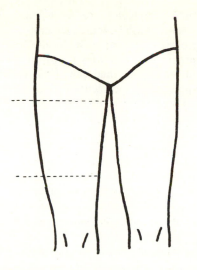

Fig. 10-13. Sites for measuring thigh circumference.

first without resistance, curls the affected leg. Gradually, resistance is added until the strength of the hamstring group has been developed to the extent of being 50% to 60% that of the quadriceps group (Fig. 10-9, *B* and *C*).

Isotonic progressive resistance exercises usually represent the final exercise stage for the reconditioning of the knee. By the use of resistance applied to the ankle or foot of the affected side, the person extends the leg through a full range of movement (Fig. 10-12). The quadriceps and hamstring groups and the gastrocnemius must be given equal attention for the restoration of full joint function.

Weight bearing parallels the return of muscle function and joint stability. As the students become reconditioned, they gradually progress from inability to bear weight to crutch walking and full mobility. The criteria often used to determine recovery from knee derangement are the return of strength and flexibility equal to or exceeding that of the unaffected side, restoration of normal circumference (Fig. 10-13), and the ability to move easily without favoring the part.

A general problem related to derangement of the knee illustrates how a program might be developed for persons who fall within the restrictions of P.L. 94-142 and for others who might have similar

needs but who would not qualify for the federally mandated program for handicapped persons. Both programs could be selected from the materials presented in this text and the accompanying laboratory manual[4] to satisfy the needs of an individual with such an acute disorder.

Evaluation techniques include any or all of the following:

1. Physician's examination, diagnosis, and advice relative to an activity and exercise program.
2. Measurement of the girth of the thigh to be compared with that of the other leg and/or the change in size of the affected leg.
3. Measurement of range of motion of the affected joint (goniometer).
4. Measurement of muscle strength of selected muscle groups before and after the completion of an exercise regimen.[5]

Performance objectives can be selected based on any or all of the data obtained from the previously listed tests. Examples of each are presented.

I. Physician's examination
   A. The physician finds quadriceps muscle strain and suggests 1 week of rest followed by quadriceps setting and leg swing exercises and, after 2 weeks, a progressive resistance exercise program for 16 weeks. Suggested objectives:
      1. The individual will be able to perform 15 quadriceps setting exercises three times a day by the end of the fifth day.
      2. The individual will be able to perform 10 repetitions of leg swings through full range of motion by the end of the third week.
      3. The individual will be able to complete 15 repetitions of No. 21, knee extensor exercise (Fig. 5-21) with 15 pounds of resistance by the end of the fifteenth week.
II. Measurement of range of motion of the affected joint
   A. The adapted physical education teacher or physical or recreational therapist tests with a goniometer to find limitations in both flexion and extension of the knee joint.
      1. The individual will increase joint flexibility in both flexion and extension by at least 15 degrees by the end of the sixth week (goniometer) (Fig. 20-23, *A*).
      2. The individual will increase joint flexibility in both flexion and extension by at least 15 degrees by the end of the eighth week, as

measured with tracings made by the instructor or therapist at the beginning and the end of the program for comparison (Fig. 20-23, *B* and *C*).

III. Measurement of the girth of the thigh
   A. The adapted physical education teacher or recreational therapist measures the girth of the thigh at the beginning and at the end of the assigned exercise program.
      1. The individual will increase the circumference measurements of the thigh by at least $1\frac{1}{2}$ inches by the end of the eighth week (Figs. 10-13 and 20-21).
      2. The individual will increase the circumference measurements of the thigh so that they are equal to or larger than those of the other thigh by the end of the tenth week (Figs. 10-13 and 20-21).

IV. Measurement of strength of selected muscle groups
   A. The adapted physical educator or recreational therapist measures the strength of the quadriceps muscle group before and after a selected exercise program.
      1. The individual will be able to complete 15 repetitions of No. 21 (Fig. 5-21) with 20 pounds of resistance by the end of the tenth week.
      2. The individual will be able to increase the number of pounds lifted by 30 as measured with a leg and back dynamometer by the end of the twelfth week.
      3. The individual will be able to increase the score on a cable tensiometer by 25 pounds by the end of the fourteenth week.

V. Selection of exercise and activity programs for improvement of a deranged knee
   A. For flexibility and mild exercise soon after sustaining an injury the following exercises should be assigned.
      1. Quadriceps setting (no. 16, Figs. 5-16 and 10-6)
      2. Hip flexion (Figs. 10-7 and 10-9)
      3. Hip extension (Figs. 10-7 and 10-9)
      4. Toe lifting (No. 30, Figs. 5-33 and 10-10)
      5. Leg swings (Fig. 10-11)
   B. More advanced exercises to follow when assigned by the instructor include the following.
      1. Foot drag (No. 17, Fig. 5-20)
      2. Knee extension (No. 18, Figs. 5-21 and 10-12)
      3. Knee flexion (Figs. 10-9 and 10-11)
      4. Half knee bends
      5. Isokinetic or universal exercise machines

Depending upon the type and extent of the knee derangement, the instructor or therapist can select the appropriate techniques to be used, can plan a sound program of activities based on accepted assessment techniques, and can show accountability with appropriate postactivity assessment techniques. Teachers, students, and parents should be satisfied with such a program based on student and instructor accountability.

Osgood-Schlatter condition

Many terms have been applied to the Osgood-Schlatter condition; the most prevalent are *apophysitis, osteochondritis,* and *epiphysitis of the tibial tubercle.* It is not considered a disease entity, but the result of a separation of the tibial tubercle at the epiphyseal junction (Fig. 10-14). The cause of this condition is idiopathic, with direct injury or long-term irritation thought to be the main inciting factor. Direct trauma as in a blow, osteochondritis, or an excessive strain of the patellar tendon as it attaches to the tibial tubercle may result in evulsion at the epiphyseal cartilage junction. Disruption of the blood supply to the epiphysis results in enlargement of the tibial tubercle, joint tenderness, and pain on contraction of the quadriceps. It usually occurs in active adolescent boys and girls between the ages of 10 and 15 years who are in a rapid growth period. If it is not properly cared for, de-

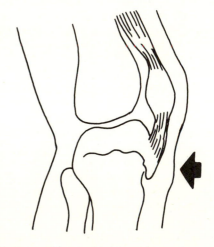

Fig. 10-14. Osgood-Schlatter condition of the knee.

formity and a defective extensor mechanism may result; however, it may not necessarily be associated with pain or discomfort. In most cases, Osgood-Schlatter condition is acute, is self-limiting, and does not exceed a few months' duration.

Local inflammation is accentuated by leg activity and ameliorated by rest. The individual may be unable to kneel or engage in flexion and extension movements without pain. Even after arrest of symptoms, Osgood-Schlatter condition tends to recur after irritation.

The physical educator may, from the complaints of the student, be the one to detect this condition, for which immediate physician referral should be made. Early detection may reveal a slight condition in which the individual can continue a normal activity routine, excluding overexposure to strenuous running, jumping, and falling on the affected leg. All physical education activities must be modified to avoid quadriceps strain, while, at the same time, preparing for general physical fitness.

Complete abstinence of all knee joint movement must be maintained when the inflammatory state persists. Forced inactivity, provided by a plaster cast, may be the only answer to keeping the overactive adolescent from using the affected leg. While immobilized in the cast, the individual is greatly restricted; weight bearing may be held to a minimum, with signs of pain at the affected part closely watched by the physician.

Reconditioning

Although Osgood-Schlatter condition is self-limiting and temporary, exercise is an important factor in the full recovery of the individual. Physical education activities should emphasize the capabilities of the upper body and nonaffected leg to prevent their deconditioning.

After arrest of the condition and removal from immobilization, the individual is given a graduated reconditioning program. The major objectives at this time are reeducation in proper walking patterns and restoration of normal strength and flexibility of the knee joint. Strenuous knee movement is avoided for at least 5 weeks and the demanding requirements of regular physical education classes may be postponed for 6 months or longer, depending on the physician's recommendations. Although the period of rehabilitation places emphasis on the affected leg, it must also include a program for the entire body.

The criteria for the individual to return to regular physical education would be as follows:

1. Normal range of movement of the knee
2. Quadriceps strength equal to that of the unaffected leg
3. Asymptomatic evidence of the Osgood-Schlatter condition
4. The ability to move freely without favoring the affected part

Following recovery, the student should avoid all activities that would tend to contuse, or in any way irritate again, the tibial tuberosity.

THE HIP AND PELVIS

The hip is an extremely powerful joint with great bony, ligamentous, and muscular strength. It serves as the main supporting structure of the body in the upright position. Without proper integrity of the hip joint and its associated structures, ambulation becomes difficult or even impossible. Although designed to withstand great and repeated stress, the hip is vulnerable to epiphyseal separations in the early growth stages and to fractures in old age. Dislocations of the hip are more prevalent than fractures in young active individuals because they have more viable and elastic tissue about the joint, compared with the porous and degenerative hip of elderly persons. Sprains, dislocations, and fractures will be considered in this section, whereas congenital and degenerative conditions are discussed in Chapter 11.

Sprains and dislocations

Any movement that exceeds the hip's normal range can result in injury. A torsion force with the foot planted and the body twisting on its long axis can result in sprain or dislocation. A direct force to the knee while the thigh is flexed and adducted, such as striking the dashboard in an auto accident, can result in fracture and dislocation of the femoral head. A common complication of the hip dislocation or fracture, particularly in older individuals, is injury to the sciatic nerve or disruption of the ligamentum teres carrying the main nutrient artery to the head of the humerus.

THE SPINE

The spine is composed of individual vertebral segments consisting of a sacrum, a coccyx, and 7 cervical, 12 thoracic, and 5 lumbar vertebrae. Although each vertebral region has individual features, in general, they are designed for weight bearing, protection of the spinal cord, muscle attachment, and trunk and head mobility. Vertebrae become increasingly large as they progress downward to accommodate for the upright posture. Adding to the complexities of the spinal column are the cervical, dorsal, and lumbar curves that accommodate gravity while the individual is in the erect position.

Many authorities consider the vertebral column as still being in an evolutionary stage of adaptation. This assumption is reached because of the inadequate way the individual adjusts to the various forces applied to the spine. In essence, the spine must function as both stationary support and a dynamic unit.[3]

Gross movement of the spine consists of the combined articulations of each vertebra. Between two vertebrae are articular facets that form joints. Each articular facet has a synovial membrane and is joined together by ligamentous tissue. Between the bodies of each vertebra are fibrocartilaginous discs composed of a hard outer fibrocartilage and a gelatinous center, the *nucleus pulposus,* which provides shock-absorbing qualities to the entire spine. Gross movement of the spine is initiated by a gliding action of the individual joints, combined with the adaption of the intervertebral cartilages. The cervical region is permitted free flexion and extension, whereas head tilting takes place with the combined movement of rotation and torsion. The thoracic spine moves laterally more easily than it flexes and extends because of its bony limitations. Although lateral bending and rotary movement are limited in the lumbar spine, flexion and extension are permitted.

Spine injuries

Back disorders, primarily of the lower back and neck, are becoming increasingly more prevalent in today's population. Cailliet[3] estimates that 80% of the human race will complain of back pain, particularly in the low back region. Lack of exercise and poor muscle tone, combined with the hazards of modern living, serve to predispose individuals to acute back problems. Pathological problems of the back fall mainly into three categories: congenital, mechanical, and traumatic. Congenital and mechanical affections are considered in Chapters 9 and 11, respectively.

The back regions that are most susceptible to musculotendinous ligamentous injury are the cervical and low back regions, each being unique in its potential to injury. The neck, as the result of its flexibility, is able to withstand a great deal of traumatic force applied to it. However, sudden twists, forced hyperextension, or a quick snap of the head can produce varying degrees of damage. The primary muscles involved are the upper trapezius and the sternocleidomastoid. A strain of the neck musculature may appear as wryneck or acute torticollis. Deeper injury may affect ligamentous supporting structures or may result in herniation of the cervical intervertebral disc. Automobile accidents involving rear-end collisions are producing increasingly greater numbers of *whiplash* injuries, in which the recipient's head is snapped forcefully forward and back, tearing and stretching supporting tissue.

The individual with various anatomical weaknesses, congenital or acquired, in the low back region is prone to acute conditions. The individual with poor abdominal muscle tone or faulty vertebral alignment, with its concomitant muscular imbalance, has the stage set for future injury and chronic low back pain. Whether it is acute or of gradual onset, trauma plays a primary role in low back affections. The sequence of injury usually occurs after a sudden trunk twist or bending from the waist that places acute stress on inflexible atonic musculature or structurally deformed low back vertebrae. The low back injury may be reflected in a dull ache, pain radiating down a leg, muscle spasm, or restricted movement. Occurring from the same mechanisms as the lumbosacral sprain is the herniated lumbar disc (intervertebral disc syndrome). Often, the herniated disc is a product of gradual degeneration over a period of time. A sudden strain to the lumbar region increases the internal pressure of the intervertebral disc, forcing the nucleus pulposus to push outward, usually posteri-

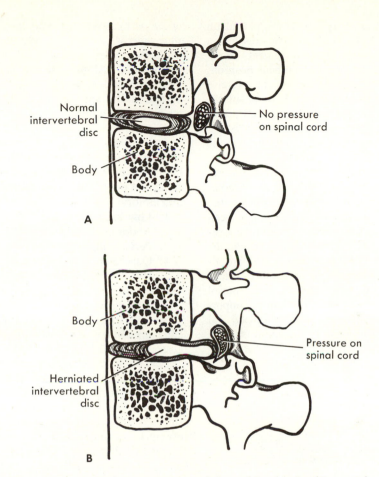

Normal intervertebral disc

No pressure on spinal cord

Body

A

Body

Pressure on spinal cord

Herniated intervertebral disc

B

Fig. 10-15. Sagittal section showing: **A,** a normal disc and **B,** a herniated intervertebral disc.

orly (Fig. 10-15). The protruding nucleus pulposus may cause pressure on adjacent nerves, resulting in pain and incapacitation.

Dislocations of the vertebral column have the highest incidence in the cervical region. A hyperextension or severe torsion force can result in dislocation or cervical fracture. Torque of the head or neck places most stress on the cervical atlas and axis and, if of great enough intensity, can lead to spinal cord damage, paralysis, or even death.

Violent hyperflexion of the trunk, or falling from a height and landing of the feet or buttocks, can produce a vertebral fracture, particularly in the lumbar or dorsal region. Bony fragments may lac-erate spinal nerves or even the cord, causing partial or complete paralysis of the lower limbs.

Reconditioning

Severe acute neck conditions, such as are incurred in dislocations or fractures, are immobilized by a cast or skeletal traction. This procedure may be carried on for weeks or even months. In lesser injuries such as whiplash the neck may be immobilized by a cervical collar. The period of neck splinting allows healing to take place without aggravation by neck movement. During this period of immobilization, general conditioning exercises should be carried out for all unaffected parts of the body. Emphasis particularly should be placed on the upper extremities to avoid contractures and a loss of shoulder joint range of movement. If the student is required to be in a recumbent position, muscle tensing and range of movement exercise must be carried out to all the major joints several times a day. When the student is permitted active neck movement, mobility in all directions is the first concern and then a graded strength program is initiated.

Reconditioning of acute low back problems requires an understanding of the anatomical complexities involved. Rest is often prescribed through the acute stages. If corrective surgery has been given, a muscle setting program should be executed several times a day while the patient is in the recumbent position. When active exercises are allowed, a program of stretching, strength development, and reeducation is initiated. Postural control and good body alignment are of the utmost importance. Abdominal strength must be developed and lumbosacral flexibility must be acquired so that proper pelvic alignment is reestablished. *Because*

of the pull placed on the lumbar curve by the iliopsoas muscle, double straight leg raising exercises while the student is in the supine position are contraindicated. Along with the graded exercise program, the student should be taught how to carry on normal daily activities such as sitting, standing, walking, or running without undue stress and tension in the low back region.[8]

The following exercises, divided into seven basic categories, are often given to persons with low back problems associated with faulty lumbar spine and pelvic alignment, muscle imbalance, and inflexibility:

1. Low back stretching
2. Abdominal strengthening
3. Pelvic rolling
4. Quadriceps stretching
5. Hip flexor stretching
6. Hamstring and heel cord stretching
7. Postural reeducation

Specific exercises for hamstring stretching, heel cord stretching, and postural reeducation are discussed in detail in Chapter 5.

Low back stretching is employed because a tight low back prevents normal trunk flexion. Individuals with an accentuated lordotic curve often are unable to fully round their backs. A safe exercise for sufferers of a pathological low back condition is executed from a supine position (Fig. 10-16). Knees are first pulled alternately to the chest and then, if without pain, are brought together to the chest. Each stretch should be statically held for at least 30 seconds and then gradually released. Variations of this stretch are sitting in a chair curl-

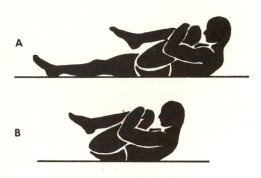

Fig. 10-16. Stretching the low back.

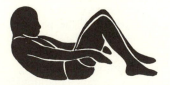

Fig. 10-17. Abdominal strengthening using an abdominal curl.

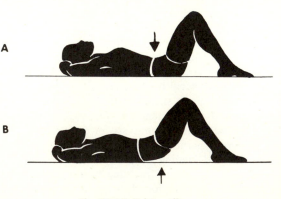

Fig. 10-18. Pelvic rolling.

ing the trunk into flexion, and touching the heels with the fingertips and allowing the head to slowly move between the legs.

Abdominal strengthening is necessary because, as discussed in Chapters 5 and 9, weak abdominal muscles are often associated with pain and disorder of the low back region. Strengthening should be executed without strain being placed on the lumbar spine and, specifically, the iliopsoas muscle. An effective exercise is the abdominal curl (Fig. 10-17). The subject assumes a hook lying position with the arms extended forward. Maintaining the hips and knees in a flexed position, the person slowly curls the trunk, starting with the chin on the chest and executing 5 to 10 repetitions of the exercise. The trunk should curl up to a position no greater than a 30-degree angle with the supporting surface to reduce hip flexor action.

The *pelvic rolling* exercise is designed to strengthen the lower abdominal muscles, stretch the lumbosacral muscles, and educate the subject to proper pelvic positioning, as discussed in Chapters 5 and 9. The subject assumes a hook lying position with hands folded behind the head (Fig. 10-18). The lordotic curve is flattened by rolling the pelvis backward. Holding the flattened position, the subject contracts the gluteal muscles (pinches the buttocks together) and raises the tailbone from the mat approximately 3 inches, holding the position for 10 seconds, executing 5 to 10 repetitions of the exercise.

Quadriceps and hip flexor stretching is important because tight quadriceps, primarily the rectus femoris, and tight hip flexors (iliopsoas muscles) are often associated with lordosis and low back pain. Stretching of these areas is difficult and requires very exact positioning. Two stretches are suggested. The first stretch is conducted from a supine position. The subject pulls the knee of one leg to the chest while the other leg is maintained in an extended position (Fig. 10-19, *A* and *B*). Caution must be taken that the extended leg does not rise from the floor. A longer stretch can be achieved if the extended leg's knee is allowed to bend back under the end of a table or bed. The stretch position should be held for 30 seconds and then the

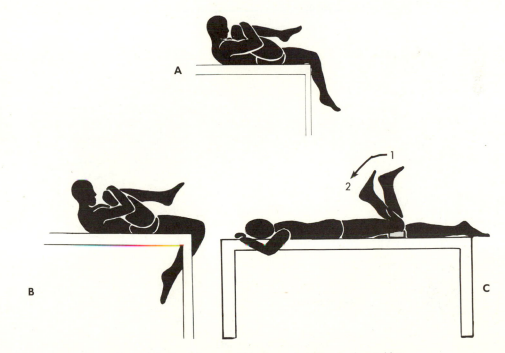

Fig. 10-19. Quadriceps and hip flexor stretching for leg and hip.

legs should be alternated. The subject must be advised to keep the low back flat while stretching. A second stretch is conducted in the prone position on the floor or on a wide plinth or table. A pad 1 to 3 inches thick is placed under the thigh of the leg to be stretched, just above the knee. The pelvis should be kept in a backward or upward tilt and flat on the supporting surface so the iliopsoas and rectus femoris muscles are at maximum stretch. Additional stretch can be placed on the rectus femoris if the knee of the affected leg is flexed. The stretch time should be gradually increased as the individual accommodates to the increased flexibility (Fig. 10-19, *C*).

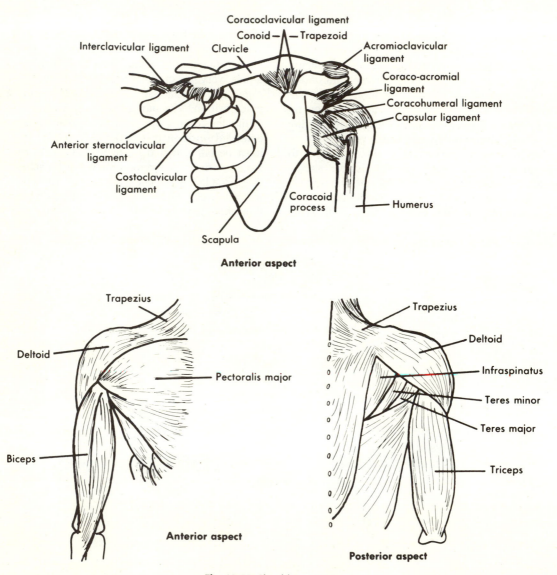

Fig. 10-20. Shoulder anatomy.

THE SHOULDER COMPLEX

The shoulder complex or girdle, in contrast to the stable pelvis, is designed to provide free mobility. It is formed by the clavicle, scapula, humerus, and associated ligaments and muscles (Fig. 10-20). The clavicle, as it joins the sternum, forms the only skeletal contact the shoulder complex has with the thorax. It forms a strut or bridge to the scapula, which, in turn, holds the head of the humerus. The shoulder complex is composed of four separate articulations that allow scapulohumeral movement to take place: the glenohumeral, coracoclavicular, acromioclavicular, and sternoclavicular articulations.

Shoulder articulations

The *glenohumeral articulation* is classified as enarthrodial, or ball and socket, and is formed by the round head of the humerus joining the shallow concavity of the glenoid fossa. A loose synovial capsule surrounds the joint, which is reinforced by ligaments. Tendons crossing the joint serve to strengthen and reinforce the ligamentous arrangement.

The *coracoclavicular articulation* allows for only slight movement of a syndesmotic type. Its prime function is to suspend the scapula and the clavicle, which are held together by the strong coracoclavicular ligaments.

A gliding joint, the *acromioclavicular articulation,* is composed of the lateral end of the clavicle and the acromion process, forming a very weak union. Its primary support is produced by a joint capsule reinforced by superior and inferior ligaments.

The clavicle, at its medial end, articulates with the outer angle of the manubrium called the *sternoclavicular articulation*. It is held in place on the sternum by strong ligamentous bands.

The dynamics of the shoulder complex are extremely lengthy and complicated; therefore, we intend to provide a description of those motions that are pertinent to specific injuries and their restoration.

Shoulder injuries

Because of the shoulder complex's structural design, which provides mobility with little articular strength, it is extremely vulnerable to trauma. Falls on the outstretched hand, a severe torsion of the humerus, or a direct blow to the shoulder girdle can result in various pathological conditions. The more prevalent injuries to the shoulder complex include strains, sprains and dislocations, and fractures.

Strains to the shoulder complex are primarily in the region of the glenohumeral joint. Overstretching of the musculotendinous unit through throwing activities, as in baseball, or torsional stress, as received in wrestling, are common mechanisms of strain. The small intrinsic muscles of the *rotator cuff* (subscapularis, supraspinatus, infraspinatus, and teres minor) are commonly traumatized through forceful overstretch of the arm in the abducted position.

Sprains and dislocations can occur at any joint in the shoulder complex. A disruption of the sternoclavicular joint occurs from a fall on the outstretched hand or from a direct inward blow, such as may be received in football. The acromioclavicular sprain or dislocation can arise from forces upward or downward against the acromion process. The partial or complete glenohumeral dislocation represents one of the most often received when the arm is abducted and externally rotated.

Shoulder *fractures* most commonly involve the clavicle; however, the upper humerus is vulnerable to fracture and epiphyseal separation in active youths. Anatomically, the clavicle lacks support at its middle third and, consequently, receives most fractures at that site. Clavicular fractures of the greenstick type are received most often by junior and senior high school students.

Reconditioning

Injuries to the shoulder complex often lead to muscle contractures, with a subsequent lack of range of movement, particularly when immobilization is imposed, as in a sling or cast. Severe damage may require surgical intervention, prolonged immobilization, or both. In such situations, muscle tone must be maintained by muscle setting exercises of the affected part and full range of movement exercise must be provided for adjacent areas such as the elbow, wrist, and hand. Although each disorder of the shoulder must be considered

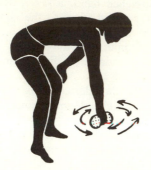

Fig. 10-21. Pendulum exercise for the shoulder (Codman).

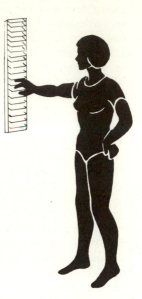

Fig. 10-22. Wall finger walking.

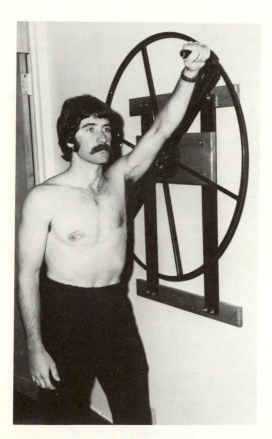

Fig. 10-23. Shoulder wheel. (Courtesy of California State University, Audio Visual Center, Long Beach, Calif.)

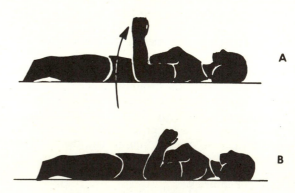

Fig. 10-24. Active shoulder rotation.

unique for each person, the majority require some form of graded exercise that will restore maximum mobility and strength within individual limitations. Several exercises are specifically designed for shoulder complex reconditioning, including the Codman's pendulum exercise, the wall finger walking exercise, the shoulder wheel, and active rotation.

The *Codman's pendulum exercise* (Fig. 10-21) is conducted in a stooped position to reduce the effect of the force of gravity. It is designed to mobilize and free the contracted glenohumeral joint capsule. The participant bends from the waist the affected arm hanging down; in this position, the shoulder movements of flexion, extension, adduction, abduction, and circumduction can be performed in either direction. Within the limits of pain and fatigue, movement arcs are at first made small, gradually being extended along with an increase in executions until 10 have been reached.

The *wall finger walking exercise* (Fig. 10-22) is designed to provide the participant with an increased range of shoulder movement. In this exercise, the student attempts to walk up the wall with the fingers of the affected arm. Each attempt that is higher than the last is recorded on the wall. Shoulder flexion and/or abduction range of motion can be increased depending on whether the individual is facing the wall or the side is toward the wall.

The *shoulder wheel* (Fig. 10-23) is a machine that is very popular in centers for reconditioning. It is a metal wheel mounted on the wall, with the center axis adjustable to the patient's shoulder level. A wing nut can be tightened in the center to provide the correct resistance for each person. An adjustable handle is affixed to one of the wheel's spokes at a point approximating the patient's arm length. The shoulder wheel allows the patient to engage in circumduction exercises while facing the wheel and in flexion-extension exercises while standing sideways to the wheel.

Active rotation from a supine position (Fig. 10-24) allows mobilization of the glenohumeral joint without extraneous movements of the other shoulder complex articulations. Rotation is first executed with the arm flexed and the elbow positioned next to the body. External and internal rotation is then attempted. As the patient gains full range of move-

ment, with the elbow held next to the body, the arm is gradually abducted from the body. The rotation movements can be assisted by the physical eduator or therapist or resisted by pulley or dumbbell weights (Chapter 5).

A number of pieces of equipment are used for developing shoulder function. A length of rope, a towel, or a wand approximately 36 inches long and held at either end provides an excellent means for increasing shoulder girdle function. Such equipment as parallel or horizontal bars and climbing ladders provide the patient with more advanced exercise opportuities (Chapters 5 and 20).

THE ELBOW

The elbow is composed of three articulations, consisting of those between the radius and the humerus, the radius and the ulna, and the ulna and the humerus. The movement of flexion and extension is provided for in the ulnohumeral joint, whereas forearm rotation takes place at the proximal flat circular head of the radius. Strong collateral ligaments stabilize the elbow laterally and medially, whereas the upper end of the radius is supported by an articular capsule called the angular ring (Fig. 10-25). Adding to the stability of the elbow are the flexor muscles, the biceps, the brachialis, the brachioradialis, and the triceps extensor muscle.

Elbow injuries

Although basically designed as a strong articulation, the elbow is subject to various acute conditions in active young persons. The injury often results from a fall on the outstretched hand, from an abnormal force to the joint, or from repeated overstretching, as in throwing activities.

A fall on the outstretched hand, a forcing of the elbow joint into a position of hyperextension, or severe torsion while in the flexed position can cause musculotendinous injury, ligamentous stretching, fracture, or dislocation. A dislocation appears as backward, forward, or lateral displacement of the ulna or radius. Repeated acute insults to the tissue of the elbow, as occur in throwing or striking types of activities, often cause an accumulation of inflammation and subsequent scarring. Activities such as pitching, serving in tennis,

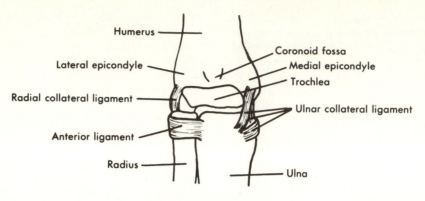

Fig. 10-25. Elbow anatomy.

swinging a golf club, or throwing a javelin commonly cause strain to the elbow joint.

Reconditioning

The elbow, having received injury involving articular structures, has a great propensity for contractures, myositis ossificans, and varying degrees of ankylosis. Therefore, a concentrated reconditioning program must be offered in the early stages of injury. Shoulder movements, together with active hand and wrist exercises, are encouraged. When free movement is permitted by the physician, active assistive movements of flexion, extension, and rotation are encouraged several times a day within the limits of pain and fatigue. After restrictive tissues have been lengthened satisfactorily, a progressive resistive program may be instituted. The student may be encouraged to carry books with the affected arm to facilitate stretching. It should be noted, however, that a contracted elbow should never be forced into full extension. Tissue aggravation only encourages the chronic condition of myositis ossificans, often with permanently disabling results.

THE FOREARM, WRIST, AND HAND

The forearm bones consist of the ulna and the radius. The ulna extends directly from the humerus to the carpal region. In contrast, the proximal head of the radius is held by a strong network of ligamentous tissue. Considered an extension of the hand, the radius, compared with the ulna, is much thicker at its distal end than at its proximal end.

Architecturally, the wrist is structured to produce great flexibility and to promote hand dexterity. The carpal bones are arranged in two rows and are held together by a strong network of ligaments Although individually the carpal bones move slightly, combined they create great flexibility in the region of the wrist. Anatomically, the hand represents a highly versatile and intricate organ. The 27 bones forming the hand include the 8 carpal bones, the 5 metacarpal bones, and the 14 phalanges (Fig. 10-26).

A complex system of muscles helps carry out the motions of the wrist and hand. Flexors of the wrist and phalanges consist of superficial and deep muscles. The deep flexor muscles stem from the ulna, the radius, and the interossei and the superficial flexors stem from the internal condyle of the humerus. Wrist and finger extensor muscles originate at the external condyle of the humerus.

Forearm, wrist, and hand injuries

In general, the lower arm is highly susceptible to trauma, with strains, sprains, dislocations, and fractures prevalent among physically active children and young adults.

With the numerous musculotendinous units associated with the lower arm, strains are a common problem. Sudden overstretching or abnormal and repetitive stress activities, such as throwing a baseball, swinging a golf club, or stroking a tennis racket, may lead to varying degrees of acute, subacute, or chronic lower arm strains.

A joint disruption caused by trauma occurs often

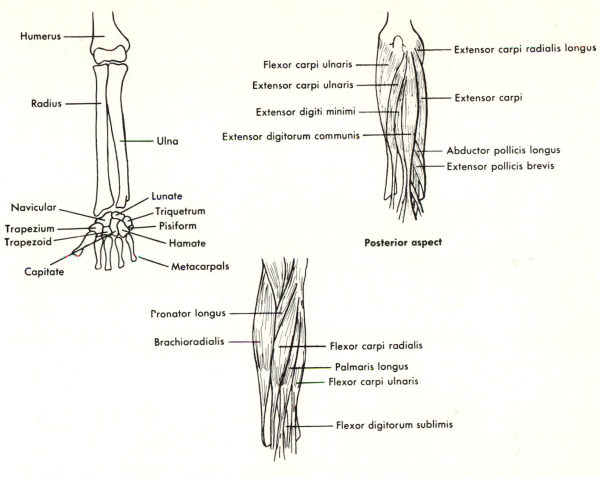

Posterior aspect

Anterior aspect

Fig. 10-26. Forearm and wrist anatomy.

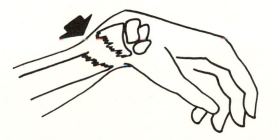

Fig. 10-27. Colles' fracture.

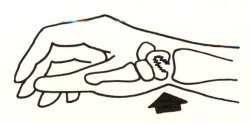

Fig. 10-28. Navicular fracture.

to wrist and fingers. Wrist injuries are commonly the result of a fall on the outstretched hand or a sudden twist. What is commonly thought to be wrist sprain is often tendon strain. A severe wrist sprain may, in actuality, be a fracture of the navicular bone. A navicular fracture occurs when force is applied, as in sudden hyperextension of the wrist. The most common dislocation of the wrist is that of the lunate carpal bone. The cause of a lunate dislocation is a forceful hyperextension of the wrist as the radius exerts pressure downward. Stretching of the dorsal carpal ligament allows the lunate to slip forward and out of its bed.

Because of their mobility and the fact that their main support is provided by ligaments, the carpometacarpals are easily subjected to sprain. The metacarpophalangeal joint is more mobile than the carpometacarpal joint and more subject to sprain when in an abducted position. Immobilization, up to 3 weeks in duration, is a standard procedure for a thumb sprain or dislocation. The need for a functional and intact thumb demands proper care and rehabilitation procedures.

Sprains and dislocations of fingers are often caused by hyperextension to the extent that ligament and capsular tissues are stretched or torn. Following splinting in a partially flexed position for a period of time with restorative exercises is the usual sequence of care.

The same mechanism that results in sprain and dislocation about the wrist and fingers aso causes fractures. The fall on the outstretched hand may produce either the common Colles' fracture or fracture to the navicular bone. A Colles' fracture (Fig. 10-27) can be described as a forward displacement of the radius at its distal end. A navicular fracture, as described earlier, is usually a consequence of wrist hyperextension and compression of the radius and second row of carpal bones (Fig. 10-28). Improper diagnosis and inadequate wrist immobilization in the navicular fracture may lead to a condition of aseptic necrosis and bone degeneration, with subsequent permanent wrist damage. An x-ray examination should lead to proper treatment of these two fractures.

Reconditioning

Fine motor function is of primary importance to the lower arm. Consequently, restoration means forearm rotation, wrist flexibility, and dexterity of fingers. As with the other parts of the body, whenever one part is immobilized, the other parts must be exercised to maintain function. Such activities as squeezing a small ball or a piece of sponge rubber, wringing a towel (Chapter 5), or rolling a piece of paper into a small ball are excellent exercises to reestablish hand strength and facility. Ball squeezing and towel wringing may be added to the exercise routine when range of movement has been reestablished.

REFERENCES

1. Accident facts, 1975, Chicago, 1975, National Safety Council.
2. Anderson, W. A. D., and Scotti, T. M.: Synopsis of pathology, ed. 10, St. Louis, 1980, The C. V. Mosby Co.
3. Cailliet, R.: Low back pain syndrome, ed. 2, Philadelphia, 1968, F. A. Davis Co.
4. Crowe, W. C., Arnheim, D. D., and Auxter, D.: Laboratory manual in adapted physical education and recreation, St. Louis, 1977, The C. V. Mosby Co.
5. Daniels, L., Williams S. M., and Worthingham, C.: Muscle testing, Philadelphia, 1965, W. B. Saunders Co.
6. deVries, H. A.: Physiology of exercise for physical education and athletics, Dubuque, Iowa, 1974, William C. Brown Co., Publishers.
7. Klafs, C. E., and Arnheim, D. D.: Modern principles of athletic training: the science of sports injury prevention and management, ed. 5, St. Louis, 1981, The C. V. Mosby Co.
8. Licht, S., editor: Therapeutic exercises, ed. 2, New Haven, Conn., 1961, Elizabeth Licht, Publisher.
9. O'Donoghue, D. H.: Treatment of injuries to athletes, Philadelphia, 1976, W. B. Saunders Co.
10. Paul, W. D., and Soderberg, G. L.: The shin splints confusion, Proceedings of the Eighth National Conference on the Medical Aspects of Sports Medicine, Chicago, 1967, American Medical Association.
11. Raney, R. B., Sr., and Brashear, H. R.: Shands' handbook of orthopaedic surgery, ed. 8, St. Louis, 1971, The C. V. Mosby Co.

RECOMMENDED READINGS

Cailliet, R.: Foot and ankle pain, Philadelphia, 1968, F. A. Davis Co.
Cailliet, R.: Neck and arm pain, Philadelphia, 1964, F. A. Davis Co.
Cailliet, R.: Shoulder pain, Philadelphia, 1966, F. A. Davis Co.
Klein, K. K., and Allman, F. L., Jr.: The knee in sports, New York, 1969, The Pemberton Press.
Krusen, F. H., editor: Handbook of physical medicine and rehabilitation, Philadelphia, 1971, W. B. Saunders Co.
McLaughlin, H. L.: Trauma, Philadelphia, 1959, W. B. Saunders Co.
Olson, O. C.: Prevention of football injuries, Philadelphia, 1971, Lea & Febiger.
Rusk, H.: Rehabilitation medicine, ed. 4, St. Louis, 1977, The C. V. Mosby Co.

11

Musculoskeletal disorders

Chronic and congenital

Orthopedic impairments constitute a major challenge to physical education, with an estimated 2.4 million orthopedically impaired individuals under 21 years of age in the United States.[24] It also has been determined that children with congenital malformations constitute about 30% of all the crippled children in the United States.[24]

The term *chronic* is defined as a condition having a very gradual onset and a duration longer than 3 months, whereas *congenital* affections refer to those disorders that are present at birth. This chapter is concerned with the most prevalent of those conditions commonly found in children and young adults. They consist of amputations, arthritis, developmental hip dislocation, epiphyseal hip affections, muscular dystrophy, spina bifida, talipes, and torticollis.

Persons with disabilities described in this chapter should qualify for aid under P.L. 94-142 as orthopedically impaired or other health impaired. As such, they could be mainstreamed or placed in special classes or schools depending upon the severity of their disabilities. Evaluation procedures and exercise and activity plans for use by physical educators and therapists are presented in later sections of this chapter.

AMPUTATIONS

Amputation refers to the removal of some member, part, or body organ through surgery, trauma, or some congenital malformations. Adams[2] points out that there are over 300,000 amputees in the United States; 32% of their amputations involve the upper extremities and 68% involve the lower limbs. Amputations may be categorized as congenital, traumatic, or elective. The *congenital amputation* is one in which a body part fails to develop properly during the prenatal period. A *traumatic amputation* occurs as the result of some violence to the body, whereas the *elective amputation* is one in which surgery is performed to ameliorate a disease condition or to correct a congenital or traumatic condition. Commonly, elective surgery is conducted for vascular impairments, infection, or, more often, for malignant tumors in children.[1]

Wherever there is an amputation, a prosthetic appliance must be considered. To employ a prosthesis, a stump must be both free from irritation and functional. Therefore, sites of amputations become extremely important. An optimum site for lower extremity amputation is based on the location and extent of normal tissue, type of function required, placement of prosthesis, and stump appearance.[4] Besides these factors, the person's future needs and individual personality must be taken into consideration.

Lower extremity amputations

The successful surgical amputation requires good circulation to ensure proper healing; it also requires enough remaining stump that a prosthesis may fit properly. The main requirement for a lower limb stump is that it is able to bear the body weight with an artificial limb and allow for maximum function. A limb that is improperly prepared by the surgeon may evoke constant irritation by the prosthesis. Abnormal irritation and pressure points by the artificial limb while weight bearing will develop into skin lesions and additional incapacitation.

The lower limb prosthesis consists of a socket for the stump and, depending on the level of amputation, an artificial knee joint, ankle joint, and segmented foot (Fig. 11-1). A conventional artificial foot allows for plantar flexion and dorsiflexion, with rubber bumpers to simulate the action of the gastrocnemius and anterior tibialis muscles. After the fitting of the artificial leg, gait training is performed. The type of prosthesis to be used is determined by the level of the amputated part. Lower limb amputations are categorized primarily into below-knee (BK) and above-knee (AK) types. The most common BK prosthesis used today is the patellar tendon bearing (PTB) with a sack foot. This

prosthesis provides the wearer with a closed socket by which the stump fits snugly at its distal end to provide good proprioception.[22] AK amputees who are young and have good stump musculature will generally be fitted with a quadrilateral suction socket prosthesis. The individual with a hip disarticulation requires a prosthesis that is controlled by the action of the pelvis. The Canadian type of hip disarticulation prosthesis provides the user with maximum stabilization and mobility.

Upper extremity amputations

The loss of any part of an upper extremity is often accompanied by severe functional and emotional consequences. Prehension, tactile sense, and balance are affected.

Because of the great variance in upper extremity amputations, classification is extremely difficult. With some exceptions in the hand amputation, a long stump is desirable in order to provide for

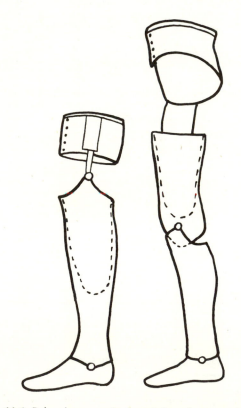

Fig. 11-1. Below-knee prosthesis and above-knee prosthesis.

adaptability in fitting a prosthetic appliance. No single artificial arm can fill all the requirements of the amputee. A choice must be made as to which need will be satisfied: cosmetic, heavy labor, or dexterity. Every effort is made by the surgeon to reconstruct hand function and to maintain prehension and sense of touch. In an effort to replace some semblance of hand function, various terminal devices have been made for the amputee. The two most common devices are the cosmetic prosthetic hand, having some prehension, and the more useful and adjustable split hooks (Fig. 11-2). Control of the artificial upper limb is frequently provided by steel cables and a shoulder harness.

Children with amputations

Children with amputations, whether acquired or congenital, should be provided with a prosthesis according to their particular growth and development demand.[18] Most authorities indicate that the sooner a child is provided with an appliance, the sooner proper habits of locomotion or dexterity can be acquired. Children with congenital amputations

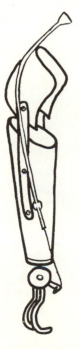

Fig. 11-2. Upper limb prosthesis.

are now being fitted with prostheses as early as 3 months of age. As the child grows, constant attention is given to the function and fit of the prosthesis. Functioning capabilities of appliances fitted early in life are gradually increased to take advantage of the child's developing neuromuscular abilities. An improper fit may result in poor movement pattern development.[6]

Therapeutic management

After surgery, the patient's stump is usually placed in good alignment. Since the leg stump tends to go into abduction, flexion, and external rotation, it is positioned parallel to the mattress. General postural alignment and good body mechanics are disrupted with the loss of a major extremity, a factor to be considered in the total rehabilitative process.

An elastic bandage is applied early after surgery to control hemorrhage and to shrink, toughen, and shape the stump in its preparation for the prosthesis. Swelling caused by edema is prevented by the compression of the elastic bandage and elevation of the part. Stump hygiene becomes the utmost importance in preventing skin problems. A daily routine of cleansing the stump, the elastic bandage, the stump sock, and the socket of the prosthesis must be carried out.

Phantom pain is a normal phenomenon that occurs after the loss of an extremity. Sensations such as numbness and "pins and needles" in the lost limb are common complaints. The reasons for such a phenomenon are various and obscure.

Exercise plays an important part in the management of amputees. Gullickson[7] described the therapeutic exercise needs of the amputee as follows:

1. To increase joint range of movement
2. To correct or prevent contractures
3. To establish proper body alignment and mechanics
4. To provide proper stump circulation
5. To maintain a balance of muscle power, endurance, and coordination
6. To prevent atrophy
7. To toughen the stump for use in a prosthesis
8. To improve the general physical fitness of the amputee

Maximum physical fitness must be established by amputees if they are to be able to withstand prolonged recumbency and the effect the amputation will have on their body mechanics. Ideally, a general program of conditioning should be started in the preoperative stage; however, in most cases this is not feasible unless the amputation is elective and planned well in advance of surgery. Immediately after amputation, a bed exercise regimen should be started that includes muscle setting of the affected limb and isotonic movement of all other major joints to prevent atrophy and contractures. Stoner has presented excellent discussions of patient evaluation and treatment and the selection and use of orthotic and prosthetic devices for all types of amputations.[11]

Implications for physical educators and therapists

The amputee poses a real challenge to the physical educator. Because of the varied types and sites of amputation as well as the different personalities involved, physical education programs must be individualized. The pupil should be encouraged to engage in and learn as many different activities as the condition will permit. Of major concern to the pupil is the maintenance of proper postural alignment, good general body balance, proficient use of a prosthesis, a high level of physical fitness, and therapeutic and personal confidence.

Physical education and therapeutic recreation offer the amputee opportunities for development toward independence. The amputee should be encouraged to engage in all types of physical activities. Swimming and gymnastics are particularly important in developing the full potential of the amputee. A physical education class or recreation program is an excellent place for the amputee to acquire a positive self-concept. Embarrassment by the student about the missing body part can be lessened by an understanding teacher or therapist and the person's acceptance as an equal participant in physical activities by peers (see Chapters 5 and 8).

ARTHRITIS

The term *arthritis* is derived from the two Greek roots *arthro-,* meaning joint, and *-itis,* meaning inflammation. It has been estimated that over 12 million persons in the United States are afflicted with

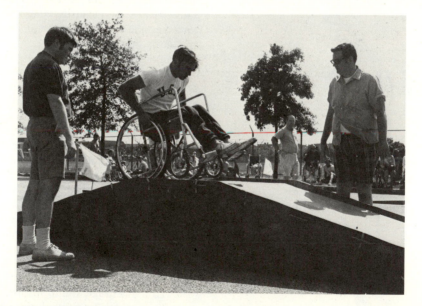

Fig. 11-3. A program of therapeutic management requires that persons confined to a wheelchair be able to control movement up and down ramps. (Courtesy of Julian Stein, American Alliance for Health, Physical Education, Recreation, and Dance and Rehabilitation Education Center, University of Illinois, Champaign-Urbana, Ill.)

some form of rheumatic disease. The importance of this statistic is magnified by the knowledge that with the medical conquest of infectious diseases being so successful, the sharply rising incidence of chronic and degenerative diseases is even more significant. Also, since arthritides inflict a low mortality and high morbidity, the potential for increasing numbers of those afflicted and disabled by them is great.[17]

It is difficult to agree on a classification of the many arthritides, primarily because of the lack of accurate knowledge of their etiology. The American Rheumatism Association indicated that the three forms of arthritis most prevalent are arthritis from infection, arthritis from rheumatic fever, and rheumatoid arthritis. Arthritis after trauma and osteoarthritis or degenerative joint disease of the aging also have a high incidence among the general population.

Infectious arthritis

The occurrence and extent of infectious arthritis has been greatly reduced with the advent of antibiotics. Various pyogenic microorganisms, for example, streptococci, staphylococci, gonococci, pneumococci, and meningococci, have been identified as causative agents of infectious arthritis. The disease appears as an acute inflammatory condition of the synovial membrane and hyaline cartilage, with joints becoming swollen, hot, red, and painful. Associated muscle tendons may also become inflamed, resulting in contractures, inactivity, and, subsequently, muscle atrophy. Uncontrolled infection will eventually result in bony deterioration.

Rheumatic fever and arthritis present an involvement of many joints, but without the chronic effect of degeneration of articular tissue. Having its highest incidence in childhood, rheumatic fever is associated with the group A beta-hemolytic streptococcus of the upper respiratory tract. After a general systemic reaction of sore throat and fever, a transitory polyarthritis travels from one joint to another. Carditis may later be detected by the appearance of murmurs, tachycardia, and chest pain (see Chapter 12).

Rheumatoid arthritis

Rheumatoid arthritis represents the nation's number one crippler, afflicting over 3 million per-

sons. It is a systemic disease of unknown cause. Seventy-five percent of the cases occur between the ages of 25 and 50 years and in a ratio of 3:1, women to men. A type of rheumatoid arthritis called *Still's disease,* or juvenile arthritis, attacks children before the age of 7 years. An infection theory postulates that a microorganism may play an important role. However, there is a great variance in expert opinion as to the exact cause of the disease. Hughes[9] indicated that a great many factors may predispose acquisition. Major contributors could be infection, heredity, environmental stress, dietary deficiencies, trauma, and organic or emotional disturbance.

The disease progesses in the patient, gradually resulting in general fatigue, weight loss, and muscular stiffness. Aticular involvement is symmetrical and characteristically found, in its earliest stages, in the small joints of the hand and feet. Tenderness and pain may occur in tendons and muscular tissue near inflamed joints. As the inflammation in the joints becomes progressively chronic, degenerative and proliferative changes occur to the synovial tendons, ligaments, and articular cartilages. If not arrested in its early stages, joints become ankylosed and muscles atrophy and contract, eventually causing a twisted and deformed limb.

The majority of persons afflicted with rheumatoid arthritis recover almost totally with only minor residual effects. However, it has been estimated that about 10% to 15% of cases become crippled to the point of invalid status. The course of the disease, for the most part, is unpredictable, with spontaneous remissions and exacerbations.

Treatment

Medical treatment of the rheumatoid arthritic involves proper diet, rest, drug therapy, and physical therapy. Because of its debilitating effect, prolonged bed rest is discouraged, although daily rest sessions are required to avoid undue fatigue. A number of drugs may be given to the patient by the physician, depending on individual needs; for example, salicylates such as aspirin relieve pain, gold compounds may be used for arresting the acute inflammatory stage, and adrenocortical steroids may be employed for the control of the degenerative process.[17,19] Physical therapy is primarily concerned with preventing conctracture deformities and muscle atrophy by the use of heat, massage, and graded exercise.

Accompanying chronic rheumatoid arthritis are psychological, social, and economic problems. Psychosocial problems can be as difficult to resolve as those manifested by the disease. The arthritic may feel sensitive about the condition, particularly when deformity is apparent. The theory has been advanced that the rheumatoid arthritic often displays extreme dependence, insecurity, feelings of inadequacy, and an inability to cope successfully with the demands of the environment. The following eight personality characteristics of rheumatoid arthritics have been proposed:[16]

1. Leading quiet lives
2. Being shy and feeling inadequate
3. Having marked feelings of inferiority
4. Being self-sacrificing
5. Being overconscientious
6. Having a strong need to serve others
7. Being obsessive-compulsive
8. Having a tendency toward depression

Peer adjustment may pose a serious problem for the afflicted adolescent. However, as with any reaction to a disease entity, adjustment is personal and individual.

Wolff[27] discusses the development of drugless ways of controlling pain in arthritics. Although admitting that these techniques are still on the "fringes of medicine," he states that the relentless pain of arthritis can often be controlled effectively with nonchemical techniques such as biofeedback, self-hypnosis, behavior modification, and transcutaneous nerve stimulation. Such techniques are often used as an adjunct to other more traditional types of treatment.

Exercise requirements

The exercise requirements for the arthritic fall into three major categories: those that prevent deformity, those that prevent muscle atrophy, and those that maintain joint amplitude and basic function. The physical educator can use gradual or static stretching, isometric muscle contraction, and graded isotonic exercises to advantage.

Preventing deformity is a major concern of the arthritic. In the acute stage, when muscle contractures are prevalent, splinting is a common practice. While lying in bed and splinted, the patient is en-

couraged to engage in muscle tensing exercises numerous times during the day. Such a program tends to prevent general weakness and maintains a balance of strength.

Preventing muscle weakness from inactivity is very important if the arthritic is to maintain joint function. Muscle setting exercises, isometrics, and isotonic exercises must be employed throughout the convalescence of the patient. Particular emphasis is paid to the gluteus and knee extensor muscles, which are extensively used in ambulation.

Maintenance of normal joint range of movement is of prime importance for establishing a functional joint. Stretching is first employed passively by the therapist and is then gradually undertaken by the patient (see Chapter 5).

Implications for physical educators and therapists

An individual with arthritis may need rest periods during the day. These should be combined with a well-planned exercise program. Activity should never increase pain or so tire an individual that normal recovery is not obtained by the next day.

Because of the nature of arthritis, an activity program must be based on the particular requirements of the indiviual. If the disease has been arrested from the acute stage, a variety of sports and game activities may be initiated; however, abnormal physical stress or injury must be avoided at all costs. Swimming is an excellent activity for the arthritic; however, the water must not be chilling. Additional sports might include archery, golf, badminton, tennis, or weight training. Exercises that improve joint range of movement should be conducted daily. Posture training and good body alignment must be stressed in all aspects of the arthritic's daily living (see Chapters 5, 8, and 9).

HIP AFFECTIONS
Developmental hip dislocation

The developmental hip dislocation, commonly called the *congenital hip,* refers to a partially or completely displaced femoral head in relation to the acetabulum (Fig. 11-4). Haas[8] estimated that it occurs six times more often in females than in males; it may be bilateral or unilateral, occurring most often in the left hip.

The cause of the congenital hip dislocation is idiopathic or unknown, with various reasons proposed. Heredity seems to be a primary causative factor in faulty hip development and subsequent dysplasia. Faulty prenatal development as the result of an abnormal in utero position or injury from the birth process is a possible additional cause. The practice of a physician holding a newborn child by the feet or binding the infant in swaddling clothes, with thighs adducted or internally rotated, may force the hip to become dislocated. Michele[12] cited that only about 2% of developmental hip dislocations are, in actuality, congenital and, therefore, produced by a defective germ cell.

Generally, the acetabulum is shallower than the nonaffected side and the femoral head is displaced upward and backward in relation to the ilium. Ligaments and muscles become deranged, resulting in a shortening of the rectus femoris, hamstring, and adductor thigh muscles and affecting the small intrinsic muscles of the hip. Prolonged malpositioning of the femoral head produces a chronic weakness of the gluteus medius and minimus.[12] A primary factor in stabilizing the hip in the upright posture is the iliopasoas muscle. In the developmental dislocated hip, the iliopsoas muscle serves to displace the femoral head upward; this will eventually cause the lumbar vertebrae to become lordotic and scoliotic.

Detection of the hip dislocation may not occur until the child begins to bear weight or walk. Early recognition of this condition may be accomplished by observing asymmetrical fat folds on the infant's legs and by restricted hip abduction on the affected side. A positive *Trendelenburg test* (Fig. 11-5) reveals that the child is unable to maintain the pelvis level while standing on the affected leg. In such cases, weak abductor muscles of the affected leg allow the pelvis to tilt downward on the nonaffected side. The child walks with a decided limp in unilateral cases and with a waddle in bilateral cases. No discomfort or pain is normally experienced by the child, but fatigue tolerance to physical activity is very low. Pain and discomfort become more apparent as the individual becomes older and as postural deformities become more structural. Medical treatment of the developmental hip dislocation depends on the age of the child and the extent of displacement. Young babies with a mild involvement may have the condition remedied through gradual abduction of the femur by a pillow splint, whereas more complicated cases may require traction, casting, or surgery to restore proper hip continuity.

Exercise therapy is given as soon as the splint

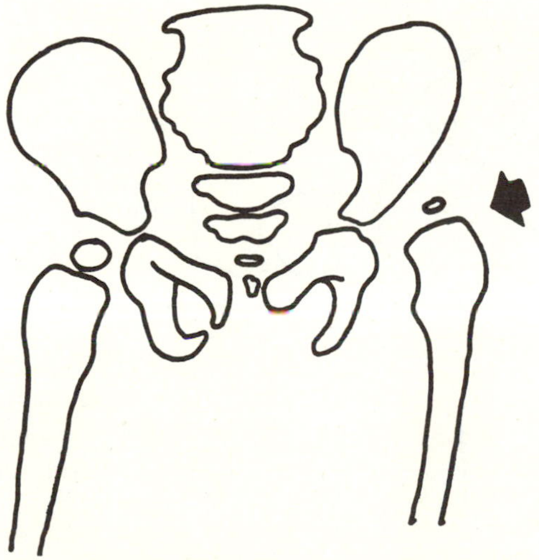

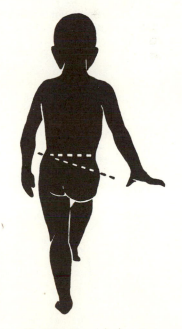

Fig. 11-4. Developmental hip dislocation.

Fig. 11-5. Trendelenburg test.

for fixation of the femur in the adducted position is removed. Slowly, the thigh is returned to a normal position. Heat and massage are given to encourage circulation. Active exercise is permitted, along with passive stretching to contracted tissue. Primary concern is paid to reconditioning the movement of hip extension and abduction. When adequate muscle strength has been gained in the hip region, a program of ambulation is conducted, with particular attention paid to walking without a lateral pelvic tilt[12] (see Chapter 5).

Implications for physical educators and therapists

A child in the adapted physical education or therapeutic recreation program with a history of developmental hip dislocation will, in most instances, require specific postural training, conditioning of the hip region, continual gait training, and general body mechanics. Swimming is an excellent activity for general conditioning for the hip and it is highly recommended. Activities should not be engaged in to the point of discomfort or fatigue.

Coxa plana

Coxa plana is the result of chondromalacia or osteochondritis dissecans, an abnormal softening, of the femoral head. It is a condition identified early in the twentieth century independently by Legg of Boston, Calvé of France, and Perthes of Germany. Its gross signs reflect a flattening of the head of the femur (Fig. 11-6, *A*) and it is found predominantly in boys between the ages of 3 and 12 years. It has been variously termed *osteochondritis deformans juvenilis, pseudocoxalgia,* and *Legg-Calvé-Perthes disease*. The exact cause is not known; trauma, infection, and endocrine imbalance have been suggested as possible causes.

This condition is characterized by necrosis and degeneration of the capital epiphysis of the femoral head. Osteoporosis, or bone rarefaction, results in a flattened and deformed femoral head. Later development may also reveal a widening femoral head and a thickened femoral neck. The last stage of coxa plana may be reflected by a self-limiting course in which there is a regeneration and an almost complete return of the normal epiphysis within 3 to 4 years. However, recovery is not always complete and there is often some residual deformity present. The younger child with coxa plana has the best outlook for complete recovery.

The first outward sign of this condition is often a limp favoring the affected leg, with a pain referred to the knee region. Further investigation by the physician may show pain on passive movement and restricted motion in internal rotation and abduction. X-ray examination will provide the defin-

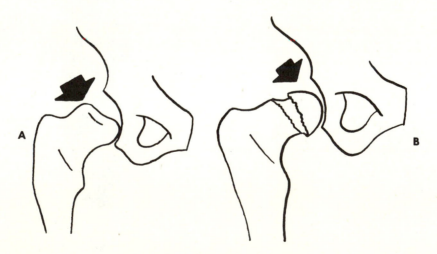

Fig. 11-6. A, Coxa plana. **B,** Coxa vara.

itive signs of degeneration. The physical educator or therapist may be the first person to observe the gross signs of coxa plana and bring it to the attention of parents or physician.

Treatment of coxa plana primarily entails the removal of stress placed on the femoral head by weight bearing. Bed rest is often employed in the acute stages, with ambulation and non–weight-bearing devices used for the remaining period of incapacitation. The sling and crutch method for non–weight bearing is widely used for this condition (Fig. 11-7).

Coxa vara and coxa valga

The adult femoral head or neck of the femur is at a normal angle of inclination of about 128 degrees. An abnormal increase in this angle is termed *coxa valga* and a decrease is called *coxa vara* (Fig.

11-6, *B*). Coxa vara and coxa valga are disturbances in the proximal cartilage or epiphyseal plate of the femur that result in alteration in the angle of the shaft as it relates to the neck of the femur. Steindler[20] describes the pathomechanics of coxa vara and coxa valga as resulting from the combined stresses of an abnormal increase or decrease in weight bearing. A variation of more than 10 to 15 degrees can produce a significantly shortened or lengthened extremity.[20]

Coxa valga and coxa vara can result from many etiological factors, for example, hip injury, paralysis, non–weight bearing, or congenital malformation. Coxa vara and coxa valga are described according to where the structural changes have occurred in the femur, that is, neck (cervical), head (epiphyseal), or combined head and neck (cervicoepiphyseal). Two types of conditions have been recognized: the congenital and the acquired. The congenital type may be associated with the developmental hip. The acquired coxa vara is, by far, the most prevalent and occurs most often in adolescent boys between 10 and 16 years of age. It is commonly termed *adolescent coxa vara*.

Adolescent coxa vara is found in boys who have received a displacement of the upper femoral epiphysis. Boys who are most prone to adolescent coxa vara have been found to be obese and sexually immature or tall and lanky, having experienced a rapid growing phase. Trauma, such as is incurred in a hip fracture or dislocation, may result in an acute coxa vara. More often, through constant stress, a gradual displacement may take place. Whatever the mechanism of injury, the individual experiences progressive fatigue and pain on weight bearing and progressive stiffness, combined with a limited range of movement. As in coxa plana, a limp is apparent, which reflects weakness in the hip abductor muscles and pain referred to the region of the knee. With displacement of the epiphyseal plate, the affected limb tends to rotate externally and to abduct when placed in flexion.

Management in the early stages of coxa vara involves crutch walking and the prevention of weight bearing to allow revascularization of the epiphyseal plate. Where deformity, displacement, and limb shortening are apparent, corrective surgery may be elected by the physician.

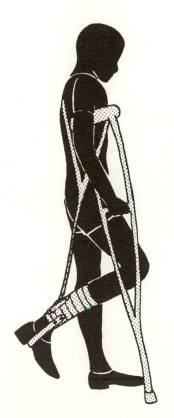

Fig. 11-7. Sling and crutch for hip conditions.

Implications for physical educators and therapists

The individual with an epiphyseal affection of the hip presents a problem of muscular and skeletal stability and joint range of movement. Stability of the hip region requires skeletal continuity and a balance of muscle strength, primarily in the muscles of hip extension and abduction. Prolonged limited motion and non–weight bearing may result in contractures of tissues surrounding the hip joint and an inability to walk or run with ease. Abnormal weakness of the hip extensors and abductors causes the individual to display a positive Trendelenburg sign.

A program of exercise must be carried on by the individual to prevent muscle atrophy and general deconditioning caused by lack of activity. Muscle-tensing exercises for muscles of the hip region when movement is prohibited are conducted, together with isotonic exercises for the upper extremities, trunk, ankles, and feet.

When the hip becomes asymptomatic, a progressive isotonic non–weight-bearing program is first initiated for the hip region. Active movement emphasizing hip extension and abduction is recommended. Swimming is an excellent adjunct to the regular exercise program. When the physician considers the patient free from a pathological joint condition, weight-bearing exercises can commence. Program dosage should never exceed the point of pain or fatigue until full recovery is accomplished. A general physical fitness program emphasizing weight control and body mechanics will aid the student in preparing for a return to a

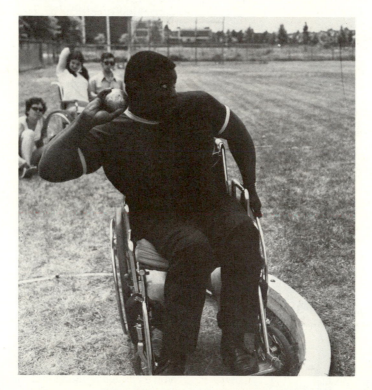

Fig. 11-8. Some persons are not able to return to the full program. They are in need of special consideration when participating in special sport events. (Courtesy of Julian Stein, American Alliance for Health, Physical Education, Recreation, and Dance and Rehabilitation Education Center, University of Illinois, Champaign-Urbana, Ill.)

full program of physical education and recreation activities (see Chapters 5 and 8).

MUSCULAR DYSTROPHY

Muscular dystrophies are chronic, progressive, degenerative, noncontagious diseases of the muscular system, characterized by weakness and atrophy of the muscles of the body. Muscular dystrophy is probably the most serious disabling condition that can occur in childhood. Although not fatal in itself, the disease contributes to premature death in most known cases because of its progressive nature. Late in the disease, connective tissue replaces most of the muscle tissue. In some cases, deposits of fat give the appearance of well-developed muscle. Despite the muscle atrophy, there is no apparent central nervous system involvement in the disease.

Although the exact incidence of muscular dystrophy is unknown, estimates place the number afflicted with the disorder in excess of 200,000 in the United States. It is estimated that more than half those cases known fall within the age range of 3 to 13 years.

The exact cause of muscular dystrophy is not known. Speculation regarding etiology includes faulty metabolism (related to inability to utilize vitamin E), endocrine disorders, and deficiencies in the peripheral nerves. There is some indication that an inherited abnormality causes the body's chemistry to be unable to carry on proper muscle metabolism. Wallace[26] indicated that heredity influences the severity of the disease and that the distribution of the affected muscles in individual patients is determined primarily by the linkage of a faulty gene.

There are numerous classifications of muscular dystrophy, with regard to the muscle groups affected and the age of onset. However, four main clinical types of muscular dystrophy have been identified. They are the pseudohypertrophic type, the facioscapulohumeral type, the juvenile type, and the mixed type.

Pseudohypertrophic type

The pseudohypertrophic type is the most prevalent type of muscular dystrophy and is usually recognized between the ages of 4 and 7 years. It is largely confined to males. Symptoms that give an indication of the disease are the following:

1. Decreased physical activity, compared with children of commensurate age
2. Delay in the age at which the child walks
3. Poor motor development in walking and stair climbing
4. Little muscular endurance
5. A waddling gait with the legs carried far apart
6. Walking on tiptoe
7. Moving to all fours when changing from a prone to a standing position
8. Weakness in anterior abdominal muscles
9. Weakness in neck muscles, which makes it difficult to sit erect
10. Pseudohypertrophy of muscles, particularly in the calves of the leg, which are enlarged and firm on palpation
11. Pronounced lordosis and gradual weakness of lower extremities

As the disease progresses, imbalance of muscle strength in various parts of the body occurs. Deformities develop in flexion at the hip and knees. The spine, pelvis, and shoulder girdle also eventually become atrophied. Contractures and involvement of the heart may develop with the progressive degeneration of the disease. In general, the later the age at which the disease is observed, the slower it progresses. Consequently, persons who are afflicted later may perform functional activities longer.

Facioscapulohumeral type

The facioscapulohumeral type of muscular dystrophy is the second most common. The onset of symptoms or signs of the facioscapulohumeral type is usually recognized between the ages of 3 and 20 years, with the most common age of onset between 3 and 15 years. This form of muscular dystrophy affects the shoulder and upper arm and the person may have trouble in raising the arms above the head. There is also a weakness in the facial muscles and the child may lack the ability to shut the eyes, close the eyes completely when sleeping, whistle, or drink through a straw. A child with this type of disease often appears to have a masklike face that lacks expression. Later, involvements of the muscles that move the humerus and scapula will be noticed. Weakness usually appears later in the abdominal, pelvic, and hip musculature and anomalies such as scoliosis and lordosis develop in the spine (see Chapter 9). This type of muscular dystrophy is often milder than the pseudohypertrophic type, and some persons with it have been able to live useful lives. Facioscapulohumeral muscular dystrophy usually progresses slowly.

Juvenile type

The juvenile type begins in late childhood, adolescence, or early adult life. Muscle atrophy is more general, with the muscles of the shoulder girdle being affected first. The progression is usually slower than in the types mentioned previously and persons afflicted with this type live longer.

Mixed type

The mixed version of muscular dystrophy may occur between the ages of 30 and 50 years. Involvement is most likely to appear in the area of the scapula and pelvis. This type may take on many of the characteristics that appear in the pseudohypertrophic type.

Implications for physical educators and therapists

The age of onset of muscular dystrophy is of importance to the total development of the children. Those who contract the disease after having had an opportunity to secure an education, or part of an education, and develop social and psychological strengths are better able to cope with their environments than are those who are afflicted with the disease prior to the acquisition of basic skills.

Although the characteristics of patients with muscular dystrophy will vary according to the stage that the disease has reached, some general characteristics are as follows:

1. There is a tendency to tire quickly.
2. There may be a tendency to lose fine manual dexterity.
3. Truitt[23] and Ripley et al.[15] concluded that children with muscular dystrophy have normal intelligence but lack motivation to learn because of isolation from social contacts and limited educational opportunities.
4. Progressive weakness tends to produce adverse postural changes.
5. Emotional disturbance may be prevalent because of the progressive nature of the illness

and the resulting restrictions placed on opportunities for socialization.[23]

Nothing currently known will arrest muscular dystrophy once it begins. Because of the negativism prevalent in some cases as a result of the inability of these children to serve a social purpose, this lack of knowledge has been a serious deterrent to expansion of educational plans for patients with muscular dystrophy. However, it is worth noting that scientific research may be close to solving unanswered questions regarding the disease, and eventually the progressive deterioration of muscles may be halted.

Inactivity seems to contribute to the progressive weakening of the muscles of those with muscular dystrophy. Exercise of muscles involved in the activities of daily living to increase strength may permit greater functional use of the body. Furthermore, exercise may assist in reducing excessive weight, which is a burden to those who have muscular dystrophy. The diet should be closely monitored.

Control of excess weight is essential to the success of a rehabilitation program of those with progressive muscular dystrophy. For individuals whose strength is marginal, any extra weight throws an added burden on ambulation and on activities for daily living[17] (see Chapter 7).

One must recognize that the dystrophies cannot all be considered the same; therefore, the physical and social benefits that children can derive from physical education and recreation programs are different. Those who have milder forms of muscular dystrophy, which progress slowly, can derive many benefits from well-constructed adapted physical education and therapeutic programs, and children should be allowed to play as long as they can.

A great deal can be done to prevent deformities and loss of muscle strength from inactivity. If a specific program is outlined during each stage of the disease, it is possible that the child may extend the ability to care for most daily needs for many additional years. In addition to the administration of specific developmental exercises for the involved muscles, exercises should include development of walking patterns, posture control, muscular coordination, and stretching of contractures involved in disuse atrophy. It should be noted, however, that all exercises should be under the direction

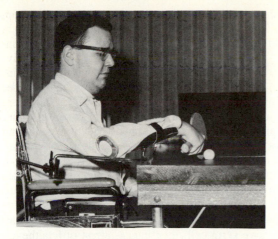

Fig. 11-9. A student with muscular dystrophy finds Ping-Pong enjoyable. (Courtesy of the American Alliance for Health, Physical Education, Recreation, and Dance.)

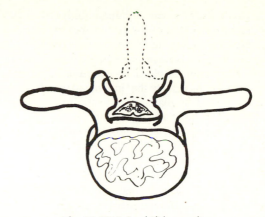

Fig. 11-10. Spina bifida occulta.

of a physician, as should the program of ambulation. Rusk[17] stresses that variations in prognosis affect the ambulatory and exercise needs of the muscular dystrophy patient. He lists eight stages of disability with suggested ambulatory activities and restrictions that should help educators and therapists in program planning. In an attempt to achieve social and emotional progress from activities, it may be desirable to blueprint the activities around the remaining positive strengths so that enjoyment and success can be achieved (Fig. 11-9).

The progressive weakness and muscle deterioration make the child with muscular dystrophy particularly susceptible to respiratory infections.[11] Therefore, the physical educator and therapist should be particularly alert not to expose these children to damp environments or to situations that are conducive to respiratory infections.

CONGENITAL SPINAL COLUMN MALFORMATIONS
Spina bifida

Of the dysplastic congenital defects occurring to the spine, spina bifida is the most common. Spina bifida implies congenital malformation of the posterior aspect of the spinal column, in which some portion of the vertebral arch fails to form over the spinal cord. It has been estimated that spina bifida occurs in 1 of 1,000 infants born, of which 80%

do not survive the first year. Spina bifida might appear as an external herniation of meninges, meningocele, or myelomeningocele or, more commonly, as spina bifida occulta without an external sac (Fig. 11-10). In any type of spina bifida, spinal cord involvement may occur and produce varying degrees of neurological impairment ranging from mild muscle imbalance and sensory loss in the lower limbs to complete paraplegia. In almost half the children with myelomeningocele, a hydrocephalic condition also exists. In these cases, shunting is mandated to prevent irreversible brain damage.[18] However, neurological disturbances may be completely absent in spina bifida occulta or may not become symptomatic until later in life.[9] "Spina bifida occulta is the unfused condition of vertebral arches without any cystic distension of the meninges. There may or may not be changes in the overlying skin, neurological signs, or pathological changes in the spinal cord."[21]

Children who are paraplegic from spina bifida are often able to move about with the aid of braces and crutches. Of considerable concern is the prevention of contractures and associated foot deformities, for example, equinovarus, through daily passive flexibility exercises.[11]

Implications for physical educators and therapists

No particular program of physical education or therapy can be directly assigned to the student with spina bifida. Some students have no physical reaction and discover the condition only by chance through x-ray examination for another problem. On the other hand, a student may have extensive neuromuscular involvement requiring constant medical care. A program of physical education or therapeutic exercise based on the individual needs of the person should be planned, but activities that could distress placement of any shunts and/or put pressure on sensitive areas of the spine must be avoided.

Spondylolysis and spondylolisthesis

Spondyloloysis and spondylolisthesis result from a congenital malformation of one or both of the neural arches of the fifth lumbar vertebra or, less frequently, of the fourth lumbar vertebra. Spondylolisthesis is contrasted to spondylolysis on account of its anterior displacement of the fifth lumbar on the sacrum. Foward displacement may occur as a result of a sudden trauma to the lumbar region. The vertebrae are moved anteriorly because there is an absence of bony continuity of the neural arch and the main support is derived from its ligamentous arrangement. In such cases, individuals often appear to have a severe lordosis.[20]

Many individuals have spondylolysis, or even spondylolisthesis, without symptoms of any kind, but a mild twist or blow may set off a whole series of low back complaints with localized discomfort or pain radiating down one or both sides. The pathological condition may eventually become so extensive that surgical intervention will be required.

Implications for physical educators and therapists

Proper therapy can provide the person with a painful low back because of spondylolysis or spondylolisthesis with a graduated exercise program that may help prevent further aggravation and, in some cases, remove many symptoms characteristic of the condition. A program should be initiated similar to that of ameliorating the postural malalignment of lordosis (with primary concentration on the strengthening of abdominal muscles), the lengthening of low back muscles, and the segmental realignment of legs, pelvis, and spine (Chapters 5 and 9). Games and sports that overextend, fatigue, or severely twist and bend the low back should be avoided. In most cases, the physician will advise against contact sports and heavy weight lifting.

TALIPES (CLUBFOOT)

One of the most common deformities of the lower extremities is talipes or clubfoot. *Talipes* is a term derived from the Latin *talus* meaning ankle, and *pes,* meaning foot. This defect can be acquired or congenital. The acquired clubfoot can develop from a spastic paralysis, as in cerebral palsy or other neuromuscular disease, which may eventuate in bone and soft tissue changes. A congenital clubfoot is by far the most prevalent type. However, the pathogenesis is not clearly understood. A defective germ cell, inheritance, arrest of fetal development, muscle imbalance, or faulty in utero position have been advanced as possible causes.

A clubfoot deformity is characterized by the position in which the foot is formed and may be described as *equinus* (plantar flexion), *calcaneus* (dorsiflexion), *varus* (inversion), or *valgus* (eversion). The clubfoot deformity, if not corrected, would force the individual to walk on the side of the foot or on the ankle rather than on the sole of the foot.

Talipes equinovarus

Talipes equinovarus has the highest incidence, amounting to 70%, among the congenital forms of clubfoot. Adams[1] described talipes equinovarus as being adducted and inverted at the subtalar, midtarsal, and anterior tarsal joints, while contracted tissue pulls the foot into a plantar flexed position (Fig. 11-11, *A*). The calcaneus fails to grow, remaining small or underdeveloped. If not corrected early in life, the individual with talipes equinovarus develops an awkward gait and walks on the outside of the foot and ankle.

Therapeutic management

Treatment of the clubfoot may be conservative or operative. If the deformity is recognized soon after birth, a plaster cast is employed to retain the foot in an overcorrected position. Special clubfoot shoes with a ridged steel pole may be employed for the prewalker to help maintain the proper position of the foot. Various corrective shoes may be

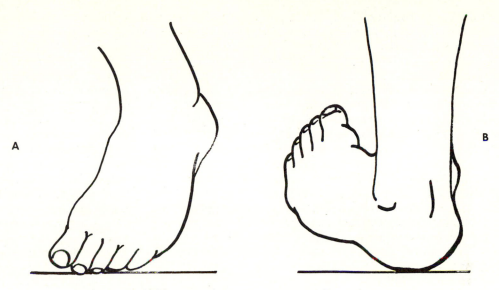

Fig. 11-11. Clubfoot. **A,** Talipes equinovarus. **B,** Talipes calcaneovarus.

worn and splints applied to continue the development of proper foot alignment until amelioration is achieved.

Implications for physical educators and therapists

The pupil's limitations and capabilities will depend on the extent of residual derangement and deformity. A handicapped child with a severe malformation may be restricted from standing for long periods or may be unable to walk without fatigue. Activities requiring running and jumping must be modified.

Exercise cannot be considered a means for correcting a clubfoot. However, a graded program should be given the pupil that will maintain or improve muscle tone, improve ambulation, and develop good body mechanics (Chapters 5 and 9). Team and individual sports activities are beneficial for the pupil with clubfoot, but they may have to be adapted to prevent the deleterious effects of extensive running, jumping, and kicking (Chapter 8).

TORTICOLLIS

Torticollis, or wryneck, is an acquired or congenital neck deformity characterized, most often,

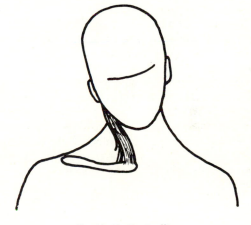

Fig. 11-12. Torticollis.

by a shortening of the sternocleidomastoid muscle (Fig. 11-12) and, occasionally, the scalenus, platysma, splenius, and trapezius muscles. It appears as a flexion and tilting of the head, together with rotation toward one side.[14]

Acquired torticollis may develop from an acute, subacute, or chronic inflammatory process resulting from strains, sprains, or wounds. Habit patterns such as those developed by defective eyesight or hearing difficulties may tend to produce a postural torticollis. Other acquired conditions may be psychogenic in nature and can be produced by a psychoneurotic tic, which contributes to a chronic torticollis.[5]

Congenital torticollis can result from malposition of the head in utero, defective cervical vertebral development, or disruption of circulation to the neck muscles. Continuous muscle shortening eventually leads to scar development and contractures. As the child grows older, facial deformity may be noted. The face on the contracted side becomes flattened, with the eye and mouth distorted downward. It is thus important for physical educators and therapists to recognize and make proper referrals for this condition at the earliest possible time.

Therapeutic management

Medical care for the acute wryneck involves rest, traction, heat, massage, mild manipulation, and, in some cases, a Thomas collar for immobilization and support, depending on the patient's requirements.[5] Chronic and congenital torticollis requires more extensive and prolonged medical management than does acquired torticollis. In mild cases, stretching exercises or bracing may be employed. However, with the more complicated conditions, surgery with bracing might be the treatment of choice, followed by an extensive physical therapy program. The total psychological, sociological, and medical implications of the pupil must be kept in mind. Often, grave psychological problems arise from bodily disfigurement.

Implications for physical educators and therapists

The reactions to this condition are individual and depend on the child's psychological makeup. Lack of feelings of personal worth or self-esteem may occur as a result of an unusual appearance and the negative reaction of peers. The physical educator or therapist should provide an atmosphere of acceptance and encouragement for the child.

An individual with torticollis is not usually limited in physical activity. When permitted by the physician, a program of graded exercises should be employed to increase the strength of weakened neck musculature and to stretch contracted tissue. In some cases, topical heat applied to the shortened area will aid muscular relaxation and elongation. Wale[25] suggested that active exercises for torticollis should include head side flexion away from the contracted side, with rotation movement in the direction of the affected side.

Because students are usually capable of a great variety of sports activities, they should be introduced to as many as possible. For students whose torticollis is psychogenic in origin, low-tension activities such as swimming, golf, and tennis and appropriate tension reduction exercise programs are suggested (see Chapters 6 and 8).

REFERENCES

1. Adams, J. C.: Outline of orthopaedics, Baltimore, 1966, The Williams & Wilkins Co.
2. Adams, R. C., et al.: Games, sports, and exercises for the physically handicapped, Philadelphia, 1972, Lea & Febiger.
3. Anderson, W. A. D., and Scotti, T. M.: Synopsis of pathology, ed. 10, St. Louis, 1980, The C. V. Mosby Co.
4. Burnham, P. J.: Amputation of the lower extremity, Ciba Clin. Symp. No. 16, 1964.
5. Cailliet, R.: Neck and arm pain, Philadelphia, 1964, F. A. Davis Co.
6. Daniels, A. S., and Davies, E. A.: Adaptive physical education, New York, 1975, Harper & Row, Publishers.
7. Gullickson, G., Jr.: Exercises for amputee. In Licht, S., editor: Therapeutic exercise, ed. 2, New Haven, Conn., 1961, Elizabeth Licht, Publisher.
8. Haas, H.: Therapeutic dislocation of the hip, Springfield, Ill., 1963, Charles C Thomas, Publisher.
9. Hughes, J. G.: Synopsis of pediatrics, ed. 5, St. Louis, 1979, The C. V. Mosby Co.
10. Klafs, C. E., and Arnheim, D. D.: Modern principles of athletic training: the science of sports injury prevention and management, ed. 5, St. Louis, 1981, The C. V. Mosby Co.
11. Krusen, F. H., editor: Handbook of physical medicine and rehabilitation, Philadelphia, 1971, W. B. Saunders Co.
12. Michele, A. A.: Iliopsoas, Springfield, Ill., 1962, Charles C Thomas, Publisher.
13. Prior, J. A., and Silberstein, J. S.: Physical diagnosis: the history and examination of the patient, ed. 5, St. Louis, 1977, The C. V. Mosby Co.
14. Raney, R. B., Sr., and Brashear, H. R.: Shands' handbook of orthopaedic surgery, ed. 8, St. Louis, 1977, The C. V. Mosby Co.
15. Ripley, H. S. et al.: Personality factors in patients with muscular dystrophy, Am. J. Psychiatry **99:**781-787, 1943.
16. Rotstein, J.: Arthritis performance, Philadelphia, 1965, W. B. Saunders Co.
17. Rusk, H. A.: Rehabilitation medicine, ed. 4, St. Louis, 1977, The C. V. Mosby Co.

18. Salter, R. B.: Disorders and injuries of the musculoskeletal system, Baltimore, 1970, The Williams & Wilkins Co.
19. Stecher, P. G., editor: The Merck index, ed. 8, Rahway, N.J., 1968, Merck & Co., Inc.
20. Steindler, A.: Kinesiology of the human body, Springfield, Ill., 1955, Charles C Thomas, Publisher.
21. Swinyard, C. A., editor: Comprehensive care of the child with spina bifida manifesta, New York University, Rehabil. Monogr. No. 31, 1966.
22. Tosberg, W. A.: Upper and lower extremity prosthesis, Springfield, Ill., 1962, Charles C Thomas, Publisher.
23. Truitt, C. J.: Personal and social adjustments of children with muscular dystrophy, Am. J. Phys. Med. **34:**124-128, 1955.
24. U.S. Department of Health: Welfare services for crippled children, Public Health Services Publication No. 2137, Washington, D.C., 1971, U.S. Government Printing Office.
25. Wale, J. O., editor: Tidy's massage and remedial exercises, Baltimore, 1961, The Williams & Wilkins Co.
26. Wallace, H. M.: The muscular dystrophies. In Framptom, M. E., editor: The physically handicapped and special health problems, Boston, 1955, Porter Sargent, Publisher.
27. Wolff, B. B.: Arthritis alerter, San Diego, 1979, Arthritis Foundation.

RECOMMENDED READINGS

Am. J. Phys. Med., vol. 46, February 1967.
Cailliett, R.: Foot and ankle pain, Philadelphia, 1968, F. A. Davis Co.
Cailliett, R.: Low back pain syndrome, ed. 2, Philadelphia, 1968, F. A. Davis Co.
Cailliett, R.: Shoulder pain, Philadelphia, 1966, F. A. Davis Co.
Licht, S., editor: Therapeutic exercise, ed. 2, New Haven, Conn., 1965, Elizabeth Licht, Publisher.

12

Cardiorespiratory disorders

The term *cardiovascular* includes all diseases of the heart and the blood vessels throughout the body. This includes rheumatic and congenital heart conditions, coronary heart disease, hypertensive heart disease, and cerebrovascular disease. The rheumatic and congenital heart conditions are the primary heart disorders found in the public schools. Moreover, 25 million Americans live with some type of heart or blood vessel disease.[1] This chapter is concerned with fundamental principles of establishing physical education programs for children with heart disease of the congenital and rheumatic types and physical education programs that may help in delaying the degeneration of the cardiovascular system in regard to coronary heart disease and hypertensive heart disease. Heart disease in children is a major problem and commands the attention of the physical educator. It is imperative that teachers have a general understanding of the heart and circulatory system (Figs. 12-1 to 12-3) and of the major kinds of deviations of the cardiovascular system. Furthermore, Individual Education Programs must be developed and implemented for many children with heart conditions.

Cardiovascular diseases are estimated to cause more than 54.3% of all deaths in the United States.[1] Compared with other disabilities, heart conditions cause the greatest number of restrictions in physical activity. Congenital heart disease and rheumatic fever are the heart disorders that occur most often in children of school age. It is estimated that there are about 500,000 children in this country suffering from rheumatic fever[19] and that rheumatic fever and rheumatic heart disease account for approximately two thirds of all heart disease in children.[35] Furthermore, Ross and O'Rourke[36] estimate that rheumatic valvular heart disease is responsible for about 15,000 deaths each year in the United States in people under 65 years of age.

CLASSIFICATION OF HEART MURMURS

When the blood flows past the valves of the heart, sounds are made that are easily detected by a stethoscope. Heart murmurs are of two types. The first is a functional murmur, which is believed to result from a physiological disturbance. In these cases, there is usually no sign of heart disease. The murmur may disappear on another examination.

The second type of murmur is the organic murmur, which is usually a result of some defect of the heart. Organic murmurs may be either acquired (caused by disease) or congenital (present at birth). On many occasions, the mitral and aortic valves are afflicted. Valve affliction may cause either regurgitation (imperfect closure of the valve, permitting a backflow) or stenosis (incomplete opening of a valve, which restricts the flow of blood). The organic murmur usually warrants the close supervision of the physical educator, for this type of murmur generally is associated with some form of cardiac disease.

MAJOR TYPES OF CARDIOVASCULAR DISEASE

The American Heart Association[19] listed four major types of cardiovascular disease:

1. Rheumatic heart disease, which damages the heart and its valves, muscles, and blood vessels by scar tissue and is caused by rheumatic fever
2. Congenital heart disease, which is a malfunction of the heart occurring in fetal life
3. Hypertensive heart, commonly known as high blood pressure, which places a prolonged stress on the heart and major arteries
4. Coronary heart disease, or arteriosclerosis of the coronary arteries, a condition in which the coronary arteries become sclerotic or hardened and narrowed and the passage of blood through the channels becomes more difficult. The chief cause of coronary heart disease is atherosclerosis, that is, the formation of atheromas or fat masses on the lining surface of the coronary arteries (Fig. 12-4).

The first two of these conditions, rheumatic heart disease and congenital heart disease, are commonly found in school-aged children. The latter two are the result of a degenerative cardiovas-

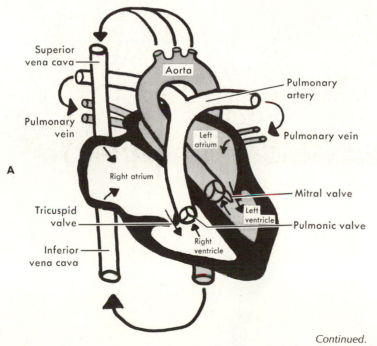

Continued.

Fig. 12-1. A, Blood flow through the normal heart. **B,** Blood flow through the heart. *1,* Blood enters right atrium; *2,* then flows to right ventricle; *3,* goes to the lungs through the pulmonary artery; *4,* returns from the lungs to the left atrium; *5,* then goes to the left ventricle; and *6,* flows through the aorta into the body.

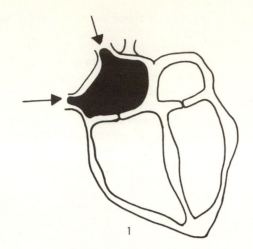
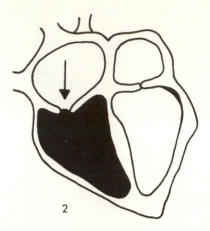
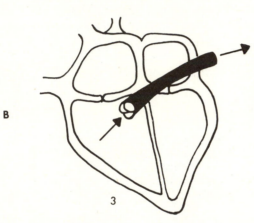
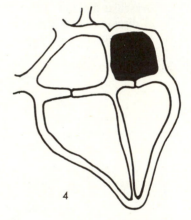
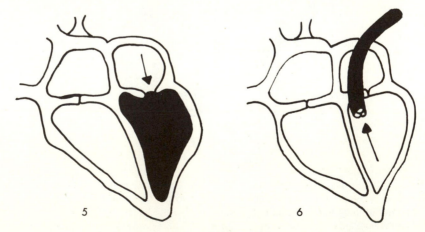

Fig. 12-1, cont'd. For legend see p. 309.

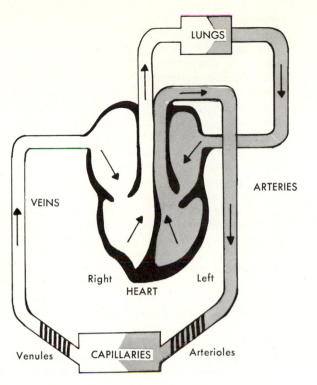

Fig. 12-2. Circulation to the lungs and body.

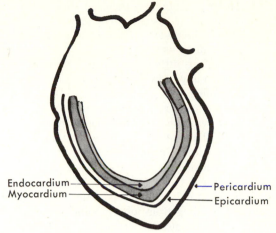

Fig. 12-3. Layers of the heart.

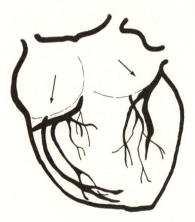

Fig. 12-4. Arrows indicate coronary arteries.

cular system and are prevalent among the aging population, but often have their origins in poor health practices of younger persons.

Rheumatic fever

Rheumatic fever is a disease that school-aged children may contract. Rheumatic fever ranks first in causes of death in children and adolescents from 5 to 19 years of age. Consequently, it presents a great problem to physical education teachers.

Although the direct cause of rheumatic fever is not known, the disease is an acute infection related to a hemolytic streptococcus. There are three main phases in the development of rheumatic fever. In the first stage, the youngster has a sore throat caused by a streptococcus infection. The child then recovers, in the second phase, for 1 to 4 weeks; the third phase begins when the child contracts acute rheumatic fever, which may last for weeks or months. The following are warning signals that may be of use to the educator, school nurse, or physician:

1. Failure to gain weight
2. Pallor
3. Fatigue
4. Poor appetite
5. Frequent colds and sore throats
6. Tonsil or adenoid problems
7. Scarlet fever or any known streptococcal infection
8. Unexplained nosebleeds
9. Unexplained fever
10. Pains in arms, legs, or joints
11. Unusual restlessness, irritability, twitching, or jerky motions

12. History of previous rheumatic fever
13. Behavior and personality changes
14. Poor schoolwork by a child who has previously done well
15. Breathing difficulties, rapid breathing, exceptionally slow breathing, or arrhythmical breathing

During the acute attack of rheumatic fever, there are usually symptoms that are caused by the localization of inflammation. The inflammation may be in the joints; in the skin, in the form of a rash; in the brain, causing Saint Vitus's dance; and in the heart, causing a faulty closure of the heart valves. There is also marked fever and migration of heat, pain, and swelling from joint to joint. In many instances, the first attack of rheumatic fever is very mild and difficult to diagnose. Consequently, most of the children who have contracted rheumatic fever escape the first time with little or no heart damage. However, no immunity can be built up to rheumatic fever. On the contrary, there is a strong tendency for the disease to recur. Therefore, it is vital that the initial attack of rheumatic fever be diagnosed as such so that precautions can be taken to withstand or prevent a second attack.

Through the administration of antibiotics that destroy the streptococcus bacteria, effective prevention of recurring attacks of rheumatic fever can be achieved. Without prophylactic medication, second attacks occur in from 50% to 70% of children who have had one attack.[28] Once the initial attack

of rheumatic fever has manifested itself, primary interest is not so much in the heart or in the amount of physical activity in which the child is engaged, unless severe damage has occurred, but in the practice of preventing streptococcal infection. In the event that a child is in a preventive program against rheumatic fever and contracts a streptococcal infection, more often than not, penicillin will eradicate the infection. Therefore, the American Heart Association has listed the following guides to assist persons in identifying possible streptococcal infections:

1. Did the sore throat come on suddenly?
2. Does the youngster complain that the throat hurts most when he or she swallows?
3. Does it hurt the child under the angle of the jaw when it is pressed gently with the fingers? Are the lymph glands swollen?
4. Does the child have fever? How much? (Streptococcal infections bring on fever between 101° and 104° F.)
5. Does the child complain of headache?
6. Is the child nauseated?
7. Has the child been in contact with anyone who has had scarlet fever or a sore throat?

When deterrents of the recurring attacks of rheumatic fever are not successful, in many instances, the heart is permanently injured. Injury affects one or both of the valves on the left side of the heart. The valves heal by means of scars, which leave the heart rough or deformed. This deformity may pre-

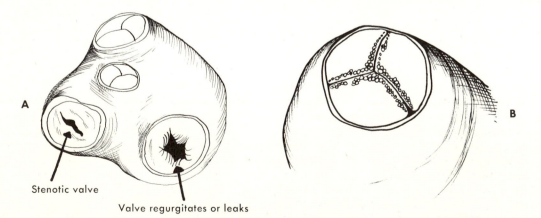

A

Stenotic valve

Valve regurgitates or leaks

B

Fig. 12-5. A, Rheumatic disease of heart valves. **B,** Rheumatic disease along cusps of aortic valve.

vent the valves from functioning properly. The valves may also become narrowed (stenosed). Recurring attacks of rheumatic fever usually subside during adolescence (Fig. 12-5).

Congenital heart disease

The range in the severity of congenital heart disease is great. The defect can be so mild that it in no way affects the child, or it can be so severe that the consequence is death. It is a disease that occurs in many combinations as a result of defective fetal development of the heart and vessels of the circulatory system. Sherrill[38] indicates that one half of all congenital heart defects are caused by the following conditions: ventricular septal defects (22%), patent ductus arteriosus (17%), and tetralogy of Fallot (11%). Thirty-two percent are caused by the following conditions: transposition of the great vessels (8%), atrial septal defect (7%), pulmonary stenosis (7%), coarctation of the aorta (6%), and aortic and subaortic stenoses (4%). The remaining 18% are caused rare conditions. Some of the causes of congenital heart disease have been associated with metabolic and endocrine disturbances, infectious virus, or vitamin deficiencies during the first 3 months of pregnancy. German measles during the first trimester of pregnancy has been believed to contribute to possible congenital heart disease. Great advances in heart surgery during the past few years have made it possible to correct congenital heart defects that would formerly have resulted in death so that the child may live. However, it should be noted that not all children with congenital heart defects can benefit by operation.

The following are some of the specific disorders of congenital heart disease:

1. Patent ductus arteriosus, in which the passageway between the pulmonary artery and the aorta remains open after birth and some of the blood that should go through the aorta is short-circuited to the lungs. This works to the disadvantage of both the pulmonary and the general circulations.
2. Tetralogy of Fallot ("blue baby"), congenital abnormalities that consist of an opening of the septum between the ventricles and abnormal positioning of the aorta to the right in such a manner that it lies over a defect of the septum of the left ventricle so that some

blood leaves the aorta, which results in enlargement of the right ventricle and a decreased amount of the blood going to the lungs for reoxygenation (Fig. 12-6).

3. Coarctation of the aorta (constriction of the aorta), generally after the arteries branch off to the head and arms. This causes limitation of blood to the tissues and organs of the body together with high blood prssure in the upper extremities and low blood pressure in the lower extremities, which, if not corrected, lead to later complications (Fig. 12-7).

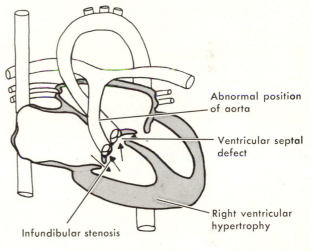
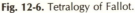

Abnormal position of aorta

Ventricular septal defect

Right ventricular hypertrophy

Infundibular stenosis

Fig. 12-6. Tetralogy of Fallot.

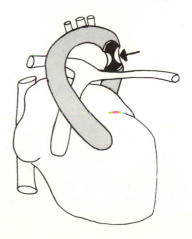

Fig. 12-7. Arrow indicates coarctation of aorta.

CLASSIFICATION OF CARDIAC DISEASES

The approval of the activity program for a child with a cardiac disorder must come from the physician. Therefore, most diagnostic referral forms that come from medical personnel use the standard classification procedures developed by the American Heart Association. The classification represents an estimate as to what the person can do in response to effort. This classification provides enough information for a teacher so that a child with a cardiac disorder will not be unduly restricted from physical activity. The classification of patients with diseases of the heart is as follows:

Class I: Patients with heart disease, but without resulting limitation of physical activity. Ordinary physical activity does not cause undue fatigue, palpitation, dyspnea, or anginal pain.

Class II: Patients with cardiac disease resulting in slight limitation of physical activity. They are comfortable at rest. Ordinary physical activity results in fatigue, palpitation, dyspnea, or anginal pain.

Class III: Patients with cardiac disease resulting in marked limitation of physical activity. They are comfortable at rest. Less than ordinary activity causes fatigue, palpitation, dyspnea, or anginal pain.

Class IV: Patients with cardiac disease resulting in inability to engage in any physical activity without discomfort. Symptoms of cardiac insufficiency or of the anginal syndrome are present even at rest. If any physical activity is undertaken, discomfort is increased.

The complementary classification is as follows:

Class A: Patients wih a cardiac disease whose ordinary physical activity need not be restricted.

Class B: Patients with cardiac disease whose ordinary physical activity needed not be restricted but who should be advised against severe or competitive physical efforts.

Class C: Patients with cardiac disease whose ordinary physical activity should be moderately restricted and whose more strenuous efforts should be discontinued.

Class D: Patients with cardiac disease whose ordinary physical activity should be considerably restricted.

Class E: Patients with cardiac disease who should be at complete rest, confined to a bed or a chair.

In addition to the classification of children with cardiac disorders for the purpose of assisting teachers in the administration of physical activity, the Ohio State Department of Education has stated some general rules for administering activity to children who have cardiac disease. These rules are as follows:

1. The children should be observed and reclassified at regular intervals.
2. They should have their temperatures taken daily.
3. They should have rest periods, with frequency depending on the severity of the condition.
4. Perhaps the best guide for determining limitations is the response to exercise and the frequency with which shortness of breath occurs.

MEDICAL DIAGNOSTIC PROBLEMS

Medical personnel assume the responsibility of defining the limits of physical activity for the child with heart disease. Diagnostic difficulties are encountered when attempting to determine the limits of physical activity for the child. The following are some of the problems that face diagnosticians. First, the physician's experience in cardiac practice may be limited. Many advances have been made and are currently being made in the research of heart disease. Consequently, the physician must be aware of the most recent evidence for proper diagnosis.[5] Second, the physician's own attitudes toward heart disease may prompt inactivity. Some physicians are cautious in their diagnoses and wish to protect their patients as well as themselves professionally. As a result, there is a tendency to "overdiagnose."[12] Furthermore, Vodola[45] indicates that, for many years, some physicians have disapproved of physical activity for patients exhibiting circulorespiratory problems.

Recent trends indicate that physicians are inclined to include graded activities for patients who have cardiac disease after careful evaluation of the limits to be imposed. Improved diagnostic techniques are also available to the physician.

NATURE AND NEEDS OF THE PERSON WITH CARDIAC DISABILITY

Persons with cardiovascular disabilities must not overstep their bounds in either the physical or the emotional dimension of living, for doing so can mean disaster. These restrictions can cause both emotional disturbance and psychic disorders. Furthermore, cardiovascular impairment in some is dynamic, with the persons either deteriorating or being rehabilitated so that they can live more fully functioning lives. Persons living under these circumstances must constantly make adjustments to their environment to maintain the balance between their capabilities with respect to the heart. This also confronts persons with psychological and emotional problems. They may withdraw and underestimate their capabilities, thereby unnecessarily placing substantial obstacles in their way to independent living. They may suppress the seriousness of the condition and perform acts that may jeopardize their lives.

Cardiovascular disability also stands in the way of fulfillment of optimal vocational experiences, for schoolwork is often missed and experiences may be few, narrow, and distorted. Therefore, it is of the utmost importance that education be concerned with the establishment of orderly progression and increasing standards of performance and achievement for these children.

The child with cardiac disability in physical education

Because heart disease is complicated and not well understood among physical education professionals dealing with persons who have cardiac disease, fears and apprehensions have long interfered with the educational management of such persons. The role of the physical educator in dealing with children who have cardiac disease is to create a protective environment and yet to provide activities that keep the children from feeling different. Children with cardiovascular impairment require the same educational opportunities and have the same needs as typical children. Therefore, the principle of the Individual Education Program in the least restrictive environment also applies to these children.

There is little doubt that the needs of children with heart disease are great. Therefore, there are two alternatives for educational placement of these children in the public schools—a regular class or a special class. The present tendency is to integrate children with cardiac difficulties with peers in regular classes, for every child wants to be like other children. Some suggestions for teachers of these children are as follows:

1. Provide opportunities in physical activities for biological and sociological development of the children.

2. Take special precautions to counter ill health, for example, colds and streptococcal infections.
3. Appraise the physical status of the children.
4. Correct remediable defects.
5. Develop in each child a positive attitude toward body care.
6. Base educational practices on data incorporated in the Individual Education Programs.
7. Provide opportunity for a balanced program of activities and recreation in an atmosphere free from tension and strain.
8. Take an interest in planning to meet the recreational needs for the children in the community.
9. Maintain a positive attitude toward the children's disabilities and try to create this attitude in the rest of the students.

Children's feelings about themselves and their physical conditions are often more important than the conditions themselves.

When a child or adolescent has been separated from a normal environment as a result of restricted experience because of cardiovascular deficiency, a lower performance level and general immaturity and dependency may be found. Unnecessary restriction of physical activities for such a child gradually gives way to the individualization of treatment to suit the needs of the child. Individualization is the keynote for physical activity for such a child because there are considerable differences between types of heart disease.

There is impressive evidence that, in many cases, physical training can enhance some elements of cardiovascular functioning in some patients with heart conditions, when approved by the physician. Examples of physical training for such persons have been reported by Trap-Jensen and Clausen,[43] who state that physical training causes striking improvements in exercise tolerance of patients with angina pectoris. In addition, Frick, Katila, and Sjögren[15] indicate a trend toward larger stroke volume of physically trained patients with cardiac disease as compared with controls. Other effects of training on the cardiovascular system are a reduction of blood pressure and serum lipids and a lower heart rate. All of these factors may reduce the demands on the heart. Thus, it appears that physical training under proper guidance can be of value to the patient. The rehabilitation movement has demonstrated that the traditional practice of permanent bed rest for most of these patients was not only unnecessary, but a mistake from both psychological and physiological standpoints. Kraus and Raab[26] state that the courage to take a calculated risk has already been proved fully justified and, today, physicians who recommend carefully graded exercise practices for their patients with heart conditions no longer expose themselves to the dangers of being condemned by their clientele and their colleagues.

IMPLICATIONS FOR PHYSICAL EDUCATORS AND THERAPISTS

There is great variability among children who have cardiac disorders. Therefore, the amount and kind of exercise to be prescribed for a child with a cardiovascular disability must take into account the individual and the particular disability. Once the program has been prescribed for a child, with the consent of the doctor, the teacher must be a keen observer and impress on the patient the importance of staying within the prescribed limits of exercise. Activities should be discontinued immediately in the event that the child shows stress. Perhaps the best indicators of a stressful situation involving physical activity are heart rate and blood pressure.

The following are some of the controls that should be used as a guide to keep the child with cardiac disability within his or her capabilities:

1. Reduce the cadence of the exercise.
2. When using progressive exercises, start in a lying position, then a sitting position, and finally a standing position.
3. Keep the number of repetitions low.
4. Be sure to check for cardiac stress; check heart rate and blood pressure and watch for shotness of breath.
5. Make the dosage congruent with the reaction of the student to the exercise.
6. Aerobic exercise, within the establshed physical bounds of the child, should provide for maximum improvement.

Types of formal exercise, in most cases, can be

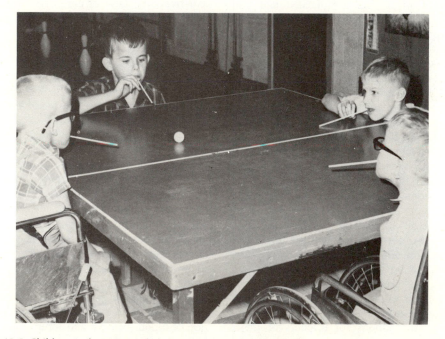

Fig. 12-8. Children performing a task that requires respiratory capability. (Courtesy of Julian Stein, American Alliance for Health, Physical Education, Recreation, and Dance and University Hospital School, University of Iowa, Iowa City, Iowa.)

adapted to the individual's condition. However, it is suggested that competitive games of a highly emotional nature and of considerable intensity, for example, football, basketball, baseball, or soccer, should be carefully evaluated before including them in the program for the child with cardiovascular impairment. Situations that involve high intensity with regard to physical activity and highly charged emotional situations should be avoided. Activities that involve hill or rope climbing should be closely evaluated in regard to the capabilities of such a child; the energy expended during these activities is considerably more than the energy expended during activities on level ground. Greater stress may be placed on the heart as a result of such activities.

A physical education program should be designed to meet the needs of children with cardiac conditions on all school levels. The cost of oxygen to the heart is the real key to a choice of activities or exercises. An aerobic program can thus be planned within the bounds of the patient. There are many games that are a part of the elementary school physical education curriculum that are acceptable with regard to physical dosage for children of moderate cardiac disability. Games that do not require sustained activity and that allow for rest between activities are permissible for the child with moderate disability. At the outset, the activities of the physical education program should be modified with respect to distance traveled, duration of the exercise, and dosage of exercise until both the instructor and the student are aware of the student's capacities. It is best to abstain from activity that is severe or of long duration. The student should not swim or run for distances or at high speeds unless he or she has proved that this intensity of activity is within his or her capabilities.

Progressive exercise is an important feature of a rehabilitation program or a person with cardiovascular disability. The following basic progressive procedures are suggested:

1. All exercise should be short and slow in the beginning of the program, with increasing rhythm and longer duration as the program progresses.
2. The first phase of activity should involve the exercise of individual limbs from a lying position only.

3. Later, the student may exercise from a sitting position, then standing, and then progress to walking exercises or exercises that involve mild mobility, followed by light developmental activities.
4. Breathing exercises and relaxation training may be indicated by the physician.

An example of a progressive exercise program is the system of progressive walking and hill climbing developed by Oertel.[11] The system involves progressive walking and hill climbing in which the work load is extended by the distance walked or the height of the hill climbed.

EXERCISE PROGRAMS FOR PATIENTS WITH CARDIAC DISEASE
Prerequisites

There are several prerequisites needed for the effective utilization of exercise treatment programs for persons who have heart conditions. Some of them are as follows:

1. An activity sequence in which a patient can be placed at the present level of educational performance.
2. Evaluation procedures to determine the level of the individual's functioning and activity capability
3. Individual prescriptions of activity for each person
4. Objectives and goals for each person

Prior to entering an activity program, the participants should be medically screened and then should be informed of the benefits and risks of such a program. Information should be provided on potential risks and on the effects of training and fitness on cardiovascular function. Physicians should direct cardiac programs for persons who are at risk.

It is important that goals be set prior to the initiation of the activity program in order to facilitate measuring the progress of the learner. The goals to which the programmer may project are increases in the parameters of measurable laboratory functioning (oxygen uptake) and the behavioral capability of the performer to produce greater amounts of activity as a result of progression through the program. When objectives are set for an exercise program, it should be possible to measure progress toward the preformulated objectives.

Cardiovascular assessment

Cardiovascular assessment is an essential feature of the total exercise program. It is important that cardiac contraindications be identified. These may be ascertained through medical physical examinations, chest x-ray films, biochemical assays, metabolic tests, electrocardiograms, and stress testing. As a rule, the administration of these tests will detect cardiac murmurs, arrhythmias, hypertrophy, intraventricular blocking, hypertension, congenital anomalies, diabetes, hypercholesterolemia, heavy smoking, signs of myocardial insufficiency, and other risk factors. In addition, it is advisable to test under dynamic conditions. Thus, the physiological competence of the individual is assured in relation to physiological parameters that indicate the presence of current functioning of the individual. A steady state of the heart rate during bicycle ergometer exercise or a steady recovery rate from step or treadmill tests is not enough to furnish an adequate index of initial level of physical conditioning for the patient.

Physical training and coronary heart disease

The goal of physical training is to attain physical fitness conducive to good cardiovascular function and good health. The attainment of the desired level of fitness should occur in orderly fashion, usually at a restrained rate of progress. This is necessary if programming is to be beneficial for persons who possess great variability in cardiovascular functioning.

Recently, a number of deaths have been reported in subjects undergoing currently popular "do-it-yourself" jogging programs.[20] The incidence of death in the natural course of programming, regardless of the level of physical activity, makes it impossible to exclude deaths from any regimen. It would, therefore, be unreasonable to discontinue programs where the occurrence of death and myocardial infarction are not increased. Instead, specific steps must be takn to educate subjects and professional staffs in the proper use of this modality. The statement made by the American Heart Association's Committee on Exercise emphasizes this by stating:

For the sedentary individual there is serious risk in the sudden unregulated and injudicious use of strenuous exercise.But it is a risk that can be minimized and perhaps even eliminated through proper preliminary testing and the individualized prescribing of exercise programs.[2]

To clarify the term *risk* the following definitions are suggested:

1. Persons *at risk* or *at high risk* are those who have a few, a majority, or all of the established risk factors pointing toward the potential development of coronary heart disease. An exercise testing and conditioning program, properly supervised, should prove useful in reducing these risks.
2. If used freely, the term *risk* or *high risk* is synonymous with *hazard,* indicating an existing potential danger of unhealthy occurrences when individuals are physically stressed.

Before beginning unrestricted exercise, a sedentary person should have a thorough medical examination to exclude contraindications. This should include orthopedic, respiratory, and cardiovascular evaluation. It should also include an assessment of physical fitness. Other sources[2] offer details of contraindications to exercise testing.

TESTS OF PHYSICAL CONDITION

Most exercise tests for an evaluation of physical work capacity or, more specifically, maximal oxygen uptake, are based on a linear increase in heart rate with increasing oxygen uptake or work load. However, all predictions from submaximal tests should be done with caution. When persons of different age groups are tested, some sort of correction factor must be included, since the maximal heart rate declines with age.[3] Even when the tests are carried out under standardized conditions, the methodological error in a prediction of the maximal aerobic power is considerable (standard deviation = 10% to 15%). However, submaximal tests can be used for screening the functional capacity of the oxygen-transporting system.

Objective tests to determine the effect of training on different functions are important. Such tests may be an aid in the development of the program and may encourage the individual to continue training. The submaximal bicycle ergometer test is a simple, inexpensive, and reliable test. At the very least, indirect measurements (or prediction) can give an indication of the person's physiological fitness for endurance-type work, and periodic retesting can give an indication of improvement. Such evaluation also constitutes a strong motivational tool for the participant.

Exercise prescription

A maximum heart rate can be determined from standard tables, after which exercise prescriptions can be started somewhere below the 60% level and then can be gradually increased. The prescription of exercise follows certain basic guidelines that are applicable to all persons, regardless of age, state of health, or functional capacity. To be meaningful, the exercise prescription must include the type(s) of physical activity, the *intensity*, the *duration*, and the *frequency*. The task of exercise prescription is much more difficult for sedentary persons, for older persons, for those who have risk factors, and particularly for those who are symptomatic. Thus, for each individual, the degree of risk associated with exercise involves the following interdependent variables:

1. The severity of the exercise relative to the habitual intensity of exercise performed
2. Age
3. Functional capacity
4. Health
5. Risk factors
6. Symptomatology

The target level for training is defined as that level at which or below which progressive abnormalities occur. Target levels for training should be used only as guidelines. These levels must be adjusted for each subject individually, with the aid of clinical observations and response to the initial effort test to arrive at an ''actual'' target level. This actual target level may vary somewhat from day to day, depending on daily fluctuations in the subject's other activities.

One *met* is the equivalent of a resting oxygen consumption, which is approximately 3.5 ml/kg/minute. Mets during exercise are determined by dividing work metabolic rate by resting metabolic rate. The met cost of treadmill work is dependent on body weight, but the met cost of bicycle ergometry is independent of body weight.

The intensity of the exercise may be prescribed by mets or by heart rate.

Exercise prescription by mets

The peak and average intensities of exercise may be estimated by determining 90% and 70% of the individual's functional capacity. Thus, for a person with a maximum functional capacity of 8 mets, intensity would be calculated as follows:

Peak conditioning intensity = $0.9 \times 8 = 7.2$ mets

Average conditioning intensity = $0.7 \times 8 = 5.6$ mets

There is an alternative method that sets a sliding scale for estimating the average conditioning intensity.[2] The sliding scale allows for the variability resulting from known differences in the intensity that can be tolerated by persons with different functional capacities. The baseline intensity is established at less than 60% of the functional capacity in mets.

Mets may be estimated from the work load performed (Table 12-1) or by calculating oxygen intake from measurements of minute ventilation and expired gas composition. Either estimate of mets may be used effectively by the physical educator for exercise prescription.

In supervised exercise programs, it would appear that the greatest hazard might lie in the subject's overactivity, above and beyond that which is appropriate at any given time. This factor is control-

Table 12-1. Energy expenditure in mets during stepping at different rates on steps of different heights*

Step height		Steps/minute			
Centimeters	Inches	12	18	24	30
0	0	1.2	1.8	2.0	2.4
4	1.6	2.1	2.5	2.9	3.7
8	3.2	2.4	3.0	3.5	4.5
12	4.7	2.8	3.5	4.1	5.3
16	6.3	3.1	4.0	4.7	6.1
20	7.9	3.4	4.5	5.4	7.0
24	9.4	3.8	5.0	6.0	7.8
28	11.0	4.1	5.5	6.7	8.6
32	12.6	4.4	6.0	7.3	9.4
36	14.2	4.8	6.5	8.0	10.3
40	15.8	5.1	7.0	8.7	11.7

*From American College of Sports Medicine: Guidelines for graded exercise testing and prescription, Philadelphia, 1975, Lea & Febiger.

lable with proper supervision of the training sessions.

In the untrained, progressively greater restrictions need to be placed on exercise regimens. This frequently means that, in the beginning, subjects are trained at paces that are less demanding than those they themselves might choose. The initial workout should not exceed 2 or 3 mets for a sedentary person, with 1 met as the increment of step size.

Intensity of exercise

The most difficult problem in designing exercise programs is the prescription of the appropriate exercise intensity. The percentage of functional capacity a given individual is able to sustain for a given conditioning period is quite variable. Consideration must be given to the fact that the capacity for performing routine or conditioning work is relatively less in persons with low functional capacities (6 mets or less) than it is in those with high functional capacities. One group indicates that reasonable estimates for exercise prescription are that during conditioning sessions, *peak efforts* should not exceed 90% of functional capacity and *average intensity* should approximate 70% of functional capacity. The duration can then be set empirically on the basis that the participant recovers fully.[2]

In the early stages of a conditioning program, precise control of effort is necessary to ensure that participants do not create difficulty by expending too much effort. Peak efforts may need to be lowered to less than 60% of functional capacity and then gradually increased. These controls continue to be useful at all stages of a conditioning program because they enable the participant to expend the most energy per unit of time. Furthermore, improvements, plateaus, or regressions in performance can be evaluated quickly and efficiently.

Target levels for training

Exercise prescriptions for persons at risk are determined largely by the heart rate and electrocardiogram (ECG) response to the initial effort test. The purpose of the initial exercise test is to determine the target level for training and to provide a basis for future comparative fitness measurements.

Patterns of exercise for symptomatic subjects do not differ greatly from those for nonsymptomatic subjects, except for the factors that determine peak severity. For nonsymptomatic subjects with normal response to exercise tests, these would include a predetermined heart rate; for those who respond abnormally, these would include the level at which progressive abnormality occurs; for example, some untoward event occurs and thus places an upper limit on exercise. As work capacity increases, exercise programs are changed to challenge the individual and thus the target range is increased.

PRINCIPLES FOR TRAINING

An adaptation to a given load takes place gradually; in order to achieve further improvement, the training intensity has to be increased. There is, however, no linear relationship between the amount of training and the training effect. For instance, 2 hours of training each week may cause an increase in maximal oxygen uptake by 0.4 liter/minute. The rate and magnitude of the increase varies from one individual to the next. It is important to ascertain what amount of training may produce a satisfactory result. Less effort is needed to

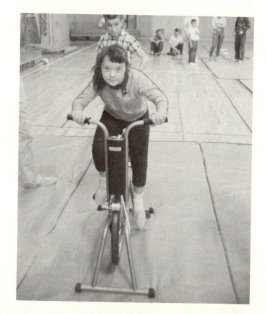

Fig. 12-9. A bicycle can be used in training students for cardiovascular endurance. (Courtesy of Julian Stein, American Alliance for Health, Physical Education, Recreation, and Dance and University of South Dakota, Vermillion, S.D.)

maintain a reasonable degree of physical condition than to attain it after a period of prolonged activity. Since maximal oxygen uptake and cardiac output can be attained at a submaximal speed, this lower speed is probably optimal as a training stimulus. As pointed out, even work loads demanding only a submaximal oxygen uptake do improve the physical condition for *very* untrained individuals.

Potential hazards in prescriptions for cardiac patients

Some factors or practices frequently associated with physical training sessions of normal persons should be specifically prohibited or extreme caution used with the cardiac patient. Close supervision is essential until the subject and the physician have been educated as to the pattern, progression, and regression of abnormalities and a study has been made of the coronary arterial circulation.

Improvements in work tolerance may be associated with gross changes in the anatomy of the coronary arterial system, as characterized by coronary arteriograms.

Features that constitute additional stresses to the cardiovascular systems, and that therefore should be avoided, are as follows:

1. It is well known that thermal stress (extremes of heat and cold) can evoke considerable strain.
2. Sudden death when snow shovelling is caused by a combination of the effects of cold exposure and sudden severe effort in an unconditioned subject. Care should be taken to be preconditioned, enter the cold gradually, keep the chest covered, and intersperse work with rest periods.
3. The ingestion of fluids at extreme temperatures is known to produce cardiac arrhythmias, but fluids are needed to prevent dehydration.
4. Large meals tend to divert a greater portion of the cardiac output to mesenteric vascular beds.

Guidelines for exercise testing and prescriptions for cardiac patients

1. When properly prescribed, physical activity is beneficial, since it maintains or increases functional capacity and may modify some risk factors associated with atherosclerotic disease.

2. Initial prescription, including upper limits of exertion, and subsequent modifications can be safely determined from knowledge generated from repeated graded exercise tests given under medical supervision.
3. The attainment and maintenance of functional capacity and work loads commensurate with ability is a concern of professionals, particularly for those individuals considered *at risk* from an injudicious increase in their physical activity levels.
4. Fitness is relative and must be individualized.
5. Subject's symptoms can be useful in assessing limitations in physical training.

In summary, the minimal amount and type of exercise required to achieve optimal physical fitness and to protect against lethal coronary attacks need to be better delineated. There is also a need to demonstrate whether or not physical reconditioning after a coronary attack actually reduces the propensity to recurrence and prolongs life. The hazards as well as the benefits of carefully supervised exercise programs need to be ascertained, but there is much to suggest that the potential benefits far exceed the hazards. More discrete guidelines and criteria are needed to delineate the indications and contraindications and to ensure safety and efficacy.

RESPIRATORY DISORDERS

Respiratory disorders (particularly asthma), like cardiovascular disorders, often impair the opportunity for individuals to participate in self-fulfilling physical activity. Research attempting to determine the relationship between physiological parameters and specific, individually planned instruction on respiratory function is not as well documented as is research in the cardiovascular area. However, there are many authorities who do affirm the positive benefits of physical activity for the individual with asthma.* Until there is further substantiation of the therapeutic value of physical activity for those suffering from respiratory disorders, caution is advised.

Allergies and asthma

Allergy is a term used to designate the hypersensitive reactions of some persons when exposed to

_____
*See references 6, 7, 21, and 31.

certain foreign substances called *allergens*. These substances are harmless in similar amounts to most other persons. Allergies are estimated to affect about 16 million persons in the United States.[22] Persons may be allergic to many different substances that affect them in varying degrees. Among these substances are the following:

1. Foods (strawberries, eggs, chocolate, wheat, pork, nuts, citrus fruits, etc.)
2. Inhalants that attack the respiratory tract (pollens, tobacco smoke, vapors, dust, perfumes, etc.)
3. Substances that come in contact with the skin (dyes, poison ivy, poison sumac, fur, leather, animal hair, etc.)
4. Infectious agents (bacteria, viruses, fungi)
5. Drugs (vaccines, antibiotics, serums)

Forms of allergy that are of greatest consequence to the physical educator are probably those caused by inhalants such as pollens and dust particles that affect the respiratory tract. In the United States, there are 13.5 million victims of hay fever, the most common indication of allergy. Hay fever and asthma are of particular consequence to the physical educator since, because of them, endurance in physical activity is seriously curtailed. Inhalation of certain pollens, grasses, dust, or particles in the environment or in the gymnasium is a common cause of allergy.

Treatment

The treatment of allergies is a medical problem. In some instances, physical educators may be able to identify such cases. In the event that allergies are identified among their students, referrals should be made to the physician. There are four possible approaches in treating conditions of allergies:

1. *Avoiding the substance causing the allergy*. It may be possible to avoid the allergen that is causing the problem. This, of course, is dependent on locating the cause of the allergy. Possible adjustments made for children who are allergic to pollens in the fall might be prescribed, for example, indoor activity that would free them from the pollens present on the athletic field. Precautions that might be taken to assist in deterring the effects of allergens are avoidance of certain mat coverings that might contribute to allergic conditions, reduction of the dust in the gymna-

sium, a change in diet, or the withdrawal of a drug.
2. *Desensitization*. The desensitization process is carried out by injecting, in progressively increasing doses, an extract of the causative antigen. This procedure is followed in the cases of pollens, dust, vaccines, and serums.
3. *Antihistamines*. Antihistamines counter or reduce the symptoms produced by excessive release of histamine into the blood.
4. *Hormone therapy*. Adrenal or pituitary hormones often are instrumental in bringing relief to the person with an allergy.

Implications for physical educators and therapists

In many cases, children with allergies must make adjustments to the activities of their physical education classes. However, necessary adjustments vary greatly with the intensity, frequency, and duration of the allergy attack. Allergies often reduce the ability of children to withstand the onset of physical fatigue, and they may need to withdraw from an activity while their classmates continue. This affects them emotionally and socially because they appear different from their peers. Asthmatic children often fall into this category. However, these children may be helped in several ways. Some of the ways are as follows:

1. Adapt the activity to provide an opportunity for children to play with peers and develop social characteristics desirable for all children in physical education programs.
2. Improve the physical fitness of the children through progressive developmental activities.
3. Teach and improve neuromuscular skills commensurate with the children's abilities. This will enable them to participate in wholesome leisure activities in the form of carryover sports. There is evidence that programmed exercise for children with asthma is beneficial and that progressive activity increases lung capacity, which, in turn, may reduce the number and severity of asthmatic attacks. Children with asthma in the elementary grades may participate in games of low organization and movement exploration activities. As a rule, these activities enable children to perform at their own rates. However, at the junior high and high school levels, in

which competitive play is part of the program, adaptations for children with severe allergies must be taken into consideration. Activities such as dancing, specific developmental exercises, badminton, softball, shuffleboard, tennis, bowling, and golf are acceptable for children with severe allergies. However, the fundamental rule to consider when placing children with allergies in physical activity is to let each child participate in activities commensurate with current abilities.

Bronchial asthma

Bronchial asthma usually results from allergic states in which there is an obstruction of the bronchial tubes or the lungs or a combination of both. Usually the bronchial tubes are attacked by spasms of the bronchial musculature and excess mucus, which causes an insufficient amount of air to flow into the lungs. When attacks occur, mucus fills the bronchial tubes and makes it difficult to breathe. The asthmatic attacks vary in length and intensity; some last only a matter of minutes, whereas others may persist for days. Asthmatic attacks may be induced by exposure to cold air, smoke, irritating gases, pollen, and other allergy-producing substances. Asthma accounts for 11.4% of all chronic conditions in children under the age of 1 year and for 22% of all days lost from school, because of chronic conditions, by children between the ages of 6 and 16 years.

Physical activity can play an important part in enhancing the physical functioning of children with asthma. Macman and Itkin[27] point out that physical conditioning may be indicated for a large number of patients suffering from asthma as a means of increasing the usefulness of their lives. Duration and level of activity are relevant variables to consider when asthmatics are engaged in physical activity. Jones, Wharton, and Buston[24] and Taub[42] indicate that intermittent exercise, within the framework of individual capability, is appropriate for the asthmatic.

The physical educator can assist the child with asthma in the following ways:

1. Take care not to precipitate an attack through vigorous activity.
2. Attempt to develop physical fitness through activity within the student's capacity.
3. Teach motor skills that will enable the child to participate in the team games and carryover activities.
4. Instruct in relaxation skills, correct posture, and breathing exercises.
5. Provide opportunities for social growth by involving the student in adapted activities with peers.

Exercises for the asthmatic child should be concerned with full chest excursion, including the stretching of restricted musculature and the strengthening of weakened trunk muscles. Because complete expiration is difficult as a result of bronchial spasm, the student is encouraged to breathe diaphragmatically. Instructions are given to expand the abdomen with inhalation and to force exhalation as completely as possible. To emphasize the breathing-out phase, the student is told to make a sound with the mouth as in blowing out a candle. Students who find it difficult to completely empty the lungs of air may aid themselves by applying hand pressure to both sides of the chest. Breathing should be taught from all positions: reclining, sitting, and standing. Many activities aid the asthmatic child in learning to breathe properly, for example, short-distance jogging with the student breathing rhythmically by inhaling and exhaling on each step or blowing a Ping-Pong ball across a table to an opponent, emphasizing short inhalation and long, forceful exhalation. (Points may be scored by blowing the Ping-Pong ball off the other side of the table.) To increase the force and time of the exhalation, the table can be raised so that the ball must be blown up an incline. Balls can also be suspended from strings and the student then tries to blow the ball as high as possible with long, controlled exhalations.

The asthmatic child's condition should be reassessed periodically, for as the attacks become less frequent and exercise tolerance becomes greater, increased exercise dosage should be added to the program of physical activity. Conversely, if a child has recurring and more severe attacks, then further adaptive measures should be taken to ensure participation at optimal levels in the program.

Asthma and physical activity

Experimental programs have indicated that active participation in carefully planned physical education activity may have value to many children having asthma or some other respiratory disorder.[41] In the past, physical inactivity has been encouraged for children with respiratory disorders. In many cases, this pattern of suppressed physical activity leads to a life-style that prevents participation in physical activity, even when the person is free from attacks and asthmatic symptoms. As the result of this attitude, less than optimal physical and social development occurs. Because of this factor, Stein[41] considers that there should be a reexamination of the values of physical activity for the asthmatic child.

There is evidence that high levels of activity can be undertaken with the condition of asthma.[39] Stein uses the illustration of Rick Demontan, Olympic gold medal winner in swimming, and Jim Ryan, who set a world record in the mile run, both of whom achieved these feats despite asthma.[41] Many doctors now recommend that restrictions on physical activities for children with asthma be lessened and that, between attacks, they should be provided with movement opportunities commensurate with their abilities. The concept of developmental physical education maintains that there is an activity level at which all children can perform to further their physical and motor development.

Asthmatic children can gain strength, endurance, coordination of movement, and, possibly, more efficient pulmonary function as a result of engaging in physical activities. Swimming may be of particular value for persons with asthma.[9] Stein also indicates that swimming seems to provoke less exercise-induced asthma than comparable activities.[41]

There is a great need for physical educators and medical professionals to engage in cooperative efforts so that the child with a respiratory disorder may attain the full benefits of participation in physical activities. It is essential that there be dialogue between these professionals so that research can be conducted and programming can be implemented, based on the best information available concerning the nature of the activity program that should be prescribed for those with respiratory problems.

REFERENCES

1. Adams, R. C., Daniel, A. N., and Rullman, L.: Games, sports, and exercises for the physically handicapped, Philadelphia, 1972, Lea & Febiger.
2. American College of Sports Medicine: Guidelines for graded exercise testing and prescription, Philadelphia, 1975, Lea & Febiger.
3. Astrand, I., and Rodahl, K.: Textbook of work physiology, New York, 1970, McGraw-Hill Book Co.
4. Barry, A. J., et al.: Effects of physical training on patients who have had myocardial infarction, Am. J. Cardiol. **17:**1-8, 1966.
5. Becker, M. C., Vasey, C., and Kaufman, J. G.: Social aspects of cardiovascular rehabilitation, Circulation **21:**546-557, 1960.
6. Blumenthal, M. N., and Pederson, E.: Physical conditioning program for asthmatic children, J. Assoc. Phys. Ment. Rehabil. **21:**1, 1967.
7. Blumenthal, M. N., et al.: Controlling asthma through sports and counseling, Phys. Sports Med. **2:**51-54, 1974.
8. Cardiovascular diseases in the U.S.: facts and figures, New York, 1958, American Heart Association.
9. Claverie, E. D.: Changes in pulmonary efficiency and aerobic capacity of asthmatic and non-asthmatic children in a swimming program, Unpublished Master's thesis, Denton, Tex. Texas Woman's University, 1971.
10. Cureton, T. K.: Physical fitness with normal aging adults, J. Assoc. Phys. Ment. Rehabil. **11:**145-149, 1957.
11. Daniels, A. S., and Davies, E. A.: Adapted physical education, New York, 1975, Harper & Row, Publishers.
12. Durbin, E., and Goldwater, L. J.: Rehabilitation of the cardiac patient, Circulation **13:**410-418, 1956.
13. Ecstein, R. W.: Effect of exercise and coronary artery narrowing the coronary collateral circulation, Circulation Res. **5:**230, 1967.
14. Fisher, P.: Painless myocardial infarction, Northwest Med. **57:**315-318, 1958.
15. Frick, M. H., Katila, M., and Sjögren, A. L.: Cardiac function and physical training after myocardial infarction. In Larsen, A. O., and Malmborg, R. O., editors: Coronary heart disease and physical fitness, Baltimore, 1972, University Park Press.
16. Gardberg, M.: Remarks on the rehabilitation of the cardiac patient, J. Lawson Med. Soc. **109:**335-338, 1957.
17. Hanson, J. S., et al.: Long-term physical training and cardiovascular dynamics in middle-aged men, Circulation **38:**783-799, 1968.
18. Hayden, H., Suggs, A. W., and Beaty, H. W.: B is for breathing, Outlook **1:**3, 1969.
19. Heart disease in children, New York, 1956, American Heart Association.
20. Hirsch, E. Z., Hellerstein, H. K., and Macleod, C. A.: Physical training and coronary heart disease. In Mohler, I. C., editor: Exercise and the heart, New York, 1973, Academic Press, Inc.
21. Hyde, J. S., and Swarts, C. L.: Effects of an exercise program on the perennially asthmatic child. Am. J. Dis. Child. **CSVI:**383-396, 1968.
22. Johnson, W., et al.: Health concepts for college students, New York, 1962, The Ronald Press Co.
23. Jokl, E.: Safe participation in sports, J.A.M.A. **169:**97-167, 1959.
24. Jones, R. S., Wharton, M. J., and Buston, M. H.: The place of physical exercise and bronchodilator drugs in the assessment of the asthmatic child, Arch. Dis. Child. **38:**539-545, 1963.
25. Kovrigina, M.: In Carter, C., and Carter, D., editors: Can-

cer, smoking, heart disease, drinking in our two world system today, Toronto, 1958, Northern Book House.

26. Kraus, H., and Raab, W.: Hypokinetic disease, Springfield, Ill., 1961, Charles C Thomas, Publisher.

27. Macman, M., and Itkin, I. H.: Four-way study of asthma, Rehabil. Rec. **7:**14-17, 1966.

28. Marienfeld, C. J.: The cardiologist looks at the school child. In Margary, J. J., and Eichorn, J. R., editors: The exceptional child, New York, 1960, Holt, Rinehart & Winston, Inc.

29. McGlynn, D.: Exercise gets to the heart of the matter, Outlook **3:**4, 1969.

30. Naughton, J., et al.: Cardiovascular responses to exercise following myocardial infarction, Arch. Intern. Med. **117:**541-545, 1966.

31. Peterson, K. H., and McElhenny, T. R.: Effects of a physical fitness program upon asthmatic boys, Pediatrics **35:**295-299, 1965.

32. Puthoff, M.: Corrective, developmental, and recreational activities (chronic respiratory conditions), Proceedings of the First Statewide Conference on Physical Education for Handicapped Children and Youth, Brockport, N.Y., October 1972, State University of New York at Brockport.

33. Puthoff, M.: New dimensions in physical activity for children with asthma and other respiratory conditions, Health Phys. Educ. Rec. **43:**75-80, 1972.

34. Rechnitzer, P. A.: Effects of a 24-week exercise program on normal adults and patients with previous myocardial infarction, Br. Med. J. **1:**734, 1967.

35. Rosenson, L., and DeRegniers, S.: The cardiopathic-rheumatic fever. In Frampton, M. E., and Gall, E. D., editors: Special education for the exceptional, Boston, 1960, Porter Sargent, Publisher.

36. Ross, J., and O'Rourke, R. A.: Understanding the heart and its disease, New York, 1976, McGraw-Hill Book Co.

37. Rowell, L.: Human cardiovascular responses to exercise. In Mohler, I. C., editor: Exercise and the heart, New York, 1973, Academic Press, Inc.

38. Sherrill, C.: Adapted physical education: a multidisciplinary approach, Dubuque, Iowa, 1976, Wm. C. Brown Co.

39. Sinclair, W. A.: Physical education and asthma are compatible, Calif. Assoc. Health Phys. Educ. Rec. J. **36:**19, 1973.

40. Sloman, G., et al.: Effect of a graded physical training program on the working capacity of patients with heart disease, Med. J. Aust. **1:**4, 1965.

41. Stein, J.: Effects of physical activity and excise upon asthmatic children, Report to U.S. Office of Education. In Physical education and recreation for the handicapped: programs for the handicapped, Washington, D.C., 1975, American Association for Health, Physical Education, and Recreation.

42. Taub, S. J.: Effects of physical therapy evaluated in chronically asthmatic children, Eye Ear Nose Throat Mon. **41:**105-106, 1968.

43. Trap-Jensen, J., and Clausen, J. P.: Effect of training on the relation of heart rate and blood pressure on the onset of pain in effort angina pectoris. In Larsen, L. A., and Malmbor, R. O., editors: Coronary heart disease and physical fitness, Baltimore, 1970, University Park Press.

44. Turner, R. W. D.: Diagnosis and treatment of essential hypertension, Lancet **1:**897-903, 953-958, 1959.

45. Vodola, T. M.: Individualized physical education program for handicapped children, Englewood Cliffs, N.J., 1973, Prentice-Hall, Inc.

46. Whitehouse, F. A.: Cardiovascular disability. In Garrett, J. F., and Levine, E. S., editors: Psychological practices with the physically disabled, New York, 1962, Columbia University Press.

13

Neurological dysfunctions

This chapter presents a discussion of some of the major dysfunctions within the central nervous system and their implications for adapted physical education. Because of the complex nature of the central nervous system, a brief overview of its anatomy and selected functions will be given.

ORGANIZATION OF THE NERVOUS SYSTEM

The nervous system is ''a system of extremely delicate nerve cells, elaborately interlaced with each other, collectively consisting of the brain, cranial nerves, spinal cord, spinal nerves, autonomic ganglion, ganglionated trunks and nerves, maintaining the vital function of reception and response to stimuli.''[22] It governs and coordinates all activities of the body, providing a means by which changes in the body's internal and external environment can be accomplished. Those changes are the result of stimuli that cause impulses to occur in specific receptor organs such as those found in the skin, joints, muscles, eyes, ears, and organs of taste and smell. Generally speaking, the nervous system is categorized into the central nervous system (CNS), which is composed of the spinal cord and brain; the peripheral nervous system, which is made up of the cranial and spinal nerves and the organs of the special senses; and the autonomic nervous system, which is concerned with the involuntary control of the body's internal function.[17]

The major centers of the CNS (Fig. 13-1, *A*), ranging from the less to the more complex, are the spinal cord, brain stem, cerebellum, diencephalon, and telencephalon. The functioning of the CNS follows a hierarchy of complexity beginning in the spinal cord and ending at the uppermost aspect of the telencephalon, or cerebral cortex. Reflex responses and servomechanisms (feedback loops) also become progressively more complex as growth, development, and maturation take place. As maturation and development occur within the normal nervous system, inhibition of neutral responses takes precedence over those responses concerned with excitation.[22]

The *spinal cord* is divided into the cervical, thoracic, lumbar, and sacral levels and receives all the bodily sensations below the face. It contains centers that deal with sensorimotor integration, autonomic responses, ascending and descending nerve pathways, receptive and expressive neurons for receiving and responding to both visceral and somatic stimuli, and inter- and intraspinal nerve pathways. It is also a center for the less complicated primitive reflexes.

The *brain stem* is subdivided into the medulla, the pons, and the midbrain (Fig. 13-1, *B*). In general, the brain stem contains ascending and descending nerve pathway centers that are mainly concerned with the degree of an individual's alertness and the ability to stay awake for a prolonged period of time. This arousal system is known as the reticular system and can be found throughout the CNS, but it is concentrated in the brain stem. The brain stem also regulates sensory and motor neurons, integrates muscle tone, and controls the reflex functions of breathing and heart action. Emanating from the brain stem are 10 of the 12 cranial nerves concerned with facial functions.

The *cerebellum* is considered by many to both directly and indirectly received impulses from all the senses of the body, integrating and coordinating their function. For example, it maintains muscle tone and control of synchronous muscle action. The cerebellum is concerned with the functions of the vestibular system, especially with the functions of body balance and those reflexes that maintain the body's major segments in proper relationship. Moore[22] described the cerebellum as '''the monitor and integrater for past, present, and future neuromuscular behavior.''

The *diencephalon,* or interbrain, lies between the brain stem and the telencephalon. It is made up of the thalamus, hypothalamus, epithalamus, metathalamus, and other structures. Basically, the diencephalon is a complex for sensory integration and serves as a relay nerve center leading to and from the major senses, with the exception of the sense of smell. On the other hand, the hypothalamus is the master controller of the endocrine and autonomic nervous systems.

The *telencephalon* is the uppermost aspect of the CNS and is composed of three important regions: the basal ganglion, the limbic system, and the cerebral cortex. The basal ganglion provides integration of the sensorimotor centers concerned with unconscious stereotyped behavior such as the maintenance of muscle tone that is required for the upright posture. It also facilitates and inhibits automatic reflex behavior that is exhibited in the cross pattern arm swing during walking. The basal ganglion is the major storage center for "learned," or semiautomatic, reflexes commonly seen in games and sports activities or in the routine activities of typing, writing, dressing, and eating. On

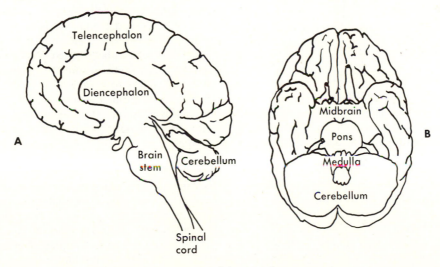

Fig. 13-1. Major regions of the central nervous system.

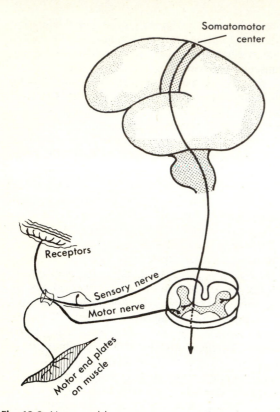

Fig. 13-2. Upper and lower motor neuron. From the motor area of the cerebrum, an impulse is conveyed by an upper motor neuron that is essential for voluntary movement. The lower motor neuron originates from the anterior gray column of the brain stem or spinal cord with its axon penetrating motor end plates of a muscle by a peripheral nerve, allowing for muscular activity.

the other hand, the limbic region seems to be primarily concerned with controlling the emotions and personality as well as memory storage. It should be noted, however, that memory and reflex behavior are not confined to any one area of the nervous system. The highest level of sensorimotor behavior is found in the cerebral cortex, which is a main center for learning communication. It has receptive and expressive areas as well as centers that are primarily concerned with association, perception, memory, and personality. In general, the cerebral cortex makes it possible for humans to recognize a stimulus, associate it to some past events, and create new patterns of behavior that may be used immediately or may be stored for future use.

The terms *sensory* and *motor* are commonly referred to in the movement sciences. They, in all probability, should not be separated into two words, but should be referred to as *sensorimotor* because sensation is usually followed by a response (Fig. 13-2). The body receives sensations from three primary sources, namely, exteroceptors, interoceptors, and proprioceptors.[20] The *exteroceptors* receive sensations that indicate pain, temperature, and feeling from outside of the body through the special senses of seeing, hearing, smelling, testing, and maintaining equilibrium. The *interoceptors* receive sensations that indicate hunger, pain, abnormal muscle shortening, and cramping from the interior of the body. The receptors that deal with movement and body posture are the *proprioceptors* found in muscles, tendons, joints, fasciae, and the vestibular labyrinth organ. It should be noted that the proprioceptors also provide the human organism with a body position sense known as kinesthesia. A fourth set of receptors might be added to this list of sensory sources; they would be called the *exteroproprioceptors*. They are concerned with vibratory sense and fine tactile discrimination necessary for object identification through manipulation (stereognosis).

NERVOUS SYSTEM LESIONS AND DYSFUNCTIONS

Because of the complexity of the nervous system, complete understanding of all the factors that adversely affect it is impossible at this time. However, this section is concerned with those conditions with which the adapted physical educator or therapist may come in direct contact. The term *lesion* here refers to a specific pathological site that can be identified on examination. Dysfunction does not necessarily refer to a lesion, but, more generally, to the absence of complete or normal functioning.

Nerve and spinal cord disorders

An injury to a peripheral nerve is followed by varying degrees of functional loss, up to and including a complete paralysis. Proprioception, skin sensation, and various tendon reflexes may be partially or completely disrupted. Pathology in the spinal cord also can produce a variety of problems involving both the sensory and motor systems. For example, acute poliomyelitis is a viral disease that attacks the anterior horn cells of the spinal cord, preventing nerve impulses from reaching a muscle via a peripheral nerve. Destruction or disruption of the anterior horn cell can result in a flaccid type of paralysis, followed by atrophy of that muscle. Degenerative conditions occur in the spinal cord, creating varying degrees of dysfunctions, for example, in muscular dystrophy. Trauma to the spinal cord can also create numerous adverse conditions, including partial or complete paralysis, depending on the extent of nerve cell damage. Paralysis is usually named for the number of parts of the body affected; for example, monoplegia refers to paralysis of one limb; diplegia, two limbs; triplegia, three limbs; and quadiplegia, four limbs. Hemiplegia refers to paralysis of one half of the body. The reader should also note that peripheral nerves have the capacity to regenerate about 1 to 2 mm/day, whereas nerve fibers and cells within the CNS do not effectively regenerate.

Brain stem disorders

Disorders that emanate from the brain stem region can produce many different abnormal symptoms, depending on the sensory or motor pathways affected. Generally speaking, lesions in the brain stem can result in muscle spasticity or hypotonicity and deficits in tactile discrimination such as pain or temperature alterations. Postural and/or survival reflexes such as swallowing, breathing, and heart function may also be adversely affected.

Cerebellar disorders

Dysfunctions within the cerebellum can create severe problems in the motor system, five of which predominate, namely, ataxia, hypotonia, asthenia, tremor, and nystagmus. *Ataxia* may be manifested in a number of ways, for example, disturbance in balance, posture, and locomotion; inability to synchronize movement patterns that may involve several joints; *dysmetria,* or inability to stop a movement at a certain desired point; and *dysdiadochokinesia,* or inability to make rapid or opposite movements such as finger tapping or fast alteration of the forearm in pronation and supination. *Hypotonia,* a result of a cerebellar disorder, may be reflected by a decrease in tendon reflexes as well as *asthenia* or paresis in which skeletal muscles may tire readily after only minor activity. *Tremor* may also be present in cerebellar dysfunction. This con-

dition impairs the execution of purposeful movement. *Nystagmus* implies a constant involuntary movement of the eyeball when it is moved away from the center resting position. Besides these impairments, cerebellar dysfunction can also produce *dysarthria,* in which there occurs speech that is slurred and, often, difficult to understand.

Cerebral disorders

Gatz[17] considers the cerebral cortex the final center for the integration of neural function. Although there are specific areas within the cerebrum that can be pinpointed as having specialized functions, there are many other functions that cannot be clearly delineated. However, Brodmann's cortex areas are presented here for descriptive purposes (Fig. 13-3).[17] For example, Brodmann's motor strip (area 4), which is located in the frontal lobe of the brain, provides fine and gross motor control. Dysfunction within this area can result in alternating involuntary muscle contraction and relaxation (clonic contraction) or in the violent muscular contraction that characterizes the grand mal epileptic seizure. On the other hand, the premotor area (area 6, lying just in front of area 4) provides supplementary gross motor control and ability in learning new movement skills. Lesions in the premotor area alone may produce muscle spasticity, whereas lesions in area 4 alone may result in a flaccid paralysis or a floppy muscle. The remaining sections of the prefrontal lobe are considered by many professionals to be essential for abstract thinking and judgment. Dysfunction in this region often produces bizarre, and sometimes unpredictable, personality behaviors.

Dysfunctions within the primary sensory and associative regions of the cortex may create a variety of symptoms; for example, a lesion in Brodmann's area 17 may prevent stimuli from coming to the cortex via the eyes, whereas, dysfunction in area 18 may prevent a visual stimulus from being analyzed by an individual. The process of *knowing,* or gnosis, involves the comparison of a stimulus with some past experience. Inability to recognize or associate sensory data is known as agnosia. Therefore, a dysfunction in the region of the parietal lobe of the cerebral cortex may result in a condition in which the individual is unable to identify common objects through the combined senses for feel and manipulation *(astereognosis).* The person

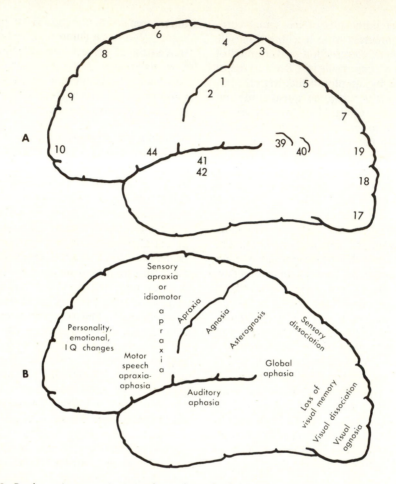

Fig. 13-3. Brodmann's areas. **A,** Areas located on the left cerebral hemisphere. **B,** Dysfunction in relation to Brodmann's disease.

with dysfunction in the sensory and associative regions of the cortex may find it extremely difficult to identify the sides of the body *(laterality),* revealing subsequent disturbances in body image. Of great importance to all movement therapists is the general condition of *apraxia,* or the inability to initiate purposive motor acts. In this condition, the sensory and motor systems could be functioning normally; however, dysfunction in associative fibers going to the motor cortex makes effective motor planning difficult or impossible.

Abnormal reflex behavior

Reflexes are bodily responses that are mechanical and automatic in nature and are essential for human development. The normal infant has, at birth, the critical reflexes necessary for survival, such as breathing and digestion, in addition to the reflexes of sneezing, coughing, sucking, and rooting.[24] The foundations for adaptive and postural reactions are also present, together with those reflexes that direct visual, auditory, skin, and deep tendon responses. The newborn displays gross muscular reactions when startled or placed in body positions that require postural adjustments. Fiorentino[15] states:

From birth onward, we are activated by powerful afferents. These come from the outside world through exteroceptors such as eyes, ears, skin; internally, from interoceptors and proprioceptors.

[Although] the entire nervous system is involved in all reflexes to a greater or lesser degree, reflexes in the infant, for the most part, are dominated by the spinal cord and brain stem.[15]

Gradually, as maturation takes place, the primitive reflexes diminish in strength, becoming inhibitive or superimposed by a higher order of reflex behavior. Higher level motor skills are made possible only when the primitive reflex behavior has satisfactorily been overcome and maturation of the higher CNS has taken place[15] (see Chapters 2 and 3).

Dysfunction within the CNS can delay the inhibitory control of higher centers over primitive reflexes, preventing the integration of more complex motor behavior. Brain injury at birth may prevent the individual from ever fully overcoming primitive reflexes. On the other hand, a brain injury in later life might cause a loss of the once acquired inhibitory responses, reverting back to a more primitive reflex behavior. The brain-injured person often displays immature postures and movement patterns that may be further disrupted by abnormal muscle tonus in various parts of the body.

Spinal reflexes predominate during the first 2 months of life. They are considered *phasic,* coordinating the muscles of the extremities in patterns of total extension or flexion.[14,15] Reflexes at the brain stem level are usually present in the infant from the first 4 to 6 months of life and have mainly to do with postural changes that the infant negotiates while in a reclining position. The midbrain reflexes, on the other hand, assist the infant up to about 12 months of age, helping to establish head-body relationships and the beginning locomotor skills of rolling over, sitting up, and raising the body up to an all-fours position on the hands and knees. Final reflex control is accomplished at the cortical level, gradually emerging after 6 months and continuing throughout life. Cortical level reflexes are primarily concerned with the dynamics of equilibrium in the upright bipedal position.

SEVERE NEUROMOTOR DISORDERS

The term *cerebral palsy* is used to denote conditions that stem from brain injury. Cerebral palsy includes mental retardation, convulsive disorders, and impulsive disorders such as hyperkinetic behavior, minimal cerebral dysfunction, and visual, auditory, and perceptual problems.[11]

Cerebral palsy is a condition, rather than a disease. It denotes a number of types of neuromuscular disabilities characterized by disturbances of voluntary motor function. The degree of motor involvement of children with cerebral palsy may range from those who have serious physically disabling effects to those who have little physical disability.

Statistical estimates indicate that approximately 1 in 14,000 births in the United States results in severe brain injury.[1] This points to a need for continuing emphasis on a search for programs and techniques in education that will provide for optimal living potential in the adult years.

Conditions that give rise to neuromotor disorders may be operative during the prenatal, natal, or postnatal periods. Authorities believe that approximately 30% of the cases occur during the prenatal period, 60% during the natal period, and the remaining 10% from postnatal causes. Prenatal causes may be maternal infection such as rubella, syphilis, and toxoplasma; metabolic malfunctioning; toxemia; diabetes; placental abnormalities such as fetal anoxia; and excessive radiation.

Natal causes fall into two basic categories: compression of the head with unusual pressures and trauma and inadequate air exchange in the newborn. Conditions that may give rise to neuromotor disorders from unusual pressure may be the following: breech extraction, contracted pelvis of mother, difficult forceps delivery, prolonged labor, precipitated delivery, placenta previa, and separation of the placenta.

Postnatal causes may be trauma; infection such as encephalitis, meningitis, and brain abscesses; anoxia; neoplasms; toxic poisons; hyperpyrexia; vascular accidents; and blood group incompatibility.

Since the extent of the brain damage that results in neuromotor dysfunction varies greatly, diagnosis is related to the amount of dysfunction and associated motor involvement that has occurred. Severe brain injury may be evident shortly after birth. However, children with cerebral dysfunction who have slight brain damage and little motor involvement may be difficult to diagnose. In the milder cases, developmental lag in the motor and intellectual tasks required to meet environmental demands may not be detected until the children are 3 or 4 years old. As a rule, the clinical signs and symptoms of cerebral palsy reach their maximum degree of severity at the age of 2 to 4 years. In some cases, children with cerebral dysfunction who have a minor motor involvement and who are not severely handicapped have the greatest difficulties adjusting to their environments. They deviate from normative behavior to the extent that they are different and set apart from their peers. However, the impairments are mild enough that special services for adjustments are not solicited.

Hard signs of neuromotor disorders

The different clinical types of cerebral dysfunction display various obvious motor patterns, commonly known as *hard signs*. Therefore, it is important that the physical educator know the classifications and their characteristic motor patterns in order to implement physical education programs for children with cerebral palsy. In 1954, the Nomenclature Committee of the American Academy for Cerebral Palsy adopted a classification that was derived from observable symptoms. There were six clinical classifications: spasticity, athetosis, rigidity, ataxia, tremor, and atonia. Of those with cerebral palsy, 50% are clinically classified as spastic, 25% athetoid, 13% rigid, and the remaining 12% are divided among ataxic, atonic, tremulous, and mixed and undiagnosed cerebral palsy conditions.[2]

Spasticity

Muscular spasticity is greatest in prevalence among the types of cerebral palsy. One of the physical characteristics of spasticity is that muscle contractures that restrict muscular movement give the appearance of stiffness to affected limbs. This makes muscle movement jerky and uncertain. Spastic children have exaggerated stretch reflexes that cause them to respond to rapid passive stimulation with vigorous muscular contractions. Tendon reflexes are also hyperactive in the part involved. In the event the spastic condition involves the lower extremities, the legs may be rotated inward and flexed at the hips, knees may be flexed, and a contracted gastrocnemius holds the heel off the ground. Lower leg deficiency contributes to a scissors gait that is common among persons with this type of cerebral palsy. When the upper extremities are involved, the characteristic forms of physical deviation in the person with spastic cerebral palsy include flexion at the elbows, forearm pronation, and wrist and finger flexion.

Spasticity is most common in the antigravity muscles of the body. In children with spastic cerebral palsy, contractures are more common than in children with any of the other types of cerebral palsy. In the event contractures are not remedied or programmed for, permanent contractures may result. Consequently, the maintenance of good posture is extremely difficult. Because of poor balance among reciprocal muscle groups, innervation of muscles for functional motor patterns is often difficult. Mental impairment is associated with spasticity more than with any other clinical type of cerebral palsy, so the incidence of mental retardation among this group is high.

Athetosis

Athetosis is the second most prevalent clinical type of severe cerebral dysfunction. The distinguishing characteristic of the athetoid individual is recognizable incoordinate movements of voluntary muscles. These movements take the form of worm-like motions that involve trunk, arms, legs, tongue, or muscle twitches of the face. The unrhythmical, uncontrollable, involuntary movements seem to increase with voluntary motion and emotional or environmental stimulus. Because of the athetoid individual's inability to control muscles voluntarily, posture is unpredictable and poses a problem. Involvement in the muscular control of hands, speech, and swallowing often accompanies athetosis.

Rigidity

A central feature of the rigid type of cerebral palsy is the functional incoordination of reciprocal muscle groups. There is great resistance to slow motion and the stretch reflex is impaired. Mental retardation often accompanies this clinical type of cerebral palsy.

Ataxia

The outstanding characteristic of the ataxic type of cerebral palsy is a disturbance of equilibrium, which impairs the ability to maintain balance. This impairment in balance becomes evident in the walking gait. The gait of the person with ataxic cerebral palsy is unstable, which causes weaving about during locomotion. Standing is often a problem. Kinesthetic awareness seems to be lacking in the ataxic individual. Also, the ability to locate objects in three-dimensional space is often impaired. Muscle tone, as a rule, is poor in persons with ataxic cerebral palsy.

Tremor

Tremor is evidenced by a rhythmic movement that is usually caused by alternating contractions between flexor and extensor muscles. Tremors appear as uncontrollable pendular movements.

Atonia (flaccidity)

Atonia is characterized by a lack of muscle tone. The muscles of the atonic person are often so weak that the activities of daily living are severely hampered.

Alternate systems of classification

Another means of classifying persons with cerebral palsy is in regard to the limbs that are affected. The classifications are as follows:
1. Paraplegia—legs only
2. Diplegia—legs mainly, arms slightly
3. Quadriplegia—all four extremities
4. Hemiplegia—one half of the body or the limbs on one side of the body
5. Triplegia—both legs and one arm, or both arms and one leg
6. Monoplegia—one extremity

A third way in which individuals with cerebral palsy are classified is based on the anatomical part that contributes to the palsy. There are three primary classifications, including the following:
1. Pyramidal—usually resulting in spasticity
2. Extrapyramidal or basonuclear—when this part of the nervous system is affected, athetosis, tremors, and rigidity are manifested
3. Cerebellar—resulting in ataxia

General characteristics

Although persons with cerebral palsy are usually classified on the basis of motor involvement, damage to the brain generally involves other sensory and psychological impairments. Some of the secondary impairments that may accompany motor involvement are mental retardation, hearing and vi-

sion loss, emotional disturbance, loss of perceptual ability, and inability to make psychological adjustments.

Studies also have shown that a substantial number of persons with brain injury are visually handicapped. According to Denhoff and Robinault,[12] "various authors agree that over 50% of the cerebral palsied children have ocular-motor defects." In other words, brain-injured children often have difficulty in coordinating their eye movements. The implications of this condition for physical activities that are highly loaded with oculomotor tracking of projectiles point to a need for programs that train for ocular control.[11]

Loss of hearing is often concomitant with cerebral palsy; however, there is disagreement among investigators as to the incidence of hearing loss among individuals with cerebral palsy. Fish[16] found that 20% of children with brain injury had hearing losses. When clinical types were compared, children with athetoid type had the greatest incidence of hearing loss. Although it is apparent that there is greater hearing loss among individuals with cerebral palsy than among a comparable normative population, it is still worth noting that the hearing impairments do not occur with as much frequency as do visual problems.

Persons with cerebral palsy are also affected with perceptual handicaps to a greater extent than is the typical population. Many gross perceptual distortions have been recorded among the cerebral palsied population that are associated with loss of the sense modes, especially losses of vision and hearing.

Emotional disturbances are another concomitant disorder to cerebral palsy. Children with cerebral dysfunction are often afflicted with significant physical impairment that may deprive them of opportunities for ordinary social experience and thus impair their normal social maturation.[5] Interrelated with maldevelopment in the physical and social spheres may be retarded emotional development. The basic needs of the child with cerebral palsy require fulfillment. These basic needs are recognition, esteem, and independence, all of which are an integral part of participation in the experiences of childhood.[2] Block[6] listed traits that thwart the underlying drives toward approval, acceptance, and self-actualization and that cause or give rise to major psychological problems. They are as follows:

1. Unresolved dependency feelings and excessive need for affection
2. Excessive submissiveness and compliance, which hide underlying hostility
3. Egocentricity with emphasis on expansive self-concepts
4. Compensation for feelings of inferiority and inadequacy by fantasy
5. Resignation, rather than recognition of limitations imposed by the disability
6. Superficial conscious recognition of the handicap and unconscious rejection of the self

Treatment of severe neuromotor disorders

There is no treatment for the repair of a damaged brain. However, the portion of the nervous system that remains intact can be made functional through a well-managed training program. Intervention by the physical educator and other liaison personnel is needed to build functional developmental motor patterns with the operative parts of the body. Each child should be evaluated closely and programs should be formulated utilizing those functional abilities of the child that remedy the disabilities that can be corrected and that circumvent those disabilities that are nonremediable. The specific child should be considered when determining the dosage of exercise. The athetoid child, because of numerous involuntary muscular activities, is much more active than are the spastic, ataxic, and rigid children, who are inhibited regarding physical activity.

The four prevalent procedures in medical treatment are bracing, drugs, surgery, and rehabilitation. Braces are important as an aid in teaching joint function as well as in assisting in the locomotion of patients who are severely handicapped. Another use for bracing is the prevention of deforming contractures. Drug administration usually serves two functions: aiding in exercise therapy by assisting with relaxation of muscle groups when neuromuscular education is attempted, and controlling epileptic seizures through the use of anticonvulsant drugs.

There are differing opinions as to the value of orthopedic surgery for person's with cerebral palsy. Certain types of operative procedures have met with considerable success, especially with par-

ticular types of cerebral palsy. Physical growth of children affects the efficiency of muscle and tendon surgery; however, surgery, for the most part, is not curative, but, rather, gives assistance in the functional activities of daily living. Tenotomies (or tendon surgery) of the hip adductor and hamstring muscles seem to be the most valuable surgical procedures for adults.

Implications for physical educators and therapists

One of the great problems that has interfered in the successful education of children with cerebral palsy is the lack of acceptance by general educators of the emotional, intellectual, and physical disabilities in learning areas. The multitude of behavioral differences displayed by these children indicates a need for Individual Education Programs.

A number of educational facilities are designed to cope with educational problems of children with brain injury. Some of these sources of education are the following:

1. Home instruction for severely physically disabled children with cerebral palsy who cannot attend school
2. Hospital schools that serve children with the more severe handicaps
3. Institutions for the mentally retarded, for those children with cerebral palsy who have subaverage intelligence
4. Sheltered care facilities for near-normal children with cerebral palsy who have severe physical handicaps
5. Special schools, or classes in public schools, that are organized for crippled children
6. Placement into regular school classes

In many instances, the teacher has more opportunity to meet the total needs of the child with cerebral palsy than do other professional personnel. There are often various related services that also work on behalf of the child. The planning process of the Individual Education Program should coordinate the related services with the physical education program and with other therapeutic endeavors. The new federal legislation focuses on the education of the child. Therefore, the related services or therapies should assist cerebral palsied children to benefit from direct physical education services.

One of the main responsibilities of the teacher of

the child with severe brain injury is to provide an environment that will afford opportunities for maximal personal adjustment and the development of mental health. A prerequisite for creating this type of environment is for such teachers to be well-adjusted themselves, for there are many instances in which problems that the child encounters will be reflected in behavioral problems for the teacher. Therefore, it is critical that teachers be warm and understanding and have a genuine interest in each child, regardless of the problems the child may present. Rejection of the child by the teacher does not provide an atmosphere conducive to personal adjustment.

Even though children with neuromotor disorders may differ physically, they want to have social re-

spect from their peers. Therefore, the teacher should attempt to provide opportunities for brain-injured children to learn in an environment in which they can enjoy normal experiences, as do their nonhandicapped classmates. This requires highly specialized and individualized techniques and demands ingenuity, inventiveness, and patience on the part of the teacher.

Children with brain injury, in addition to motor involvement, often have perceptual problems that necessitate instructional adjustment (Fig. 13-4). There are many areas of perceptual disturbance; therefore, it is necessary to identify particular perceptual dimensions that are not functioning properly for a child. Cruickshank[9] identified specific areas of perceptual disability: (1) distinguishing

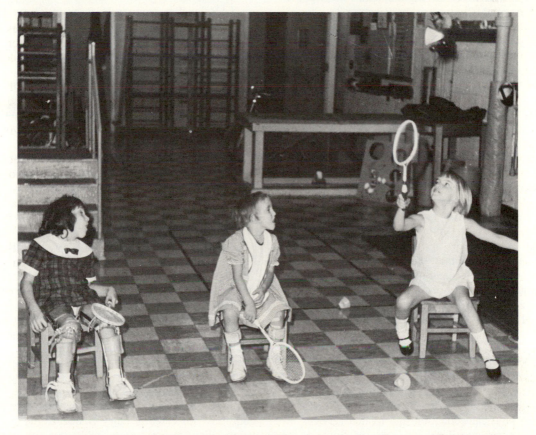

Fig. 13-4. Cerebral palsied children with different abilities playing together. They may differ physically, but they want to engage in activities with their peers. (Courtesy of Julian Stein, American Alliance for Health, Physical Education, Recreation, and Dance.)

form and color, (2) recognizing spatial relationships, (3) differentiating between high and low or loud and soft sounds, (4) seeing the whole, and (5) following simple directions. There is growing evidence that some of the perceptual characteristics mentioned can be improved through training.[19] Perceptual training techniques are developed primarily through visuomotor and sensorimotor training programs. The aspects of such a program include developing locomotor patterns, balancing, bouncing, performing actively to rhythm, developing ocular control, and using devices that detect form perception. All of these perceptual activities are inherent in most physical education programs. However, the quality of physical education programs could be improved by identifying and implementing programs of activities that might enhance these particular perceptual characteristics (Chapter 3).

Typical children bring with them to school a broad experiential history of activities that have accrued during their preschool years. This experiential history lays the background for later, more complex skills. However, in the case of the child with severe brain injury who has been handicapped in the acquisition of motor experience, a program of readiness for the more complex skills should be implemented by going further back in the stages of motor development. The purposes of such a readiness program may be to provide developmental experiences, to develop satisfactory motor perception, and to build proficiency in motor skills. The readiness period may take considerable time in order to prepare the child with cerebral palsy socially, emotionally, and physically for the more complex learnings that will give meaning to leisure time, vocational pursuits, and adult living. The prerequisites to administering physical activity or teaching physical skills are psychological, sociological, and physiological readiness for specific activity.

Physical education for the severely neurologically impaired

The Individual Education Program is designed to meet the unique needs of each child. Therefore, special physical education and related services include many types of physical activity. Some of the therapeutic activities and techniques include the following:

1. Muscle stretching to relieve muscle contractures, prevent deformities, and permit fuller range of active motion
2. Gravity exercises that involve lifting the weight of the body or body part against gravity
3. Muscle awareness exercises to control specific muscles or muscle groups in movement
4. Neuromuscular reeducation exercises, that is, movements performed through their current range to stimulate the proprioceptors and return the muscles to greater functional use
5. Reciprocal exercises to stimulate and strengthen the action of the protagonist
6. Tonic exercises to prevent atrophy or to maintain organic efficiency
7. Relaxation training to assist in the remediation of muscle contractures, rigidity, and spasms
8. Postural alignment to maintain proper alignment of musculature
9. Gait training to educate or reeducate walking patterns
10. Body mechanics and lifting techniques to obtain maximum use of the large muscle groups of the body
11. Proprioceptive facilitation exercises to bring about maximal excitation of motor units of a muscle with each voluntary effort to overcome motor functioning paralysis
12. Ramp climbing techniques to improve ambulation and increase balance, a form of progressive, resistive exercise for the purpose of developing strength

There is impressive evidence that motor skills, muscular endurance, and strength can be developed in these children through progressive exercise and activity in an adapted physical education program. In many instances, the environment of enforced inactivity in which brain-injured children have developed has left them short of their potential development. The opportunities for adapted physical education to enhance maximum physical development of these children are great. Furthermore, children with cerebral palsy frequently do not develop adequate basic motor skills because of their limited play experiences.

When the child participates in group activity, it

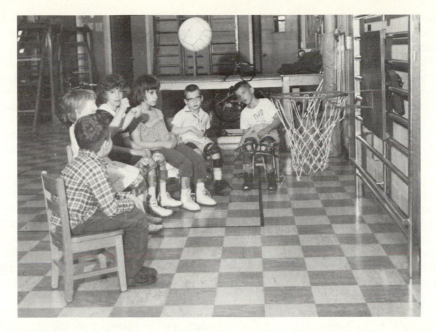

Fig. 13-5. Activity can be modified to accommodate neurologically impaired children. (Courtesy of Julian Stein, American Alliance for Health, Physical Education, Recreation, and Dance and University Hospital School, University of Iowa, Iowa City, Iowa.)

may be necessary to adapt the activity to the child's abilities or to modify the rules of the game. An example of rule adaptation for the handicapped child in soccer would be narrowing the goal area that must be defended. Another strategy of activity adaptation might be to require the child with cerebral palsy to play in a position that requires a slower pace or demands less activity than does some other position in the game. An example of this might be the goalkeeper in a soccer game. This position is usually less active than are the other positions on the team. Positions in many sports vary in the degree of mobility required to play them (see Chapter 8).

In addition to using rule modification and adaptation of activity, the program must consider the capabilities of each individual child. Children with spasticity, athetosis, and ataxia differ greatly in function. For instance, the spastic child finds it easier to engage in activities in which motion is continuous. However, in the case of the athetoid child, relaxation between movements is extremely important to prevent involuntary muscular contrac-

tions that may thwart the development of skills. Ataxic children have a different motor problem: they are usually severely handicapped in all activities that require balance. The motor composition of the basic types of cerebral palsy, as well as of each individual child, is an important variable in the selection of activities. Rest periods should be frequent for children with cerebral palsy. The length and frequency of the rest periods should vary with the nature of the activity and the severity of the handicap. The development of a sequence of activities varying in degree of difficulty is important. This provides an opportunity to place each child in an activity that is commensurate with his or her ability and proposes a subsequent goal to work for.

Physical activities described under the definition of physical education in P.L. 94-142 are appropriate for cerebral palsied children. At the elementary level, appropriate activities might include fundamental motor patterns such as walking, running, jumping, skipping, and hopping and fundamental motor skills such as throwing, kicking, and catching. The junior high school level curriculum should be in keeping with the activities of the peer group of the child with cerebral palsy. Such activities may include developmental exercises, the development of body mechanics, and games that lead up to highly organized sports activities. In the high school program it is important that children with cerebral palsy learn carryover sports such as bowling, archery, badminton, rhythms, swimming, shuffleboard, and golf. These activities provide the media of social interaction and worthy fulfillment of leisure time in postschool years.

For optimal development in motor skills, physical education should be extended to the individual with cerebral palsy beyond formal education because it usually takes such children longer to acquire skills than it does typical children. Furthermore, recreational services that are commensurate with their abilities should be provided for these persons in the postschool years. To date, the greater emphasis has been placed on recreational services for young children with cerebral palsy rather than on the adult population.

MINIMAL NEUROMOTOR DISORDERS
Soft signs of neuromotor disorders

As discussed earlier, brain injury and its resultant dysfunction appear to be on a continuum, with symptoms ranging from the more obvious *hard signs* to the less obvious, and sometimes subtle, *soft signs*. Another expression commonly given to the large area of minor neurological problems is *minimal nervous system dysfunction*. The individual classified under this heading, besides displaying coordination difficulties, may demonstrate emotional outbursts that are not reasonably expected.[7] Other problems that may be associated with minimal nervous system dysfunction may be in the areas of perception, conception, memory, speech, language, and the cognitive skills required in reading, writing, and arithmetic.[15] Those individuals deemed to have minimal gross and fine motor control may be considered physically awkward or clumsy. Touwen and Prechtl[26] have identified seven factors that can be found in children classified as having a minimal nervous system dysfunction, namely, hemisyndrome, dyskinesia, synkinetic or associated movement, balance disturbances, auditory-perceptual disturbances, problems in emotional behavior, and the inability to perform a fast sequential or rhythmical movement.

A hemisyndrome refers to a weakness and a decrease in muscle tone on one side of the body, making gross motor activities difficult. Dyskinesia is reflected by movements that are jerky, slow, or irregular, usually when attempting fine or small muscle skills. Synkinesia becomes apparent when a movement is attempted on one side of the body and is mirrored on the other. The ability to effectively perform static or dynamic balance such as standing on one foot or walking heel-to-toe on a balance beam may also be disrupted. Auditory-perceptual problems such as difficulty in responding to verbal commands or inability to understand or remember directions may also be associated with minimal cerebral dysfunction. Other characteristics are problems in performing rhythmical movements such as marching or dancing. Children may also display an inability to make quick, repeated movement changes such as are required in tapping a finger or foot. Emotional problems may stem directly from the cerebral dysfunction or may result from difficulty in coping with the demands of the environment.

The physical educator and therapist should note that a child having a number of neuromotor soft signs may be considered a "klutz" in our society.[4] Unable to play effectively with other children, the clumsy child is often an unfulfilled and unhappy person. However, there is evidence that if such a child's neuromotor dysfunctions can be pinpointed and appropriate intervention programs can be instituted, the child can overcome the lack of movement efficiency and progress within normal functioning expectations.[21]

Minimal motor deficits are often a result of (1) persisting primitive reflexes that cause a child to move in a clumsy, awkward manner; (2) lack of development of equilibrium reflexes and inadequate vestibular functioning that make keeping one's balance very difficult; and (3) insufficient tactile and/or kinesthetic information to the somatosensory area of the cerebral cortex, which results in inefficient motor planning.[13]

Programs of physical education and recreation can aid the individual with minimal motor deficits by including some of the following activities: bouncing and jumping to inhibit some primitive reflexes; tug-of-war and wrestling games to facilitate equilibrium reflexes; spinning, rolling, turning, and scooter games to stimulate vestibular reactions;

and large movements while wearing wrist and ankle weights to facilitate kinesthetic sensations.

Problems in arousal

Managing the level of arousal when confronted with a given stimulus has been primarily assigned to the reticular system found throughout the CNS. Dysfunction in this system can result in two major problem areas: hyperactivity and hypoactivity.

Hyperkinetic impulse disorders may be caused by some organic cerebral dysfunction, may have a genetic antecedent, or may reflect a lag in the maturation and development of the nervous system. As a result of the problem, the child may display a number of behavioral characteristics such as impulsivity, distractibility, disorganization, explosiveness, or an inability to delay gratification. Often, the hyperactive child is described as behaving as would a much younger child or one that is ''driven'' and out of control. It has been suggested that hyperkinetic activity is the result of an inability to properly filter out and monitor stimuli; the individual is therefore bombarded by unselected stimulation from the environment.[11]

There have been many strategies and methods suggested for treatment of the hyperactive child. These have met with varying success. In general, these approaches can be classified into the following: medications, behavior modifications, environmental engineering, and movement methods.

Since as early as 1937, CNS stimulants have been used to benefit the hyperkinetic child. In more recent years, amphetamines such as methylphenidate (Ritalin) have been used increasingly with countless children deemed hyperactive. Under the guidance of a competent physician trained in the area of learning and behavioral problems, appropriate medications may be a useful tool. However, abuse of these drugs may create problems that have yet to be determined.

The use of positive reinforcement techniques in the home and school environments has found some success in helping the hyperactive child gain self-control. In contrast to punishment, reinforcement by reward has been found to be more successful, especially in keeping to a minimum the child's feelings of degradation and worthlessness, often associated with hyperactivity.[8]

Engineering the environment has been found to be successful with some children. By eliminating distracting influences from the environment and helping the child focus on one type of stimulus at a time, concentration may be improved.

Assisting the hyperactive child through selected movement methods has also been found to be beneficial by many educators and movement therapists. For example, it has been found that neural inhibition occurs following the application of slow, repetitive activities. Inhibition and relaxation are produced by sending inhibitory impulses to the bulbar section of the brain, which contains a large grouping of reticular nerve fibers. Slow stroking of the skin, neutral warmth such as that in a tepid bath, gentle rhythmical rocking, and soft sounds in a slow rhythmical pattern will inhibit the arousal system.[23] Relaxation training such as the Jacobson technique (Chapter 6) assists in reducing the aroused state. Other movement methods that have been found very successful in helping the hyperactive child gain self-control are games requiring rhythm, a well-defined and structured motor response, and gross and fine muscle coordination.[8]

Hypokinesis, or hypoactivity, implies less than average activity. The hypoactive child is one in whom there is too little arousal, lethargy, and, sometimes, sleepiness. Unlike the child with hyperkinetic impulse disorders, the child who is hypokinetic is often in the background, causing no problems for the parent or teacher. Other characteristics might be having poor coordination, being disliked by peers, being a poor player, having poor muscle tone, and being sloppy. Once medical implications such as endocrine dysfunction or disease have been discounted, a program for the underaroused individual can be instituted. Mainly, those activities that stimulate the nervous system should be used, for example, in fast and irregular rhythms or activities that stimulate the child's vestibular system: bouncing, fast rolling, spinning, tilting, and swinging. Exercising against a resistance should also be considered a major body stimulator and activities that involve quick muscle stretching will produce a stimulation to those muscles being stretched.

CONVULSIVE DISORDERS

The term *convulsive disorders*, or *epilepsy*, refers to a clinical syndrome in which the central features, seizures or convulsions, are a result, in part, of a disturbance in the electrochemical activity of

the brain. There are recurrent disturbances of consciousness that may or may not be accompanied by muscular involvement. There is a relatively high incidence of convulsions in children; however, convulsions are not necessarily indicative of epilepsy. Convulsive disorders are grossly misunderstood by the lay public in that associations are often made between epilepsy and mental defect and emotional disturbance. Consequently, the lay public may often view the disorder with fear and prejudice. Although these fears are unfounded, it cannot be denied that epilepsy can affect alertness, vitality, and social and emotional adjustment; this may make children less effective in an educational setting.

A physical education teacher may have occasion to serve an epileptic child and it is important that the teacher be familiar with the disorder. However, it must be remembered that children with epilepsy are children first and may differ from other children only in that they have the potential for occasional seizures. More often than not, if there is maldevelopment in personality variables, it is the result of psychosocial conditions, rather than epilepsy itself.

It is difficult to arrive at an accurate reporting procedure to determine the prevalence of epilepsy because of the fear some persons have about letting others know of the disorder. However, there are an estimated 1,860,000 persons with epilepsy in the United States.[19]

Although epilepsy is widespread, drugs have been developed that can control epileptic seizures in approximately 80% of the cases. Unfortunately, less than 50% of all epilespy patients receive effective treatment.

There is speculation concerning the cause of epilepsy; however, there is no thorough understanding regarding the cause. Although epilepsy may not be said to be inherited, the predisposition to the disorder appears to be inherited, for there is a tendency for epilepsy to run in families. Epileptics are classified into two main categories, according to cause: unknown causes (idiopathic) and known causes (symptomatic).

Idiopathic epilepsy includes all those cases in which no structural damage in the nervous system can be found. Approximately 60% to 70% of the cases of epilepsy fall within this group.

Symptomatic convulsive disorders may be caused by a host of factors, among which may be acute infection to the brain, trauma, allergies, abnormality of prenatal conditions, emotional instability, malnutrition, birth injuries, cardiovascular disorders, and infections such as encephalitis and meningitis.

Classification of seizures

Many classifications of seizures have been suggested in the literature regarding epilepsy. Perhaps the classification most beneficial to the physical educator is that of six groupings that have been proposed, based on the physical appearance of the child during the seizure, electroencephalographic findings, and the effects of drugs in controlling the seizures. The classifications are as follows:

1. Jacksonian seizures
2. Convulsive seizures
3. Grand mal seizures
4. Psychomotor seizures
5. Petit mal seizures
6. Autonomic seizures

The principal features of these six types of seizures can be summarized as follows: in the first type, symptoms are localized; in the second, excessive movements are the main feature; in the third, transient loss of consciousness is the main characteristic; in the fourth, the central feature is amnesia; in the fifth, there is a brief loss of consciousness; and the last type is manifested by functionally independent, spontaneous symptoms.

Jacksonian seizures

Jacksonian seizure patterns are characterized by an upward march from an extremity such as an arm or a foot. The attack may start at the finger and spread progressively to the wrist, arm, and shoulder, where it is maintained unless it spreads to other body parts. It may then become a grand mal seizure and is often associated with organic lesions of the brain. It may be accompanied by a feeling of numbness and there may be alternate contraction and relaxation of muscles.

Convulsive seizures

Convulsive seizures usually localize on one side of the body or a single extremity but do not march. The attack is often initiated by alternate contraction

and relaxation movements of the face or of an extremity. It is also common for the hands and eyes to turn to one side.

Grand mal seizures

The grand mal seizure is the most common type of attack. It is estimated that approximately 50% of those who have grand mal seizures experience a warning period in which dizziness and numbness occur; this is called an *aura*. When the warning precedes the attack for several hours, the term *prodrome* is applied to the warning.[25] The warning allows the person to lie down and prepare for the seizure. In some instances, an epileptic child may go through the aura period without going into a full seizure. The physical educator should be aware of the aura so as to prepare to assist during the attack.

A person who has never witnessed a grand mal seizure may find the first attack traumatic. When persons undergo a seizure of the grand mal type, they may drop to the floor; convulse with body stiffening, writhing, and twisting; experience alternating contractions and relaxations; drool; lose bladder and bowel control; fall into unconsciousness; and then usually enter a deep sleep.

Psychomotor seizures

It is important that the physical education teacher have knowledge of the psychomotor seizure because it takes the form of abnormal behavior patterns and might be misinterpreted as warranting punishment. This seizure is characterized by a period of amnesia and tonic spasm may or may not be present. When muscular hyperactivity is present, it may be accompanied by a bluish coloring of the skin and drooling. The child may lose partial contact with reality or may be completely out of contact with the surroundings. The child may be inactive or hyperactive during the seizure. Other characteristics of the psychomotor seizure might be the child's making unconscious sucking noises with the mouth or aimless movements with the hands, striking another child, tearing up paper, moving about the room in a daze, or performing other bizarre psychic behaviors. Consciousness is not lost during this attack; however, the child has no memory of these happenings. This type of seizure, because of the different forms that it takes, often leads to mistaken psychological diagnoses.

Petit mal seizures

There are no overt convulsions during the petit mal seizure; however, consciousness is lost for a few seconds. A child may continue an ongoing activity, but motor activity is minimal and there may be a few flickering movements of the eyelids and face or mild rhythmical jerkings of the hands and arms. The seizure begins abruptly and, after it is over, the trend of conversation or the activity is resumed by the child as if nothing had happened. Petit mal seizures are more frequent in children than in adults and attacks range in frequency from 1 to 200 a day. During the seizure, the child is inattentive and displays a blank look on the face. This type of seizure is difficult for the educators to diagnose, for the unknowing teacher may consider the child a daydreamer or inattentive. The seizure may be accompanied by myoclonic jerks in which a single jerk of an arm or trunk muscle occurs without apparent loss of consciousness. It may also be accompanied by a sudden postural collapse of muscles with consequent nodding of the head; if the collapse is generalized, the child may even fall down.

Autonomic seizures

The autonomic seizure is rare. This seizure consists of periods of flushing, sweating, fast heartbeat, gagging, heightened blood pressure, or fear that occurs without obvious cause. Unconsciousness is absent.

Psychosocial adjustment

Many persons regard epilepsy with fear because they do not understand the nature of the disorder. Consequently, there is great social and economic prejudice expressed toward epileptics by the nonhandicapped majority. As a result, the social handicap manifested by the disorder is often more important than the physical deficiency itself. Much of the prejudice displayed toward epilepsy is caused by inadequate information about the disorder. Many misinformed lay persons often develop a stereotyped concept of the epileptic personality. Attitudes unconsciously reflect ancient beliefs that were attributed to the seizures and that led to the social degradation of persons with epilepsy. These views of the nonhandicapped majority have great implications for the social, psychological, educational, and vocational problems of the epileptic's adjustment.

Convulsive disorders in childhood must be considered as having psychological significance in the development and formation of personality. It is assumed that fear of social embarrassment through a seizure, in the case of the more obvious seizure types, and concern over the etiology of the illness are great deterrents to the healthful personality development of epileptic children.

Inasmuch as public misconceptions regarding epilepsy still prevail in many communities, the educational opportunities for epileptic children, in many cases, are lacking. Usually, epileptic children can attend school and participate in regular physical education activities with their peers, but they are often confronted with prejudice that may adversely affect their schooling. Hopefully, in the ensuing years, this prejudice against epilepsy will be thwarted to the extent that the deprivation of opportunity in education will not still prevail. Physical educators can assist in breaking down stereotyped concepts that lead to prejudice toward children having this disorder. If gains can be made in reducing public prejudice, personality development among epileptics will possibly be enhanced.

Characteristics of epileptics

Considerable research has been done on the intellectual abilities of children with epilepsy. A summary of the literature on the characteristics of epileptics would suggest the following:

1. Categorically, epilepsy does not significantly affect intelligence. There are epileptics who are in the upper ranges of intellectual functioning and epileptics who are mentally retarded. Epileptics who are mentally retarded may be retarded for the same reasons that nonepileptics are retarded, and epileptics of higher levels of intelligence may function as such for the same reasons nonepileptics do so.
2. Epileptics, as a group, appear to be within the normal range of intellignece, but are slightly below the mean.
3. There is an apparent lack of data that indicate progressive mental deterioration of epileptics.
4. Mental impairment in epileptics may be caused by adverse social and psychological

factors associated with the disorder and these factors may deter cognitive development.
5. The development of anticonvulsant medication provides opportunities for increased socialization and development of sound mental health in the epileptic.
6. It is unlikely that anticonvulsant medication results in significantly impaired psychological functioning.
7. It is unlikely that anticonvulsant medication results in significantly impaired intellectual functioning.

The prejudiced views of the nonhandicapped majority of persons often precipitate stresses, which, in turn, can be responsible for emotional conflict within an epileptic person. Therefore, it is not uncommon to find those with convulsive disorders who encounter emotional problems exceeding those of the typical population. The physical and motor characteristics of epileptic children are as variable as with so-called typical children. However, it may be hypothesized that variability among this population in motor and physical characteristics is great. It would be anticipated that there are epileptics highly skilled and highly developed in the motor and physical areas as well as epileptics who are poorly skilled and poorly developed in the same areas.

Treatment of convulsive disorders
Drug therapy

Medical advances, through the development of anticonvulsant drugs, have made it possible for most children with epilepsy to attend regular classes. It is estimated that approximately 80% of epileptics can, with guidance, secure an education in regular classes and engage in vocations with success. Drugs reduce both the frequency and the severity of the seizures to socially acceptable levels. Drugs are usually administered under the direction of a physician on the basis of the type and nature of the seizure. Some of the common anticonvulsant drugs that are used to control seizures are phenobarbital, phenytoin (Dilantin), trimethadione (Tridione), paramethadione (Paradione), methylphenylethyl hydantoin (Mesantoin), and phenacemide (Phenurone). Drug administration must be supervised carefully because of side effects that might occur. Anticonvulsant drugs apparently work in one of two ways: either they depress the function of nervous tissue or they replace a chemical substance that is lacking and thus raise the convulsive threshold to above its normal level. Dosages are usually reduced for patients who have been free of seizures for a given period of time.

Surgical treatment

Surgical techniques for the removal of defective areas of the brain can be beneficial in controlling seizures. Conditions that may indicate surgery are brain tumors, abscesses, scar tissue, or depressed fracture of the skull. There are, however, relatively few convulsive disorders requiring neurosurgery.

Psychological treatment

Some form of psychological treatment is often indicated for children suffering from epilepsy. The form of such treatment varies from one individual to another. Lack of treatment often results in perpetuation of the handicap, for it usually affects social and emotional behaviors. Such treatment seems warranted because there is impressive evidence showing a relationhip between seizures and psychological variants such as fear, frustration, and unacceptable interpersonal relationships.

An environment conducive to optimal growth of physical and mental health is most helpful. To achieve this end, good personal hygiene and regular meals with a balanced diet are essential. Regular periods of physical activity, conducted in an atmosphere that exposes the child to a minimum of emotional stress and promotes productivity and normal behavior, are of great benefit. Also, there should be a structured life-style, with regular times for sleeping, eating, and physical activity.

Teacher's role during a seizure

The poise of the teacher during a student's seizure is of tremendous importance, for the teacher can properly manage the situation so that there is maximum understanding on the part of the other students and minimum disruption of the class. It is suggested that the teacher convey to the students the nature and possibilities of a seizure. The children can then cope with the situation more easily.

It is important that the teacher know the kind of seizure to expect from a given child, the medication the child is receiving, and the restrictions that the physician has ordered. In the case of the grand mal seizure, the child may experience an aura that involves nausea, trembling, dizziness, or pain in the extremities or stomach. If the aura can be detected, it will give the teacher the opportunity to place the student in a safe place and prepare the class for the ensuing experience. This will also give the teacher time to lower the student to the floor and thus prevent possible injury from falling when the seizure occurs. The teacher should loosen any apparel that may constrict the student's movement and should not try to restrain the student from the convulsive stage of the seizure. A soft object such as a folded handkerchief should be placed between the back teeth when the student's mouth opens to prevent the student from biting the tongue or cheek. After the attack, the child should be moved to a quiet room until full consciousness is regained. In the event that sleep follows the seizure, the child should not be awakened.

Implications for physical education

It is now accepted that general physical activity is beneficial to children with epilepsy (Fig. 13-6). This is a result partly of the psychological therapy that play and activity have for children and partly of the physiological benefits of such activity. Vigorous activiity seems to enhance drug therapy and resistance to seizures. Physical activity is also instrumental in the development of cardiovascular fitness. The capacities for physical activity and the nature of seizures among the epileptic population vary considerably. Therefore, the physical education program should be planned on an individual basis.

Like any other child, handicapped or nonhandicapped, an assessment of educational needs must be made and then subsequent programs must be implemented to meet these needs. However, in the case of epileptic children who have controlled seizures and who are enrolled in regular classes, there is little reason why they cannot participate in the same type of physical activity as their classmates. Epilepsy itself does not necessarily contraindicate competitive and contact sports or the use of gymnastic apparatus.[3]

Swimming does not seem to be an activity that is contraindicated in even the most severe cases of epilepsy. However, a buddy system employed in the case of the child with epilepsy enhances the safety factor. There is consensus that epileptics should not perform physical activities where a fall would result if a seizure were experienced without warning. Such activities would include rope climb-

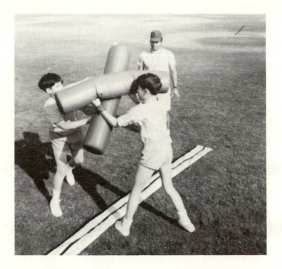

Fig. 13-6. Children with epilepsy need programs of vigorous physical exercise.

ing and gymnastics that involves parallel bars, trampolines, and so forth. However, individual consideration remains the basic determinant. Body contact sports for children with epilepsy should be considered on the basis of individual evaluation. It cannot be denied that there is some risk associated with some of these activities. If the physical, social, and emotional objectives of a physical education program can become a reality to a child, then a small risk may be warranted. To fulfill the needs of an epileptic child in the physical education program, it is imperative that the instructor know the nature, limits, and implications of the epilepsy of a particular child and obtain a recommendation from the child's physician.

THE MULTIHANDICAPPED CHILD

The multihandicapped child is one who is afflicted with several handicapping conditions. Combinations of sensory, emotional, mental, perceptual, neurological, physical, and motor handicaps may be present. Although it is important for the physical educator to attend to the individual's total development, this section is primarily concerned with the aspect of programming over which the instructor has the greatest control: the physical edu-

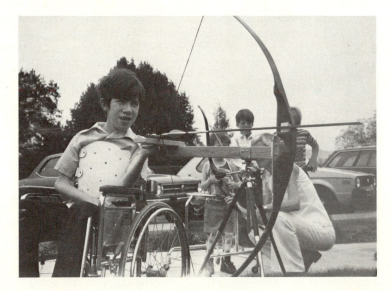

Fig. 13-7. Multihandicapped persons can participate in modified physical activity. (Courtesy of Julian Stein, American Alliance for Health, Physical Education, Recreation, and Dance.)

cation curriculum as defined in P.L. 94-142. The aspects of growth and development are purported to be interrelated. Thus, it may be possible through physical and motor improvement of the multihandicapped to effect positively concomitant aspects of development.

If muscles are weak, progressive techniques in the development of strength should be applied. These techniques in progression are passive exercise, active-assistive exercise, active exercise, and progressive-resistive exercise. The increments of a progressive-resistive exercise program should be small and gradual and, since there may be spasticity in muscle groups, attention should be given to the coordination of particular movements. All remaining neuromuscular units should be integrated into the movement pattern.

In the case of severe damage to motor cells, it may be necessary to design programs that assist movement prerequisites that enhance the acitivities of daily living. Daily living skills increase the individual's ability to function independently. These training programs might include the development of such fundamental motor patterns as standing, walking, stair climbing, and rotary diagonal movement patterns such as feeding, grooming, and other self-help activities. In the case of persons who are severely impaired, functional training is a long process requiring a great deal of patience. The medical profession and special instructional staff are usually required to plan and implement functional training programs of motor activity that are not incorporated in the physical education curriculum of P. L. 94-142.

Activity programs that will enhance the development of strength, endurance, and coordination will be of invaluable aid to the child. It is necessary to remember that each multihandicapped child is different. Therefore, there can be no one program for all children. A full assessment in areas of specific educational need must be made to develop an Individual Education Program to meet each child's needs. However, certain considerations common to all multihandicapped children who participate in the physical education program should be taken into account. In general, activities should be selected that represent the widest range of activities appropriate to the child's age group and the program constructed should fit each pupil's indi-vidual needs. When the program is being constructed, it should be determined whether the activities might create muscular imbalance by strengthening one group of muscles at a faster rate than the antagonistic group. Selection of activities also involves finding the game or activity that can circumvent the disability. For instance, if there is involvement in the legs, it is possible to select activities that can be accomplished through proficiency with the arms.

The multihandicapped pupil may be afflicted with paralysis, weak antigravity muscles, and tight reciprocal muscles. The consequences of these atypical aspects of physical development may contribute to abnormal patterns of motion and faulty body alignment. Therefore, the restoration and the maintenance of correct body alignment and movement patterns are of great importance to the prevention of malalignment. Particular attention should be paid to weakened antigravity muscles such as the abdominal muscles, the extensors of the spine, the hip extensors, the trapezius, and the gastrosoleus muscles. There are cases in which the antigravity muscle groups are beyond repair for functional use. In such cases, it may be necessary for the physician to prescribe supporting appliances such as braces.

More often than not, because multihandicapped youngsters are handicapped physically, they have had little opportunity to participate in recreational activities. It is necessary to remember that recreation is derived from the meaning that the child attaches to the activity. It must be fulfilling and it must bring fun, self-expression, and socialization into the life of the child. Recreation for multihandicapped children, in general, should be activities from which they obtain pleasure or diversion from the routine of the day's activities. Usually, these will be activities in which they have developed competency; recreation, by definition, means to recreate some activity that has been performed in the past and to recreate it for the sheer pleasure that the activity brings (see Chapter 5).

Water activity is of special value to the multihandicapped child, for the water provides buoyancy that facilitates the movement of affected limbs. It also has value in that it tends to relax tensed muscles so that movement may eventually become more efficient through greater reciprocal innervation between muscle groups. It is in the water that the multihandicapped child can most closely approximate the movement ability of typical children.

In summary, physical education has a vital role in the physical restoration of multihandicapped children. The activities in which they engage should be broad in scope so that they contribute to physical, social, and recreational needs.

REFERENCES

1. Adams, R. C., et al.: Games, sports, and exercises for the physically handicapped, Philadelphia, 1972, Lea & Febiger.
2. Allen, R. M.: Cerebral palsy. In Garrett, J. F., and Levine, E. S., editors: Psychological practices with the physically disabled, New York, 1962, Columbia University Press.
3. American Academy of Pediatrics: The epileptic child and competitive school athletics, Pediatrics **42:**700-702, 1968.
4. Arnheim, D. D., and Sinclair, W. A.: The clumsy child: a program of motor therapy, ed. 2, St. Louis, 1979, The C. V. Mosby Co.
5. Bice, H. V.: Some factors that contribute to the conept of self in the child with cerebral palsy, Ment. Hyg. **38:**120-131, 1954.
6. Block, W. E.: Personality of the brain injured child, J. Exceptional Child. **21:**91-100, 1955.
7. Bryan, T. H., and Bryan, J. H.: nderstanding learning disabilities, Port Washington, N.Y., 1975, Alfred Publishing Company Inc.
8. Cratty, B. J.: Remedial motor activity for children, Philadelphia, 1975, Lea & Febiger.
9. Cruickshank, W. M., editor: Cerebral palsy, its individual and community problems, Sracuse, N.Y., 1966, Syracuse University Press.
10. Cruickshank, W. M., Bice, H. V., and Wallen, N. E.: Perception and cerebral palsy, Syracuse, N.Y., 1957, Syracuse University Press.
11. Denhoff, E.: Cerebral palsy: the preschool years, Springfield, Ill., 1967, Charles C Thomas, Publisher.
12. Denhoff, E., and Robinault, I.: Cerebral palsy and related disorders, New York, 1960, McGraw-Hill Book Co.
13. deQuiro, J. B., and Schrager, O. L., Neuropsychological fundamentals in learning disabilities, San Rafael, Calif., 1978, Academic Therapy Publications.
14. Fiorentino, M. R.: Normal and abnormal development, Springfield, Ill., 1972, Charles C Thomas, Publisher.
15. Fiorentino, M. R.: Reflex testing, methods of evaluating C.N.S. development, Springfield, Ill., 1973, Charles C Thomas, Publisher.
16. Fish, L.: Deafness in cerebral-palsied school children, Lancet **2:**370-371, 1955.
17. Gatz, A. J.: Manter's essential of clinical neuroanatomy and neurophysiology, ed. 3, Philadelphia, 1966, F. A. Davis Co.
18. Hoffly, J. E., and Angers, W. P.: Understanding the child with epilepsy, Catholic School J. **67:**27-29, 1967.
19. Kephart, N. C.: The slow learner in the classroom, Columbus, Ohio, 1960, Charles E. Merrill Books, Inc.
20. Layshon, G. A.: Programmed functional anatomy, St. Louis, 1974, The C. V. Mosby Co.
21. McLaughlin, E.: Follow-up study on children remediated for perceptual motor dysfunction, Unpublished Master's thesis, University of Kansas, 1979.
22. Moore, J. C.: Neuroanatomy simplified, Dubuque, Iowa, 1969, Kendall/Hunt Publishing Co.
23. Moore, J. C.: The nervous system, Proceedings of the Third National Workshop for Rehabilitation Personnel in Sensorimotor Treatment Techniques, St. Louis, December 10-14, 1974, University of Missouri, St. Louis.
24. Olson, W. C.: Child development, ed. 2, Boston, 1959, D.C Heath & Co.
25. Scott, D.: About epilepsy, New York, 1973, International Universities Press, Inc.
26. Touwen, B. C. L., and Prechtl, H. F. R.: The neurological examination of the child with minor nervous dysfunction, Philadelphia, 1970, J. B. Lippincott Co.

RECOMMENDED READINGS

Clarke, H. H., and Clarke, D. H.: Developmental and adapted physical education, Englewood Cliffs, N.J., 1963, Prentice-Hall, Inc.

Daniels, A. S., and Davies, E. A.: Adapted physical education, ed. 3, New York, 1975, Harper & Row, Publishers, Inc.

Fait, H. F.: Special physical education: adapted, corrective, developmental, ed. 2, Philadelphia, 1966, W. B. Saunders Co.

Wolf, J. M., editor: The multiply handicapped child, Springfield, Ill., 1969, Charles C Thomas, Publisher.

14

Sensory disorders

Sensory disorders are functional impairments that are usually permanent. Children with sensory disorders represent a unique challenge to the physical educator because, in addition to their sensory impairments, they usually demonstrate other developmental lags. Many of these children have not had opportunities to motorically explore the envi-

ronment during their early years. As a result, intact sensorimotor systems are not stimulated adequately and motor development and physical fitness levels suffer. Low vitality and perceptual-motor developmental lags often prevent the children from participating in activities not contraindicated by the primary sensory disorder.

Sensory disorders discussed in this chapter include visual and hearing impairments and aphasia. Part B of P.L. 94-142 specifically addresses the first two of these disorders, mandating physical education for those children whose impairments necessitate special eduation and related services. The children with these specific disorders who qualify for adapted/developmental physical education programs demonstrate one or more of the following:

1. Deafness that is so severe that the child is impaired in processing linguistic information through hearing with or without amplification, which adversely affects educational performance.
2. A permanent or fluctuating hearing impairment that adversely affects the child's educational performance but that is not included under the definition of deaf.
3. A visual handicap that, even with correction, adversely affects the child's educational performance. The term includes both partially seeing and blind children.
4. Deafness-blindness with concomitant hearing and visual impairments, the combination of which causes such severe communication and other developmental and educational problems that the child cannot be accommodated in special educational programs solely for deaf or blind children.[40]

BLINDNESS AND PARTIAL SIGHT

Visual impairments may have varying adverse effects on children, creating a special challenge to adapted physical educators. Attention to visual problems should not be so great that concern for the development of the whole child is lost. The development of the whole child in the normal environment with concurrent awareness of individual differences is of paramount importance. Children with visual impairments must be approached with regard to their own unique educational needs. Thus, all blind and partially sighted children should have a full preevaluation in specific areas of the physical education curriculum to determine their needs.

The child who has a loss of vision may also be impaired in the function of mobility and may be less able than are typical children in motor abilities. Therefore, there is a great need for blind children to be provided with opportunities, through adapted physical education, that will compensate for their movement deficiencies.

Children with loss of vision are, for educational purposes, classified as blind (*those who are educated through channels other than vision*) or partially sighted (*those who are able to be educated, with special aids, through the medium of vision, with consideration given to the useful vision they retain*).

Blindness is determined by visual acuity and is expressed in a ratio with normal vision in the numerator and actual measured vision in the denominator; for example, 20/30 vision means that the eye can see at the distance of 20 feet what a normal eye can see at 30 feet. The legally blind are described as those who have a visual acuity of 20/200 or less in the better eye after maximum correction or who have a visual field that subtends an angle of 20 degrees or less in the widest diameter.

There are varying degrees of blindness. If a person is not totally blind, it is still possible to make functional use of whatever vision remains. Some blind persons have little residual vision and are unable to perceive motion and discriminate light. These individuals are at the upper end of the continuum of blindness. Some blind persons, however, are capable of perceiving distance and motion, whereas others possess these capabilities and are also able to travel with the use of residual vision.

Students who are educationally blind in that they received their education through means other than vision have been known to play a skilled game of handball. In the event the ball is black and the walls of the court are of a light color, the students may perceive the motion of the handball well enough to participate in the activity. In handball doubles, a sighted person may be paired with a blind partner. The sighted player can indicate to the blind partner the direction of the ball, which can subsequently be differentiated from the light-colored wall.

The point that is to be stressed is that when a person is considered blind, it does not necessarily mean that the majority of the activities in a typical physial education program must be ruled out for participation. Rather, a person's capacity for specific activity depends on the degree of blindness as well as available skill.

The term *partially sighted* refers to persons who have less than 20/70 visual acuity in the better eye after correction, have a progressive eye disorder that will probably reduce vision below 20/70, or have peripheral vision that subtends an angle less than 20 degrees. Hathaway[16] referred to partially sighted children as those who have undergone eye operations and require physical and psychological adjustment to such conditions as *enucleation* (removal of an eye) or those who have muscle anomalies and conditions that necessitate reeducation of the abnormal eye. Each child must be considered according to his or her ability to function, regardless of the nature or degree of the visual handicap. In some instances, a child's vision may fall within the normal range, but the child may have progressive eye difficulties or a disease of the eye or body that seriously affects vision.

Visual defects

There are several defects that may cause degeneration of vision. Some of these visual defects are the following:

1. Refractive errors such as myopia, hyperopia, and astigmatism
2. Structural anomalies such as cataracts
3. Infectious diseases of the eyes
4. Impaired muscle function of the eye such as strabismus and nystagmus

Kerby[18,19] reported that 49% of the visual defects found among partially seeing children are caused by errors in refraction, the most prevalent of which are hyperopia, myopia, and astigmatism. These abnormalities of vision are concerned with the internal ciliary muscles of accommodation, which increase the curvature of the lens. *Hyperopia,* or farsightedness, is a condition in which the light rays focus behind the retina, causing an unclear image of objects closer than 20 feet from the eye. The term implies that distant objects can be seen with less strain than can near objects. *Myopia,* or nearsightedness, is a refractive error in which the rays of light focus in front of the retina when a person views an object 20 feet or more away. *Asigmatism* is a refractive error caused by an irregularity in the curvature of the cornea of the lens, causing parts of the light rays from a given object to fall behind or in front of the retina. As a result, vision may become blurred.

In addition to the internal muscles of the eye mentioned previously, there are six muscles attached to the outside of each eyeball that control the movement of the eyes. Singular binocular vision involves coordinating the separate images that enter each eye into a single image in the visual cortex of the brain. When the two eyes function in unison, the images entering each eye are matched in the visual cortex and binocular fusion results. If, however, the supply of energy to the extraocular muscles is out of balance, the eyes do not function in unison. When this ccurs, the movements of one eye deviate from those of the other eye and the separate images entering through each eye will not match in the visual cortex. The amount of visual distress experienced because of mismatched images depends on the degree of deviation of the eyes and the abilty of the CNS to "correct" the imbalance.

The two most prevalent dysfunctions of external visual muscle control are heterotropias and heterophorias. *Heterotropias* are manifest malalignments of the eyes during which one or both eyes consistently deviate from the central axis. As a consequence, the eyes do not fixate at the same point on the object of visual attention. When the eyes turn inward, such as with crossed eyes, the condition is called *esotropia;* when one or both eyes turn outward, it is called *exotropia. Hypertropia* is the name given to the condition when one or both eyes swing upward; the term *hypotropia* is used when one or both eyes turn downward. Tropias always create depth perception difficulties.

Heterophorias are tendencies toward visual malalignments. They usually do not cause serious visual distress because when slight variations in binocular fusion occur in the visual cortex, the CNS tends to "correct" the imbalance between the pull of the extraocular muscles. However, after prolonged use of the eyes, for example after reading several hours, the stronger set of muscles overcome the correction and the eyes swing out of alignment. An individual becomes aware of the malalignment when the vision of the printed page begins to blur. Phorias, like tropias, are named for the direction the eye tends to swing (*eso-* means in, toward the nose; *exo-* is a lateral drift; *hyper-* means up; and *hypo-* refers to down). Phorias create depth perception difficulties only after the "correction" is lost.

Eye specialists

There is a need for teamwork between educational, medical, and other personnel who serve children who have limited vision. Therefore, the physical educator should understand the roles of professionals who are involved with eye care and should know who is responsible for rendering specific services. Eye specialists include the following:

1. The ophthalmologist, a licensed physician who specializes in the treatment of eye diseases and optical defects
2. The optometrist, a nonmedical practitioner licensed to prescribe and fit glasses and deal with optical defects of the eyes without the use of drugs or surgery
3. The optician, a skilled technician who grinds lenses and makes up glasses
4. The orthoptist, an assistant who provides eye exercises and orthoptic training as prescribed by medical personnel

Identification of visual impairments

Vision tests are extremely important in order to identify and remedy vision disorders and to facilitate the education of visually handicapped persons. A widely used test of vision is the Snellen test, which is a measure of visual acuity. This test can be administered with expediency to a child by nonprofessional personnel and is applicable to young children. The Snellen chart can detect such conditions as myopia, astigmatism, higher degrees of hyperopia, and other eye conditions that cause imperfect visual images. However, the chart primarily measures central distance visual acuity. It does not give indications of near-point vision, peripheral vision, convergence ability, binocular fusion ability, or muscular imbalance. A thorough vision screening program must include tests supplementary to the Snellen test. Other visual screening tests that may provide additional information are the Massachusetts vision test, the Keystone Telebinocular test, and the Orthorator test. Hathaway[16] recommended the Massachusetts vision test for acquiring more data about visual disorders. This test battery consists of the illuminated Snellen E chart, a plus lens test for hyperopia, and a test for horizontal and vertical muscle balance at 20 feet as well as for horizontal muscle balance at reading distance.

Limitations in peripheral vision constitute a visual handicap, particularly in some activities involving motor skills. Consequently, knowledge of this aspect of vision may assist the physical educator in determining methods of teaching and types of activities for the visually impaired child. Peripheral vision is usually assessed in terms of degrees of visual arc and is measured by the extent to which a standard visual stimulus can be seen on a black background viewed from a distance of about 39 inches when the eye is fixed on a central point.

It is difficult to evaluate the results found on a given test of vision, for two persons with similar vision characteristics on a screening test may display different visual behavior physically, socially, and psychologically.

Although objective screening tests of vision are important, it is suggested that daily observations be made to supplement the screening tests. Daily observation for symptoms of eye trouble is of particular importance in the early primary years. Detection of visual handicaps early in development enables early intervention, which maximizes skill development. Symptoms that may indicate eye disorders and that may be observed by the physical educator are the following:

1. Eyelids that are crusted and red, in which sties or swelling appear
2. Discharges from the eyes
3. Lack of coordination in directing vision of both eyes
4. Frequent rubbing of the eyes
5. Inattention when sustained visual activity is required or when looking at distant objects
6. Tenseness of the body
7. Squinting
8. Forward thrust of the head
9. Walking overcautiously
10. Faltering or stumbling
11. Running into objects not directly in the line of vision
12. Failure to see objects readily visible to others
13. Sensitivity to normal light levels
14. Inability to distinguish colors
15. Difficulty in estimating distances
16. Bloodshot eyes

Incidence

It is difficult to assess the incidence of blindness and partial vision because of the differing definitions of blindness and the problems that exist in identification. Consequently, dependable statistics on the incidence of blindness in the United States are lacking, although there is a growing awareness that a greater incidence of blindness and vision impairment exists than had been believed previously. Kennedy and Danielson[17a] estimate that 0.1% of the population is visually handicapped. There are a considerable number of children with visual defects who are not categorized as either blind or partially sighted. Estimates indicate that approximately 20% of elementary school children and 30% of high school students have some visual defect.

Classification

There are many ways of classifying persons with loss of vision. They may be classified according to cause, topography, degree of vision loss, time of onset, or collateral effects. The underlying causes of vision loss include infectious diseases, accidents and injuries, poisoning, tumors, and prenatal influences. Prenatal causes account for 41.8% of blindness, poisoning for 19.3%, heredity for 14.3%, tumors for 5.1%, injuries for 4.9%, and infectious diseases for 7.4%.[18]

Classification by topography refers to the part of the eye affected and the nature and the location of the eye defect. These classifications include defects of the retina, the crystalline lens, and the optic nerve.

Perception of vision falls on a continuum. It is

important for the physical educator to be aware of the amount of residual vision that a partially sighted person has. The residual vision can fall on a continuum extending from slight impairment (20/70) to total blindness.

Lowenfeld[21] suggests that it is necessary to consider the time of onset of the vision loss as well as the amount of vision possessed. Lowenfeld also indicates that children who have lost their sight before ages of 5 to 7 years do not retain a useful visual imagery. In the event blindness is acquired after the preschool years of life, the children have opportunities to acquire perceptual experiences that will better enable them to cope with their environment at a later time. The early developmental period in which the child explores both the environment and his or her own physical abilities is of critical importance.

Developmental factors

Vision loss has serious implications for the general development of motor, academic, intellectual, psychological, and social characteristics.

Buell[4] indicates that the motor and physical proficiency of partially sighted children generally exceeds that of their totally blind peers. From this information, one might infer a relationship between degree of vision loss and physical and motor proficiency. Furthermore, numerous professionals observe that the posture of the visually handicapped is below normal standards.* As Scholl[34] points out, the blind infant has little motivation to hold the head up because of lack of visual stimulation. Thus, in the formative stages of postural development (head control), blind children are behind normative expectations. In many instances, intervention with training programs and adaptive measures is necessary to meet the developmental needs of the maturing child with a loss of vision. It is important to have some knowledge of how the child with vision loss may develop physically, socially, and psychologically so that the physical educator can be alert to cope with needs that may arise.

Evidence indicates that blind pupils in the public schools are educationally retarded as compared with their sighted peers of the same chronological age.[1,13] Some of the reasons may be that blind children may have a maladjustment at the onset of blindness, making it difficult to stay abreast of sighted peers, and that they need to master new tools such as braille reading and writing. Physical educators must be alert to detect educationally retarded blind children. They must not be misguided by grade placement but must assess and meet the physical, motor, and social needs of each child.

Physical activity is essential for optimum child

---

*See references 8, 14, 30, and 37.

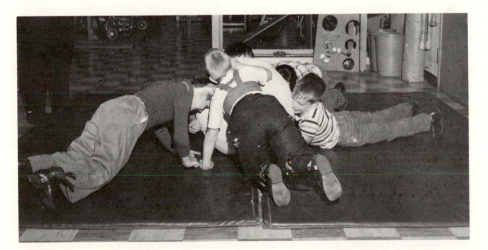

Fig. 14-1. Vision is not required to push against the cage ball. (Courtesy of Julian Stein, American Alliance for Health, Physical Education, Recreation, and Dance and University Hospital School, University of Iowa, Iowa City, Iowa.)

growth and development. Through movement experiences, children with vision losses acquire a better understanding of themselves, others, and the world around them. However, limited vision restricts physical and motor activity, which, in turn, limits the range and variety of experiences the children may encounter. They then becomes less effective in meeting the demands of the environment. Opportunities for manipulating toys and objects are extremely important in the early life of blind children because it is through touch and feeling, rather than through vision, that they learn about the physical world.

Providing an environment in which children with vision impairments can develop optimally is a great challenge. Because of the limitation in vision, blind children are often slower in learning such skills as walking, talking, prehension, feeding, and socialization unless they are given special help that will assist in developing these traits.

Norris and Brody[29] found that blind children showed delayed mastery of motor responses in tasks requiring fine motor coordination. There is impressive evidence that fine motor coordination develops with fluency only after the children have had experiences in gross motor activity. This would point to a need to provide environmental experiences for both gross and fine motor activities. Norris and Brody also stress the importance of opportunities for physical activity and express the opinion that physical development of blind children is usually normal, although the rate may be slower than for children with normal vision.

Research available regarding the social maturity of blind children reveals that, in general, they receive significantly lower social maturity scores than do children who see.[23,24,28] Physical education programs may well be an important medium for enhancing the social maturity of blind children.

Perception
Obstacle perception

When a blind person stops walking before coming to a wall or a large object that obstructs the intended path, this is called obstacle perception. Some authorities have indicated that obstacle perception can be learned.[38] It appears to be a function of audition, in which the person responds to an environmental need. Blind persons are capable of avoiding obstacles by detecting changes in pitch as

they move about in their environment and develop an awareness of objects.

Sensory perception

It was once a prevalent notion that visually limited children compensated for defective vision with supersensitive hearing, touch, taste, and smell. However, it is now accepted that the visually limited do not possess natural compensation.[35] It is possible that blind children utilize their other sensory abilities better through increased attention to them and through practice and opportunities for learning. A sighted person may be unaware of auditory stimuli in the environment, whereas a blind person would attach great significance to the stimuli; however, there may be little difference between the actual hearing abilities of the blind person and the seeing person.

Psychological and social adjustment

The emotional and social characteristics of the visually limited vary with each individual. However, Cowan, Underburg, and Verrillo[7] found that, regarding the relationship between the degree of disability and psychological and social adjustment, better adjustment was associated with greater visual disability. These findings indicate that degree of visual disability does not necessarily lead to proportionate maladjustment. Conclusions drawn from this study were that social and emotional maladjustment, as typically defined and measured, are not necessary consequences of limitations in vision and that such maladjustment that does occur is not directly proportional in severity to, or necessarily directly related to, visual limitation.

Psychological and social adjustment of the blind cannot be separated from the attitudes with which the nondisabled view them. The lack of respect of one's peers may create a need for a disproportionate amount of social and emotional adjustment. The adjustment of blind persons is not only to blindness but to their peers. The correlates of maladjustment are to be found in deficiencies of respect accorded the individual, rather than a lack of visual experience.

The uphill battle and social adjustment of the blind requires special attention; sighted persons acquire social habits through imitation, but the blind need direct instruction in everyday social adjustment. The emotional and social climate of the physical education class can be structured so that blind children will be able to function comfortably at their own levels and assist in establishing wholesome social relationships. Lack of individualized instructional procedures can contribute to frustration by creating situations that accentuate, rather than minimize, differences.

The ultimate goal of the class atmosphere for children with vision losses is to provide experiences that will assist them in adjusting to the seeing society in which they live. The selection and method of experiences in the physical education program are critical. These experiences should not be of such a nature that blind children are overprotected to the extent that growth is inhibited; rather, the experiences should provide challenge, yet remain within the range of the children's capabilities for achieving skill objectives.

The problems that confront the teacher regarding successful emotional and psychological adjustment of the visually limited involve both visually limited children and nondisabled children. Guidelines for achieving the goal of adjustment for teachers of visually handicapped children are as follows:

1. Provide opportunities for participation and enjoyment in new experiences
2. Provide Individual Education Programs in which the children are free to grow and develop at their own rates
3. Find ways in which they can best contribute to the groups that are satisfying to them
4. Help them become acquainted with their physical surroundings

Equally important in the social and psychological adjustment of visually handicapped children is the attitude of nondisabled persons toward them. Physical education teachers working with children who are visually handicapped should attempt to minimize the stereotyped manner in which the visually limited child receives an education and should encourage nonhandicapped children to accept the blind for who they are. The development of such attitudes of the nonhandicapped support the principle of normalization of the handicapped.

Mobility

One of the greatest problems caused by blindness is difficulty in moving about. Success in school and at work in later years depends on mobility. Mobility contributes to the independence of blind persons, which in turn leads to opportunities for physical, social, and psychological development.

A program of training in mobility for the blind in a gymnasium or playing area will greatly increase the degree of independence to perform in a physical education program. Orientation and training programs should help the persons cope with physical surroundings effectively. Training programs should also assist in successful interaction with peers as well as with the physical facilities and equipment. It must be remembered that some blind persons have enough vision to travel about. This vision is called *travel vision*. The individual capabilities of each child should be assessed to determine the extent of the mobility training program.

Educational placement

The physical education teacher may be requested either to instruct a class in which visually limited children are integrated with the regular class or to instruct a class composed solely of visually limited children.

There is a growing awareness that similarities are greater than differences when visually limited children are compared with seeing children. Therefore, integration of visually limited children with their nonhandicapped peers should occur to meet the new federal mandates of placement of all handicapped children in the least restrictive environment (regular class, if possible). Such placement emphasizes the positive aspects of the children and minimizes differences.

In the past, it was not uncommon for children with limited vision to be referred to and placed in residential schools. However, with the implementation of P.L. 94-142, a countertrend has grown to bring instructional aids into resource rooms and regular classrooms of community schools.[32] Such practice has created a number of service delivery alternatives for least restrictive placement. Reynolds and Birch[32] indicate the following cascade system for children with vision handicaps:

Some suggested considerations prerequisite to effective education of the visually limited child are as follows:

1. Regular class
2. Regular class with assistance by vision consultant

3. Regular class with consultation and itinerant instruction (orientation and mobility training)
4. Adapted physical education, conducted by specialist; children attend part time
5. Self-contained adapted physical education class
6. Residential schools for the blind

The itinerant teacher is a specialist who possesses specific skills to work with children of limited vision. They team with regular classroom teachers on behalf of visually handicapped children. For more information concerning the duties of this type of teacher the reader is referred to Moore and Peabody.[26]

Implications for physical education

The physical education teacher must be able to respect individuals who have atypical vision. Furthermore, attention should focus on the abilities, as well as the deficits, of visually handicapped children for the purpose of creating an environment conducive to optimal growth. An assessment of the needs, abilities, and limitations of visually limited children is necessary, with subsequent program development according to defined needs. This is a challenging task for a teacher; however, it has been pointed out by many good teachers that instructing the visually limited has enabled them to do a better job with typical children because it was necessary to plan more carefully when working with the visually limited group.

Some suggested considerations prerequisite to effective education of the visually limited child are as follows:

1. Skilled observation of motor performance and behavioral characteristics of individuals and of group participants
2. Recognition of differences in the manner in which the visually limited child learns, as compared with the typical child, followed by appropriate adaptive methodology
3. Understanding of the growth and development of physical and social competency
4. Knowledge of appropriate curricula and methods in physical education for the visually limited

High-quality physical education programs can enhance the progress of the visually limited child socially, emotionally, and physically. Loss of vision, by itself, is not a limiting condition for physical exercise. A considerable amount of developmental exercises of muscular strength and endurance can be administered to such children. Through developmental exercise, the visually limited child will develop aesthetic qualities such as good posture, graceful body movement, and good walking and sitting positions. Furthermore, physical education programs develop and maintain a

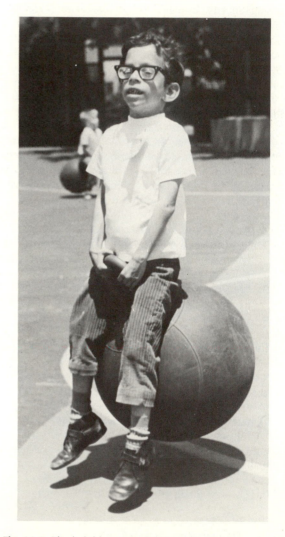

Fig. 14-2. Blind children can participate in numerous physical activities. However, they must know their constraints in space. (Courtesy of Julian Stein, American Association for Health, Physical Education, Recreation, and Dance.)

healthy, vigorous body with physical vitality and good neuromuscular coordination. In addition to physical benefits, the physical education program will contribute to such social-emotional outcomes as security and confidence on the part of the visually limited and promote acceptance of the handicapped by their sighted peers (Fig. 14-2).

Adapting methods and activities

Children with limited vision are capable of participating in numerous activities; however, the degree to which participation is possible is dependent on factors already mentioned. Therefore, it is recommended that there be available broad curriculum areas at appropriate levels of development to accommodate each child. Visually handicapped children may represent a cross section of any school population with regard to motor abilities, physical fitness characteristics, and social and emotional traits. The purpose of adapting methods and activities for the visually limited is to provide many experiences that sighted children learn primarily through visual observation. A goal of group activity in which a child with limited vision participates is to assign a role to the child that can be carried out successfully. It is undesirable for the child to be placed in the position of a bystander.

Adaptation of the physical education program for visually limited individuals should provide confidence for them to cope with their environments through increasing their physical and motor abilities. It should also produce in them a feeling of acceptance as individuals in their own right. To achieve these goals, the program should include adaptation of the general program of activities, when needed; additional or specialized activities, depending on the needs of the child; and special equipment, if needed.

The physical educator who administers activities to children with limited vision should take special safety precautions. Some considerations that may enhance the safety factor in physical education programs for the visually limited are the following:

1. To secure knowledge, through medical records and observation, of the visually limited child's limitations and capabilities
2. To orient the child to facilities and equipment
3. To provide special equipment indicating direction, such as guidelines in swimming and running events, deflated softballs, etc.

Adaptation of teaching methods

The visually limited child must depend on receiving information through sensory media other than vision. Audition is a very important sensory medium of instruction. Another sensory medium that can be used is kinesthesis through manual guidance and movement of the body parts administered by an instructor or another student. This gives assistance in comprehension of body position and body action of the visually limited student. The blind child has little understanding of spatial concepts such as location, position, direction, and distance; therefore, skin and muscular sensations give meaning to body position and postural change in motor activity. The manual guidance method (accompanied by verbal corrections) is often effective in the correction of faulty motor skills, for two senses are utilized for instruction. A technique used with some success in the integrated class is for the teacher to use the blind child in presenting a demonstration to the rest of the class by manually manipulating the child through the desired movements. This enables the visually limited child to get the tactual feel of movement and instruction to the sighted class members is not deterred.

Providing information, rules, and tests in braille for the visually limited to study in advance of a presentation in class may be helpful. Advance study enables the visually limited child to better understand the presentation.

Instructional aids that may be applicable for the physical education teacher are the following:

1. Teachers should be alert to the behavioral signs and physical symptoms of visual difficulties in all children.
2. Teachers should not let visually limited children exploit their visual limitations to the extent that they withdraw from participation or underachieve in motor performance.
3. Teachers should arrange seating with regard to the child's range of vision. Glare should be reduced and accommodations should be made for appropriate light contrasts between figure and ground when presenting instructional materials.
4. Teachers should develop a respect for the particular way in which the child learns, such as tactual-kinesthetic methods and use of auditory cues for direction in space.
5. Teachers must learn respect for individual

differences and take time and effort to accept these differences and cope with them (Chapter 8).

Adaptation of skill activities

One of the chief problems to be confronted in the social and psychological adjustment of the visually limited person is the lack of opportunity for social participation with sighted persons. Recreational opportunities provide a possible outlet for making social contact with the sighted population and also provide self-expression for the visually limited individual (Chapter 8).

Because of the great visual content included in the components of certain games, some skill activities are more difficult to adapt to the visually limited than are others. In the case of the more severely handicapped, participation in the more complex activities may be extremely difficult to modify. However, the skills comprising a game may be taught and lead-up games with appropriate modifications will usually be within the grasp of the child. Some adaptations to basic sports skills are discussed in this section.

Basketball

1. *Passing—additional use of audition*
   a. A sighted person should call the visually limited child's name when the ball is to be passed to the visually limited child.
   b. Sighted classmates may snap their fingers with their hands raised to guide the height of a pass executed by visually limited children.
   c. When a ball is passed to a visually limited person, it should be done so with a bounce pass so that the speed and direction of the ball can be detected.
2. *Dribbling—additional use of kinesthesis*
   a. Teaching progression in the dribble is important. The child should first bounce the ball with two hands in a stationary position, then bounce it with one hand in a stationary position, and then move forward and backward while bouncing the ball.
   b. The child should take short steps when dribbling on the move. This will enable the student to push the ball downward instead of outward to achieve greater control of the ball.
3. *Shooting—additional use of kinesthesis and audition*
   a. The teacher should use verbal instruction and manual guidance. Manual guidance is an efficient method when a gradient response is needed by the participant.

   b. Direction and distance of a shot can be aided if a classmate stands under the basket and talks or calls to the visually limited child.
4. *Guarding—increased space*
   a. The visually limited child should be provided with more space in which to move when executing guarding drills.
5. *Game participation—increased tactility*
   a. The teacher should have the visually limited child play with a sighted player in each position during the early teaching of the game.
   b. A scoreboard that can be read tactually can be constructed from fiberboard to inform blind persons of the score of the game, fouls, time remaining, etc.

Baseball

1. *Decreased space*
   a. The baselines should be shortened; the more severe the handicap, the shorter the baselines should be.
   b. For a totally blind batter, the ball containing a noisemaker can be pitched by rolling it on the ground. The batter should swing the bat parallel to the ground. The more severe the handicap, the larger the ball should be.
2. *Tactile aid*
   a. In the case of an integrated class, sighted children can guide the runners in the base paths. An additional aid to the runner is to station sighted class members at each base for further guidance of the visually limited runners.
3. *Adaptation of the rules of the game*
   a. If a totally blind person picks up a grounder, the runner is automatically out if between bases.

Football

1. *Adaptation of position*
   a. Children who have the greatest visual handicaps should be placed in the line. End positions and backfield positions are more difficult for the visually limited child because of visual factors inherent in the positions.
2. *Adaptation of the rules of the game*
   a. When playing touch football, modify the game so that potential violent contact is minimized, perhaps requiring only one hand touch anywhere on the runner for the more severely handicapped. More difficult tags can be required for the less handicapped.
3. *Adaptation of space per pupil*
   a. The number of contestants on each team should be reduced so that collisions will be less likely to occur.

Soccer

1. *Adaptation of position in accord with ability*
   a. Persons with greater loss of vision are more able to play the defense and goal positions than the front line positions.
2. *Modify equipment*
   a. The ball should be modified so that it is softer in order to minimize the danger of being struck. Deflate the ball slightly to retard the rolling progress of the ball when teaching special classes for the blind.
   b. Skills should be emphasized in the form of lead-up games.

Track and field

1. *Participation*
   a. All events are feasible for participation by the blind, with the exception of hurdling.
2. *Additional use of kinesthesis*
   a. Cables should be strung between track lanes to guide runners with severe vision loss.
3. *Adaptation of position*
   a. The child with a visual limitation should be given the outside lane when running against a sighted child. In the special class, those with greatest vision loss should be placed in the outside running lanes to avoid their being in proximity to two persons.
4. *Auditory aid*
   a. In the integrated class, sighted students can run ahead of the visually limited child and call his or her name in the longer races.
   b. In endurance running in the integrated class, a sighted student may run beside the visually limited child and use his or her voice as an orientation device for the visually limited child. The position of the visually limited child should be maintained without touching the partner.
   c. The more severely handicapped children may use the standing high jump instead of the running high jump. However, if the running high jump is attempted, a square piece of tin may be taped to the floor of the takeoff point, which, on contact, will convey to the jumper that he or she is taking off at the right distance from the bar.
   d. The visually limited child can perform the running broad jump with the assistance of one sighted child at the far end of the broad jump pit to give an auditory signal for direction. A second child can run with the visually limited child to inform him or her when it is time to jump.
5. *Tactile aid*
   a. In relay racing, the child with severe vision loss can run first to avoid receiving the baton. A sighted student should run as a guide with the child when the exchange of the baton is made to the next person.

Field hockey

1. *Kinesthetic aid*
   a. Dribble: The visually limited child should tap the ball a short distance and in a straight line. If the ball is lost on the dribble, small circular movements that become progressively larger should be made with the stick until the ball is located. When the ball is too far away, the visually limited child should be notified.
   b. Bullies: The player keeps the stick in contact with the ball and takes the bully in the same manner as do sighted children.
2. *Auditory aid*
   a. Passing: Teammates should give audible sounds when they wish to receive a pass.

Bowling

1. *Kinesthetic aid*
   a. A guide rail should be placed beside the approach so that the visually limited person may receive aid in direction when delivering the ball.

Gymnastics

1. *Participation*
   a. Gymnastics and work on the apparatus are activities that can be performed by totally blind children.
2. *Adaptation of position*
   a. Provisions should be made for adequate space for performance for the visually limited child.
3. *Tactual orientation*
   a. Each piece of apparatus should be tactually observed before participation.
4. *Tactual observation*
   a. Tactual observation of the stunts to be performed is desirable.

Trampoline

1. *Auditory aid*
   a. Removal of the center cables from the mat of the trampoline will assist in centering the bounce of the child. The voice of the instructor should be used to center the bounce. Verbal direction can be given with respect to the position of the person bouncing.
2. *Kinesthetic aid*
   a. The teacher should jump with the child and then inform him or her of the correct time to execute the seat drop.
   b. The child should first assume a position of land-

ing, then begin a drop from the hands and knees, progress to the feet, and, finally, execute the front drop.

Locomotor skills

1. *Aid by increase of space*
   a. Adequate room should be provided for performance. The child should be assured that there are no obstacles.
2. *Kinesthetic aid*
   a. Hopping and jumping may be taught by having the visually limited child feel the upward and downward movements of a classmate.
   b. The visually limited child should link arms with two classmates who skip forward until the rhythm of the movement is developed and it becomes possible for the child to skip alone.

Swimming

1. *Kinesthetic aid*
   a. As in land skills, kinesthetic orientation is a good instructional tool for achieving proficiency in most of the swimming skills.
   b. Manual guidance of the participant's body and limbs and tactual observation of a sighted swimmer's skills are valuable instructional tools. When teaching swimming to the visually limited, adaptive and lead-up techniques are useful.
   c. Walking in the water is a lead-up activity to the "flutter kick."
   d. The "dog paddle," as a lead-up activity to the "American crawl," provides tactual stimulation of both arms and legs throughout the entire stroke.
   e. Kickboards and flotation devices are of great value, for they give support to the body and make it possible for the child with a vision loss to explore the environment in the water.
   f. The child should be supported under the shoulder blades to assist floating on the back.
   g. A slide provides assistance for entry into the water.
   h. Guide ropes assist swimmers in staying in their lanes and prevent them from bumping the edge of the pool.
   i. Handrails are useful for orientation when mounted near the sidewalls.
   j. The diving board should be covered with nonslippery material.
2. *Auditory aid*
   a. Auditory cues should be used to inform the visually limited child when to make a turn while swimming.
   b. Belt flotation devices or support around the waist gives confidence to the child when treading water.
   c. In water entries, the visual limitation of a student

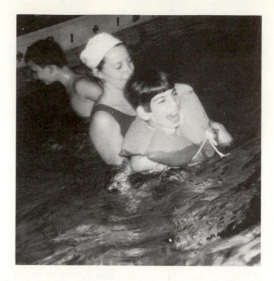

Fig. 14-3. Kinesthetic aid to assist in orienting a person to the water. (Courtesy of Carolyn Williams, Handicapped Swim Program, Slippery Rock State College, Slippery Rock, Penn.)

requires that the progression necessary for achievement of a successful dive be in small increments. The first step should be an attempted entry from the steps of the pool, followed by a jump from the deck, and then a headfirst entry with the instructor holding both hands of the diver with one hand and holding correct head position with the other hand. This should be followed by the unassisted headfirst entry.

DEAFNESS AND IMPAIRED HEARING

Hearing is one of the strongest lines of communication between persons and the world in which they live. Children who have permanent hearing impairments are afflicted with handicaps that often have an impact on their total development, adjustment, and personality. The responsibility of meeting the special needs of such children requires the cooperation and skills of many disciplines. The purpose of this section is to provide a background into the nature and needs of those who are deaf and hard-of-hearing and to discuss the role of physical education in meeting these needs as part of the total educational process.

Hearing is subjective in that two persons experiencing the same sound will attach different meanings to the sound. Similarly, the meanings attached to impaired hearing by scientists and by educators who work with deaf and hard-of-hearing individuals differ. Therefore, it seems desirable to examine the implications of hearing loss as viewed by these two disciplines.

Science's concern for hearing loss is with regard to two objective measures that can be recorded by the audiometer. These measures are *pitch* (or tone) and *intensity* as measured by the decibel (dB).

Hearing loss plotted in decibels on a linear scale does not represent the limits of human audition. However, quantitative degrees of hearing loss may be of some value to the physical educator.

The degree of hearing impairment, in many cases, is associated with quantitative hearing loss as measured by the decibel. The following is an example of what might be expected from persons placed on various points of a hearing-loss continuum:

Loss not in excess of 15 dB does not represent any severe impairment. However, if the hearing loss is in the range of 30 dB, some impairment in communication may be evident. In the event the deficit is in the range of 50 dB, serious impairment in communication may be expected. Speech can be heard only through amplification if the decibel measurement is in the range of 75 dB loss. When the decibel range reaches 90 dB loss in the better ear, the individual is close to total deafness.[27]

The acquisition of speech and language development is basic to the subsequent development of the individual. Therefore, the time of onset of deafness is a critical factor in determining the effects that it may have on the learning situation. A child who is afflicted with a hearing loss early in development progresses more slowly than does one who is afflicted with a loss later in the developmental process.

Relevant to the education of children with auditory handicaps is the classification of hearing losses established by the Conference of Executives of American Schools for the Deaf.[6] These groupings, which have been made primarily to lay a foundation for education, are listed as follows:

1. *The deaf:* Those in whom the sense of hearing is nonfunctional for the ordinary purposes of life. This general group is made up of two distinct classes, based entirely on the time the loss of hearing occurred.
   a. *The congenitally deaf:* Those who were born deaf.
   b. *The adventitious deaf:* Those who were born with normal hearing but in whom the sense of hearing became nonfunctional later through illness or accident.
2. *The hard-of-hearing:* Those in whom the sense of hearing, although deficient, is functional with, or without, a hearing aid.[6]

Proper diagnosis of a hearing defect is very important, for the educational program may be dependent on it. Categories of deafness that should be considered in the educational planning of the student are the following:

1. *Psychogenic deafness:* A condition in which the receptive organs function adequately and there is no damage to the nervous system, but, for emotional reasons, the person does not respond to sound.
2. *Central deafness:* A condition in which the receiving mechanism of hearing is functioning properly, but an abnormality in the CNS prevents the person from hearing. This disorder is often referred to as auditory or sensory aphasia, or word deafness.
3. *Perceptive or sensorineural deafness:* A condition caused by a defect of the inner ear or of the auditory nerve in transmitting the impulse to the brain.
4. *Conductive loss:* A condition in which the intensity of sound is reduced before reaching the inner ear, where the auditory nerve begins. Since hearing loss is a problem that is multidimensional in nature, it is important that the educator form no generalized concept regarding the deaf or hard-of-hearing child without considering such relevant factors as degree of hearing loss, age of onset, and type of hearing loss.

Incidence

In the United States, there are approximately 18 million hearing-impaired individuals, 3 million of whom are children. Also, it has been estimated that 5% of school-aged children have some hearing deficiency with 1 or 2 out of 10 of this group requiring special educational attention.[35] This means that adaptive procedures must be considered in cases of hearing loss, but only a few hearing loss cases will require completely altered educational methods.

There is evidence that hearing loss is on the increase. This increase may be the result of the following factors.

1. The lengthening of the life span, accompa-

nied by deterioration of the sensory processes among the aged

2. An increase of hearing loss among infants whose lives have been saved by modern medicine but who were born with a defective hearing mechanism
3. The impairment of the hearing mechanism by the loud noises of modern technology
4. The use of more thorough identification and screening procedures to detect hearing loss among the population at large

Causes

Deafness may occur before birth, at birth, or after birth. Some hearing defects are acquired, whereas other hearing defects are hereditary in nature. Myklebust[28] found 39.1% of the incidence of deafness to be acquired, 22.6% to be hereditary, and 38.8% to be of unknown origin.

Various types of hearing impairment may result from particular causes, which may be listed as follows:

1. *Psychogenic deafness:* Personality inadequacies generally associated with neuroses or psychoses.
2. *Central deafness* (affecting the auditory pathways within the CNS): Diseases of the brain affecting the auditory pathways, such as cerebral tumor or abscess, arteriosclerosis, cerebral hemorrhage, and multiple sclerosis. Another form of central deafness is auditory aphasia, which is caused by a lesion in the cortex and association paths of the brain, preventing comprehension, concept formation, and symbolization through audition.
3. *Sensorineural impairment:* Sensorineural impairment may be a result of prenatal, natal, or postnatal causes.

Hearing tests

There are two purposes in the assessment of hearing loss. One purpose is to determine how well the person's hearing serves the process of communication; the other is to see what can be done in terms of auditory rehabilitation. The educator is mainly concerned with hearing tests for the first reason. It is desirable to have children diagnosed at the earliest possible age so that correctable defects may be cared for adequately. If this is done, the impairment will not interfere greatly with the development of the child. Gesell and Amatruda[11] have suggested the following list of signs of hearing loss:

1. *Hearing and comprehension of speech:* (a) General indifference to sound; (b) lack of response to the spoken word; (c) response to noises as opposed to words.
2. *Vocalization and sound production:* (a) Monotonal quality; (b) indistinct speech; (c) lessened laughter; (d) meager experimental sound play; (e) vocal play for vibratory sensation; (f) head banging, foot stamping for vibratory sensation; (g) yelling, screeching to express pleasure or need.
3. *Visual attention:* (a) Augmented visual vigilance and attentiveness; (b) alertness to gesture and movement; (c) marked imiativeness in play; (d) vehemence of gestures.
4. *Social rapport and adaptation:* (a) Subnormal rapport in vocal games; (b) intensified preoccupation with things rather than persons; (c) puzzled and unhappy episodes in social situations; (d) suspiciousness and alertness, alternating with cooperation; (e) marked reaction to praise and affection.
5. *Emotional behavior:* (a) Tantrums to call attention to self or need; (b) tensions, tantrums, resistance, due to lack of comprehension; (c) frequent obstinacies, irritability at not making self understood.[11]

Informal methods

The electric audiometer is the most refined instrument for the detection of hearing loss. However, informal methods may still be of use for the rough appraisal of a child's hearing. Some of the tests are as follows:

1. *The watch tick test:* A watch is brought progressively closer to the child's ear until he or she acknowledges the sound of the watch.
2. *The coin click test:* A coin is brought in contact with a hard surface that is placed progressively closer to the child's ear. It is for the purpose of detecting high-frequency losses.
3. *The conversational test:* The child is placed 20 feet from the teacher and is spoken to in a regular conversational tone. In the event the child cannot hear the examiner, the examiner moves closer and closer. If the child has difficulty hearing at 10 to 20 feet, he or she should be referred for a more thorough examination.

4. *The whisper test:* This test is administered in a manner similar to the conversational test except that the examiner uses a whisper.

The electric audiometer

Thorough assessment of auditory acuity requires the investigation of a number of different aspects of hearing. Some of the aspects of hearing evaluation are the following:

1. Testing the ability to discriminate pitch and loudness
2. Determining the ability to hear and understand speech
3. Checking sensitivity to increases in loudness
4. Determining the ability to tolerate loudness
5. Considering the possibility of functional or sensory impairment

The assessment of comprehensive hearing characteristics is beyond the training of the educator. However, the "sweep check" test, a screening test using a standard pure tone audiometer, can be administered by a nonspecialist. Six pitches (300; 500; 1,000; 2,000; 4,000; 8,000 cycles/second) are presented to the subject at an intensity of 10 to 15 dB. Failure to hear at least five of the six tones indicates a need for referral. It is possible to examine 15 to 20 persons an hour by administering this test.

Characteristics

Meyerson[27] states that most samplings in a study of deaf children revealed considerably lower scores on measures of intelligence, educational achievement, and personality than did the groups with which they were compared. However, he cautions that this should not be interpreted as convincing evidence that hearing impairment is directly or necessarily related to intelligence, educational achievement, or personality. It also has been stated that deaf children are generally from 2 to 4 years retarded educationally and that the majority of them do not complete the eighth grade. This is supported by Fusfeld,[10] who found that of 134 applicants to Gallaudet College (a college for the deaf), the median grade achievement on the Stanford achievement test was grade 9.2. It is difficult to assign meaning to much research in the education of the deaf because of the inability to control such variables as experiential and social deprivations,

institutionalization, and methods of instruction. The sensory deficit of hearing often creates a deprived environment that gives rise to unequal opportunities to explore the environment and develop and pursue interests. These inequalities probably place the child with hearing impairment in a disadvantageous position as compared with a typical child.

Developmental factors

Hearing loss that afflicts youngsters in the early phases of development impairs the total developmental process. One of the effects of deafness is to limit the children's play experience with other children. Play in the preschool years is important in learning social skills and in the development of motor skills. In play situations, deaf children are often uncertain as to the part they should play in the game, and therefore they often withdraw from participation. Thus, the role of play, which is so important to the social, psychological, and motor aspects of development in typical children, is usually limited in deaf children.

The socializing effects of play that are experienced by typical children are not experienced to the same degree by deaf children. Consequently, slower social development occurs in deaf children. It is in social maturation that the handicap of deafness is most apparent.[28] Studies have indicated that the average deaf child is retarded in social maturity as compared with the average hearing child of the same age. This retardation is probably partially caused by language inadequacy that results from the hearing loss.

Deaf children, because of their impaired ability to function socially with their peers and because of the limitations imposed on them by their restricted developmental experiences, are likely to be subjected to more strain than are hearing children. Therefore, young deaf children may be less emotionally mature than hearing children of the same age because of the greater number of frustrations they have experienced. Heider and Heider[17] report a study in which deaf and hearing children were compared in a game situation. It was observed that in situations in which pairs of typical children and pairs of deaf children interacted, there was more tendency for a hearing child to dominate the activity than for a deaf child to dominate. The games

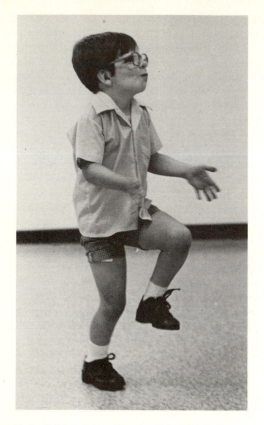

Fig. 14-4. Children with all types of handicaps need gross motor activity. (Courtesy of the Special Education Early Childhood Intervention Program, University of Kansas, Lawrence.)

played were also classified with respect to structuralization. Again, it was indicated that those of the hearing group were more highly organized and showed greater continuity of structure. These findings were interpreted as meaning that hearing children have more effective means of communication to control social situations. This study is indicative of the effects of the inability to communicate in a play situation and the resulting effect on some aspects of personality.

The age of onset of the hearing deficiency is relevant to the total developmental processes. If children do not lose their hearing until after speech has developed, they have some concept of the process of communication. However, if children are born with severe hearing impairments, they lack a valuable tool for learning and their developmental progress is usually retarded.

Case history

Case histories often provide valuable information about children with limited hearing. The following information may be of relevance to the educational process:

1. Type, amount of loss, cause, and age of onset involved in impairment
2. Psychological impact of the onset on the student and the family
3. Student's major modes of communication and problems arising from communicative limitations
4. Effects of the disability in the social, educational, recreational, and domestic spheres
5. Behavior, attitudes, achievements, and aspiration of the student
6. History of diagnostic experiences and rehabilitative measures, including special education
7. Attitudes, motivations, and problems concerning education
8. Presence of other disabilities (visual defects and organic brain damage)
9. Health and medical problems

These data, if obtainable, should provide comprehensive information and may assist the future educational and rehabilitative program.

Parent education

Parent participation in the education of a child who has a hearing loss is very important. Many parents who face rearing a child with a severe hearing impairment have little knowledge of what they can do. After the child is in school, it is important for the parents to have a general idea of how the child's hearing is developing, how basic education is progressing, and how certain aspects of the school program can be extended to the home. The purpose of parent education is to assist the parent in gaining a more realistic outlook regarding the child's future. There is general agreement that parent educational programs are necessary and that orientation is an essential part of any program for the child with impaired hearing.

Rehabilitation

Great individual differences exist among the deaf and hard-of-hearing regarding their response to various stimuli. The educational limitations caused by these individual differences must be taken into consideration. For example, persons with tinnitus (a ringing in the ears) are highly sensitive to noise and vibration and may not perform well in a noisy educational facility such as the gymnasium. Deaf children with impaired semicircular canals, which affect balance, should not climb to high places to perform. Also, some children with hearing loss should not participate in activity where there is excessive dampness, dust, or change in temperature.

Methods of training

There are two prevalent methods of educating deaf persons. They are known as *oralism* and *manualism*. The oral method involves the media of lip reading and facial gestures for communication, with no associated use of hand signs. The manual method makes use of hand signals (signing) to express thoughts. Some educators of those who are deaf and/or hard-of-hearing have stressed the importance of *total communication*. Thus, the child is taught to use the avenues of communication: lip reading, facial and body gestures, and hand signs (with verbalization, when possible).

Children with a hearing loss should be taught to make as much use of their residual hearing as possible. Teaching children with hearing loss to use what hearing they have is called *auditory training* and consists of improving listening skill. This type of training systematically develops the children's discrimination of gross sounds and rhythm patterns of speech. In addition to auditory training, which is designed to enhance the communicative process, lip reading and speech training are also used. Special skills training, as a rule, takes up little of the program time. However, some authorities believe that this form of compensatory education is the most important part of the plan to prepare hard-of-hearing children for life in a hearing world and that more time should be devoted to such programs.

A number of hard-of-hearing children are enrolled in regular physical education classes, and adaptation in instructional techniques should be made for optimal learning. Many hard-of-hearing children wear hearing aids. If this is the case, it may be best to remove the aids when vigorous physical activity is scheduled. However, once the hearing aid is removed, the students are handicapped in audition and learning, particularly through the verbal medium, so that instructional adjustments are necessary. One adjustment that can be made easily is to place the children close to the instructor so that greater amplification of speech is received. A second adjustment that may help is for the instructor to keep the face in view of the hard-of-hearing children.

When one sensory avenue to gathering information is impaired, it is necessary to rely more on other senses. In the case of children with hearing loss, visual aids are of great significance in instruction. Visual demonstrations, blackboard work, films, and slides are important instructional aids for the deaf. To get the attention of the class, waving the hands or turning off and on lights has proved effective in some instances.

Implications for physical education

The objectives in a physical education program for hard-of-hearing children are the same as those for normal children. However, loss of hearing, which impairs the ability to communicate effectively with others, is a great social handicap. Therefore, an objective that should be given priority is the provision of opportunity for social interaction through games with other students. Also, deaf children tend to have poor body mechanics and poor patterns of locomotion. Although the activities in physical education for deaf and hard-of-hearing persons are similar to those in the regular program and although deaf and hard-of-hearing persons may function well in regular programs, there is an obvious need for special and compensatory attention to those who are deaf to fulfill the objectives of the physical education program (Chapters 4 and 8).

In the preschool and early elementary school levels, suggested activities for the deaf are those that develop basic motor skills and rhythm activities. Valuable instruments for such rhythmical activities are percussion instruments such as cymbals, triangles, drums, and tambourines, for these instru-

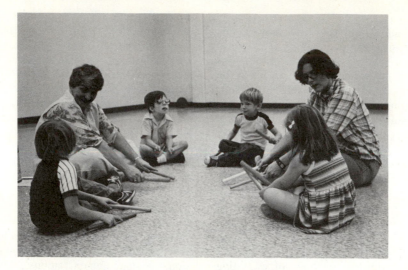

Fig. 14-5. An activity that could be used in training students for auditory perception. (Courtesy of the Special Education Early Childhood Intervention Program, University of Kansas, Lawrence.)

ments are capable of producing vibrations to which the deaf child can respond.

Deaf and hard-of-hearing children do not, as a rule, need a different set of activities from typical children. However, in many instances, because of the limitations imposed by the hearing disorder, physical and motor development may be retarded. Therefore, it is wise to be aware of possible physical underdevelopment and poor motor coordination among deaf and hard-of-hearing persons. If some children have these deficiencies, the program should try to remedy or ameliorate them. The physical education program for those who are deaf and hard-of-hearing should provide for developmental activities that have been defined in the regulations of P.L. 94-142. In addition to this curriculum, the sense of balance should be assessed carefully because, in some instances, the function of the vestibular mechanism, which is responsible for balance, may be damaged. A balance program should be designed for such students and their progress should be assessed. If children are unable to progress in overcoming this difficulty, it may be necessary to plan a program that would partially circumvent the impairment of balance. These children are often unable to hear auditory signals that

give them warnings of impending danger. It is necessary to use visual signals of warning in this instance (Chapter 3).

APHASIA (SEVERE ORAL LANGUAGE HANDICAP)

Aphasia refers to a disturbance in language behavior having an organic base. It is a defect or loss of the power of expression by speech, writing, or signs or of the power of comprehension of speech or written language. Since language behavior involves visual, perceptual, and symbolic processes, interference with any of these processes may have an effect on language. The central focus of this discussion will be on the visuomotor aspects of human development and its effects on the acquisition of language.

Aphasia can occur in both children and adults. It may be incurred (1) through trauma as the result of a direct blow to the head, (2) by a cerebral vascular accident (CVA), commonly called a *stroke,* (3) by a tumor, or (4) from a disease. In addition, severe emotional or physical trauma, excessive rejection, or total isolation can become the basis of an emotional withdrawal and can cause aphasia.

Aphasia may be reflected in perceptual disorganization, disturbance in learning, problems in secondary motor functioning, and limitations in abstracting specific language symbols.

Characteristics

Aphasic children often have difficulty in the discrimination of sound that is to be organized into words. In addition to the problems of converting auditory information into meaningful symbols, other symptoms such as impaired laterality, restlessness, inattention, emotional outbursts, distractibility, hyperactivity, hypoactivity, short attention span, aggressiveness, unusual fears, excessive gregariousness, severe to mild emotional problems, catastrophic reactions, unpredictable behavior, and unusual compulsions may be present. However, it is not uncommon for the aphasic child to demonstrate a considerable number of motor competencies.

Although in a great many severely aphasic persons extremely poor motor coordination may be present, motor difficulties often manifest themselves in poor eye-hand coordination, a failure to perform specific complex movement tasks, and awkwardness in the fundamental motor skills.

Behavioral disorders often thwart the development of language and those abilities that are prerequisite to language. Some children with aphasia show signs of distractibility and perseveration. This disintegrated behavior must be dealt with before language or the prerequisites of language can be effectively developed. For the aphasic child, it is important that the environment be constructed so that effective perception and language behaviors can be developed. These procedures are discussed in Chapter 13.

The physical educator can make a contribution to the child with aphaia through a motor development program that has the capability of assisting in the correction of perceptual distortions and motor retardation.

Maturational milestones and motor correlates

Lenneberg[20] has drawn a parallel in graphic form between language stages and motor development (Table 14-1). Motor correlates with an increase in speech capability may be associated with greater movement potential of the child. The parallel is most interesting. However, there is little scientific information on causal relationships between speech and motor development.

Implications for physical education

Children with any disorder should be permitted to participate in physical activity that is commensurate with their abilities. In the case of aphasic children, on many occasions, the physical prerequisites for participation in activity are present. If this is the case, then vigorous activity to enhance the physical motor and perceptual capabilities should be employed by the physical educator.

The nature of the handicapping condition of aphasia is one that primarily involves communicative skills. An important part of the teaching process utilized by the teacher to aid the aphasic learner involves the use of precise symbols for communication. The following teaching suggestions are made to the instructor of the aphasic child:

1. Use a few simple words with gestures to communicate objectives.
2. Specify what the child is to do with precision.
3. Use a multisensory approach to communicate with the child.
4. Be consistent with the signaling system. In the event that this is not done, there may be a discrepancy between inputs that require the same behavior on different occasions.
5. Repeat the instruction of tasks to be learned, if necessary.
6. Provide opportunity and time for the child to process information and do not expect quick responses to instructions.

Programming

The physical education program for the aphasic child should be designed for perceptual-motor development and the development of language through physical activity or movement. The child should also learn the concepts and ideas that stand for the word or words relating to a specific activity or movement.

The perceptual-motor evaluation can be of assistance for an educational therapist in the remediation of language disorders. Many assessment tools

Table 14-1. Maturational milestones, motor correlates, and language development

Age (months)	Language stage	Motor development
3 to 4	Coos and chuckles.	Supports head in prone position. Responds to human sounds by turning head in direction of sound source.
6	Exhibits babbling, resembling one-syllable utterance. Makes identifiable combinations such as "ma," "da," "di," "du."	Sits without props, uses hands for support.
8	Exhibits some echolalia.	Stands by holding onto object. Grasps with thumb opposition.
10	Exhibits distinct echolalia, which approximates sounds heard. Responds differentially to verbal sounds.	Creeps efficiently. Pulls to standing position. May take a side step while holding on to a fixed object.
12	Reduplicates sounds in echolalia, possibly first words for identification. Responds appropriately to simple sounds.	Crawls. May stand alone. May walk when held by one hand or may even take steps.
18	Possesses repertoire of 3 to 50 words, some two-word phrases. Reveals intonational patterns through vocalizations. Experiences great increase in understanding of language.	Walks with ease. Runs. Can build two-block tower. Begins to show hand preference.
24	Possesses vocabulary of 50 or more words for naming and for bringing about events. Utilizes two-word phrases of own formulation.	Can walk up or down stairs. Plants both feet on each step.
30	Experiences vocabulary growth proportionately greater than at any other period of life. Speaks with clear communicative intent. Makes conventional sentences (syntax) of three, four, and five words. Still includes many infantilisms in articulation. Exhibits good comprehension of speakers in surroundings.	Can jump. Can stand on one foot. Exhibits good hand and finger coordination. Can build six-block tower.
36	Possesses vocabulary that may exceed 1,000 words. Demonstrates syntax much like that of older person in surroundings.	Runs proficiently. Walks up and down stairs alternating feet. Has established hand preference.
48	Demonstrates linquistic system essentially like that of adults in environment, except for articulation (phenomic production). May begin to develop own "rhetorical" style of favorite words and phrases.	Can hop on one foot (usually right). Can throw a ball to an intended receiver. Can catch a ball in the arms.

Modified from Lenneberg, E. H.: Biological foundations of language, New York, 1966, John Wiley & Sons, Inc.

may overlap in their design. Some tests that may be of value are the following:

1. *Goodenough Draw-A-Man Test*[12]*:* The child is scored on the details of drawing a man.
2. *The Purdue Perceptual Motor Survey*[33]*:* The child performs gross motor activities that assess the body schema, copy-of-design tests, and oculomotor ability.
3. *The Oseretsky tests*[31]*:* This scale is composed of six separate items with chronological age norms. The scale measures general static coordination, dynamic coordination of the hands, general dynamic coordination, motor speed, simultaneous voluntary movements, and asynkinesia (inability to perform without overflow or superfluous movements).
4. Luria's[23] dynamic organization of movements, which include (a) motor tests of the

ability to reproduce rhythm, (b) tests of the ability to shift from one motor pattern to another, (c) bimanual tasks of simultaneous relationships of two hands, and (d) body image tasks.

Selected activities

There are several types of physical activity that may be used to assist postulated prerequisites of speech development. These include gross motor and fine motor skills that involve auditory, visual, and tactile stimulation. The training activities listed here may provide a base for sequential programming. For a program to become effective, it must possess a sequence of activities capable of reaching learners at their present levels of educational performance. Instructional programming techniques may be applied to most of the activities discussed in this section.

Gross motor activities. Gross motor activities may include any of the following fundamental motor patterns and skills:

1. Running, skipping, hopping, or leaping to auditory inputs
2. Jumping over obstacles or on patterns with a specific command
3. Executing locomotor tasks with the eyes closed
4. Executing balancing tasks with the eyes closed
5. Starting and stopping on command
6. Ascending stairs to an auditory beat
7. Throwing and catching on command
8. Kicking and throwing for accuracy

Visual memory tasks. Visual memory tasks may include either of the following:

1. Superimposing cut-out body parts with a corresponding outline and drawing them in on a blank circle
2. Reassembling an outlined figure that has been cut apart

Identification of body parts. Identification of body parts may include any of the following:

1. Kicking a ball with the foot
2. Slapping a ball with the hand
3. Rolling a ball up the arm
4. Tapping a ball with the fingers
5. Dropping a ball on the toes

Training children with impaired perceptions

For the majority of children with aphasia, it is desirable to include activities that involve conversation. Activities should involve small groups of children and simple motor patterns that will initiate conversation before, during, and after the actual activity or movement.

It has been suggested that a basic or fundamental list of words (minimum of 35 words to be sufficient) be developed or worked on with the aphasic child. This basic list consists of words such as *over, under, across, top, bottom, right, left, up, down, forward, backward, front, back, side, through, around, slow,* and *fast*. It is also recommended that these words be posted on a bulletin board or written on the blackboard so that certain words may be assigned on a particular day.

Using this basic word list, the child can then be asked such things as "Tell me how many," "How are you moving?" "Who is moving?" Once the aphasic child can understand and demonstrate these fundamental words and clearly understand their meaning, it is time to build on this basic list of words. Additional words can then be added to the list, increasing the complexity of the phrases, for example, (1) rub hands, (2) rub hands fast, (3) rub hand very fast, (4) John, rub your hands very fast, and (5) John, I want you to rub your hands very fast. A child might be asked to (1) stand up, (2) walk to the door, (3) jump up and down three times, (4) come back to the chair, and (5) sit down.

Visual perceptual training. The aphasic child must be able (1) to form visual relationships to change direction when needed in motor performance, (2) to organize and synthesize the peripheral and focal visual fields, and (3) to translate into movement that which is perceived. Some suggested activities to achieve these goals are stacking blocks, stringing beads, performing pegboard activities, stacking rings on pegs, turning the pages of a book, pulling off socks, and lacing a shoe.

Tactile perceptual training. The inability to recognize objects through the sense of touch impairs comprehension of the environment through other sensory avenues. Some children need training in identifying objects by touch. Education in this modality will assist the total learning process.

Some suggested activities might involve identifying blocks of different shapes by having the child look at and feel each of several differently shaped blocks and, with closed eyes, identifying objects by touch. This may be done by using a ball, a doll, a top, a toy train, a piece of fruit, etc. Other activities involve tracing with the finger (guided by the teacher) around a form and then pointing to the matching space in a form board. This may be done first with the eyes open and then with the eyes closed.

Auditory perception and memory training

The motor-aphasic child may find it difficult to execute the movements indicated by spoken words because of a loss of memory in recalling the motor patterns described by speech. In such cases, there is a need to relearn word-motor patterns.

Training children with impaired auditory perception in listening and interpreting sound or speech is important. It is necessary to train first awareness and then discrimination of gross sounds. If the child has little difficulty, the teacher should proceed first to awareness and discrimination of finer sounds and then to awareness and discrimination of voice and speech. These children usually need "alerting" in responding to auditory stimuli; they must understand thoroughly what is expected of them and they need intensive practice. Some specific techniques are described below. The educator should place the children in front of a mirror so that they may watch themselves and others practice words being formed. Learning may take place by watching and imitating others. The mirror provides visual feedback that may assist in establishing relationships between the motor and auditory aspects of speech behavior. Some children may also need the assistance of a mirror or manual manipulation to learn how it feels to say the words.

The following are a few of the types of questions that might be asked of a group:

1. The children may be asked to "run and touch the fence." While the children are participating, questions may be asked such as "What are we doing?" "How are we moving?" and "Can you touch me?"
2. One or two children may be chosen to lead exercises and may be asked, "Will you do your favorite exercise?" "What exercise are we doing?" "Are we moving fast or slow?"
3. Hoops may be used and children may be asked, "Can you jump through the hoop" "Can you jump in the hoop?" "What color is the hoop?"
4. Awareness of persons in a group should be encouraged by asking, "Who is next to you?" "How many people are in the group?"
5. Perceptual questions may be asked, such as "Can you show me 'in'?" "Can you show me 'out'?" "Are you hopping on one foot or two?" "Can you tell me what you are doing?" "Can you show me 'forward' and 'backward'?"

These activities offer specific examples and demonstrate actual teaching techniques now used to help the aphasic child. A well-balanced program for the aphasic child cannot and should not be overlooked. The program should not only include activities involving language training and retraining but also activities that build and improve on the child's physical conditioning and fitness.[5]

REFERENCES

1. Adair, M.: Working with the slow-learning blind child, Int. J. Educ. Blind **17**:37-39, 1951.
2. American Foundation for the Blind: Am. Foundation Blind Bull. Legislation ser. **13**:5, 1959.
3. Bradway, K. V.: Social competence of exceptional children. III. The deaf, the blind and the crippled, J. Exceptional Child. **4**:69, 1937.
4. Buell, C. E.: Physical education and recreation for the visually handicapped, Washington, D.C., 1973, American Association for Health, Physical Education, and Recreation.
5. Carpenter, R. D.: Why can't I learn? Glendale, Calif., 1972, Regal Books.
6. Committee on Nomenclature, Conference of Executives of American Schools for the Deaf, Am. Ann. Deaf **83**:1-3, 1938.
7. Cowan, E. L., Underburg, R., and Verrillo, F. G.: Adjustment to visual disability in adolescence, New York, 1961, American Foundation for the Blind.
8. Cratty, B. J.: Movement and spatial awareness in blind children and youth, Springfield, Ill., 1971, Charles C Thomas, Publisher.
9. Facts on the major killing and crippling diseases in the United States, New York, 1971, National Health Education Committee.
10. Fusfeld, I.: The academic programs of schools for the deaf, Volta Rev. **57**:63-70, 1955.
11. Gesell, A., and Amatruda, C. S.: Developmental diagnosis, New York, 1957, Harper & Row, Publishers.

12. Goodenough, F. L.: Draw-A-Man Test, Chicago, 1934, World Book Encyclopedia Co.
13. Greaves, J. R.: Helping the retarded blind, Int. J. Blind **23:**163-164, 1953.
14. Hanninen, K. A.: Teaching the visually handicapped, Columbus, Ohio, 1975, Charles E. Merrill Company.
15. Hatfield, E. M.: Estimates of blindness in the United States, Sight Sav. Rev. **43:**69-80, 1973.
16. Hathaway, W.: Education and health of the partially seeing child, ed. 4, New York, 1950, Columbia University Press.
17. Heider, F., and Heider, G.: Studies in the psychology of the deaf, Psychol. Monogr. **53:**158-169, 1941.
17a. Kennedy, M. M., and Danielson, L. C.: Where are unserved handicapped children? Educ. Train. Ment. Retarded **13:**408-413, December 1978.
18. Kerby, C. E.: Causes and prevention of blindness in children of school age, New York, 1952, National Society for the Prevention of Blindness.
19. Kerby, C. E.: Causes of blindness in children of school age, Sight Sav. Rev. **28:**10-21, 1958.
20. Lenneberg, E. H.: Biological foundations of language, New York, 1966, John Wiley & Sons, Inc.
21. Lowenfeld, B.: Creative and mental growth, New York, 1952, Macmillan Publishing Co., Inc.
22. Lowenfeld, B., editor: The visually handicapped child in school, New York, 1973, John Day Company.
23. Luria, A.: Higher cortical functions in man, New York, 1966, Basic Books, Inc., Publishers.
24. Maxfield, K. E., and Field, H.: The social maturity of the visually handicapped preschool child, Child Dev. **13:**1-27, 1942.
25. Menninger, C. A.: Mental effects of deafness, Psycholanal. Rev. **11:**144-155, 1924.
26. Moore, M. W., and Peabody, R. L.: A functional description of the itinerant teacher of visually handicapped children in the Commonwealth of Pennsylvania, Pittsburgh, 1976, School of Education, University of Pittsburgh.
27. Meyerson, L.: A psychology of impaired hearing. In Cruickshank, W. M. editor: Psychology of exceptional children in youth, Englewood Cliffs, N.J., 1955, Prentice-Hall, Inc.
28. Myklebust, H. R.: The psychology of deafness, New York, 1960, Grune & Stratton, Inc.
29. Norris, M. S., and Brody, R. H.: Blindness in children, Chicago, 1957, University of Chicago Press.
30. Oliver, J. N.: Blindness and the child's sequence of development, J. Health Phys. Educ. Rec. **41:**37-39, 1970.
31. Oseretsky, N. A.: Metric scale for studying the motor capacity of children. In Lassner, R.: Annotated bibliography of the Oseretsky test of motor proficiency, J. Consult. Clin. Psychol. **12:**37-47, 1948.
32. Reynolds, M., and Birch, J.: Teaching exceptional children in all America's schools, Reston, Va., 1977, Council for Exceptional Children.
33. Roach, C., and Kephart, N. E.: The Purdue Perceptual Motor Survey, Columbus, Ohio, 1965, Charles E. Merrill Publishing Co.
34. Scholl, G. T.: Understanding and meeting development needs. In Lowenfeld, B. editor: The visually handicapped child in school, New York, 1973, The John Day Company.
35. Seashore, C. E., and Ling, T. L.: The comparative sensitiveness of blind and seeing persons, Psychol. Monogr. **25:**148-149, 1918.
36. Sherrill, C.: Adapted physical education: a multidisciplinary approach, Dubuque, Iowa, 1976, William C. Brown Co.
37. U.S. Department of Health, Education, and Welfare, Federal Register (August 23) 1977, pp. 42474-42518.
38. Werchel, P., Mauney, J., and Andrew, J. G.: The perception of obstacles by the blind, J. Exp. Psychol. **40:**746-751, 1950.

RECOMMENDED READINGS

Agranowitz, A., and McKeown, M. R.: Aphasic handbook for adults and children, Springfield, Ill., 1964, Charles C Thomas, Publisher.
Bauman, M. K., and Yoder, N. M.: Adjustment to blindness re-viewed, Springfield, Ill., 1966, Charles C Thomas, Publisher.
Buell, C. E.: Physical education for blind children, Springfield, Ill., 1966, Charles C Thomas, Publisher.
Cruickshank, W. M., and Johnson, G. O.: Education of exceptional children and youth, Englewood Cliffs, N.J., 1971, Prentice-Hall, Inc.
Daniels, A. S., and Davies, E. A.: Adapted physical education, New York, 1975, Harper & Row, Publishers.
Haring, N. G., and Schiefelbusch, R. L., editors: Methods in special education, New York, 1975, McGraw-Hill Book Co.
Hirst, C. C., and Michaelis, E.: Developmental activities for children in special education, Springfield, Ill., 1972, Charles C Thomas, Publisher.
Kesster, J. W.: Psychopathology of childhood, Englewood Cliffs, N.J., 1966, Prentice-Hall, Inc.
Myklebust, H. R., editor: Progress in learning disabilities, New York, 1975, Grune & Stratton, Inc.
Roberts, A. C.: The aphasic child: a neurological basis for his education and rehabilitation, Springfield, Ill., 1966, Charles C Thomas, Publisher.

15

Mental retardation

It is now recognized that mental retardation is not a fixed, unalterable condition that condemns an individual to a static, deprived lifetime of failure to achieve. Rather, today we understand that cognitive, psychomotor, and affective behaviors are dy-namic processes that, if properly stimulated, can develop further than ever before imagined. Early concepts of mental retardation viewed the condition as an inherited disorder that was essentially incurable. This notion gave rise to hopelessness on the part of professionals and resulted in social and physical separation of those who were mentally retarded. After years of research and innovative programming it is now recognized that intelligence and other functions are dependent upon the readiness and experience of the child, the degree and quality of environmental stimulation, and many other variables. Given the knowledge available today, there is no justification for unilaterally relegating the mentally retarded person to a life of inactivity and isolation. However, difficulties faced by the mentally retarded population change as society changes. Thirty years ago society was more agrarian than it is today. Intellectual and social demands of the agrarian society differ markedly from a technological structure. The complexities of the modern social order make it much more difficult for the mentally retarded to cope successfully. It is becoming evident that all of our advanced knowledge and skill about enhancing functioning must be provided to prepare mentally retarded children to interact optimally in contemporary society.

DEFINITION OF MENTAL RETARDATION

In 1973 the American Association on Mental Deficiency (AAMD)[12] redefined mental retardation as follows: ''Mental retardation refers to subaverage general intellectual functioning existing concurrently with deficits in adaptive behavior, and manifested during the developmental period.''

Terms used in the definition have important implications for all educators working with the mentally retarded, because they project the dynamic nature of the condition. Specifically, the following concepts should be noted:

Mental retardation: This term implies a slowness in development rather than the static descriptors used historically, such as amentia, feeblemindedness, mental deficiency, mental subnormality, idiocy, imbecility, and moronity.

Subaverage: The mental retardate's functioning is lower than normative expectancies for the society. That is performance is more than one standard deviation below the mean of a given age group on a standarized IQ measure.

General intellectual functioning: Determination of intellectual functioning requires an assessment of overall cognitive performance on one or more of the various objective tests developed for that purpose.

Deficits in adaptive behavior: Adaptive behavior is the ability to cope with the natural and social demands of the environment. A deficit exists when a person lacks average ability to adjust responses to environmental demands. Inability to effectively modify behavior may result from any or all of the following: (1) a delay in acquiring early perceptual-motor skills that are prerequisite to commanding physical and intellectual tasks; (2) a lack of knowledge because of limited experience; and (3) a lack of understanding of social behaviors needed to maintain oneself in the community, in gainful employment, and during exchange with other members of the community.

Manifested during the developmental period: The fact that behavior is an orderly predictable sequence is acknowledged in this phrase. It is generally agreed that the developmental period refers to the first 16 years of life. Sometimes slow development is evident during infancy. Delayed sitting, crawling, and walking are often the first clues that a child may be mentally retarded. However, slowness in acquiring knowledge may not become apparent until a child reaches school age and his or her performance is compared with that of others in a structured group setting.

Inherent the 1973 definition is that mental retardation is simply a slowness to demonstrate performance levels expected from the majority of persons of a given age. Gone are the inferences that the mental retardate is ''stuck'' at a certain age level, that social interaction is undesirable, and that development of cognitive, psychomotor, and affective abilities is not possible. Rather, we are provided an image of a condition that slows the development of an individual along a continuum. Given this definition, the educator's role becomes one of utilizing appropriate techniques to ensure the greatest possible progress for the mentally retarded student.

Implications for physical education

Within the framework of the definition mentioned, the term *mental retardation* is descriptive of the current status of an individual with respect to the two basic criteria of adaptive behavior and intellectual functioning as measured by IQ. It can be seen that a person may meet these criteria of mental retardation at one time in life and not at another. This is often the case with many of the higher grade mentally retarded persons. In many instances, they are not known to be retarded before they enter school and are assimilated into society after school. It is only after they have failed to meet the academic standards set by the public schools that they are placed in special education classes and labeled retarded. After leaving school, they are often employed in the community and become relatively indistinguishable from the normative population. Under the new definition, a sharp rise in the incidence of mental retardation occurs during the school years, with a regression of incidence in the adult years, when these persons are functioning in society. The incidence is great at grade six because many children are unable to achieve an academic level beyond this point.

It is important to note that this definition requires the association of two basic criteria—adapted behavior and subaverage IQ—before a person is termed mentally retarded. The physical educator must examine the components contributing to mental retardation and remediate or ameliorate them. The physical educator can assist the adaptive behavior of the mentally retarded individual by developing and implementing perceptual-motor training programs. This is reported to enhance the utilization of the senses for better cognitive learning (Chapter 3).

Deficits in adaptive behavior

As was indicated earlier in this chapter, deficits in adaptive behavior may result from maturational delays, limited learning experience, and/or a lack of social skill. The physical educator is able to intervene in these areas and in so doing contribute to the mentally retarded person's development.

In the preschool years, the adaptive behavior criterion for mental retardation rests heavily on sensorimotor development. There is impressive evidence that early motor development is central to the whole developmental process. Kephart[15] expressed concern that modern technology is decreasing opportunities for random motor experimentation to assist in developing the senses. In addition, it has been observed that more severely mentally retarded children lack the basic motor skills and/or desire to explore their physical surroundings. It becomes increasingly apparent that sensorimotor programs designed to facilitate basic motor development are crucial to these children's ability to interact with their environments. Current trends to offer physical education programs to facilitate sensorimotor development of preschool children (particularly in culturally deprived areas where the incidence of mental retardation is relatively high) show great promise. The earlier the potentially retarded person is identified through motor evaluation techniques and appropriate intervention is implemented, the greater the motor development progress. Benefits in learning ability can also be expected to accrue.

Implications for learning

There is growing evidence that early generalized basic motor skills are the forerunners of spatial relationships and other symbolic representations that may lay the foundations for elementary school learning. If this proves to be the case, physical education in the preschool years may be crucial in the prevention of learning problems for persons who demonstrate motor development delays. Early educators of mentally retarded persons approached education through development of the senses. It was believed that by bombarding the peripheral nervous system with sensory stimuli, pathways leading to the CNS (where perception takes place) would be opened. Some of those early techniques can be found in contemporary perceptual-motor development theories; however, explanations for their use differ. Benefits are believe to result from altering thresholds of sensory receptors and/or facilitating chemical action at synaptic junctions. Regardless of the underlying belief, there is some evidence in the literature that physical education programs raise the IQ scores of the mentally retarded.[18] This would suggest a positive contribution to a child's ability to learn and hence to perform more favorably in a cognitive learning situation. Additional research of the effect of physical activity on intellectual functioning in retarded persons is needed. A direct benefit more readily observed is the value of motor proficiency in contributing to social interaction of the mentally retarded.

Implications for social adjustment

Social adjustment as a qualifying condition of mental retardation refers to the individual's ability to function independently in the community, to maintain gainful employment, and to meet personal and social responsibilities.

Because the mentally retarded will most likely use motor skills, rather than intellectual skills, in the pursuit of a vocation and because progress has been reported in the development of motor skills among the mentally retarded, motor proficiency has vocational implications for the mentally retarded. Increased motor proficiency may lead to such job possibilities as simple crafts or manual labor, domestic work, routine industrial work such as assembly and production line operations, and agricultural work. There is a need for identifying common psychomotor functions present in many vocations. Programs for the development of motor abilities that have vocational implications and would lead to a higher level of employability for those who are mentally retarded are greatly needed.

Motor proficiency also has implications for the social and recreational activities of mentally retarded persons. The physical educator is a primary source for the development of leisure skills in the mentally retarded. Typical persons have intellectual resources from which to draw for recreational experiences. These recreational experiences may include reading, opera, lectures, and social gatherings that have a high component of verbalization. On the other hand, mentally retarded persons are limited in the intellectual sphere and must draw heavily on motor activity for recreational experiences. For this reason, programs of physical education that carry over to recreational motor skills applicable to adult living are of the utmost importance for the mentally retarded. Recreational activity can contribute to the physical, social, and psychological aspects of self-satisfying living for mentally retarded individuals.

Implications for personal-social factors

The definition of mental retardation proposes by AAMD lists three personal-social factors that may contribute to the adaptive behavior criterion of mental retardation. They are impairment in interpersonal relations, responsiveness, and cultural conformity. It is well accepted among physical educators that one of the basic objectives of a physical education program is the development of personal-social aspects of living. Therefore, conscientious programs of physical education that fulfill this objective appear to be tools for ameliorating the adaptive behavior criterion of mental retardation.

Impairment in interpersonal relations reflects deficiencies in the individual's ability to relate adequately to peers or authority figures. It may also demonstrate an inability to recognize the needs of other persons in interpersonal interactions. The activities of physical education programs afford great opportunities for the development of interpersonal relations through participation in the games of our culture. It is accepted that many of the team games of current physical education programs require that an individual sacrifice personal feelings for the good of the group and to play cooperatively in order to reach common goals. It is often necessary that the individual relate to an authority figure to achieve the goals of an activity. The authority figure may be the official of the contest or the teacher. Development of these personal-social traits lies at the heart of the physical education program.

Deficient responsiveness is characterized by an inability to delay gratification of needs and to strive for long-range goals. It is also marked by unresponsiveness to stimuli other than the biological and physical stimuli of comfort or discomfort. In physical activity, it is often necessary for persons to withstand some discomfort to achieve a skill that they have never before been able to perform. This might be the case in learning to swim, tumble, catch a ball, or maintain any type of activity relating to endurance. Inability of mentally re-

tarded children to persist at a physical task was illustrated by Auxter.[2] When mentally retarded children were to sustain a maximum muscular contraction on a hand dynamometer, it was found that they were significantly less capable than were the typical children with whom they were being compared. Since psychological limits are reached more quickly than are physiological limits, it may well be that the will to sustain activity contributes more to fatigue in a task than does physiological endurance. Physical education programs for mentally retarded individuals may well provide the media for reducing their unresponsiveness and contribute to the amelioration of the adaptive behavior criterion.

Deficiencies in cultural conformity reflect behavior that does not conform to social mores or meet standards of dependency, reliability, and trustworthiness. They also refer to behavior that is persistently asocial, antisocial, or excessively hostile. Physical education programs, as well as all other programs of education, attempt to transmit desirable characteristics through their programs.

Implications for sensorimotor factors

In addition to personal-social factors contributing to the maladaptive behavior of the mentally retarded, impairment of sensorimotor factors contributes to the inability of persons to adapt their behavior. Reference to impairment in sensorimotor skills is made by the AAMD to disabilities, either gross or fine, in motor coordination. The development of sensorimotor skills of the mentally retarded individual lies within the domain of the physical educator. Indeed, this is one of the primary objectives of the physical education program. In the preschool years, motor activity plays a part in developing the senses. The development of motor skills has implications for the educational, vocational, social, and recreational activities of mentally retarded persons and is certainly a contributing factor to the criterion of impaired adaptive behavior.

Although the available research reports a discrepancy in scores between retardates and normal individuals on motor tasks, significant improvement has been reported in multiple trial motor learning tasks.[5,11,14] This leads to the speculation that physical education programs for the mentally retarded, if conscientiously constructed and implemented, may be of consequence to the amelioration of sensorimotor deficiencies that contribute to the maladaptive behavior criterion of mental retardation.

CLASSIFICATION OF MENTALLY RETARDED PERSONS

Professionals in the field of mental retardation recognize that mentally retarded persons in the generic sense are not homogeneous in nature. Consequently, physicians, psychologists, educators, and sociologists have evolved their own methods of classification. Mentally retarded persons have been classified according to psychological criteria, educational criteria, and etiology; the classification according to etiology will not be discussed here.

Psychological classifications

The psychological classification of the AAMD considers primarily different degrees in mental retardation based on psychological evaluations. These groups are identified in terms of sigma scores on a psychological examination or IQ test. The classification of AAMD using the Stanford-Binet intelligence test as a guide is as follows:

1. Profoundly retarded, IQ under 19—requires complete custodial care.
2. Severely retarded, IQ 20-35—can be trained to care for some of his bodily needs; develops some language; has great difficulty in social and occupational areas.
3. Moderately retarded, IQ 36-51—usually unable to master academic skills; can be trained to perform daily routines; can usually perform in a sheltered workshop.
4. Mildly retarded, IQ 52-68—has some degree of educability in terms of reading and writing; is educable in the area of social and occupational competence.[12]

Educational classifications

The terms *educable* and *trainable* are used to describe the mentally retarded children in special classes in the public schools. The characteristics of educable children compare favorably with those of children described as borderline and mildly retarded in the psychological classification. The IQ range may be anywhere from 50 to 80 or higher, depending on the legislation of the particular state and the administrative procedures of the particular school. The problem of differentiating between the children to be educated in regular classes and those to be placed in special classes for mentally retarded children is one of paramount importance. The current trend in legislation in some states is for inclusion of educable mentally retarded children in regular classes (mainstreaming). The integrated concept requires that physical education teachers utilize new instructional procedures to accommodate differences in learning styles and performance variability.

The IQ scores of trainable children are usually between 36 and 51 (moderately retarded). The differences between trainable and educable mentally retarded children are that many educable mentally retarded children may be expected to live independently in the community, whereas trainable children, more than likely, will work within the environment of a sheltered workshop. Educable mentally retarded children are capable of learning some academic skills, but trainable mentally retarded children are usually severely limited. Furthermore, recent legislation has declared that every child, regardless of level of functioning, has the right to an education. Therefore, many children who are profoundly and severely mentally retarded have been enrolled in public schools where their educational needs must be met. Nearly all the needs of the profoundly mentally retarded are physical and motor. Therefore, modification of the physical education curriculum and of procedures for developing trained personnel is a critical need (Fig. 15-1).

PROGRAMS FOR MENTALLY RETARDED PERSONS

Physical education programs should be based on the nature and needs of the learner. As mentioned previously, there is great variability among the mentally retarded population. This is attributable to inherent differences between high-grade and low-grade retardates, causations, and many other disorders that accompany mental retardation.

Associated disorders accompanying mental retardation may be sensory impairments such as blindness, being hard-of-hearing, or deafness; emotional disturbances; and neurological disorders such as cerebral palsy, muscular dystrophy, and problems in perception. It becomes evident that physical education programs for mentally retarded persons must meet a multitude of needs at all age levels

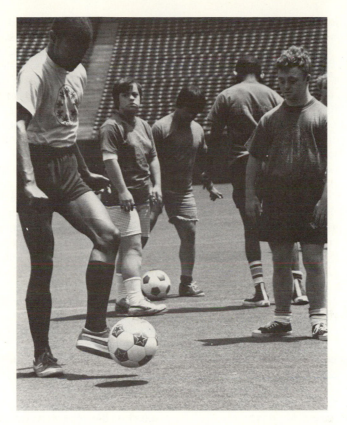

Fig. 15-1. Mentally retarded persons preparing for soccer in the Special Olympics. (Courtesy of the Joseph P. Kennedy Jr. Foundation, Special Olympics, Washington, D.C.)

and at all levels of intellectual and physical development.

Differential diagnosis

It is a prevalent practice for the placement of children in special classes to be based on IQ. However, great differences exist among children who have the same IQ. Therefore, the physical educator must be more concerned with the individual than with a tag that is designed for educational expediency. To understand the individual, the following suggested areas of diagnosis are listed:

1. *Consideration of associated disorders that accompany mental retardation:* Special educational techniques should be developed for slow learners who have partial sensory impairments and for children who are retarded deaf, retarded blind, retarded psychogenic, and retarded with cerebral palsy.

2. *Neurological evaluation:* Electroencephalogram, neurological reflexes should be checked.

3. *Psychomotor examination:* Reaction time, speed of limb movement, aim, hand steadiness, and manual and finger dexterity are evaluated.

4. *Perceptual assessment:* Perceptual disorders may be disruptive in the learning of motor skills. The Frostig developmental scales[9] and the Kephart perceptual motor survey[15] should be employed for evaluation.

5. *Physical fitness test:* AAHPER physical fitness test and Fleishman's physical fitness test may be used.

6. *Motor fitness test:* Measures that include basic motor skills such as running, jumping, and throwing are needed.
7. *Motor development scales:* The Gesell developmental scales[10] are recommended for young learners. The Bruininks-Oseretsky Test of Motor Proficiency[4] is appropriate for learners from $4^1/_2$ to $14^1/_2$ years of age.
8. *Etiology:* The individual with an organic condition may be more severely retarded in the motor sphere than the cultural-familial retarded person.

Retardation in culturally deprived areas

Special programs must be designed for preschool children who show motor or mental retardation. Infants who are slow to develop head lifting and body righting movements can benefit from exercises described in *The Baby Exercise Book*.[16] For the mentally retarded child, the baby exercises should be followed by a program of motor exploration with early training in self-help skills and locomotor development. Physical education programs to serve preschool potentially retarded persons in culturally deprived areas have been described by Kephart.[15] The Kephart programs are designed to develop generalized motor patterns, hand-eye coordination, and body image.

Programs for developing preschool motor skills

There are many mentally retarded children who function on motor skills at a preschool level. Mentally retarded children classified as trainable often fall into this group as do young educable mentally retarded children of the primary group. The basic needs of this particular group of mentally retarded children are management and control of the whole body. Therefore, the program should be directed toward building a large repertoire of movement skills. These children should be made aware of the body in relation to other parts. There is a need for a great deal of random experimentation and gross body movement, particularly the exploration of gravitational forces. Activities that have proved successful at clinics for preschool mentally retarded children at Slippery Rock State College have included climbing activities on stall bars, tumbling and walking activities on an inclined board, and bouncing activities on a miniature trampoline. Gravitational forces challenge the children and exercise control of these activities. It is important to construct environments so that the children will always achieve some degree of success and still be challenged. Failure or the infliction of pain often makes subsequent participation in the activity undesirable.

One of the basic problems encountered by children in these types of activities is learning to transfer weight from one foot to the other without losing balance. One of the primary objectives of the program involving countering gravitational forces is directed toward the enhancement of weight transfer. Another component of a program for preschool children who function at a preschool level on motor skills is the development of basic locomotor and play skills serving as the foundation for more complex skills used in sports and games. These skills include running; jumping, throwing, catching, striking, and kicking. This type of training is done with a directive purpose approach where there is a low ratio of instructors to children.

Gains can be made in ocular tracking skills of preschool retarded children by the implementation of catching activities. Objects of varying weights and sizes that travel at different rates of speed are caught by the mentally retarded children. The speed of the object can be controlled and developmental programs in tracking objects can be implemented for the purpose of developing hand-eye coordination. Rhythms also have proved popular with these children.

Some teaching suggestions for preschool mentally retarded children are the following:

1. Move body parts manually to achieve desired movement patterns. (Verbal communication is difficult or impossible with some of these children.)
2. Demonstrate the activity. This is of invaluable assistance to these children.
3. Be firm, but accept the children and use a positive approach. They often show reluctance to engage in activities; however, if the environment of the activity affords them security and if they have some measure of success, the children usually respond to the initiation of the activity at subsequent times.
4. Use strong auditory and visual cues to focus attention on the task at hand for the more se-

verely retarded. Intensity of the stimulus is important to initiate and sustain activity.

5. Consider individual abilities in attention span.
6. Give encouragement when the children meet with success. However, encouragement should not be indiscriminate.
7. Keep records of progress.
8. Aim for progression in motor and social skills.

Objectives of physical education

The objectives of physical education programs for the mentally retarded are extremely important. An examination of the priority of objectives of the total curricula for typical children reveals that intellectual or academic objectives are highest on the list. It is in these endeavors that children spend the most time. The second priority of objectives favors preparation for a vocation. Typical children are taught skills to enable them to select from a variety of occupational endeavors. The objectives apparently receiving the least attention in curricula of typical children are the social and physical objectives.

When the educational objectives for mentally retarded children are examined carefully, it becomes clear that the priority of these objectives should be inverted from that of objectives for typical children. Inasmuch as trainable mentally retarded children fail in most academic tasks and educable mentally retarded children plateau in achievement of intellectual skills at an elementary level, this objective cannot be held in the same priority as for typical children. Vocationally, mentally retarded persons are usually trained for special occupations falling within their particular capabilities.

Although occupational competency is extremely important to mentally retarded persons, there is impressive evidence that motor proficiency and social skills are more often the wherewithal of a successful occupation than are intellectual abilities. Therefore, because of the extreme importance of physical and social objectives in the education of the mentally retarded, such persons must be provided with quality physical education programs. Fulfillment of social and physical development is the substance of physical education programs.

Examination of the subgroups of the mentally re-tarded with regard to educational objectives shows that it may be that the more severe the retardation, the more significant the physical objective.

P.L. 94-142 specifically states that physical education curricula must include development of physical and motor fitness, fundamental motor skills and patterns, and skills in aquatics, dance, and individual and group games and sports (including intramural and lifetime sports). Keeping that mandate in mind, some suggested objectives of physical education for mentally retarded persons are as follows:

1. *Development of physical and motor fitness.* High fitness levels should afford the mentally retarded a better opportunity to cope with the environment and give them greater will to live full lives, approaching everyday tasks with the vigor and stamina to see them through to completion.
2. *Development of fundamental motor skills and patterns.* Basic motor skills and patterns underlie the ability to control the body during any physical activity. In the case of the more severely retarded and younger mentally retarded children, activities to promote sensorimotor and self-help skills to enable them to cope with everyday living would meet this objective. In the case of the less severely retarded and older retarded individuals, mastery of basic motor skills and patterns is prerequisite to more advanced leisure time and occupational activities.
3. *Development of skills in aquatics, dance, and individual and group games and sports (including intramural and lifetime sports).* Gone are the days when the physical educator can be permitted to teach only elementary children's games to the mentally retarded. The mentally retarded population must be afforded opportunities to participate in and enjoy all types of the physical activity.
4. *Development of social skills through social interaction.* Enhancement of both intergroup and interpersonal practices in the school and in the community is vital if normalization of our retarded population is to become a reality.
5. *Emotional development.* The ability to accept oneself and others in everyday situations and

the ability to face deterring limitations are indicators of a healthy self-concept. Every opportunity must be given the retarded to develop a healthy emotional attitude.

6. *Intellectual development.* The ability to assimilate data, organize information, and remember is vital to all individuals. Even severely retarded adults have demonstrated mastery of complex rote tasks. For severely retarded children, opportunities to discriminate among colors, sizes, shapes, and sounds and to develop perceptual abilities could well provide the basis for more advanced learning.

A diagnostic prescriptive approach

Kephart[15] points out the serious consequences of preschool children who lag behind established motor developmental scales. It has been suggested that, in the early years, motor, social, emotional, and psychological development are closely related. Early diagnosis and prognosis are recommended for all children who lag behind developmental norms in the motor sphere. The diagnosis should not be a method to pin a label on a child; it should be a description of the person's needs, characteristics, abilities, and necessary remediation.

Hints for teaching

The mentally retarded are a very heterogeneous group. Many techniques of instruction are necessary to elicit a desired response. Therefore, it is difficult to make generalizations that may be helpful in the instruction of physical education activities for mentally retarded persons. However, as a guide, some teaching hints follow:

1. Consider individual differences when selecting the activities. It is possible to play many games that account for differences in abilities among class members.
2. Select activities according to the needs of the mentally retarded.
3. Select activities to meet the children's interest levels. However, precautions should be taken against participation in one particular activity to the exclusion of others. Be aware of the development of rigid play behaviors.
4. Do not underestimate the abilities of mentally retarded children to perform skilled movements. There is a tendency to set goals too low for these children. This is particularly true when working with educable mentally retarded children from cultural backgrounds.
5. Develop recreational skills that make it possible for mentally retarded children to integrate socially with peers and members of their family now and in later life.
6. Select activities primarily on the basis of the development of motor skills. In the past, mental age and chronological age have

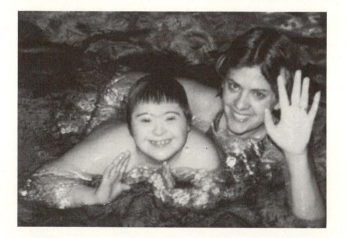

Fig. 15-2. Manual support enables a mentally retarded child to become oriented to the water. (Courtesy of Carolyn Williams, Handicapped Swim Program, Slippery Rock State College, Slippery Rock, Penn.)

played too great a part in the selection of physical activities; however, in many instances, they may be irrelevant criteria.

7. Structure the environent in which the activity takes place so that it challenges the children yet frees them from the fear of physical hurt and gives them some degree of success.

8. Lower grade mentally retarded children must be taught to play. This means that physical education is responsible for creating the play environment, developing basic motor skills that are the tools of play, and occasionally, initiating the activity.

9. The play environment must be one of safety. However, a safe play environment does not necessarily mean that the instructor should provide security to the extent that the children are unduly dependent on the instructor for physical safety.

10. Use manual guidance as a method of instruction. The proprioceptors are great teachers of movement. Manual guidance is more important in the younger and more severely mentally retarded children. The less ability the child has to communicate verbally, the greater the consideration manual guidance should have as a tool for instruction.

11. Work for progression in skill development. For preschool retardates, use the motor developmental scales; mentally retarded children functioning above the preschool level, use the progression methods commonly employed for typical children.

12. Work for active participation on the part of all mentally retarded students.

13. Adapt the activities to the abilities of *each* child. No blanket programs for the mentally retarded, as a generic group, should be used.

14. Convey to mentally retarded persons that they are persons of worth, reinforcing their strengths and minimizing their weaknesses.

15. Be patient with smaller and slower gains in more severely retarded persons. Often, gains that seem small when compared with those of typical children are tremendous for the more severely mentally retarded.

16. Use strong visual and auditory stimuli for the more severely rearded children, as these often bring the best results.

17. Have many activities available, as attention span is short.

18. Use demonstration as an effective instructional tool.

19. Keep verbal directions to a minimum. They are often ineffective when teaching more severely retarded children.

20. Provide a broad spectrum of activities that have reacreational and social significance for later life.

Physical education programs

Because of the heterogeneity of mentally retarded children, many types of programs must be developed to meet their needs. The following description of aspects of physical education programs for mentally retarded children will be broad and generalizations will be made with reference to the generic group called mentally retarded. The aspects of the physical education program to consider are development of basic skills, development of physical fitness, development of specific skills, and recreation.

Development of basic skills

The term *basic motor skills* refers to the movement patterns that occur in successive stages of development, such as crawling, creeping, walking, running, jumping, hopping, skipping, leaping, and throwing. Knowledge and application of the development of the basic skills may serve as a guide to the physical educator in identifying the current level of functioning of a particular mentally retarded child and provides information for the subsequent selection of activity.

Attention should also be given to the acquisition of gross motor movements, which, when combined, may form discernible skills. Bending, bouncing, balancing, carrying, and climbing are examples of these gross motor movements.

At the lower levels of mental retardation, the profound, severe, or moderate degree of retardation, in many cases, will determine the goals in motor development that may ultimately be achieved. In general, the more profound the retardation, the lower the limits of ultimate performance. Profoundly mentally retarded children may develop self-care skills and minimal locomotor skills.

Development of physical fitness

The development of physical fitness must occupy high priority in the objectives of a physical education program for the mentally retarded. Research has shown that the physical fitness levels of mentally retarded persons can be improved.[18] Basic components of physical fitness that have been identified and that result from vigorous physical exercise are strength, muscular endurance, flexibility, and cardiovascular endurance.

Activities contributing to the development of these characteristics of physical fitness are calisthenics, partner activities that include dual stunts, tumbling, combative games, self-testing activities, relays, games, ladders, jungle gyms, climbing ropes, jump ropes, and gymnasium apparatus.

Development of strength, muscular and cardio-

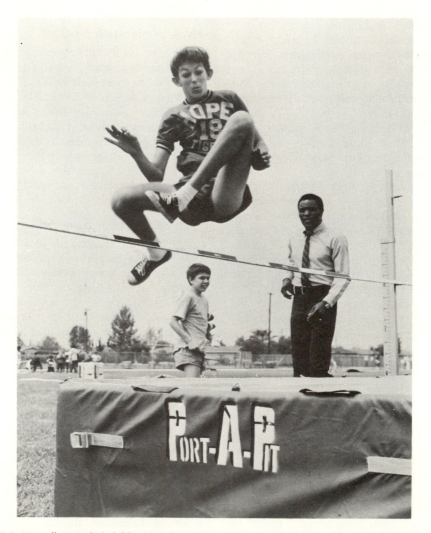

Fig 15-3. Mentally retarded children may become proficient in sports skills. (Courtesy of Western Special Olympics, California, 1971.)

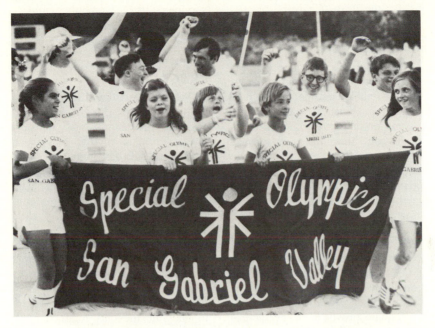

Fig. 15-4. Special Olympics receives considerable support from volunteers. (Courtesy of the Joseph P. Kennedy Jr. Foundation, Special Olympics, Washington, D.C.)

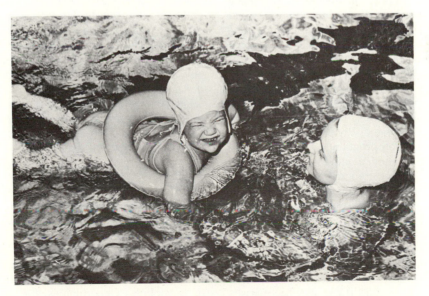

Fig. 15-5. A mentally retarded child learns what she can do in the water.

vascular endurance, and flexibility are discussed in previous sections of the text (Chapters 5, 10, and 12).

Development of specific skills

Physical education programs for mentally retarded persons should also include opportunities to develop motor skills to enable these persons to participate in sports activities. Such activities include gymnastic stunts, trampoline activity, swimming, ice skating, roller skating, bicycling, track events, wrestling, volleyball, hockey, skiing, baseball, soccer, basketball, bowling, golf, and handball. All the lead-up games that serve as forerunners to these more complex activities should be taught in small progressive units (Chapters 4 and 8).

Recreation

Recreational opportunities for mentally retarded children (Figs. 15-3 to 15-5) should be provided after the school day terminates, during school vacations, and after formal educational training. There should be adequate provision in the recreation program for vigorous activity such as sports, dancing, active games, swimming, and hiking. Intramural and community sports leagues should be provided for the purpose of using skills developed in the instructional program. In addition, winter outdoor activities such as ice skating, skiing, and snow games should be made available. Camping and outdoor education programs are other ways of affording expression of skills and interests.

In conjunction with the recreation program, special events scheduled throughout the school year serve to stimulate interests, motivate the children, and inform the community about the progress of the physical education program and about the abilities of mentally retarded children. Examples of such events are demonstrations for PTA meetings, track-and-field meets, swimming meets, play days, sports days, pass-punt-kick contests, hikes, and bicycle races.

Volunteers

When working with more severely retarded children, individual attention is often required. Volunteers trained in specific duties can be of assistance to the instructional program as well as to after-school and vacation recreation programs. Sources of recruitment for volunteers may be service clubs, women's clubs, colleges, high schools, and associations for mentally retarded persons.

SUPPLEMENTAL PHYSICAL EDUCATION PROGRAMS

Mentally retarded children should be integrated with their peers, if at all possible, in regular physical enducation classes. If they cannot participate successfully in regular classes, they should be given special developmental physical education commensurate with their capacity and needs. It is recognized that the regular physical education class may not provide adequate placement for all mentally retarded children. These children are behind the norms socially and physically to the extent that they are not motivated to participate with members of the regular class. Consequently, they are often found on the periphery of activity and do not involve themselves in the games and activities of the physical education class. An effort must be made to integrate mentally retarded persons in class activities; however, if this is not possible, special physical education programs should be adapted to the particular needs of the children.

It is also suggested that any mentally retarded children who can be successfully integrated socially in the unrestricted physical education program, but who have physical or motor deficiencies, receive supplementary physical education to remedy or ameliorate the particular diagnosed motor deficiency. Erroneous assumptions are often made relative to the physical abilities of a person labeled mentally retarded. In many instances, mentally retarded children from special classes are proficient athletes in interscholastic athletics.

EXTENDED OPPORTUNITIES BEYOND FORMAL EDUCATION

Opportunities to learn motor skills and participate in recreation utilizing those skills should be available to all persons beyond the normal years of public-sponsored education. After leaving school, children must be able to find recreation using the skills and activities taught during the formal years of schooling. Opportunities for such recreation should be available to mentally retarded persons of all ages. Physical education for the mentally retarded is a relatively recent development. Those who have been deprived of opportunities to participate and to learn motor skills should be provided with opportunities to learn these skills and to learn to utilize leisure time for physical activity. The desired aspects of physical fitness for the particular age and characteristics of a retarded person should be a part of the extended physical education program.

THE HOME PROGRAM

The amount of time that the physical educator will be involved personally with the mentally retarded children is relatively small. If maximum benefits are to be derived from programs, it is necessary to have a follow-up of activities taught in the form of a home program. Therefore, an edu-

cational program for parents describing the children's program and its purpose should be provided for implementation in the home. Parents should receive direction and assistance in methods for involving their children in physical activity taking place in the neighborhood and the home.

DEVELOPMENTAL APPROACH AND SEVERELY MENTALLY RETARDED PERSONS

Many profoundly and severely mentally retarded children, in the past, were not included in the process of public education. However, legislation and court decisions have made it mandatory that such children receive appropriate education (Chapter 1). As a result, many severely mentally impaired children with limited ability to function in motor skill

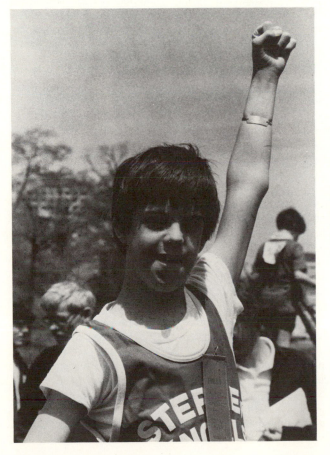

Fig. 15-6. Mentally retarded persons can achieve a sense of worth by participating in competition at their own levels of ability. (Courtesy of the Joseph P. Kennedy Foundation, Special Olympics, Washington, D.C.)

are now in our public schools. Many of these children are nonambulatory and cannot engage in self-help skills. Therefore, motor development is one of their most critical needs. Increased opportunities for physical educators to participate in the motor development of severely handicapped children constitute a great challenge.

Many severely handicapped children develop some motor skills during the first year of life. It is necessary, through assessment, to determine precisely where these childen are on a motor development continuum so that purposive programming can be structured for them.

Motor development curriculum

The curriculum for the severely handicapped child whose development progresses according to a chronological age scale in the first year of life is rather limited. For the most part, the curriculum is composed of the development of prerequisite abilities that lay the foundation for more complex skills. Often, programming involves motor behaviors determined by researchers to be landmarks in growth and development.However, before these motor landmarks can be achieved, it is necessary for the child to develop several sensorimotor prerequisites. Great precision must be exercised in the implementation of programming according to the principles of learning and development (see Chapter 3).

Accountability

The financial resources that are necessary to carry out programs for severely mentally handicapped persons are considerable. Low pupil-teacher ratios are usually required to engage these children in the instructional process. There is considerable interest in the accountability of learned behaviors of handicapped children as a result of programming. One way to account for the effects of programming on the development is to calculate as follows:

1. Administer a test to the child that can be translated in terms of rate of development.
2. Compute the rate of development (developmental age [DA] divided by chronological age [CA]).
3. Intervene with the program.
4. Compare the rate of development after the intervention with the rate at the initial evaluation for changes.

An example of this would be the following:

June, 1976 $\quad \dfrac{\text{DA 1 year}}{\text{CA 8 years}}$ OR

$$\dfrac{12 \text{ months}}{96 \text{ months}} = 0.125 \text{ rate of development}$$

June, 1977 $\quad \dfrac{\text{DA 21 months}}{\text{CA 9 years}}$ OR

$$\dfrac{21 \text{ months}}{108 \text{ months}} = 0.19 \text{ rate of development}$$

The total rate of development has increased as a result of intervention. Thus, there is a need for two types of measurement in the implementation of accountable programming. They are criterion measurement for program activities that have been achieved through programming and changes in developmental rates through intervention.

Communication of program objectives and progress

Parents and consumer advocates are concerned with the eductional progress of handicapped children. This concern is expressed in the P.L. 94-142 mandate that parents be involved in their handicapped children's Individual Educational Programs (see Chapter 1). As part of the interdisciplinary team responsible for designing the programs, the physical educator must be prepared to communicate to parents motor test results, behavioral objectives based on those test results, a proposed program of activites for the children, and progress realized. When the physical education curriculum is composed of a series of behavioral objectives linked together to achieve a desired measurable outcome, graphs simplify record keeping. Graphic information that communicates what children have gained as a result of the physical education program are easily explained to parents in behavioral terms. Such graphs also give the physical educator a pictorial indicator of the success of the intervention program. This is extremely important for personnel working with severely retarded children because it provides immediate objective information about needed program changes.

Behaviors derived from motor development scales

Bayley,[3] Gesell and Amatruda,[10] and Frankenburg and Dodds[8] have devised motor development scales and assessment tasks that indicate the developmental levels of children. The skills on these scales may be used to assess the developmental levels of severely handicapped children who function at low levels. Some of the behaviors on the developmental scales are prerequisite to others, and there is a need to identify these prerequisite behaviors so that orderly progression can be constructed within scales that can be followed in the implementation of programming.

Cephalocaudal development

Children develop from the head to the foot (cephalocaudal development).[22] The application of

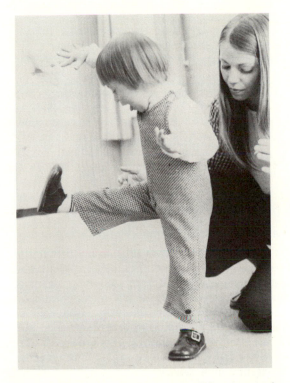

Fig. 15-7. Balancing on one foot is an ability that can be transferred to skills such as stair climbing and many other movement behaviors.

this principle of development provides guidelines to the implementation of programming for severely handicapped children because it provides the focus for programming developmental purposes. For instance, if a child can lift the head while in the prone position, it may be raised increasingly high. The increased height that the head is raised is indicative of greater development in the cephalocaudal direction because the spinal area closer to the foot is being activated. There is further need of development along this continuum when the child attempts to sit erect. It is then necessary for the child to control the musculature in the lumbar region of the spine so that the sitting behavior may be maintained. At a later point in development, control must be gained so that the hips, knees, and ankles may move with facility and locomotion may take place. Thus, strength and endurance of the musculature along the cephalocaudal continuum must be gained before the prerequisite behaviors of cephalocaudal control can be acquired. In the severely handicapped child, this is often most difficult. The skeleton and the body, which have developed through the process of maturation, often have gained weight incommensurate with the strength and endurance necessary to maintain control of the body. Therefore, programs that are designed to develop prerequisite strength and endurance are of importance (Fig. 15-7).

Proximodistal development

Another concept of development that provides guidelines for programming is the application of the principle of proximodistal development. This deals with the concept that development proceeds from the midline outward to the extremities. It is possible, through observation of children's movements, to receive information concerning the focus of where most of the programming should be directed. For instance, if most of the movement occurs at the shoulders with little movement at the elbow, the focus of the programming should be directed at the elbow, with activities that integrate the shoulder and the elbow. If the activities involve primarily movement of the elbow and shoulder, movements should be programmed that involve the wrist and that require integration of the wrist, elbow, and shoulder. Thus, the procedures involve

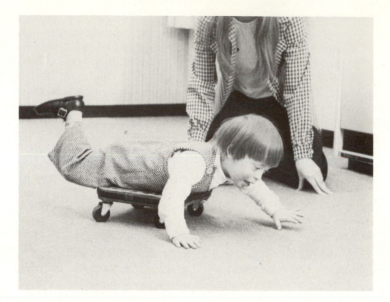

Fig. 15-8. Proximodistal development can be assessed by the movement pattern of the arms as the child moves the scooter. Some children move the scooter from the elbows, using only the shoulder muscles. Others move it with the hand, using the elbow and shoulder muscles. The more highly developed child derives force from the shoulder, elbow, and wrist. This is a higher form of proximodistal development.

observation of activity at each joint and functional integration with other joints proceeding from the proximal to the distal structures (Fig. 15-8).

Specific and general abilities. It is possible to teach specific skills that incorporate the integration of fingers, wrists, elbows, and shoulders without the application of the principle of proximodistal development. However, there may be a tendency for the skill to be specific and each such skill will have to be learned as distinct and separate. However, the development of proximodistal principles will enable the child to generalize movement patterns to acquire several skills. The facility of learning and a host of other skills will be enhanced. Therefore, there is a need to develop both specific skills and movement patterns that facilitate the development of the proximodistal principle.

Types of programs for severely handicapped children

The categories of motor programming for the severely handicapped are the following:
1. Specific skills that enable social adaptation to the environment

2. Landmark motor behaviors (crawling, creeping, sitting, rolling over, standing, walking, etc.) that serve as guidelines in development as indicated on developmental scales
3. Ability traits (strength, endurance, flexibility, balance) that serve as prerequisites for skills
4. Functional daily living skills and leisure skills that enhance life in the community.

Motor diagnosis and prescription

There must be a direct relationship between the assessment information on a target objective and the programming that will assist in reaching the stated objective. An example of diagnostic and program integrity may involve a child who has been assessed according to a developmental scale as not being able to sit erect. This becomes a target behavior and it is then necessary to direct programming that will develop the behavior of sitting. Such programming may include facilitation of the optical righting reflexes (see Chapter 3) and development of balance from a sitting position and of strength of the musculature that controls the

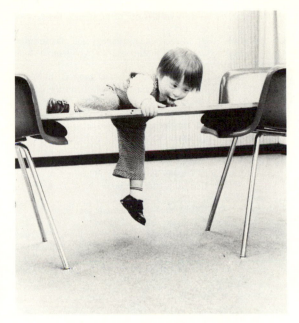

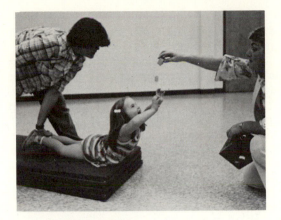

Fig. 15-10. This task is designed to develop the thoracic extensor muscles of the upper back. It is an important activity for appropriate postural development, which is lacking in many children. (Courtesy of the Special Education Early Childhood Intervention Program, University of Kansas, Lawrence.)

Fig. 15-9. The diagnosis of the ability to climb can be measured by the height of the object over which the body is to move. The programming measures increased efficiency to climb greater heights. The diagnosis and prescription must be in direct relationship to one another.

head, including thoracic and lumbar extensors of the spine. The programming would bear a direct relationship to the assessment of this particular behavior. If a child has been diagnosed as having impaired manipulative skills and cannot execute a pincer grasp, he or she should be taught to perform tasks for which the pincer grasp is used. The diagnostic test indicates the nature of the programming. The effectiveness of the programming is therefore measured by progress of the child in a positive direction from the base level performance to the target behavior (Fig. 15-10).

Hendricks[13] indicates a relationship between the development of the visual mechanism and the posturing mechanism. The development of control of the posturing mechanism enables the head to right. This affords opportunity for the visual mechanism to be appropriately placed so that it may develop. As the visual mechanism increases in capability, the posturing mechanism rights so that more environmental information may be utilized. Thus, there

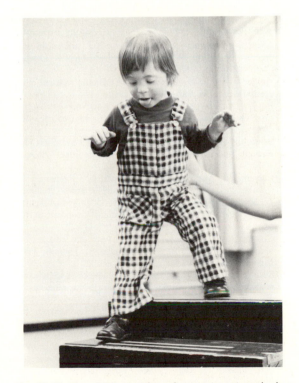

Fig. 15-11. The child's visual mechanism is activated when the eye fixates on foot placement on the stair tread.

is a need for considering the reciprocal functioning of the posturing and visual mechanism when programming (Figs. 15-11).

As the posturing mechanism is activated, it enables the visual mechanism to develop; head righting also tends to activate the manipulative activity of the child. With increased activity in the manipulation of objects, involving the hand and the eye, perceptual information about objects can be gained by pairing what is felt by the hand and what is seen by the eyes. An essential interrelationship that must be made to facilitate the development of visuomotor abilities of the severely handicapped child is the strength and endurance of the musculature that rights the body. This, in turn, places the visual mechanism where it can more efficiently function to interpret environmental objects and events. With the visual mechanism appropriately positioned, greater possibility exists for the eye to inspect the hand and for the hand to manipulate objects to gain information about the objects, leading to greater hand-eye coordination.

REFERENCES

1. Abeson, A., Bolick, H., and Hass, J.: A primer on due process: education decisions for the handicapped, Except. Child. **42**:68-74, 1975.
2. Auxter, D. M.: Muscular fatigue of mentally retarded children, Train. Sch. Bull. **63**:5-10, 1966.
3. Bayley, N.: The development of motor activities during the first three years, Monogr. Soc. Res. Child Dev. **1**:1-26, 1935.
4. Bruininks, R. H.: Examiner's manual for the Bruininks-Oseretsky Test of Motor Proficiency, Circle Pines, Minn., 1978, American Guidance Service.
5. Carrier, N., Malpass, N., and Orton, K.: Responses to learning tasks of bright, normal and retarded children, Technical bulletin, Project 578, OE-35073, Washington, D.C., 1961, U.S. Office of Education, Cooperative Research Program.
6. Cratty, B. J.: Perceptual-motor behavior and educational process, Springfield, Ill., 1969, Charles C Thomas, Publisher.
7. Delacato, C. H.: The diagnosis and treatment of speech and reading problems, Springfield, Ill., 1965, Charles C Thomas, Publisher.
8. Frankenburg, W. K., and Dodds, J. B.: The Denver Developmental Scale, Boulder, Colo., 1968, University of Colorado Medical Center.
9. Frostig, M.: Administration and scoring manual for the Marianne Frostig Developmental Test and visual perception, Palo Alto, Calif., 1964, Consulting Psychologists Press.
10. Gesell, A., and Amatruda, C. S.: Developmental diagnosis, New York, 1965, Harper & Row, Publishers.
11. Gordon, S., O'Connor, N., and Tizzard, J.: Some effects of incentives on the performance of imbeciles, Br. J. Psychol. **45**:277-287, 1955.
12. Grossman, H. J.: Manual on terminology and classification in mental retardation, Baltimore, 1973, Garamond & Pridemarks Press.
13. Hendricks, H.: The vision development process. In Wold, R. M., editor: Visual and perceptual aspects for the achieving and underachieving child, Seattle, 1969, Special Child Publications.
14. Hohman, P.: The relationship between general mental development and manual dexterity, Br. J. Psychol. **23**:279-283, 1933.
15. Kephart, N. C.: The slow learner in the classroom, Columbus, Ohio, 1961, Charles E. Merrill Publishing Co.
16. Levy, J. R.: The baby exercise book, New York, 1975, Pantheon Books.
17. Lindsley, O.: Direct measurement and prosthesis for retarded behavior, J. Educ. **148**:57-79, 1965.
18. Oliver, J. H.: The effects of physical conditioning exercises and activities on the mental characteristics of educationally subnormal boys, Br. J. Educ. Psychol. **28**:155-165, 1958.
19. Strauss, A. A., and Kephart, N. C.: Psychopathology and education of the brain-injured child, New York, 1955, Grune & Stratton, Inc.

RECOMMENDED READINGS

Bureau of Special Education, Pa.: Challenge to change program guidelines in physical education for the mentally retarded, Harrisburg, Pa., 1972, Pennsylvania Department of Education.

Cratty, B. J.: Developmental sequences of perceptual-motor tasks, Freeport, N.Y., 1967, Educational Activities, Inc.

Cruickshank, W. M., editor: Psychology of exceptional children and youth, Englewood Cliffs, N.J., 1971, Prentice-Hall, Inc.

Drowatsky, J. N.: Physical education for the mentally retarded, Philadelphia, 1971, Lea & Febiger.

Fait, H. F.: Special physical education, Philadelphia, 1972, W. B. Saunders Co.; visual, 59; auditory, 72; orthopedic, 83; cardiopathic, 97, 113-144; mentally retarded, 190; socially maladjusted, 212-225; learning disabled, 168-182.

Gallahue, D. L., Werner, P. H., and Luedke, G. C.: A conceptual approach to moving and learning, New York, 1975, John Wiley & Sons, Inc.

Hirst, C. C., and Michaelis, E.: Developmental activities for children in special education, Springfield, Ill., 1972, Charles C Thomas, Publisher.

Kirk, S. A.: Educating exceptional children, Boston, 1972, Houghton Mifflin Co.

Kirk, S. A., and Weiner, B. B.: Behavioral research on exceptional children, Reston, Va., 1963, The Council for Exceptional Children.

Recreation and physical activity for the mentally retarded, Reston, Va., 1966, The Council for Exceptional Children and American Alliance for Health, Physical Education, and Recreation.

Wedemeyer, A.: Learning games for exceptional children, Denver, 1971, Love Publishing Co.

Zwiren, M. L.: Mental retardation: how can we help? J. Am. Health Phys. Educ. Rec. **43**:79, 1972.

16

Emotional disturbances

In recent years educators have become increasingly concerned about disruption in the schools by emotionally disturbed children. It is important that educational personnel be prepared to deal with the problems of emotionally distrbed students in normal school settings.

Although the physical education teacher may provide input into the diagnosis of a child who is thought to be seriously emotionally disturbed, for the most part decisions for determining disturbances are usually made by professionals in the field of psychology. The central purpose of the physical educator is to collect the necessary data on the child's present level of physical education performance on curriculum tasks and evaluate the discrepancy between present ability and normative standards of educational performance This principle not only applies to children who are thought to be seriously emotionally disturbed but also to children who are thought to possess other handicapping conditions.

EMOTIONAL DISTURBANCE

Emotionally disturbed individuals who qualify for special services mandated by P.L. 94-142 are those whose emotional disturbance is severe enough to affect educational performance. It becomes clear after study of the definitions of handicapping conditions that the central focus of P.L. 94-142 is on the child's functioning in the class as measured against normative standards. Children whose performances are markedly below normative expectancies are entitled to special services. Thus, for every learner instructional data must be gathered that answer the following questions: (1) What is the child's present developmental level? (2) At what developmental level should the child be? and (3) What instruction should be provided to the child to rectify the deficiency?

Instructional procedures to serve handicapped children involve the following steps:

1. Gather psychometric information and case study data to determine if the child is to be considered emotionally disturbed.

389

2. If the child is considered emotionally disturbed, assess the level of physical performance necessary for success in the physical education curriculum.
3. Compare the child's present level of physical performance with normative expectancies.
4. If there is a discrepancy, implement the instructional process as mandated by P.L. 94-142 (see Chapter 4).

The function of the school is changing from the teaching of academic subjects and stimulating the intellect to meeting the total needs of children. Therefore, it is necessary for educators to cope with emotionally disturbed children, whether through integration in the regular school setting or placement in a special class for emotionally disturbed children. Children with emotional disturbances often confront physical educators with an impaired ability to learn motor skills and can thus create management problems in the gymnasium. There is an obvious need to employ methods and materials that will provide adequate classroom management in physical education programs that will optimally assist these children to lead self-satisfying, independent lives.

Criteria of disturbance, differences in diagnostic procedures, and inabilities to establish baselines of abnormality make identification of emotionally disturbed children difficult. If children beset with affectional, physical, social, and adult-model deprivations; victims of unrealistic standards; and those resorting to an antisocial code of life were added together, over 20% of the children in the public schools would be considered to have an identifiable learning or emotional disability. Obviously, educators have an opportunity to make great gains in meeting the needs of these children. P.L. 94-142 requires that educators provide services that meet the unique educational needs of emotionally disturbed children. This legislation indicates increased services for the emotionally disturbed.

The term *emotional disturbance* covers a multitude of traits, personality patterns, and behaviors. There is a difference between an emotionally disturbed child and a child whose behavior indicates a state of emotional disturbance. Whereas the latter is considered a person who is confronted with conflict and who may be in jeopardy of becoming emotionally disturbed, the former is considered a person who possesses limited, inflexible, and restricted behavior that impairs adaptation to changing environments. The subsequent results often are accompanied with a reduction of behavioral freedom.

CHARACTERISTICS OF EMOTIONALLY DISTURBED PERSONS

A child is considered emotionally disturbed if he or she exhibits one or more of the following characteristics over a long period of time to a marked degree:

1. An inability to learn that cannot be explained by intellectual, sensory, or health factors. Emotional factors play a part in the learning of the child. One might infer that inability of a child to learn at expected rate leaves the child suspect to some handicapping conditions, one of which may be emotional disturbance.
2. An inability to build and maintain satisfactory interpersonal relationships with peers and teachers. The result of an emotional disturbance may thus result in some type of antisocial or asocial behavior, which has an adverse effect on the child's interaction with others at school.
3. Inappropriate types of behavior or feelings under normal circumstances. Such characteristics indicate that an individual reacts to the environment differently than do others.
4. A general and pervasive mood of unhappiness and/or depression.
5. A tendency to develop physical symptoms or fears associated with personal and school problems.

Emotionally disturbed children, as a group, are heterogeneous. This becomes apparent when a person views the behavior of an emotionally disturbed child who is hyperactive and compares this behavior with that of an emotionally disurbed child who is withdrawn. There are many behavioral characteristics that are prevalent among the emotionally disturbed; however, all emotionally disturbed children do not possess all these characteristics.

Learning

Emotionally disturbed children are frequently deficient in abilities contributing to the learning of physical skills. Since the learning process is at the heart of education, it is important that the physical educator be aware of characteristics that emotionally disturbed children often possess. Characteristics that may interfere with the learning of motor skills and the management of physical education classes are the following:

1. Poor work habits in practicing and developing motor skills and aspects of physical fitness
2. Lack of motivation in achieving goals not of an immediate nature
3. Disruptive class behavior on the part of those who are hyperactive
4. Lack of involvement on the part of those who are withdrawn
5. Inability to follow directions or seek help despite demands for constant attention
6. Short attention span
7. Poor coordination
8. Development of physical symptoms (stomachache, headache, etc.) when confronted with physical activities with which the person is not secure

Interpersonal relationships

Emotionally disturbed children are often impaired in the ability to relate appropriately to their peers. Inability to relate to their peers is often atypical in that emotionally disturbed children become easily led by other members of their peer group and become desperate followers. On the other hand, some emotionally disturbed children attempt to express themselves in a desperate effort to become leaders. In play situations, atypical behavior may also be displayed by aggression toward others; at the opposite end of the behavioral continuum, emotionally disturbed children may withdraw from social activity and play alone. There are instances in which emotionally disturbed children want to conform to group patterns but cannot. Physical education programs can assist these children in developing appropriate interpersonal relationships.

Emotionally disturbed children are also often impaired in the ability to relate adequately to their teachers. They may demand constant attention by manifesting different types of behavior patterns. On the other hand, they may remain inconspicuous and not seek the help necessary to attain the physical abilities available for them to learn. Other characteristics displayed by some emotionally disturbed children are lack of conscience, easy loss of emotional control, and formation of superficial relationships.

Inappropriate behavior under normal conditions

Emotionally disturbed children often display atypical behavior patterns under normal conditions because of difficulty in learning appropriate emotional responses. Some inappropriate behavior patterns that may be displayed under normal conditions are displays of unhappiness or depression, inconsistencies in response, rigidity in expectations of everyday living, low capacity to delay gratification, and displays of such characteristics as carelessness, irresponsibility, and apathy.

Perceptual and motor skills

Deficiencies in perceptual and motor skills make it difficult to perform the more complex activities in which perception and motor control are important. Children impaired in these areas may find it difficult to become proficient in games involving balls or moving objects. Perceptual and motor difficulties exhibited by emotionally disturbed children are difficulty in making space and time assessments (Fig. 16-1) and poor motor coordination.

Psychological development

Emotionally disturbed children often attain physiological growth without attaining parallel emotional growth. In many situations, emotionally disturbed children have failed to learn appropriate behaviors because of abnormal play or home environments in which they find themselves. The impaired development of emotional behaviors may often mean that the classroom environment must be altered to accommodate the emotional levels of the children. The physical educator must also be aware of the effects of particular classroom settings and relationships with particular emotionally disturbed children. What is of great benefit to one child may be detrimental to another child.

BEHAVIOR AND NEEDS OF DISRUPTIVE EMOTIONALLY DISTURBED PERSONS

Califano and Berry[4] indicate that violence in schools has reached a level that places the health and safety of students and faculty in jeopardy. For instance, between 1970 and 1973 violence in the

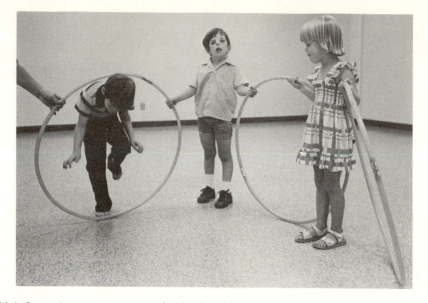

Fig. 16-1. Space time assessments may be developed by moving the body in space in relationship to objects. (Courtesy of the Special Education Early Childhood Intervention Program, University of Kansas, Lawrence.)

schools as measured by assaults on teachers and students increased 77% and 85%, respectively. Although violence is not committed by emotionally disturbed persons per se, emotional disturbance may be an influential factor in many cases.

Disruptive children do not always adhere to the rules of the school. In many instances, violation of the rules of the school interferes with the learning of other persons. Furthermore, when they behave disruptively, children are distracted from the instructional task and they do not achieve their full potential. Still another disadvantage of disruptive student behavior is the monetary cost to the school. In the state of Pennsylvania it is estimated that $1.7 million was expended in one school year for disciplinary measures.[23] Furthermore, disruptive behavior of such magnitude as to require that youths be incarcerated is estimated to cost the state $33,000 annually. Thus, the monetary cost to society and the psychological cost to disruptive students and others with whom they interact is immense.

Some state legislatures are appropriating monies for schools to experiment with alternative programs to deal with disruptive students. Testimony at congressional hearings in Pennsylvania indicates that expulsion and suspension are counterproductive[13] and that they provide endorsed vacations whenever students choose. Furthermore, expulsion and suspension tend to place stigmas on children that may make it more difficult for them to acquire appropriate education in the future.

Pup and Kennedy[21] indicate that emotionally disturbed persons who are expelled or dismissed from school often need the most attention and get the least. Poore[20] reports that recurring offenders are repeating grades two and three times. Obviously, the outlook for these children is minimal at best. Grignano[7] finds that many disruptive and emotionally disturbed persons search for educational solutions and have little success. In Pennsylvania it was found that on any school day more than 1,600 students are out of school because of suspension and nearly 400 students are expelled for the entire school year.[21]

More than a quarter of a century ago, the United States Supreme Court, in the case of *Brown vs. the Board of Education*, made the following statement:

Today education is perhaps the most important function of state and government. . . . It is the principal instrument in awakening the child to cultural values. Such an opportunity is a right which must be made available to *all* on *equal* terms. (Italics added.)

It is obvious that suspension and expulsion from school fail to provide educational opportunities for emotionally disturbed children; thus, it can in no way be considered equal education. The legitimacy of expulsion from school can be questioned. Furthermore, it is clear that suspension and expulsion are not serving as a deterrent for disruptive behavior. Rather, it is counterproductive and often is the first step toward incarceration.[16] Expulsion or suspension of emotionally disturbed children because of disruptive behavior cannot be permitted under P.L. 94-142. Individual Education Programs must be provided that will meet the children's instructional needs and cope with those behaviors that interfere with normal social living.

CAUSES OF EMOTIONAL DISTURBANCES

When teaching emotionally disturbed children, teachers sometimes find it helpful to know the causes of the emotional disturbances. This may help them to form prognoses and to be aware of circumstances that may aggravate already existing conditions. There is much speculation as to what causes emotional disturbances. Many clinicians place emphasis on locating a hypothesized environmental source of the disturbance. It is suggested that emotional blocks to learning of environmental nature might be family disorganization, parental ambitiousness, awareness of the impending birth of a sibling, or inability to adapt to a change in surroundings.

There are differing points of view regarding the predominant cause of the more severe emotional disturbances of childhood. There are many authorities who trace the cause of emotional disturbance to environmental circumstances that occur early in the life of the child. Faulty parental relationships, in particular, are believed by some authorities to account for the cause of a great portion of emotional disturbance in children. Klein[12] reports that 75% of the children he screened were from broken homes. Although it is desirable for the school to work with the parents to improve the conduct of disruptive persons, these data suggest that such cooperation may be difficult to obtain in some cases. On the other hand, there are other authorities who tend to uphold the notion that organic factors that cause a "maturational lag" make emotional compensation necessary.

IDENTIFICATION

The early identification of children who are emotionally disturbed is extremely important. It is recognized that the earlier educators and mental health specialists can attack this problem, the greater the prospect for ameliorating or remedying it. In many instances, the treatment and education of emotionally disturbed persons involve the unlearning of behavioral patterns. If identification is made early, less unlearning is necessary.

It is important that teachers know their role in screening. The purpose of screening is to determine which children are not functioning properly in a particular behavioral dimension, not to determine what caused the difficulty. The purposes of identifying children with emotional disturbances are as follows:

1. To identify children with emotional problems that impair their learning
2. To identify children with emotional problems that disrupt classroom management and prevent others from learning
3. To permit intervention in the disturbance by remedial services (special or adjunctive physical education services)
4. To place children in the educational environment in which they can best develop their potentialities

It is not easy to determine which children have problems that require special educational services. Usually, a problem in physical education classes manifests itself by disruption of the student's work, of the desirable cooperation of the group, or of the individual's ability to function adequately. A succession of disturbances that may assist educators in identifying the severity of a disturbance is described by Buhler, Smitter, and Richardson,[3] who suggest the following sequence of behavioral patterns that lead to a severe disturbance:

1. Trivial everyday disturbances such as giggling or the lack of concentration that teachers cannot study in detail. Action can be met

with counteraction to eliminate this form of disturbance.

2. Repetitious behavior that must be interpreted as a sign of deeper underlying tension.
3. Repetitious behavior accompanied by a serious single disturbance, a tantrum or breaking into tears.
4. A succession of different disturbances: talking when roll is taken, poking the person standing next to the child, staring into space, etc., on different days. This type of behavior is indicative of deep-seated tension and requires the experience of a psychologist or a psychiatrist.

There are other characteristics previously listed that will provide assistance in identifying emotionally disturbed children. More often than not, the teacher makes the initial identification of the disturbance, with subsequent referrals to the school psychologist. There is a great need for developing sensitivity to the characteristics of emotionally disturbed children in teacher training programs so that these children may be better served in a public school setting.

Behavioral description

Emotionally disturbed children possess a multitude of traits. Consequently, the label *emotionally disturbed* tells little about a particular person.

It has been traditional to classify emotionally disturbed children with a label describing their behavior. Suggested categories that may be of significance to the physical educator of emotionally disturbed children are the following:

1. *The dimension of personality afflicted:* Personality characteristics associated with emotional disturbance may be immaturity of physical, emotional, social, or psychological traits. Each trait has implications for physical education programming. Social immaturity limits the child's participation in a hierarchy of social games requiring team play and adherence to discipline with regard to obeying rules. The psychological problems are often perceptual in nature, making it difficult to match perception with motor skills that are associated with many sports activities. In many instances, the child's emotional instability may have an effect on his or her physical development.
2. *Overt behavior patterns:* Emotionally disturbed children tend to be on a continuum from hyperactivity to withdrawal. Children at each end of this continuum pose antithetical problems to the physical educator with regard to program implementation for optimal development.
3. *Degree of emotional disturbance:* Neurosis is

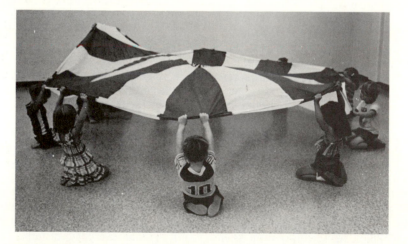

Fig. 16-2. All of the children must move together to get the parachute from the ground. (Courtesy of the Special Education Early Childhood Intervention Program, University of Kansas, Lawrence.)

a less severe form of emotional disturbance than psychosis. In the latter case, the child loses touch with reality and poses a more difficult problem for the physical educator.

4. *Associated deficiencies:* In some instances, emotional disturbance is accompanied by other disorders such as mental retardation, sensory deterioration, perceptual problems, epilepsy, and obesity.

Learning impairment

Classification according to learning impairment is mentioned to differentiate among the particular types of blocks that may impair a child's ability to learn motor skills and develop physically. In the event these particular learning blocks can be remedied or reduced in severity, greater educational benefits should be derived. Some of the fundamental psychological problems that impair the learning of motor skills are problems in relationships with others, impaired communication with others, body image problems, difficulties with vision and/or audition, and language deficiency exhibited by difficulty with articulation or syntax.

Well-implemented physical education programs may contribute to the alleviation of body image problems and problems in relating with others. However, more often than not, the other impairments mentioned will have to be circumvented in the process of teaching physical education.

THE TEACHER

The teacher of an emotionally disturbed child bears great responsibility. The teacher organizes physical activities, directs play, and, what is more critical, provides patterns of behavior for the child to emulate. It is from the teacher that immature children learn how the environment works and how persons cope.

The teacher of an emotionally disturbed child must be stable, flexible, and empathetic toward atypical behavior. However, the teacher must be able to perceive what the child is experiencing. Such a teacher provides a medium through which the child may better understand his or her own behavior and modify it. This is no easy task. Being in contact with anxiety-provoking persons often stretches the teacher's emotional capacities. Some of the behaviors that teachers often must tolerate

are implied rejection from the child, conflicting demands made by the child that may range from demanding that immediate needs be met to severe withdrawal, aggressive tactics, and immature behaviors.

Regular classroom teachers may be unaccustomed to these behaviors. However, to succeed in working with these children, teachers must understand and accept their atypical behavior patterns. It may be necessary for teachers to receive special guidance and support to prevent reaching an emotional breaking point.

THE PHYSICAL EDUCATION PROGRAM
Principles of teaching

To conduct a developmental curriculum in physical education for emotionally disturbed children, it is necessary to understand their learning characteristics in the development of motor skills and to apply principles taking these characteristics into consideration. The principles of good teaching of emotionally disturbed children in physical education are as follows:

1. *Provide the appropriate stimulation.* Many emotionally disturbed children need a strong prompt to focus their attention on the activity at hand. Use tactile stimulation in teaching if the child does not attend to the task. However, avoid overstimulation of the hyperactive emotionally disturbed child.

2. *Utilize activity and a variety of games that will accommodate their different physical, social, and emotional developmental levels.* The short attention span of these children makes it necessary to have several games on hand so that their interest can be recaptured when an initial activity is no longer productive (Fig. 16-3). Novelty in activities is a great aid in holding attention.

3. *Remove distracting objects.* The attention span can be increased if seductive objects are removed from the immediate environment because the possibilities of involvement in other activity are reduced. Bats, balls, and other play equipment should be kept out of sight until the time of use, if possible.

4. *Provide manual guidance when teaching basic skills to some emotionally disturbed*

children. This is not necessarily a good procedure for all disturbed children. A rapport must first be built between the child and the instructor before use of manual guidance or the kinesthetic method of teaching motor skills becomes effective. This method is particularly effective with *autistic* children. Manual guidance is less effective with hyperactive children than with those who are withdrawn.

5. *Impose limits with regard to use of equipment, facilities, and conduct.* Undue expectations with regard to developmental level of emotions should not be made. However, each child should adhere to behavioral limits within his or her capabilities. Action toward equipment and facilities involved in

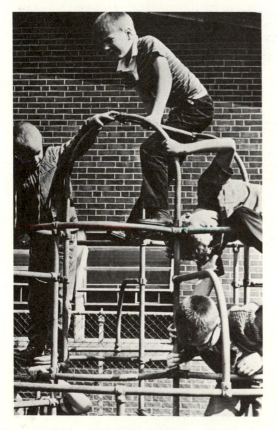

Fig. 16-3. Emotionally disturbed children at play. (Courtesy of United States Jaycees, Mental Health—Mental Retardation, Tulsa, Okla.)

play activity affords opportunities for the development of positive behavioral attitudes.

6. *Work with motor skills and games that allow some degree of success.* Every satisfying experience makes for decreased anxiety and increased confidence.

7. *Know when to encourage a child to approach, explore, and try a new activity or experience.* A new experience is often met with resistance. In such instances, it is wise to build guarantees of success into the new experience. Subsequent involvement becomes much easier for the emotionally disturbed child. The child who witnesses peers participating successfully in activities sometimes receives impetus to participate with them.

8. *Discourage stereotyped play activities that develop rigid behavioral patterns.* Emotionally disturbed children often have a tendency to respond to the same objects or activities day after day. After a skill or activity has been well mastered, it may deter initiation of other activities.

9. *Do not necessarily strive for control in all situations.* One of the major goals of education for those who are emotionally disturbed is to effect adequate social adjustment. This does not imply strict obedience to authority but the ability of the individual to adjust to situations independently of supervision. Control should be of such a nature that the preconceived goals of the Individual Education Program are being achieved.

10. *Discourage inappropriate interaction among the children.* This may result in conflicts that disrupt the whole class. It may be necessary to separate children who interact with one another in a disruptive manner.

11. *Provide activities within individual abilities and levels of development.* The instructor should know the developmental level of the child's social, emotional, and motor patterns, should be aware of how the child responds to various stimuli and activities, and should plan the program around the child's abilities and disabilities.

It is recognized that the emotionally disturbed

population is an extremely heterogeneous group that possesses varying traits. Therefore, the principles mentioned are obviously not applicable to all emotionally disturbed children. They are to serve only as a guide to the implementation of programs of physical education for the emotionally disturbed.

Objectives

The objectives of a physical education program for emotionally disturbed children are the same as those for typical children. The program for emotionally disturbed children should stress the development of motor skills and physical fitness, social competence, and personal adequacy. The objectives should be to develop personal and social competencies that will make the children aware of their own resources and potentialities to optimize the development of self. Physical activities assisting the development of desirable relationships between self and both peers and persons in authority should be provided. Physical activities should also provide constructive and positive new experiences that enhance the concept of self and provide a feeling of worth.

The approach to the education of emotionally disturbed individuals is a central problem needing resolution. The difference between medical and developmental models for emotionally disturbed children is adequately described by Hobbs.[10] Hobbs indicates that education places the emphasis on health rather than on illness, on teaching rather than on treatment, on learning rather than on fundamental personality reorganization, on the present and future rather than on the past, and on the operation of the total social system of which the child is a part rather than on the intrapsychic processes exclusively. The primary purpose of the physical educator is to deal with the process of education, not with therapeutic treatment, when implementing programs of physical education for emotionally disturbed children. This does not mean, however, that physical education programs should not and will not have therapeutic effects. On the contrary, the expectation of well-conceived educational programs should record learning gains with these children. However, the educator's goals must be broader than those of a therapist, who is primarily concerned with the mitigation of a particular disorder.

Although the general objectives for emotionally disturbed children are applicable to typical chil-

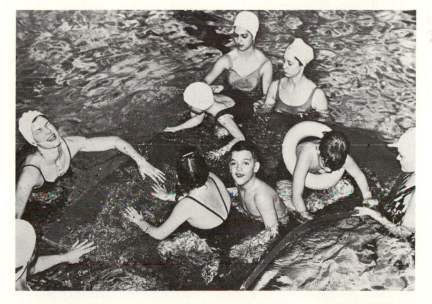

Fig. 16-4. A planned experience in water play in the Slippery Rock State College Handicapped Swim Program.

dren, there are specific objectives that may be of higher priority for the emotionally disturbed. These specific objectives include the following:

1. *The children should develop physical and motor fitness through the various organic systems of the body.* Emotionally disturbed children need to develop the ability to sustain adaptive effort, to recover from physical exertion, and to resist muscular fatigue. Hopefully, this will enable the children to become more active, demonstrate better motor performance, and become healthier in the organic systems of the body.

2. *The children should develop lifetime sport skills that provide opportunities for participation in wholesome leisure-time activity.* Motor development is also concerned with making physical movement more useful, proficient, graceful, and aesthetic. It is concerned, too, with building confidence and enhancing physical and mental health. Supplementary physical education programs should be provided for children who are deficient in lifetime sport skills.

3. *The children should be educated to get along with others by developing social competencies through numerous social experiences in games.* Emotionally disturbed children should be helped to unlearn the specific habits that caused rejection by adults and peers and to acquire the specific habits that will make them more acceptable to the important persons in their lives.

Programs of physical education must be of such a nature that all children can accomplish something at their own levels of ability. Emotionally disturbed children should not be placed in situations in which feelings of insecurity or inadequacy are reinforced by failure to perform the task (Fig. 16-4).

Educational placement

Emotionally disturbed children should be educated in the least restrictive environment. It is obvious that there is no single setting in which emotionally disturbed children are best educated. However, it is clear that their education, if possible, should be in the least restrictive environment (mainstreaming). The possible arrangements in which these children may be educated are as follows:

1. In the regular class with nonhandicapped children
2. In the regular class with a resource room teacher
3. In a segregated handicapped only class

The majority of emotionally disturbed children, and particularly the less disturbed, are educated in integrated, regular classes. There are definite social advantages to integrated placement in that these children are not set apart from their peers and do not carry an educational label that makes them different. However, under such circumstances, the individual needs of emotionally disturbed children may not be met. When emotionally disturbed children are placed in the regular class, a concerted effort must be made to meet their individual needs through the Individual Education Program.

When emotionally disturbed children cannot be mainstreamed, they may receive an assignment to a special class. Under this type of placement, the physical educator may teach the children in the same group in which they are taught throughout the day. Usually, it is necessary to consider motor differences as well as social and emotional differences because the age range of these groups may extend from early primary to junior high school grade levels. Ordinarily, special classes for the emotionally disturbed are smaller than regular physical education classes. This may provide opportunities for greater attention to individual needs.

The needs and characteristics of all children in a physical education class that contains emotionally disturbed children must be considered in the selection and implementation of physical activities. This is no easy task because of the tremendous variability in characteristics among this group. Hyperactive brain-damaged children may be adversely affected on hearing an overstimulating noise such as a drumbeat or the voice of the instructor. On the other hand, a strong stimulus may be greatly needed by other emotionally disturbed children in the same group to focus their attention on the activity at hand.

Least restrictive environment

Some of the alternative programs for disruptive emotionally disturbed children involve special, secure, very restrictive environments. Juvenile detention homes are restrictive. Some of the restrictive alternatives outside of the public school system have goals that are incongruent with the goals of education. This is not to say that under some conditions restrictive environments are not appropriate. However, under these conditions, according to P.L. 94-142, the least restrictive environment must be provided. The schools must assist the children to develop acceptable behavior patterns so that they may return to normalized settings as soon as possible. For any handicapped child who is placed in a restrictive environment, the aberrant behaviors should be identified and remedied.

Most educators are concerned with the appropriate placement of disruptive children and want to educate them.[6] However, Francis[6] indicates that the education of disruptive students must take place in an environment in which teachers have a chance of succeeding. Thus, it is clear that suspension should keep disruptive children within the school environment but under restrictions and without loss of privilege of education, with opportunities to return to more normalized educational environments.[20]

Behavioral management

Behavioral management of emotionally disturbed children, whether they are in regular or special classes, is a challenge. To cope effectively with the behavior of these children in a classroom setting, the teacher must be an astute observer and a keen psychological tactician. Management demands the analysis of the dynamic interaction of individuals and group forces acting on children during particular activities, together with the skillful application of learning principles.

Certain considerations must be made in managing the behavior of emotionally disturbed children. They must be given the leeway that typical children would be given in a learning situation. The teacher should reflect on the developmental level of the children (social, emotional, and physical) and gear expectations accordingly. It is not reasonable to expect that emotionally disturbed children will behave in the same manner as typical children. Therefore, the expectations should not be so high that teachers are adversely affected if the emotionally disturbed children do not meet preconceived standards.

It is often difficult to set limits as to when to intervene to manage atypical behavior displayed in class. The following suggestions* can serve as guidelines of intervention to control classroom behavior:

1. *Reality dangers:* The teacher should intervene if children are involved in physical activity placing them in danger.
2. *Psychological protection:* The teacher should intervene if a group gangs up on a child and uses derogatory remarks that tend to label him as a scapegoat.
3. *Protection of property:* The teacher should intervene when it is evident that school property, equipment, or facilities are in danger of being destroyed or damaged.
4. *Protection of the on-going program:* Once the class is motivated in performing a particular activity, intervene if a child who is having difficulty displays disruptive behavior.
5. *Protection against negative contagion:* The teacher should intervene if tension is mounting in an activity and a child with high social power contributes negatively to the activity.
6. *Highlighting a value area:* The teacher may want to intervene to point to an aspect of sportsmanship or rules of the game which may lie slightly below the surface of behavior.
7. *Avoiding conflicts with the outside world:* It is expected that behavior will be controlled when the public or persons other than class members are available to view the class.

Besides knowing when to intervene in the occurrence of inappropriate behaviors in the classroom, the teacher needs to know how to intervene to control such behaviors. The following discussion describes the methods designed to help teachers maintain surface behavior. Redl[22] listed 21 specific influence techniques that he has been able to identify in his work with aggressive boys. The techniques most applicable to the management of children in a physical education setting are as follows:

1. *Planned ignoring:* Much of children's behavior is designed to antagonize the teacher. If this behavior is not contagious, it may be wise to ignore the behavior and not gratify the child.
2. *Signal interference:* The teacher may use nonverbal controls such as hand clapping, eye contact, facial

*From Bulletin of the School of Education, Indiana University, July 1961.

frowns and body postures to indicate to the child the feeling of disapproval and control.

3. *Proximity control:* The teacher may stand next to a child who is having difficulty. This is to let the child know of the teacher's concern regarding the behavior.

4. *Interest boosting:* If a child's interest is waning, involve him actively in class activities of the moment and let him demonstrate the skill that is being performed or discussed.

5. *Reduction of tension through humor:* Humor is often able to penetrate a tense situation, with the end result of everyone becoming more comfortable.

6. *Hurdle lesson:* Sometimes a child is frustrated by the immediate task he is requested to perform. Instead of asking for help, he may involve his peers in disruptive activity. In this event, structure a task in which the child can be successful.

7. *Restructure the classroom program:* If the teacher feels the class is irritable, bored, or excited, a change in program may be needed.

8. *Support from routine:* Some children need more structure than others. Without these guideposts they feel insecure. Structure programs for those that need it.

9. *Direct appeal to value areas:* Appeal to certain values that children have internalized. Some of these values may be relationship between the teacher and child, reality consequences, an awareness of peer reaction, or appeal to the teacher's power of authority.

10. *Remove seductive objects:* It is difficult for the teacher to compete against balls, bats, objects that can be manipulated, or equipment that may be in the vicinity of instruction. Either the objects have to be removed, or the teacher has to accept the disorganized state of the group.

11. *Verbal removal:* When a child's behavior has reached the point where he will not respond to verbal controls, he may have to be asked to leave the room (to get a drink, wash up, or deliver a message—not as punishment).

12. *Physical restraint:* It may be necessary to restrain a child physically if he loses control and becomes violent.

TEACHER TRAINING

Discipline was rated by teachers and administrators as being of prime importance in reducing disruptive behavior in the schools. However, teachers need to be trained in the skills that enable the management and prevention of such behavior. Staley[26]

states: "I have empathy for the teacher who is expected to maintain discipline but who is not given the necessary tools to do it. . . . When demands are made that a teacher maintain discipline we should first check to see that the teacher as the means to do it." Furthermore, Bell[2] indicates that the teacher-in-training is rarely given to expect that the class will include disruptive children. There is evidence that teachers lack the necessary skills and do not understand the rights of students to secure appropriate education. Thus, considerable inservice and preservice training is needed by teachers to manage the learning of disruptive emotionally disturbed children.

EDUCATIONAL APPROACHES

There are many ways to implement educational programs for emotionally disturbed children. However, only two different educational approaches for emotionally disturbed children will be examined. Although these approaches have been used primarily in academic classroom settings, many techniques are applicable to the implementation of physical education programs. The two approaches are applied behavioral technology[9] and the planned experience approach.[24]

Applied behavioral technology

Applied behavioral technology in the education of emotionally disturbed children makes practical application of learning theory, operant conditioning, and precise objectives.[9] The major hypothesis of this approach is that emotionally disturbed children lack order or structure in the environment and in their emotional educational life, and tasks to be taught must be specified in detail. To remedy this situation, ways are sought to increase definiteness and the structure of daily classroom experiences. Factors contributing to a structured environment are identified as controlled extraneous stimulation, short-term instructional objectives, and assigned tasks with constant follow-up. The teacher's purpose is primarily to increase structure, to specify tasks to be learned, and to solidify unclear structure. Good teaching under these conditions means knowing each child well, being able to organize and manage, and having firm expectations and consistent follow-through. The implementation of this approach is expected to bring about behavior that is controlled, constructive, predictive, and orderly. It is of great importance that each moment be planned and that the child engage actively in the task.

Incorporation of learning principles into the instructional process

Legislative bodies at both the federal and state levels have identified problems associated with disruptive students in the public schools. The Law Enforcement Administration's National Crime Survey indicates that there are positive steps that can be taken to alleviate some of the problems and evinces the importance of a rational structure of incentives for positive management of behavior. Furthermore, evidence indicates that there is less violence in schools with structured programs than in schools without well-defined structure. The report points out the desirability of a structure of incentives as motivation for achievement.[4] This concept is also supported by Turner,[26] who believes that disruptive children react positively to well-organized, structured programs geared toward meeting personal needs and that most react positively to small group settings and individualized instruction. With the application of sound educational principles and techniques of learning management, disruptive children should have success in the public schools. In review, Califano and Berry[4] point out that in their study successful schools had systems of firm, consistent management. Research confirms that clearly structured, secure environments permit students to master the objectives of the program. Haring[8] indicates that "Teaching . . . necessitates finding a method of instruction which allows the child to learn. This notion is implicit in the accountability measures which are built into the individual education program." It is clear that the teacher is responsible for the students' learning. There is ample evidence that persons applying behavioral principles in education achieve specified, predetermined objectives.[2] The teaching techniques that seem most valuable are variations of the behavior modification theme.[5,8,18]

It is well established in the literature that learning potential lies within the individual. However, to maximize the effects of the Individual Education Program it is necessary to utilize available behavioral technology. Without an individualized learning model with specific short-term instructional objectives it is difficult to effectively instruct the children and manage their behavior.

Much of the foregoing discussion is based on congressional hearings that address the problems of disruption in the schools. Personnel from most aspects of the educational delivery system were requested to comment. There is some consensus as to how instruction is to be conducted. The following section describes nine principles that are relevant to the management of disruptive emotionally disturbed children in a physically education classroom.[11,12]

Nine learning principles for conducting instruction. The preconditions for the application of learning principles are as follows: there must be a precisely defined short-term instructional objective, and there must be incentives for the learner to master the objective. If either of these preconditions is not satisfied, the effect of the program will be minimized. The nine principles of learning, which are drawn from Homme,[11] are as follows:

1. Praise the correct objective.
2. Praise the correct objective immediately after it occurs.
3. Praise the correct objective after it occurs and not before.
4. Objectives should be in small steps so that there can be frequent praise.
5. Praise improvement.
6. Be fair in setting up consequences for achieving objectives.
7. Be honest and provide the agreed upon consequences.
8. Be positive so that the child may achieve success.
9. Be systematic.

Praise the correct objective. There are two ways that this learning principle can be violated by a teacher, parent, or school administrator: first, he or she may provide praise even though the objective has not been achieved; second, he or she may neglect to provide the praise even though the objective has been achieved. In the first case, the learner is being reinforced for doing less than his or her best and consequently, will have a lessened desire to put forth maximum effort on subsequent trials. In the second case, if the teacher does not deliver the agreed upon consequence (explicit or implicit), the student's desire to perform the instructional task again will be reduced.

To implement this principle effectively, persons involved with instruction (teachers, school administrators, parents, and related service personnel) must know precisely the objective or behavior that the learner is to carry out, as vague objectives confuse learners and contribute to disruptive behavior. The application of this principle must be consistent among all persons who work with the child.

Praise immediately after completion of the task. Learners need to receive feedback immediately after task performance. Homme[11] indicates that reinforcing feedback should be provided 0.05 second after the task for maximum effectiveness. Immediacy of feedback on task performance is particularly important with children functioning on a lower level. If there is a delay between task performance and feedback, the child may be confused as to what the praise is for. For example, if a child walks a balance beam correctly but confirmation of task mastery is provided late, as the child steps off the beam, the behavior of stepping off the beam may be strengthened to a greater degree than that of walking the beam, the desired objective. Thus, the timing of the feedback (immediately after the task has been completed) is important.

Praise the correct objective after it occurs and not before. If a child is praised for performing an objective before it is completed there is a good chance that he or she will expend less effort to meet the objective.

Objectives should be in small steps. Chapter 4 alluded to the necessity of arranging the learning sequence in small steps so that there can be frequent praise. If step size is small, there will be a greater rate of success, and as has been indicated, disruptive behavior may be triggered by lack of success. The principle may therefore be applied in attempts to control disruptive behavior in the classroom. Thus, if a child often exhibits many different types of disruptive behaviors, objectives can be postulated to reduce the occurrence of these disruptive behaviors in small steps. (For measurement of behaviors the reader is referred to Hall.[7a]) For handicapped children, learning by small steps permits much-needed success.

Praise improvement. The acquisition of skill toward an objective should be praised. Providing appropriate consequences for improvement may, in some instances, violate the principle of praising the correct objective. However, on tasks that cannot be broken into small steps is necessary to praise improvement. To do so, the instructor must know precisely the student's present level of educational performance; when the performance reflects an improvement on that level, the student must be reinforced with praise. Improvement means that the learner is, functioning on a higher level than before. Therefore, it is unwise to praise or provide positive consequences to students who perform at less than their best effort, because to do so may be to encourage them to contradict their potential.

Be fair in setting up consequences. When there are specific objectives to be achieved to develop skill or appropriate classroom behavior, specific consequences can be arranged to support the development of these objectives. However, if such arrangements are to be made between the learner and the teacher, there must be equity between the task and the incentives. If the learner does not have sufficient incentive to perform the tasks or to behave appropriately, he or she is unlikely to do so. This learning principle operates at very early ages.

In our clinical experience, a target objective was set for an 18-month-old boy with Down's syndrome to learn to walk. The task involved walking from one chair to another that was placed 8 feet away. If the child walked the full distance, he was allowed to play for 15 seconds the toys which were placed on top of the chairs. When this period elapsed he would then return to the task of walking a prescribed distance of 8 feet 1 inch, a short distance farther than the previous time. After a time, the child refused to participate in the activity. The child's mother suggested that he be permitted to play with the toys for 30 seconds rather than for 15 seconds. This procedure was employed and the child again engaged in the instructional task. It was inferred that the child would participate in tasks if the opportunity to play was commensurate with the effort put forth to master the objective. In our opinion, this was an example of equity between incentive and performance.

Provide the agreed upon consequence. Agreements between teachers and learners must be honored by both. If there is an implicit or explicit arrangement between the teacher and the learner and if the teacher does not follow through with the arrangement when the learner has upheld his or her end of the bargain, then the learning conditions will be seriously weakened. It is not uncommon for teachers to inadvertently forget the arrangements that have been made. Therefore, it is important for the teacher to have records of arrangements between themselves and the learner. Forgetting the preconditions between learner and teacher may have a negative impact on the pupil's learning at a subsequent time.

If the teacher requests that a learner perform a specific task, the teacher must not provide the desirable consequences unless the learner achieves the proper objective. Honest delivery of the agreed upon consequences is very similar to praise for the correct behavior. However, praise for the correct behavior usually connotes a specific short-term task, while an agreed upon consequence may involve a contractual arrangement between two parties. Principals and teachers who set policies may achieve positive results with the application of this principle.

Be positive. The objective should be phrased positively so that the learner can achieve the stated objective. An example of a positive statement would be "Walk to the end of the balance beam." An example of a negative statement would be "Don't fall off of the balance beam." In the negative instance the child is avoiding failure and there can be little value in mastering the desired behavior.

Be systematic. To make the greatest positive impact on handicapped children it is necessary to apply all of the learning principles all of the time. Inconsistency confuses the learner with regard to the material to be learned and the type of behavior to maintain during class. The consistent use of modern behavioral technology enhances a child's ability to learn desirable behaviors. This learning principle is the most difficult one for teachers of emotionally disturbed children to master.

Planned experience approach

The planned experience approach recommended by Rhodes[24] is based on the assumption that the forces of growth and the motivational effects of exploration and discovery of emotionally disturbed children are similar to those of typical children.

If children are to recognize their capabilities and resources, it is important that the experiences be planned carefully. Principles that should be applied to the preparation of experiences are as follows:

1. New experiences should be elicited in relationship to old problems. The child's responses will provide the cues to the quality and intensity of the experience and suggestions for additional preparations.

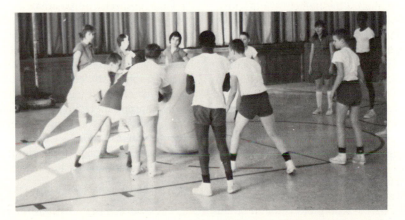

Fig. 16-5. An interesting activity that uses several sensory channels and requires some social cooperation. (Courtesy of Julian Stein, American Alliance for Health, Physical Education, Recreation, and Dance.)

2. The child must be surrounded with opportunities for new experiences that afford chances for adventure, discovery, and exploration (Fig. 16-3).
3. The child should have opportunities to express newly developed abilities.
4. The experiences should engage as many sensory channels as possible.
5. The experiences should develop new abilities channeled toward the interests of the child.
6. The experiences should include natural and immediate consequences of the child's activity.
7. The experiences should require only performances in line with the child's present abilities.
8. The teacher should find ways to help the child reflect on the experience and its meaning so that it is bound as a permanent record within the child.

These guides are most applicable to physical educators in implementing physical education programs for all children. Emotionally disturbed children are in greater need of such techniques.

COMPREHENSIVE COORDINATED PROGRAM FOR DISRUPTIVE CHILDREN

There is a need for a coordinated program that involves all of the professionals concerned with the education of disruptive emotionally disturbed children. Within the schools, the home, and the juvenile system there may be several persons who will impact on the disruptive child. Thus, comprehensive and innovative educational programs are needed. When schools operate under suspension policies, it is not uncommon for children to lose opportunity to acquire skills achieved by other members of the class. Thus, when these children return to regular class they are far behind their peers. This places more stress than ever on the children and might well elicit disruptive behavior again.

P.L. 94-142 has as a basic tenet the shared responsibility between the parents and the school. Many authorities agree that there should be increased communication among students, parents, teachers, administrators, and the community. Such communication would aid in providing effective education for disruptive children. It is interesting to note that administrators, teachers, and other professionals in the field of disruptive behavior suggest program implementation based on the principles of the Individual Education Program.

Mader[16] indicates that specific intervention with alternative programs can be beneficial to disruptive persons. He cites a study in which the rate of advancement on academic tasks was $1\frac{1}{2}$ months of progress per month in a class with alternative programs as compared with $\frac{1}{2}$ month of progress per month in a class without alternative programs. Thus, alternative programs do assist the educational progress of disruptive children without interfering with the progress of other children.

Alternative programs

There has been some experimentation with alternative programs for emotionally disturbed disruptive students. Some programs have been of a punitive nature, imposing stricter, stronger, and more forcible control over the students and employing police officers, electronic surveillance equipment, and punishment. Other programs have taken a more positive approach, providing special personal and resource rooms for specific activities or reducing the pupil-teacher ratio to 10-1. One reason for disruptive behavior by pupils may be the lack of success. If this is the case, individualized programming, which enables pupils to progress at their own rates, may provide success, which reduces disruptive behavior.

Other aspects of positive programs to counter disruption by emotionally disturbed children, as indicated by Scanlon,[25] are (1) counseling pupils on attitudes toward persons in authority (teachers, school administrators, and police) and (2) assigning disruptive students to monitor appropriate behavior of others. Sometimes individuals can determine appropriate behavior for others but fail to perceive deficiencies in their own behavior. Thus, assisting others to conduct themselves well becomes a positive experience in developing socially acceptable behavior patterns for themselves.

PLAY AND PHYSICAL ACTIVITY

Physical activity in the form of play and dance has traditionally been used by mental health specialists both as a tool in diagnosis and as therapy for emotionally disturbed persons. The qualitative aspects of play and the development of motor skills

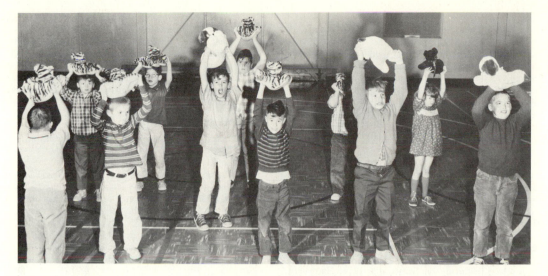

Fig. 16-6. Classroom behavior can be controlled through well-managed activity that gets children involved. (Courtesy of Julian Stein, American Alliance for Health, Physical Education, Recreation, and Dance.)

in disturbed persons have not always received a great deal of attention in the past. However, it is now recognized by educators of emotionally disturbed children that play is not an intermittent freedom from the discipline of academic tasks but is of educational value.

There is a qualitative aspect to the nature of physical activity in play that can contribute to the well-being of disturbed children. Constructive play of a higher order implies the socialization of children. Usually, emotionally disturbed children must be taught how to play and enjoy physical activity. Once constructive play is learned, it provides a medium through which the children may experiment with self-control and with the control of the environment. Play also offers opportunity for social learnings and tension release. Because emotionally disturbed children strain the educational program, they are often left out of the extracurricular and intramural activities of a regular school. This is in reverse order of their basic needs for experience in community living (Fig. 16-6).

REFERENCES

1. Becker, W., Engelmann, S., and Thomas, G.: Teaching: an applied course in psychology, Chicago, Ill., 1971, Science Research Associates.
2. Bell, R.: Testimony On the prevention of school disruption with particular reference to Senate Bill 1214, Harrisburg, Pa., 1978. (As presented to the Senate Education Committee.)
3. Buhler, C., Smitter, F., and Richardson, S.: What is a problem? In Long, H. J., editor: Conflict in the classroom, Belmont, Calif., 1965, Wadsworth Publishing Co., Inc.
4. Califano, J. A., and Berry, M. F.: Violent schools—safe schools, Harrisburg, Pa., 1977. (Study done by the United States Health, Education, and Welfare Department on Safe Schools and presented to the Senate Education Committee.)
5. Coloroso, B.: Strategies for working with troubled students. In Gearhart, B. R., and Weishahn, M. W.: The handicapped student in the regular classroom, ed. 2, St. Louis, 1980, The C. V. Mosby Co.
6. Francis, P. E.: Hearings on Senate Bill 1214, prevention of school disruption, testimony of Paul E. Francis, Harrisburg, Pa., 1978.
7. Grignano, I. A.: Testimony upon the addition of article XIX-A concerning the prevention of school disruption, Pittsburgh, 1978.
7a. Hall, R.: Managing behavior: applications in school and home, Lawrence, Kan., 1971, H. & H. Enterprises.
8. Haring, N.: Application of behavior modification techniques to the learning situation. In Cruickshank, W. M., and Hallahan, D. P., editors: Psychoeducational practices, vol. 1, Syracuse, N.Y., 1975, Syracuse University Press.
9. Haring, N. G., and Whelan, R. J.: Experimental methods in education and management. In Long, H. J., editor: Conflict in the classroom, Belmont, Calif., 1965, Wadsworth Publishing Co., Inc.
10. Hobbs, N.: How the Re-ED plan developed. In Long, H. J., editor: Conflict in the classroom, Belmont, Calif., 1965, Wadsworth Publishing Co., Inc.
11. Homme, L.: How to use contingency contracting in the classroom, Champaign, Ill., 1969, Research Press.

12. Klein, C. A.: Summary of remarks presented at the joint House-Senate Education Committee hearing, Senator Reibman, Chairperson, at 10:30 A.M., in the Ampitheater Classroom Center, Liberty High School, Bethlehem, Pa., 1978.

13. Klein, H. J.: Testimony on Senate bill 1214, Harrisburg, Pa., 1978.

14. Logan, W. R.: Testimony to the Senate Education Committee on Senate Bill 1214, Pittsburgh, 1978.

15. Lyons, D. J., and Powers, V.: Study of children exempted from Los Angeles schools. In Long, H. J., editor: Conflict in the classroom, Belmont, Calif., 1965, Wadsworth Publishing Co., Inc.

16. Mader, W.: Testimony to the Senate Education Committee on Senate bill 1214, Bethlehem, Pa., 1978.

17. Morse, W. C.: The crisis teacher. In Long, H. J., editor: Conflict in the classroom, Belmont, Calif., 1965, Wadsworth Publishing Co., Inc.

18. Morse, W. C.: The helping teacher/crisis teacher concept, Focus Except. Child. **8(4):**1-11, 1976.

19. Mosston, M.: Teaching physical education, Columbus, Ohio, 1966, Charles E. Merrill Publishing Co.

20. Poore, M.: Testimony on Senate Bill 1214, Harrisburg, Pa., 1978.

21. Pup, P. J., and Kennedy, E.: Testimony provided for the Pennsylvania Senate's Education Committee hearing on Senate bill, January 24, 1978, Woodlawn Middle School, Munhall, Pennsylvania, Harrisburg, Pa., 1978.

22. Redl, F.: Managing surface behavior of children in school. In Long, H. J., editor: Conflict in the classroom, Belmont, Calif., 1965, Wadsworth Publishing Co., Inc. (From notes abridged from N. J. Long and R. G. Newman.)

23. Reibman, J. F.: Senator Jeanette Reibman's opening remarks at the public hearings on Senate bill 1214: the prevention of School Disruption Bill, Harrisburg, Pa., 1978.

24. Rhodes, W. C.: Curriculum and disordered behavior. In Long, H. J., editor: Conflict in the classroom, Belmont, Calif., 1965, Wadsworth Publishing Co., Inc.

25. Scanlon, R. G.: School disruption update, Penn. Educ. vol. 10, April 9, 1979.

26. Staley, J. C.: Prevention of school disruption, Harrisburg, Pa., 1978. (Testimony on Senate bill 1214.)

27. Turner, Benjamin F.: Testimony: Senate bill 1214—Prevention of School Disruption Bill, Harrisburg, Pa., 1977.

28. Vaughn, J. E.: The effects of exercises and games activities upon the behavior, body image and self-image of hospitalized male psychotics, Unpublished doctoral dissertation, Springfield College, Springfield, Mass., 1966.

RECOMMENDED READINGS

Altman, L., and Linton, T.: Operant conditioning in the classroom setting: a review of the research, J. Educ. Res. **64:**277-286, 1971.

Bateman, B.: Three approaches to diagnosis and educational planning for children with learning disabilities. From proceedings of the international convocation on children and young adults with learning disabilities, Pittsburgh, 1967, Crippled Children's Home.

Brown, P., and Presbie, R.: Behavior modification skills, Hicksville, N.Y., 1973, Research Media, Inc.

Cruickshank, W. M., editor: Psychology of exceptional children and youth, Englewood Cliffs, N.J., 1971, Prentice-Hall, Inc.

Hall, R.: Managing behavior: applications in school and home, Lawrence, Kan., 1971, H. & H. Enterprises.

Haring, N. G., and Schiefelbusch, R. L., editors: Methods in special education, ed. 2, New York, 1975, McGraw-Hill Book Co.

Hewett, F. M.: The emotionally disturbed child in the classroom, Boston, 1968, Allyn & Bacon, Inc.

Long, H. J., and Newman, R. G.: Managing surface behavior of children in school. In Long, H. J., editor: Conflict in the classroom, Belmont, Calif., 1965, Wadsworth Publishing Co., Inc.

Morse, W. C.: The education of socially maladjusted and emotionally disturbed children. In Cruickshank, W. M., and Johnson, G. O., editors: Education of exceptional children and youth, Englewood Cliffs, N.J., 1958, Prentice-Hall, Inc.

Myklebust, H. R., editor: Progress in learning disabilities, New York, 1975, Grune & Stratton, Inc.

17

Other conditions

MENSTRUATION AND DYSMENORRHEA

Menstruation is a complex process that involves the endocrine glands, uterus, and ovaries. The menstrual cycle, on the average, lasts for 28 days. However, each woman has her own rhythmic cycle of menstrual function. The cycle periods usually range from 21 to 35 days, but they may occasionally be longer or shorter and still fall within the range of normality.

The average total amount of blood lost during the normal menstrual period is 3 ounces; however, a woman may lose from $1\frac{1}{2}$ to 5 ounces.[17] This blood is replaced by the active formation of blood cells in bone marrow and, consequently, does not cause anemia. On occasion, some women may have excessive menstrual flow and, in this event, a physician should be consulted. The average menstrual period is 3 to 5 days, but 2 to 7 days may be considered normal. The average age of onset of menstruation is 12.5 years, although the range of onset may be from 9 to 18 years.

Dysmenorrhea, or painful menstruation, is a common occurrence among some girls and women. The ratio may be as low as 1:4 among college women, indicating that it is the exception rather than the rule. It has been estimated that only 20% to 30% of cases of dysmenorrhea are a result of organic causes such as ovarian cysts, endocrine imbalance, or infections. Most of the causes are of functional origin such as poor posture, insufficient exercise, fatigue, weak abdominal muscles, or improper diet.

Physical activity during the menstrual period

Nolen[15] indicated, in a study of problems in menstruation, that postural deficiency may be responsible for some discomfort not just during the menstrual period but also on other days. She found that when posture was improved and good physical condition was achieved, the menses did not incapacitate girls for physical education or recreational programs.

Gilman's[10] findings indicate that activity during the menstrual period has proved helpful in the correction of dysmenorrhea. According to Clow and Sanderson,[5] many girls have discovered that if they do not have some form of exercise prior to and on the first day of their period, then they may have pain.

A number of studies report the effect of exercise on menstruation. Runge[17] studied 107 college girls who trained 15 hours each week, and Duntzer and Hellendall[8] studied 1,561 women participating in a German athletic festival. Both found that, in a majority of the cases, training was without effect on the character of menstrual activity. The activities were continued during the menstrual period without impairment to performance ability. In Duntzer and Hellendall's study, it was shown that 55% of the women suffered no decrease in efficiency, whereas 45% showed a decrease in performance either during menstruation or immediately before the onset of flow. The findings of these studies seem to indicate that menstruation affects women differently. It is suggested that menstruation does not necessarily prohibit exercise during flow, but there are exceptions to the rule.

The consensus in the literature would seem to be that excuse from physical education activity because of normal menstruation would be unwarranted.

The question has been raised as to whether girls and young women should refrain from swimming during the menstrual cycles. Phillips, Fox, and Young[16] conducted a survey among gynecologists and other physicians to determine their points of view on this issue. The menstrual period was divided into three phases: the premenstrual period (3 or 4 days prior to the actual onset of the menses), the first half of the menstrual period, and the second half of the menstrual period. The consensus among the doctors and the gynecologists was that restriction from participation in vigorous physical activity, intensive sports competition, and swimming during all phases of the menstrual period were unwarranted for girls who are free from menstrual disturbances. However, with regard to the first half of the menstrual period, there were some physicians who advised moderation with limited participation in intensive sports competition. The reason for moderation during the first half of the menstrual period is that the flow is heavier during the first 2 or 3 days and some women experience cramps during the first 2 days. Restrictions increase for women with premenstrual discomfort as the severity of the discomfort increases.[16]

Anderson[1] conducted a study on swimming and exercise during menstruation. This study showed that the incidence of discomfort associated with menstruation was less for an active group of competitive swimmers than for girls who did not participate in swimming activities. Also of interest is the study by Astrand et al.[2] of the training of 30 champions who swam a distance of 6,000 to 6,500 meters each week. They found no evidence that the strenuous swimming regimen caused menstrual disturbances.

Exercises for dysmenorrhea

The question has often been asked as to what effects exercise has on dysmenorrhea. Studies indicate that women previously suffering from moderate or severe cases of dysmenorrhea showed a decrease in severity of cramps after performing 8 weeks of prescribed abdominal exercises. These exercises, prescribed for women who had no organic causes for dysmenorrhea, provided relief of congestion in the abdominal cavity caused by gravity, poor posture, poor circulation, or poor abdominal muscle tone. Physical activity also assists relief of leg and back pains by stretching lumbar and pelvic ligaments in the fascia to minimize pressure on spinal nerves. Undue muscular tension may also have a bearing on painful menstruation; therefore, relaxation techniques and positioning of the body, accompanied by heat from a hot water bottle on the low back area, may relax tensions and consequently lessen the pain. Other relaxation techniques and exercises may also be used to reduce tension in the body (see Chapter 8).

Women who suffer from dysmenorrhea may benefit from a daily exercise program designed to alleviate this condition. The exercises should provide for improvement of posture (especially lordosis), stimulation of circulation, and stretching of tight fascia and ligaments. The exercises discussed here are suggested to alleviate the symptoms of dysmenorrhea.

Fascial stretch

The purpose of this exercise is to stretch the shortened fascial ligamentous bands that extend between the low back and the anterior aspect of the pelvis and legs. These shortened bands may result in increased pelvic tilt, which may irritate peripheral nerves passing through or near the fascia. The irritation of these nerves may be the cause of the pain. This exercise produces a stretching effect on the hip flexors and increases mobility of the hip joint[3] (Fig. 17-1).

To perform the exercise, the woman should

stand erect, with the left side of her body about the distance of the bent elbow from a wall; the feet should be together, the left forearm and palm against the wall, with the elbow at shoulder height, and the heel of the other hand placed against the posterior aspect of the hollow portion of the right hip. From this position, abdominal and gluteal muscles should be contracted strongly to tilt the pelvis backward. The hips should slowly be pushed forward and diagonally toward the wall and pressure should be applied with the right hand. This position should be held for a few counts, then slowly a return should be made to the starting position. The stretch should be performed three times on each side of the body. The exercise should be continued even after relief has been obtained from dysmenorrhea. It has been suggested that the exercise be performed three times daily. To increase motivation the girls should record the number of days and times they perform the exercise.

Abdominal pumping

The purpose of abdominal pumping is to increase circulation of the blood throughout the pelvic region. The exercise is performed by assuming a hook-lying position, placing the hands lightly on the abdomen, slowly and smoothly distending the abdomen on the count of one, then retracting the abdomen on the count of two, and relaxing. The exercise should be repeated 8 to 10 times[14] (Fig. 17-2).

Pelvic tilt with abdominal pumping

The purpose of this exercise is to increase the tone of the abdominal muscles, which may eventually contribute to relieving dysmenorrhea.[14] In a hook-lying position, with the feet and knees together, heels 1 inch apart, and hands on the abdomen, the abdominal and gluteal muscles are contracted. The pelvis is rotated so that the tip of the coccyx comes forward and upward and the hips are slightly raised from the floor. The abdomen is distended and retracted. The hips are lowered slowly, vertebra by vertebra, until the original starting position is attained. The exercise is to be repeated 8 to 10 times (Fig. 17-3).

Knee-chest position

The purpose of this exercise is to stretch the extensors of the lumbar spine and strengthen the abdominal muscles. The exercise is performed by bending forward at the hips and placing the hands and arms on a mat. The chest is lowered toward

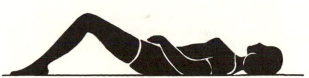

Fig. 17-2. Abdominal pumping.

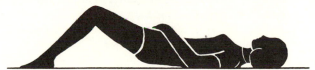

Fig. 17-3. Pelvic tilt with abdominal pumping.

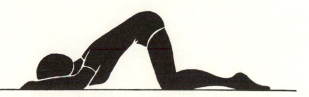

Fig. 17-4. Knee-chest position.

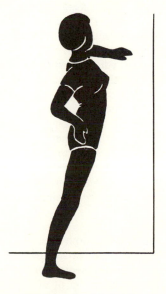

Fig. 17-1. Fascial stretch.

the mat, in a knee-chest position, and held as close to the mat as possible for 3 to 5 minutes.[11] This exercise should be performed once or twice per day (Fig. 17-4).

Implications for physical education

The conclusion reached after review of studies on the effects of physical activity on menstruation is that, for the most part, excuse from physical education class because of the menstrual cycle is not warranted. Social, professional, and athletic schedules cannot be adjusted to each woman's menstrual cycle. It is also realized that many girls and women experience discomfort with menstruation. However, by continuation of activity through the cycle, the impact of menstrual discomfort experienced often decreases.[2]

DIABETES

Diabetes mellitus is a chronic metabolic disorder, the basis of which is the inability of the cells to use glucose. The diabetic's body is unable to burn up its intake of carbohydrates because of a lack of insulin, which is produced by the pancreas. The lack of insulin in the blood prevents the storage of glucose in the cells of the liver. Consequently, blood sugar accumulates in the bloodstream in greater than usual amounts.

Combs, Hale, and Williams indicate that there are 4,000,000 diabetics in the United States. It has been estimated that approximately 65,000 new cases of diabetes develop each year and that approximately 4,750,000 persons presently residing in the United States, who are now free of diabetic symptoms, will develop diabetes during their lifetime. About 10% of the recorded cases occur among children, according to *Diabetic Fact Book,* published by the United States Public Health Service. However, there is a greater prevalence of diabetes with increasing age; approximately half the people who are afflicted with the disease are over the age of 60 years. Furthermore, there is evidence that the diabetic mother may contribute to greater prevalence of diabetic children.[12] Kogan[12] indicates that diabetic mothers have malformed children 10 times more frequently than do nondiabetic mothers.

Teachers should be aware of the symptoms of diabetes in order to help identify the disease if it should appear in any of their students, since early identification and treatment promise the best hope. Symptoms of diabetes include infections that may be slow to heal, fatigue, excessive hunger, itching, impairment in visual acuity, excessive urination and thirst, and skin infections such as boils, carbuncles, ulcers, and gangrenous sores.

The etiology of diabetes is, as yet, unknown. This condition may be caused by too much food, infection, resistance to insulin, injury, surgery, shock, pregnancy, or emotional stress.[18] There seem to be hereditary predispositions for the acquisition of the disease. Also, 70% to 90% of diagnosed diabetics have a history of obesity as a result of having a high fat and carbohydrate content in their diets. Endocrine imbalances, mental trauma, and sedentary living also appear as precipitating factors in the onset of diabetes.

Although the symptoms mentioned may be important in identifying diabetes, the most reliable method of detecting the disorder is a urinalysis by laboratory examination.

Characteristics

Overweight is one of the best-known characteristics of diabetics, particularly in adults. Reducing to normal weight often brings about definite improvement in a diabetic condition. Another characteristic of the diabetic is susceptibility to infection. Therefore, it is suggested that care and prompt treatment be exercised in the event that abrasions, blisters, cuts, or infections occur in physical education activities. Still another complication the physical educator should be cognizant of is a condition called "insulin shock." This condition occurs when the glycogen stored in the liver is depleted. The patient develops general muscular weakness, mental confusion, vertigo, profuse sweating, trembling, and either a pale or a flushed face. If there is a rapid drop in glycogen, symptoms progress to epileptic-like convulsions. When the warning symptoms appear, the patient should eat or drink something containing sugar.

Treatment

It is important that the physical educator understand diabetes treatment procedures so that cooperative efforts with the medical profession can enhance the total development of the child. Effective control of diabetes solely by diet and oral medication has long been sought. Progress toward this objective has been made in recent years through the development of therapeutic drugs that have the properties of insulin. However, another factor is important in the control of diabetes. Participation in exercise functions like insulin in that it burns glucose so less insulin is needed to convert it to glycogen for storage.[4] Insulin injections are usually self-administered by the patients, using hypodermic needles in the upper leg. The injections are generally administered either once or twice daily, depending on individual needs. Also important in the treatment of diabetes is the psychological adjustment patients must make. In addition, patients must undergo regular health checkups and have periodic urinalyses recorded by medical personnel. They must also realize that the condition still is not curable, although it can be controlled. By adjusting to the disciplines placed on them by the physician, diabetics can expect to live lives as long and productive as those of nondiabetic persons.

Insulin shock and diabetic coma

In dealing with the diabetic, the physical educator should be aware that a life-and-death situation can arise from too much or too little insulin. In an inadequate dosage of insulin, the early stages produce lassitude, uneasiness, loss of appetite, unquenchable thirst, and excessive urination. As the demand for insulin becomes greater, symptoms of vomiting, dizziness, and even a diabetic coma may result. A coma and shock condition can also occur from the opposite state of too much insulin. Insulin shock or hypoglycemia may cause a loss of consciousness and eventually, if unchecked, a comatose state. In comparing the diabetic coma with insulin shock, certain differences are apparent: insulin shock occurs rapidly, the patient's skin is moist and pale, there is seldom nausea, and the breath does not smell sweet as in cases of diabetic coma.

Exercise and diabetes

Physical exercise is an important aspect in controlling diabetes. Before the discovery of insulin in the late 1920's, diabetes was controlled primarily through diet and mild exercise. Although scanty, studies conducted before the discovery of insulin show that the number of deaths from diabetes was higher among the group of persons whose occupations were of a sedentary nature than among those with more physically active jobs. From these findings, it might be inferred that exercise was a variable in the longevity of the diabetic. Exercise has been considered so valuable to diabetics that it should be looked on as a duty and incorporated into their daily lives. Walking and mild exercise were thought to be of sufficient value. Yahraes'[21] findings suggest that there might be a relationship between exercise and efficient control of diabetes.

Diabetes does not prevent persons from improving their physical fitness through exercise. Zankle[22] demonstrated that it is possible, through exercise, to increase the Rogers physical fitness index. Furthermore, Engerbretson[9] found that daily insulin dosages in diabetic patients could be reduced when accompanied by exercise. Also, the diabetic control improves during the period of training. In addition, motor fitness of an experimental group subjected to exercise increased during the training period, whereas a nonexercising control group of subjects decreased in motor fitness.

Regular exercise programs are of value to children with diabetes, for exercise may help to stimulate pancreatic secretion as well as contribute to overall body health and assist in maintaining optimal weight, which is a problem for many diabetics. The child with diabetes can participate, in general, in the activities of the unrestricted class. However, in many cases, diabetic patients are more susceptible to fatigue than their nonhandicapped peers. Therefore, the physical educator should be understanding in the event the diabetic cannot withstand prolonged bouts of more strenuous exercise. Adaptations to particular inabilities should be considered.

Implications for physical education

School medical records should be examined in an effort to locate children with diabetes as well as other conditions that may impair their education. After the location of such students, programs of exercise should be established (with medical counsel) according to the needs of each student. The limits to the activity each diabetic child can perform vary. Continuous evaluation must be made to determine the capabilities and limitations of each diabetic child in the performance of physical and motor activity. The physical education program for the diabetic child, as all other physical education programs, should follow specific progressive sequences ranging from light to intense and simple to complex with regard to the development of physical characteristics and motor skills. It is suggested that the initial capability of the child be identified precisely so that no exercise will be prescribed that is more intense or difficult than the child's capabilities permit. Such a situation could be physiologically and psychologically damaging and might retard the child's receptivity to subsequent activity. The setting most suitable for the child with diabetes is in a regular physical education class. In the event that the condition warrants adaptation of exercise and games, these adaptations should be made. The social values accrued from participation with peers seem to far outweigh the possible slight stigma that may be placed on the child because of the adaptations in the physical education program.

KIDNEY DISORDERS

The kidneys and their related structures are the primary organs for excretion in the body, for they remove nitrogenous wastes and various other substances. In addition, the kidneys also eliminate water and help control the water content and osmotic pressure of the blood; they eliminate excess salts to keep proper salt concentration in the blood and

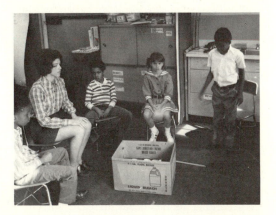

Fig. 17-5. Several handicapping conditions require limited physical activity. (Provided through Unit on Programs for the Handicapped, American Alliance for Health, Physical Education, Recreation, and Dance.)

they control acid-base balance by secreting an excess of either acid or alkaline residues. Thus, the kidneys play an important role in the maintenance of the health of the body.

The rate of kidney secretion is influenced by the pressure of the blood passing through the kidneys. Strenuous and vigorous exercise may cause the blood pressure to increase, thus augmenting the rate of urine excretion. Under conditions of vigorous exercise or high temperature, there is a loss of water and salts. In the event that the salt loss is great, the water content in the tissues will be decreased and the restoration of normal levels of salt will be difficult to achieve. Therefore, in the case of kidney disorders, vigorous exercise may be contraindicated. However, the best procedure to follow with a person who has a kidney disorder is to implement the recommendations of the physician with respect to dosage, duration, and intensity of exercise.

Perhaps the most prevalent kidney disorder that occurs in children and young adults is *chronic nephritis*. This disorder often follows acute infections such as scarlet fever, tonsillitis, diphtheria, or even colds. The symptoms for chronic nephritis may be pain in the lumbar region of the spine, fever, frequent and painful urination, and the presence of blood in the urine. If a student has such a disorder, vigorous exercise is usually contraindicated because chronic nephritis usually yields to rest, proper medical care, and, in some instances, antibiotic treatment.

Turner[19] indicates that "hollow-back posture" may sometimes interfere with normal kidney function and produce albumin in the urine. Also, severe and prolonged chilling of the body, especially after vigorous exercise, may cause congestion and injury to the kidneys. Precaution is particularly important if the child already has a kidney disorder.

A child who has contracted chronic nephritis should take part in programs of physical education within the current limits of functioning. However, the treatment and activities to be included in the program should be under the direction of the physician.

INGUINAL HERNIA

A hernia is a protrusion of an organ through an abnormal opening. The most prevalent site is in the abdominal region. Millions of persons in the United States suffer from some type of hernia, the majority of which are of the inguinal type. However, along with inguinal hernia, there is a high incidence of femoral and umbilical hernias. Generally, the inguinal hernia is more prevalent in males and occurs most often in childhood, whereas the femoral hernia is most prevalent in females.

The inguinal canal is found in the lower abdomen just above Poupart's ligament and serves as a passageway for the spermatic vessels and the vas deferens in the male and the round ligament in the female. It extends about $1\frac{1}{2}$ inches in length, with a downward and inward direction. The canal's internal and external openings are termed the internal and external abdominal rings.

There are two types of inguinal hernias: congenital and acquired. The congenital or direct hernia is primarily associated with the descent of the testes before birth and is often discovered soon after birth. Many congenital hernias close spontaneously with application of a truss, which is a mechanical device that aids in reducing the hernia by placing external pressure at the site; however, surgery for the congenital inginal hernia is the choice of many physicians.[8]

The second type of inguinal hernia occurs be-

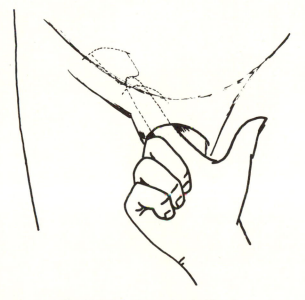

Fig. 17-6. Palpating an inguinal hernia.

tween the ages of 16 and 20 years[8] and is categorized as acquired or indirect. This is best described as a sac protruding through the internal inguinal abdominal ring. An incomplete hernia would still be in the inguinal canal, whereas a complete hernia extends past the subcutaneous external ring and descends into the scrotum.

The femoral hernia, unlike the inguinal hernia, is associated with the female sex. A portion of the lower intestine protrudes through the femoral ring that is provided for the femoral vessels leading to the upper thigh.

There are many reasons attributed to the occurrence of hernia. Some common congenital causes may be inherited weakness of the lower abdomen, faulty descent of the testes, or abnormal enlargement of the internal inguinal ring. An acquired hernia can stem from trauma (as from a blow or lifting a heavy object), from pregnancy, or from degeneration. In general, the anatomy of a hernia may be divided into three parts: the mouth, the hernial ring, and the body. The body of the hernia consists of a sac that protrudes outside the abdominal cavity, often containing a portion of the abdominal viscera.

Early symptoms of the hernia are indicated by a swelling in the area of the internal inguinal ring that expands while the abdomen is under strain and contracts under slight pressure (Fig. 17-6). Pain on exertion may also be elicited in the region of the groin.

The inguinal hernia, besides causing discomfort and aggravation, can also be a serious threat to health. A number of complications may aggravate hernial conditions; these include infection, incarceration, and strangulation. The incarcerated hernia is an irreducible hernial sac. An incarcerated hernia, if not treated promptly, may become strangulated and result in tissue damage, severe pain, and shock.

The student with a hernial condition should be aware of the inherent dangers and should be encouraged to obtain corrective surgery as soon as feasible. While in the preoperative situation, a restrictive physical education program must be afforded. Activities that produce extreme fatigue or intra-abdominal strain, such as weight lifting, gymnastics, track and field, and breath-holding activities, must be avoided. Programming emphasis should be placed on proper body mechanics, mild to moderate exercises, and voluntary lower limb movement while in a sitting or lying position.

INFECTIOUS DISEASES

There are several infectious diseases that may be contracted by schoolchildren. In many cases, modification of activity is necessary to meet the temporary needs and abilities of these children. Some of the infectious diseases that may require the special attention of the physical educator are tuberculosis, pneumonia, streptococcal infections, infectious encephalitis, meningitis, and mononucleosis.

Tuberculosis

Tuberculosis is a disease of the lungs caused by the tubercle bacillus. Predisposing factors are generally conducive for the development of the disease. These factors may include emotional or physical lowering of resistance, alcoholism, a chronic debilitating disease, poor nutrition and hygiene, or a combination of these factors.

No age group is exempt from the disease, but the greatest prevalence of tuberculosis is found among young adults and middle-aged persons.

It is difficult to identify tuberculosis. Perhaps the first indication that such an infection exists may come from a routine x-ray examination of the chest. However, other minor symptoms that may be associated with the onset of the disorder are symptoms of fatigue, failure to gain weight during growth, low fever, cough, chest pain, or a mild case of influenza.

There is great variability in degree, stage, and type of tuberculosis. Since each case of tuberculosis is different, there are many complex factors that must be resolved by the physician when treating the disease. Usually, complete bed rest is required in active cases until the disease can be brought under control. With the resumption of activities of daily living, general strength and endurance may be developed by the implementation of progressive exercise. Also included in the treatment is a nutritious diet and activities that contribute to both physical and mental health. The child who is returning to school after an attack of tuberculosis is usually unable to engage in the unrestricted physical education program. The activities must be adapted to the child's present level of educational performance. Frequent periods of rest must be afforded so that the child will not become unduly fatigued. The physical education program for the child recovering from tuberculosis should be under the direction of the physician.

The activity program should be mild at first and contain the element that all good programs contain, which is progression commensurate with the abilities of the afflicted person. Care should be taken to involve the student in activities that do not cause undue fatigue. The milder recreational activities such as swimming, archery, bowling, camping, or golf provide opportunities for the student to participate.

Pneumonia

Pneumonia is an infection of the air spaces of the lung. Usually, bacteria causing pneumonia gain a foothold through the lowered resistance of a person. There are several types of pneumonia. Some of the most prevalent types are lobar, viral, bronchial, and foreign body.

The lobar pneumonia is often manifested with chills, fever, chest pain, coughing, shortness of breath, and inability to withstand the onset of fatigue. The temperature often reaches 104° to 105° F; consequently, bluish discoloration of the lips and skin occurs.

The viral pneumonia, which generally occurs in the younger and middle-aged groups, possesses symptoms that are often difficult to identify because of gradual onset. On the other hand, pneumonia may also appear very abruptly after an upper respiratory tract infection. The most prevalent symptoms indicating viral pneumonia are generalized muscular pains and a slight cough. At times, however, the symptoms may be similar to the more explosive lobar pneumonia.

Bronchopneumonia occurs often in children. The lungs are usually inflamed and there is often an inability to withstand the onset of fatigue. A cold is also present.

Foreign bodies may also cause pneumonia, for they often precipitate a cough or low fever. In many instances, through the identification of the specific organism responsible for pneumonia, antibiotic treatment will control the disease effectively. An effort should be made to maintain a balanced, nutritious diet. The physical educator should see that a child who has returned to school after an occurrence of pneumonia is not exposed to environmental conditions that would lower resistance and provoke another attack. Also, progressive exercise, starting with activity at the student's present level of educational performance, should be administered.

Streptococcal infections

The streptococcal bacteria cause a wide variety of diseases. The diseases differ with regard to the portal of entry and the tissues on which the infectious agent acts. Some of the more important conditions caused by the streptococcal bacteria are scarlet fever and streptococcal sore throat such as tonsilitis and pharyngitis. Other diseases include mastoiditis, osteomyelitis, otitis media, impetigo, and other skin and wound infections.

Sources of the streptococcal infections are acutely ill or convalescent patients; discharges from the nose, the throat, and purulent lesions; or objects contaminated with such discharges. The transmission of the bacteria is by direct contact with the carrier, by indirect contact with objects handled, or by the spreading of droplets whereby the bacteria can be inhaled. Repeated attacks of streptococcal infections of the throat by different types of streptococci are frequent. It appears that neither active nor passive immunization against the streptococcus itself can be accomplished satisfactorily.

When a student is recovering from a streptococcal infection, caution should be exercised with assignment to an unrestricted physical education program. The same procedures for implementing exercise for the person recovering from streptococcal sore throat are applicable to other illnesses: progressive exercise in accordance with the student's present abilities. Care must be taken to place the student in an environment that will not cause a lowering of resistance, thereby increasing vulnerability to recurring streptococcal infections. Streptococcal infections are particularly dangerous for children who have had rheumatic fever. Consequently, the fact cannot be overemphasized that a child who has been afflicted with rheumatic heart disease should be guarded judiciously against streptococcal infections, which could conceivably further impair heart function. Antibiotic injections can be administered periodically to persons who tend to have recurrent streptococcal infections. This constitutes special risks in that the body may build an immunity to the antibiotic; however, for individuals who have had recurring rheumatic fever, antibiotic treatment may be necessary to avoid subsequent streptococcal infections that may prove damaging to the heart (see Chapter 12).

Infectious encephalitis

Among the many forms of encephalitis, there are two major types: (1) acute nonsuppurative encephalitis that follows or is a part of some infectious disease and (2) the arthropod-borne viral encephalitis.

Nonsuppurative encephalitis

Acute nonsuppurative encephalitis is an acute inflammatory condition of the brain that occurs as a result of complications of various infectious diseases and is characterized by some manifestation of cerebral dysfunction. The condition itself is not contagious, but it may complicate any acute infectious disease, even the common cold. Consequently, the cerebral symptoms may become more prominent than the primary disease. This form of encephalitis may attack all age groups, although children under 10 years of age are more frequently affected than adults.

Symptoms that may give an indication of acute nonsuppurative encephalitis may be headache, visual disturbances (particulary double vision), vertigo nausea, and general weakness. Observable symptoms may include change in sensory media and inattentiveness to ongoing activity. It is not uncommon to find such symptoms as convulsions, muscle twitchings or spasms, tremors, ataxias, and aphasia with the disease. Recovery from encephalitis is usually rapid and apparently complete on the surface, but, in many instances, the nervous system is permanently impaired because of degenerative changes that have occurred as a result of the disease.

Arthropod-borne encephalitis

Although there are many forms of the arthropod-borne viral encephalitis, all types produce an almost identical clinical picture. The symptoms that may be present are headache, tight hamstring muscles, stiff neck and back, fever, disorientation, stupor, coma, tremors, and spasticity. The symptoms may occur abruptly or may develop over a period of 1 week or more. When adults contract the disease, tendon and skin reflexes usually remain normal.

Implications for physical education

The physical educator should be aware of changes that may occur in a student who has had infectious encephalitis. In many instances, particularly if there has been degeneration of the nervous system, the mental as well as the physical needs of the individual may be different on return to class as compared with performance prior to the attack. The physical education teacher should know the limits of activity for each child and should be sensitive to adapting the activities so that the child may make a satisfactory adjustment to regular school activities. Characteristics that may be manifested after the attack are fatigue, impaired motor coordination, and a decrement of strength.

Meningitis

Meningitis is an acute contagious disease characterized by the inflammation of the meninges of the spinal cord. The severity with which persons are attacked by the disease varies greatly. Epidemics of meningitis occur with greater frequency in rural areas as opposed to urban areas. The disease occurs at any age; however, 40% of the meningitis cases occur in children under 10 years of age. There is also a great prevalence of meningitis in older children and young adults. Epidemics of meningitis are more prevalent in the winter and spring seasons of the year.

The onset of meningitis is usually abrupt and accompanied by severe headache and chills, followed soon by fever and vomiting. Other characteristics indicating the presence of the disease may be irritability, delirium, stupor, coma, convulsions, constipation or diarrhea, rash, infections of the ear such as mastoiditis or otitis media, difficulty in hearing, or eye conditions such as conjunctivitis, optic neuritis, diplopia, and strabismus. Meningitis is a serious disease because many complications may be associated with it. These complications are pneumonia, otitis media and mastoiditis, arthritis, hydrocephalus, ocular conditions such as conjunc-

tivitis and optic neuritis, cystitis, endocarditis, or pericarditis.

Many forms of meningitis can be classified within four major types. Several subheadings fall under each of the major types. The main classifications are meningococcus meningitis, lymphocytic choriomeningitis, influenzal meningitis, and purulent meningitis. Each form needs to be diagnosed differentially for medical treatment.

Implications for the physical educator

Usually, the convalescent period for meningitis is not as long as for some other communicable diseases. Therefore, it may be possible to involve the child more quickly in a graded program of activity than is possible in the case of other illnesses.

AUTISM

Autism is a condition in which a person is dominated by subjective, self-centered trends of thought and behavior. Two different autistic syndromes have been identified. *Early autism* appears during the first year of life. These children walk before they develop useful language, and they often never demonstrate meaningful communication skills. They develop bizarre behaviors, avoid eye contact with others, and are withdrawn. Because of their lack of social interaction and seeming cognitive defects, retarded mental development appears progressive. Both sexes are equally affected. The second form of autism, *autistic psychopathy,* begins in the third year, after useful communication skills have developed. Bizarre behaviors and avoidance of eye contact are also demonstrated by these children (mostly boys); however, prompt professional attention often alleviates social interaction difficulties.[6] In addition to inappropriate communication and social and physical behaviors, autistic children also have difficulties developing motor, visual, and auditory perception.

Motor traits of autistic children

There is considerable information concerning the abilities of autistic children. However, the data from the literature conflict with respect to general aptitude on specific motor traits. However, there is agreement that autistic children usually possess limited motor abilities as compared with other children of the same chronological age. There is some evidence, although scanty, that autistic children possess greater variance in profiles of abilities than do normal children. For instance, DesLaurlers and Carlson[7] report that autistic children have poor gross motor coordination but well-developed fine motor skills. Autistic children, in many instances, possess uneven profiles of abilities and tend to convert their assets into obvious talents, whereas other aspects of their behavior may become poorly developed.

Gross motor ability

For the most part, autistic children possess abnormalities in gross motor development. They are often clumsy and poorly coordinated. However, there are indications that through proper application of learning principles and developmental curricula, autistic children can be taught to learn gross motor activity. This has been demonstrated by Kozloff,[13] who taught autistic children physical activity through a shaping procedure of increasing the frequency and duration of episodes of self-initiated play.

Perceptual-motor ability

There is information that autistic children possess distinct limitations in matching perceptual inputs with motor outputs. Some of the limitations are as follows:

1. Inability to clap hands to music, reflecting auditory-motor disability
2. Inability to manipulate objects, the result of visuomotor disability
3. Inability to translate imitation of movement into similar motor patterns, a further example of visuomotor disability
4. Inability to perform self-help skills, the result of impairment in gross and fine motor skills

The autistic child, as a rule, possesses a set of limited motor characteristics. The physical educator thus has a challenge in the development of a most worthy aspect of the functions of everyday living. The application of physical training programs to autistic children possesses great possibilities of exploration.

Socialization and play

The autistic child often is out of touch with reality and therefore finds it difficult to socialize with other children. It has been hypothesized that stereotyped activity prevents the optimal development of skills. With limitation of skills, it is often difficult for the autistic child to engage in social activities with others. Team or group interaction depends on the severity of the disability and acquisition of skills. Competitive situations are often frightening and demoralizing to the child and tend to increase withdrawal.

Instructional activities that enable the autistic child to play effectively are essential. A clear, systematic instructional system is needed in which skills for socialization can be developed with full knowledge of missing prerequisite behaviors and of programming to provide the necessary motor skills that will enable success in social living.

Some characteristics of the autistic child that reduce social opportunities are as follows:

1. *Social withdrawal and unresponsiveness:* These behaviors often make autistic children inaccessible to their peers, their parents, and other adults.
2. *Behavioral inflexibility:* These children appear to function best in highly structured environments in which predictable routines are established. Changes in routine or in the environment tend to upset many autistic children.
3. *Stereotyped behavior:* Many autistic children engage in stereotyped behaviors in which a specific act is repeated over and over. These behaviors often are bizarre and further reduce the social acceptance of the children by others.
4. *Self-mutilating behavior:* These behaviors involve acts that injure the children. Some examples of such activity are head banging and biting and hitting oneself. All these behaviors make it more difficult for the children to engage in social activity.

Wing[20] indicates that, in normal play, rules that most children pick up easily cause autistic children great difficulty. Many such children have difficulty in adopting social play behaviors appropriate to the situation, which often results in a withdrawal. Thus, there is a need for a systematic planning of social interaction with others.

Inasmuch as play is a medium in which the inabilities of autistic children can be identified, it may be a medium through which these children may facilitate positive social behavior. There are social sequences of play and prescriptive techniques for facilitation of the social behavior in microsocial environments. These techniques are worthy of trial with autistic children.

There should be concerted efforts made to move autistic children from adult-initiated and side-by-side play to cooperative play with others. This is a formidable challenge. The play of autistic children weakens without the presence of novelty in the environment. Novelty can be introduced in several ways to foster the play behavior; some of these ways are as follows:

1. Skills within the ability levels of the children can be developed so that they may invent novel ways of manipulating the environment.
2. New playthings may be added to the environment.
3. The children can be introduced to different social settings.
4. Different environmental events may be structured.

Novelty can be added in other ways. To foster play development, it is important to pair the play materials with the skill levels of the children. Otherwise, there may be considerable difficulty in motivating the children to interact with the play materials so that skill and social development may occur.

Instructional factors

The literature indicates that if accepted principles of learning are applied to the instruction of children with autism and if target objectives are within their capabilities, progress in learning tasks is feasible. The effective use of shaping procedures in the teaching of a motor skill to autistic children has already been mentioned (Chapter 16). Wing[20] suggests the use of sequential activities for programming for autistic children. The children are then moved at their own rates through the sequence. Another technique that utilizes the principles of learning is the modeling of visual movement to communicate to the children tasks that they are to perform. The use of aversive stimuli, that is, an avoidance type of learning, may be successful but should be used as a last resort. Therefore, with the proper application of learning principles to pro-

gramming, productive positive learning results are possible with autistic children.

There are indications that tasks that are rather complex and that require complicated processing of information by the learner often are too difficult for the autistic child. Activities that require quick decisions and changing situations are, more often than not, too advanced for the autistic child. Therefore, when selecting tasks for the child, it is desirable to perform an analysis of the task according to its complexity in relationship to the ability of the child.

Several instructional techniques can be used with autistic children. However, directions should be presented in a clear, concise, and simple manner with a multisensory approach. Also, activities should be presented in such a way that there is not a reversal or mirror image effect, that is, the instructor should plan to present visual information so that children view the behavior from the rear of the instructor.

REFERENCES

1. Anderson, T. W.: Swimming and exercise during menstruation, J. Health Phys. Educ. Rec. **36**:66-68, 1965.
2. Astrand, P. O., et al.: Girl swimmers with special reference to respiratory and circulatory adaptation and gynaecological and psychiatric aspects, Acta Paediatr. (Suppl.) **147**:1-71, 1963.
3. Billig, H. E., Jr., and Lowendahl, E.: Mobilization of the human body, Stanford, Calif., 1949, Stanford University Press.
4. Bleck, E., and Nagel, W.: Physically handicapped children: a medical atlas for teachers, New York, 1975, Grune & Stratton, Inc.
5. Clow, A. E., and Sanderson, M.: Effect of physical exercise on menstruation, Mind Body **30**:19-21, 1923.
5a. Combs, B. J., Hale, D. R., and Williams, B. K.: An invitation to health, Menlo Park, Calif., 1980, Benjamin/Cummings Publishing Co.
6. de Quiros, J. B., and Schrager, O. L.: Neuropsychological fundamentals in learning disabilities, 1978, San Rafael, Calif., Academic Therapy Publications.
7. DesLaurlers, A. M., and Carlson, C. F.: Your child is asleep; early infantile autism: etiology, treatment, parental influences, Homeward, Ill., 1969, Dorsey Press.
8. Duntzer, E., and Hellendall, M.: Munch. Med. Wochenschr. **76**:1835, 1929.
9. Engerbretson, D. L.: The effects of internal training on the insulin dosage, sugar levels and other indexes of physical fitness in three diabetic subjects, Unpublished master's thesis, University of Illinois, Urbana, Ill., 1962.
10. Gilman, E.: Exercise program for correction of dysmenorrhea, J. Health Phys. Educ. Rec. **15**:377-381, 1944.

11. Kelly, E. D.: Adapted and corrective physical education, New York, 1965, The Ronald Press Co.
12. Kogan, B.: Health, New York, 1967, Harcourt Brace Jovanovich, Inc.
13. Kozloff, M.: Reaching the autistic child, Champaign, Ill., 1973, Research Press.
14. Mosher, C. D.: Dysmenorrhea, J.A.M.A. **62:**1297, 1914.
15. Nolen, J.: Problems of menstruation, J. Health Phys. Educ. Rec. **36:**12, 1965.
16. Phillips, M., Fox, K., and Young, O.: Sports activity for girls, J. Health Phys. Educ. Rec. **30:**23-25, 1959.
17. Runge, H.: Effects of bodily exercise on menstruation, J.A.M.A. **129:**68-72, 1928.
18. Schmitt, G. F.: Diabetes for diabetics: a practical guide, Miami, 1973, The Diabetes Press of America, Inc.
19. Turner, C. E.: Personal and community health, ed. 14, St. Louis, 1971, The C. V. Mosby Co.
20. Wing, J. K.: Early childhood autism, Colorado Springs, Colo, 1966, Maxwell Publishers.
21. Yahraes, H.: Good news about diabetes, Public affairs pamphlet no. 138, New York, 1948, Public Affairs Committee, Inc.
22. Zankle, H. T.: Physical fitness index of diabetic patients, J. Assoc. Phys. Ment. Rehabil. **10:**14-17, 1956.

RECOMMENDED READINGS

Clarke, H. H., and Clarke, D. H.: Developmental and adapted physical education, Englewood Cliffs, N.J., 1963, Prentice-Hall, Inc.
Daniels, A. S., and Davies, E. A.: Adapted physical education, ed. 3, New York, 1975, Harper & Row, Publishers.
Fait, H. F.: Special physical education: adapted, corrective, developmental, ed. 3, Philadelphia, 1975, W. B. Saunders Co.
Muscular dystrophy—the facts, New York, 1959, Muscular Dystrophy Association of America, Inc.
Wallace, H. M.: The muscular dystrophies. In Frampton, M. E., editor: The physically handicapped and special health problems. Boston 1955. Porter Sargent, Publisher.

PART FOUR

Organization and administration

Teachers and therapists need to be knowledgeable about plans for district and school programs of adapted physical education. They should know how to plan the curriculum, organize a class, and write Individual Education Programs. Special facility and equipment needs of the handicapped should be a part of teacher preparation programs. These topics are discussed in Part Four.

18

Program organization and administration

No one type of adapted physical education program is suitable for all school levels or for all school districts. Possibly, this is why there is a very limited amount of material written about the organization and administration of physical education for the handicapped. Good organization and administration are essential if handicapped children are to be included in increasing numbers in our schools and colleges and if they are to grow and flourish at a time when educational costs are rising and when pressures exist to examine carefully the total curricular offerings at all school levels.

If one believes in the importance of providing worthwhile physical education programs for all students at all school levels, it is then equally important to offer athletic and extramural activities for gifted students, regular physical education and intramural sports for average students, and adapted physical education for physically handicapped students. This last group, who probably need physical education and recreation experiences more than either of the other two, have in the past, been provided with inadequate experiences.

State and federal legislation, culminating in P.L. 94-142, should provide quality educational experiences in most states for handicapped persons from the ages of 4 to 21 years. Adapted physical education teachers at all school levels should plan to include special programs for the handicapped in their curricula to satisfy this mandate. Teacher education institutions must also include information on procedures to be followed for their students specializing in physical education and recreation so

that they are prepared to teach classes and offer programs for all types of disabled persons in both adapted and regular physical education classes.

Adapted physical education is traditionally offered in one or more ways in districts across the United States. Prior to the signing of P.L. 94-142, many states provided adapted physical education classes for their handicapped students under a state-supported plan. Other plans were supported by the local school district and still others were under the sponsorship of the county. Ideally, these various agencies should offer a cooperative program designed to meet the needs of all handicapped persons.

In the final analysis, each state, county, and local district must now face up to the problem of how best to meet their mandated obligation to the disabled student. In any case, the goals, principles, and objectives of such programs are similar.

In 1951, the American Association for Health, Physical Education, and Recreation and the Joint Committee on Health Problems in Education of the American Medical Association and the National Education Association prepared an excellent set of principles that should prove worthwhile to persons interested in organizing, promoting, and evaluating programs of adapted physical education.

GUIDING PRINCIPLES OF ADAPTED PHYSICAL EDUCATION IN ELEMENTARY AND SECONDARY SCHOOLS AND COLLEGES*

It is the responsibility of the school to contribute to the fullest possible development of the potentialities of each individual entrusted to its care. This is a basic tenet of our democratic faith.

1. There is need for common understanding regarding the nature of adapted physical education.

2. There is need for adapted physical education in schools and colleges. . . .

3. Adapted physical education has much to offer the individual who faces the combined problem of seeking an education and living most effectively with a handicap.

Through adapted physical education the individual can: (a) Be observed and referred when the need for

medical or other services is suspected; (b) Be guided in avoidance of situations which would aggravate the condition. or subject him to unnecessary risks or injury; (c) Improve neuromuscular skills, general strength and endurance following convalescence from acute illness or injury; (d) Be provided with opportunities for improved psychological adjustment and social development.

4. The direct and related services essential for the proper conduct of adapted physical education should be available to our schools.

These services should include: (a) Adequate and periodic health examination; (b) Classification for physical education based on the health examination and other pertinent tests and observations; (c) Guidance of individuals needing special consideration with respect to physical activity, general health practices, recreational pursuits, vocational planning, psychological adjustment, and social development; (d) Arrangement of appropriate adapted physical education programs; (e) Evaluation and recording of progress through observations, appropriate measurements and consultations; (f) Integrated relationships with other school personnel, medical and its auxiliary services, and the family to assure continuous guidance and supervisory services; (g) Cumulative records for each individual, which should be transferred from school to school.

5. It is essential that adequate medical guidance be available for teachers of adapted physical education.

The possibility of serious pathology requires that programs of adapted physical education should not be attempted without the diagnosis, written recommendation, and supervision of a physician. The planned program of activities must be predicated upon medical findings and accomplished by competent teachers working with medical supervision and guidance. There should be an effective referral service between physicians, physical educators, and parents aimed at proper safeguards and maximum student benefits. School administrators, alert to the special needs of handicapped children, should make every effort to provide adequate staff and facilities necessary for a program of adapted physical education.

6. Teachers of adapted physical education have a great responsibility as well as an unusual opportunity.

Physical educators engaged in teaching adapted physical education should: (a) Have adequate professional education to implement the recommendations provided by medical personnel; (b) Be motivated by the highest ideals with respect to the importance of total student development and satisfactory human relationships; (c) Develop the ability to establish rapport with students who may exhibit social maladjustment as a result of a disability; (d) Be aware of a student's attitude toward his disability; (e) Be objective in relationships with students; (f)

---

*Presented by permission of the Committee on Adapted Physical Education, American Alliance for Health, Physical Education, and Recreation.

Be prepared to give the time and effort necessary to help a student overcome a difficulty; (g) Consider as strictly confidential information related to personal problems of the student; (h) Stress similarities rather than deviations, and abilities instead of disabilities.

7. Adapted physical education is necessary at all school levels.

The student with a disability faces the dual problem of overcoming a handicap and acquiring an education which will enable him to take his place in society as a respected citizen. Failure to assist a student with problems may retard the growth and development process.

Offering adapted physical education in the elementary grades, and continuing through the secondary school and college, will assist the individual to improve function and make adequate psychological and social adjustments. It will be a factor in attaining maximum growth and development within the limits of the disability. It will minimize attitudes of defect and fears of insecurity. It will help the student face the future with confidence.

Content areas for physical education for the handicapped are indicated in the regulations of P.L. 94-142 (see Chapter 2). The objectives should represent definite behaviors that are attainable by students in the program; however, all students would not be expected to attain all the objectives. An adapted physical education program organized so that all of the objectives are provided for makes it possible for all students to meet those objectives of special importance to their particular needs and interests.

ADAPTED PHYSICAL EDUCATION FOR THE HANDICAPPED AND NONHANDICAPPED

The legal obligations to handicapped children are different than those to nonhandicapped children. In the past, adapted physical education programs have been developed to accommodate students who have temporary injuries (such as pre- and postoperative cases), weak musculature, or problems with posture or body mechanics. Many of these students are *not* handicapped. Thus, obligations for altering existing administrative structures for these persons to accommodate federal statutes do not apply. However, handicapped students are to be provided with Individual Education Programs in the least restrictive environment or the regular class, if possible.

OBJECTIVES OF ADAPTED PHYSICAL EDUCATION

The aim of physical education for the handicapped is to aid them to achieve physical, mental, emotional, and social growth commensurate with their potential through carefully planned programs of regular and special physical education activities.

Specific objectives to help the student accomplish this are as follows:

1. To help students correct conditions that can be improved
2. To help students protect themselves and any conditions that would be aggravated through certain physical activities
3. To provide students with an opportunity to learn and to participate in a number of appropriate recreational and leisure-time sports and activities
4. To help students understand their physical and mental limitations
5. To help students make social adjustments and develop a feeling of self-worth and value
6. To aid students in developing knowledge and appreciation relative to good body mechanics
7. To help students understand and appreciate a variety of sports that they can enjoy as nonparticipants or spectators

Many government programs and state laws currently require that program administrators and teachers state their program goals and objectives in behavioral or performance terms. This provides for more accurate assessment and accountability of programs, teachers, and students. A meaningfully stated objective is one that succeeds exactly in communicating to the reader the writer's instructional intent. Performance objectives must include the following:

1. A statement of who is going to demonstrate (the performer)
2. A statement of what exactly is included (knowledge, skills, and/or behavior)
3. A statement of the conditions under which the performance will be done
4. A statement identifying the standard of achievement (how *well* and/or how *much*)
5. A statement indicating how the performance will be measured (with what instruments, used by whom)

Chapter 4 of this text includes a more complete discussion of this topic with numerous examples given. Examples are also given in Chapter 5. Three examples are given here to help clarify the technique of writing performance objectives.

Example 1: For an obese girl assigned to an adapted physical education class to lose weight: "Jill Jones will lose $1/2$ pound of body weight each week during the 15-week fall semester."

Example 2: For a boy with cerebral palsy who wishes to improve his ability and skill in swimming: "Mike Moon will demonstrate his ability to swim a distance of 50 yards using each of two different swimming strokes (with no time limit) by the end of the spring semester."

Example 3: For a trainable mentally retarded person with severe perceptual-motor problems: "Alex Brooks will demonstrate his ability to roll over from a prone to a supine position and to crawl and creep one body length on a mat by the end of the fall quarter."

Physical education programs are influenced by a number of practical factors that vary from district to district and even among schools located in the same district. These factors include the following:

1. Community and administrative support
2. Adequacy of the budget
3. Available facilities and equipment
4. Availability of qualified supervisory and teaching personnel
5. Student interest and support

Thus, based on sound aims, objectives, and principles and conditioned by practical factors that may influence the curriculum of a school, physical education for the handicapped must be planned so that it operates most effectively for the students, teachers, and administrators of the particular school or district. Subsequent sections of this chapter should provide helpful suggestions toward this end.

ORGANIZATION OF THE PROGRAM

There should be a long-range plan of organization, whether a new program is being formulated or a well-established one is being evaluated and change suggested for it. Responsibility for the program should be delegated to one person, usually a supervisor at the district level or a well-qualified teacher if one school is being considered. In either case, this person should be aided by an advisory committee or council. This committee helps in such matters as establishment of policy, formation of long-range plans, selection and release of students (at the school level), and interpretation and promotion of the program.

The supervisor and the teacher

The person in charge of the program, together with the teachers, constitutes the program's most important single aspect. For this reason, the supervisor or teacher should be selected because of outstanding qualifications, including personality, experience, training, and knowledge of local, state, and federal regulations.

The traditional role of adapted physical education was to provide opportunities for handicapped persons to successfully participate in the activities of the physical education program. There are two different aspects to the adapted physical education program. One is accommodation of the handicapped child in handicapped-only classes; the other involves making provisions for the Individual Education Program in the least restrictive environment or the regular class. The supervisor of physical education for the handicapped should be competent in both roles.

Interpersonal skill

Interpersonal skill is a most important quality for a teacher and is doubly important for the supervisor-teacher of adapted physical education. The very nature of the position, involving as it does both teaching and administration, requires close contact with administrators, counselors, medical personnel, teachers, and students. Students with special needs require a superior teacher, one who can establish close rapport with students, teach effectively, and work diplomatically with physicians, nurses, administrators, and other teachers. These qualities are necessary to ensure success in an adapted physical education program.

Experience

Prior teaching experience with competency for implementing the Individual Education Programs is a necessary prerequisite for the person who assumes the leadership of an adapted physical education program. Techniques and procedures used in teaching special physical education vary somewhat from those used in teaching regular physical education classes. Generally, more individual teaching and counseling are done with the handicapped and a closer bond is established between teacher and pupil. Special skills and knowledge also are necessary to deal effectively with physicians, nurses, and other medical personnel.

Training

It is desirable that the person heading the adapted physical education program have, as minimum qualifications, special training in life and physical sciences, psychology, applied anatomy and physiology, and adapted physical education. Graduate training in adapted or corrective physical education, corrective therapy, or physical therapy would strengthen this background so that expert leadership can be given to members of the adapted physical education teaching faculty and to students in the program.

Federal and state legislation has allowed for the expansion of educational programs for the handicapped. To provide better instructional programs for these persons, teacher education institutions have had to expand their training programs to meet this need. Special credentials, certificates, and degrees are granted to persons who complete advanced specialized programs in preparation for their work with handicapped individuals. Extensive field work, internship, and/or student teaching assignments should be part of such advanced training.

The American Association for Health, Physical Education, and Recreation in cooperation with the Bureau of Education for the Handicapped, United States Department of Health, Education, and Welfare published *Guidelines for Professional Preparation Programs for Personnel Involved in Physical Education and Recreation for the Handicapped*. The guidelines elaborate on the preparation necessary for persons to enter programs of training to work with the handicapped and outline the qualifications that teachers and therapists should possess on completion of their training. This information has been briefly summarized as follows:

The minimum prerequisite for enrollment in any program preparing a specialist in physical education for impaired, disabled, and handicapped persons should be an undergraduate degree and/or certification in physical education. Individuals with preparation in related professions or disciplines should be considered for graduate specialist programs only if their previous training and experience are supplemented with *essential* professional competencies of the physical education teacher. Ideally every adapted physical education specialist should possess and be able to teach skills and knowledges in a variety of physical activities, to promote a love of activity and participation in a given age group, and to understand and appreciate why such participation is important and vital to all, including impaired, disabled, and handicapped persons.

The specialist in adapted physical education should be able to perform these functions:

1. Assess and evaluate the physical and motor status of individuals with a variety of handicapping conditions.
2. Develop (design, plan), implement (conduct), and evaluate diversified programs of physical education for individuals and groups with any of a variety of handicapping conditions.
3. Participate in interprofessional situations providing special programs or services for individuals or groups, including coordination of such services for a program. *

The advisory committee

The advisory committee may be district-wide or may be set up to advise relative to the program at one particular school.

An advisory committee at the district level might consist of the school district physician, a key administrator at the district level, a district or school nurse, the supervisor of adapted physical education, the special education teacher, a specialist, and, possibly, a representative from each of the following groups:

1. The regular physical education teachers
2. The teachers who do not teach physical education

---

*From Guidelines for professional preparation programs for personnel involved in physical education and recreation for the handicapped, Washington, D.C., 1973, American Association for Health, Physical Education and Recreation and Bureau of Education for the Handicapped, U.S. Department of Health, Education, and Welfare.

3. The Parent-Teacher Association or other parents' group
4. Representatives of other community groups that are closely associated with handicapped children.

This committee is advisory in nature and aids the supervisor in the establishment and interpretation of policy, in fostering good public relations, in procuring funds for the program, and in dealing with physicians', nurses', and parents' groups in the community.

An advisory committee at the school level has responsibilities similar to those of the district committe. It should advise and support the teachers of adapted physical education. It is concerned with interpretation of the program and with public relations at the school level. Members of this committee usually include the school physician, the school nurse, an administrator, teachers of adapted physical education for girls and/or for boys, and, often, one or more of the following persons: a teacher from an area other than physical education, a parent or Parent-Teacher Association member, a counselor, a student, the health coordinator, or a representative of the health teachers.

The supervisor and the teachers of adapted physical education will find that the adapted physical education committee can give them invaluable aid in planning for and interpreting this specialized type of program. The members of these committees must therefore be selected with great care.

Interpreting the program

Promoting an adapted physical education program in either a school or a school district requires excellence in program planning and teaching, demonstrating that positive results can be obtained through the conduct of a *quality* program.

Prior to the passage of P.L. 94-142, it was often necessary for the physical educator to promote programs for handicapped children. However, physical education is an entitlement of every handicapped child. Extensive child identification procedures were a part of P.L. 94-142 in the mid-1970's. Once the handicapped children were identified, they were comprehensively assessed in specific areas of educational need. Thus, at present, each local school district should have detailed data on the physical education needs of each handi-

capped child. These can be presented to school boards, administrators, parents' and teachers' groups, and students to inform them of the need for and value of adapted physical education.

The survey

A survey of a school or district for the purpose of showing a need for adapted physical education should include information about the following factors:

1. The availability of teachers and their background of education and experience
2. The time allotment necessary for the program
3. The cost of the program
4. Existing facilities and equipment and amount of additional space and supplies needed
5. Special problems concerning related services
6. Special problems involved in counseling these students and scheduling them for classes at special hours during the day

The caliber of the adapted physical education teacher is the single most important factor of those listed. Money, equipment, support from related service care providers, and other teachers all are important, but an enthusiastic, well-qualified teacher is a necessity. The teacher of physically, mentally, or emotionally handicapped children must not only be a good instructor, but must also have the understanding and the ability to establish rapport with students who are seeking an education despite their disabilities.

Because the adapted physical education program involves special classes for only a portion of the total student enrollment of a school and because class size should often be limited to allow for considerable individual instruction, scheduling problems sometimes result. School administrators and counselors must be convinced that this group of students, who have a special need, should be scheduled or programmed into the physical education class early in the selection of their class schedule. The Individual Education Program requires that each handicapped child receive instruction that meets his or her specific needs. Furthermore, the placement of the child (where the instruction is to take place) is cooperatively decided by the parents and the school. Therefore, the scheduling of handicapped children in physical education activity must be flexible.

An adapted physical education program does cost a school or school district additional money. Small classes, special equipment, a special room, and additional related services increase costs over what is spent on regular physical education classes. These costs need not be exorbitant, however. An excellent program can be provided with a minimum of special equipment and even without a special room if one is not available. To help meet the excess expenses, district, state, and federal funds should be made available for classes for handicapped students who have need for special attention in physical education.

Adequate equipment and a well-planned adapted physical education room facilitate positive teacher performance and add enjoyment to the program for the student. The teacher who has adequate facilities and equipment can do a better job of meeting the needs of the special student.

The school physician and the nurse play an important role in the adapted physical education program. The support and active backing of these persons are essential if a top-quality program is to be presented. The initial screening is often performed by medical and psychological personnel. This information indicates whether the child is handicapped and provides data concerning contraindicated activity for a specific handicapping condition. However, once the program is under way, revision of the program must be done with the cooperation of the parents and the persons providing the related services.

Considerable data are available to substantiate the importance of providing physical education classes for all students enrolled in school, extending from kindergarten through college or university. Local districts; the American Medical Association; the California Association for Health, Physical Education, and Recreation; the American Alliance for Health, Physical Education, Recreation, and Dance; and the President's Council on Physical Fitness have gathered valuable data to substantiate the need for physical education at all school levels. Published materials recommending special programs of adapted physical education in our schools are numerous.[2-12] P.L. 94-142, discussed in Chapters 1, 4, and 19, mandates the inclusion of equal educational opportunity for handicapped persons.

Teacher and student schedules

Because the adapted physical education class requires a teacher with special training, certain problems may develop in scheduling the classes of that teacher. In a small school, classes may be offered only one or two periods during the day. If more than one class is offered, it is advantageous to have them scheduled consecutively. This will facilitate opening the special adapted physical education room, providing the special equipment necessary, and obtaining the medical records and the exercise and activity cards. It will also give the teacher time between the two periods to counsel students in need of special help. These same advantages prevail for a single class if it is scheduled the first period in the morning, before or after lunch, or the last period in the afternoon.

Some important factors in student scheduling were discussed earlier in this chapter; however, there are some additional matters that also should be considered.

If the special exercise room, the pool, or the special game areas used by the adapted physical education classes are available only during certain periods of the day, the schedule should be arranged so that the adapted classes can be held in as many of these areas as possible during the course of the year. Often, adapted classes will be held in the gymnasium, the dance studio, or the gymnastic, weight-training, or wrestling room. When this is done, it should be a part of the master schedule of this particular facility. These rooms may be used in lieu of a special adapted room, or they may be used as a facility for one of the activities offered in the adapted sports and activity program.

The adapted sports and activity program can usually be quite flexible and can be organized to permit facilities to be used when they are not needed by the other physical education classes that meet during the same period. It is important, however, that a block of time be provided for the adapted class for each activity area, including the pool, so that students in this program have a rich and varied experience in a wide range of physical education activities.

If possible, adapted physical education classes for the boys and for the girls should be coeducational classes or should be scheduled at the same time of day. Thus, coeducational classes can be offered or coeducational activities can be arranged for the students in this program when the time and the activities permit.

RELATIONSHIP WITH ADMINISTRATORS, RELATED SERVICE PERSONNEL, AND PARENTS

The support of five persons or groups of persons is essential if a school or school district is to have a quality program in adapted physical education. They are the administrator, the teacher, related service personnel, the parents, and the student. The teacher's role has already been discussed and the student's role will vary with the particular handicap involved.

The administrator

The support of the administrator is necessary if the program is to receive its share of district and school resources. The administrator can help in the following ways:

1. Giving enthusiastic support to the total program
2. Providing an adequate budget

YOURNAME HIGH SCHOOL
LONG BEACH, CALIFORNIA

Alan Walters, M. D.

Dear Dr. Walters,

    In order that we may better serve the health needs of our students, the Yourname High School wishes to acquaint the medical profession with the service it is prepared to render through its physical education departments.

    As you know, physical education is required, by law, for all students attending high school in California.

    Classes for girls/boys are conducted by specially trained teachers and include special programs as follows:

Posture and body mechanics:	Preventive and corrective exercise programs for feet, ankles, knees, spinal curvatures, and other postural problems.
Weak musculature:	Developmental exercises and activities for the subfit student.
Restricted activities:	Adapted sports and activities for those students in need of a limited activity program (cardiac, asthma, etc.).
Pre- and post-operative:	Special exercise programs as prescribed by the physician.
Dysmenorrhea: (girls)	Counseling and exercise and activity programs as advised by the physician.
Rest:	Quiet games and activities, relaxation techniques, or rest as prescribed.

    Classes are small and individual attention is given each student. Your suggestions and your interest in this program are solicited.

Sincerely yours,

Marie Carol M. D.
School physician

Approved: J. Officer
           Principal

A

Fig. 18-1. A, Letter to the private physician from the school doctor.

3. Requiring adequately trained teachers
4. Supporting necessary student schedule changes
5. Providing auxiliary services such as medical aid, nursing, transportation, and maintenance

Related service personnel

Related service personnel play a very important role in physical education programs for the handicapped. In addition to providing services that will assist the children to benefit from the physical education program, they may also enhance the program in the following ways:

1. Interpreting the program to medical personnel in the district, to parents, and to the total school population (Fig. 18-1)
2. Handling or making referrals of students with special problems

3. Fully informing the adapted physical education instructors of the students' conditions and recommending exercises and activities (Fig. 18-2)

The parents

Parents are specifically informed as to their children's level of developmental progress and the specific skills that they will be able to perform by the end of the year. Such information must be contained in a written document. Many schools provide an information sheet or brochure to the parents of each student. This gives an overview of the general rules and regulations of the physical education departments. It may also include information about the adapted program, its aims, its objectives, its activity offerings, and its admission and dismissal procedures. It should be described as an

B

Date _____

To: _____
            School physician

_____ High School

From: _____, M.D.

Subject: Recommendations re: Physical Education for my patient,

_____

            Based on my examination of _____, his/her

physical education assignment should be as follows:

Diagnosis _____

Temporary _____ (How long) _____

All activities except (please list) _____

_____

Only the following activities (please list) _____

_____

Special exercises for (please list) _____

_____

Date _____ Signed _____, M.D.
                                Personal physician

Continued.

Fig. 18-1, cont'd. B, Letter from the private physician to the school.

YOURNAME HIGH SCHOOL

PHYSICAL EDUCATION DEPARTMENTS

Date _Jan 15th_

Dear _Mr Hunter_,

Your ~~daughter~~/son _Michael_ , by recommendation

of _Alan Walter, M.D._ has been assigned to the Adapted

Physical Education program because _of cardiac_

problems and poor posture.

Yourname High School's Adapted Physical Education program

offers each student in the class an opportunity to either correct,

improve, or compensate for physical or organic problems he might

have. Each student is given individual attention in accordance

with the recommendations of a family doctor or a school physician.

Every effort is made to make the time spent in this class safe

and profitable for your child.

Sincerely yours,

Approved:
Chris Steffy, M.D.   _David Walter Daniels_
School Physician   Adapted Physical Education Instructor

- -

I would like to have a conference with the Adapted Physical

Education Teacher. Day _____ Time _____. (You

may call for an appointment if you would prefer.)

Signed

_____
Parent or Guardian

Telephone number: 437-0007
437-0707

Fig. 18-1, cont'd. C, Letter to parents from the physical education instructor.

extension and an integral part of the total physical education program, open to any student in the school during a time of special need. The scope of the program can be described to the parent as including provisions for the following:

1. A physically, emotionally, or mentally handicapped person
2. A person who has been injured recently
3. A preoperative or postoperative patient
4. A person who is convalescing from serious illness

5. A person in need of special instruction to improve physical fitness or to ameliorate a postural problem

All of these matters can also be covered if the school provides an orientation day for parents or offers a special program during the year to inform the parents about the curricular offerings of each of the departments in the school. Another way to inform parents about the adapted program is through a form letter from the adapted physical education teacher (Fig. 18-1, *C*).

LONG BEACH STATE COLLEGE

Division of Health, Physical Education, and Recreation

A PLAN OF COORDINATION BETWEEN THE DEPARTMENT OF PHYSICAL
EDUCATION AND THE STUDENT HEALTH SERVICE

Every entering or re-entering student will be given a medical examination by the student health service. At the conclusion of this examination, the student will be classified by the examining physician for physical education activities according to the classifications listed below.

Class A--No restrictions

Class B--Minor restrictions in activity where a student might be excused
from one or two hazardous types of sports but would be cleared
for all others.

Class C--Limited (adapted) physical education. The physician should state
reason and briefly describe the types of exercises or activities
that would benefit the student. Assignment to a special class
might be necessary. Use code below where possible and indicate
approximate length of time for restriction.

CODE

1) Output of energy to be reduced: Not to exercise severely enough to become
much out of breath, nor long enough to become much fatigued. This class
will include persons with heart disease, diabetes, severe asthma, hyper-
thyroidism, neurocirculatory asthenia, etc., or convalescing from recent
illness.
2) Protect from physical trauma: Should be used for cases too severe or complicated to be safely handled under a simple "B" classification. Atrophied
limbs, recurrent dislocations, damaged brains, and progressive high myopia
are examples.
3) Avoid close contact with other students or with mats: Cases in which there
is mildly infectious or a repulsive skin condition, such as severe acne or
eczema. Infectious cases should be excluded from physical education entirely, until cured. Persons who have a C-3 classification should also be
placed in a "B--no swimming" class.
4) Not to use legs more than necessary: For persons otherwise OK who have
foot strain, varicose veins, old leg injuries, healed thrombophlebitis, and
similar conditions, which are severe enough to cause them some trouble.
5) Epileptic: MUST BE KEPT OUT OF POOL AND OFF OF HIGH PLACES.
6) Adapt activity to some deformity: Students who are blind or deaf or who
have amputated limbs are often not especially fragile, and do very well in
many activities if given proper assistance.
7) Hernia: Avoid anything that causes increased intra-abdominal pressure,
such as heavy lifting or straining, and anything else that causes pain
at the site of the hernia.
8) Recommended for certain activity only. Specify.
9) Has some physical condition which, while not disabling, may be benefited
by special corrective physical exercises. Examples are spinal curvatures,
foot strain, certain recurrent dislocations, and general muscular underdevelopment.

ACCIDENT OR ILLNESS REQUIRING A CHANGE OF CLASSIFICATION

A student who becomes ill or is injured may require a change in medical
classification. These students should report to the Student Health Service upon
their return to school for a check-up by the attending physician who may or may
not change the student's classification. If a change is necessary, the doctor
should fill out form #HPER 20 which will be attached to the student's permanent
record card in the Department of Physical Education. If no change is necessary,
a re-admittance slip should be filled out to clear the student for full activity
in physical education classes.

Physical Education instructors must not admit a student to an activity class
unless the student has a medical classification card on file in the Physical Education office, nor should he admit a student to re-enter class if he has been
ill, without either a "readmittance slip" or a "change of medical classification
card."

The health and safety of each student at Long Beach State College can best
be guaranteed by close cooperation between the Health Service and the Division
of Health, Physical Education, and Recreation. Close observance of these procedures will make this possible.

Fig. 18-2. Explanation of the code used on the medical report cards from the physician to the physical education department.

SELECTION AND ASSIGNMENT OF STUDENTS

The selection of students for adapted physical education and their assignment to the proper type of activity are two very important phases of the program. Students can be identified through a physical examination, through observation of students in classroom or activity situations, and through special testing procedures that are administered by members of the physical education department.

The physical examination

There are several purposes of giving each student in the school a physical examination. Ideally, the physical examination should identify pupils who have pathological conditions, provide teachers with information concerning students' growth and health status, and identify students who can benefit from the Individual Education Program. The examination must be sufficiently personalized to form a desirable constructive educative experience for the students and their parents and provide the examining physician with an opportunity to engage in a worthwhile physician-student relationship.

It is more important that the examination be comprehensive and painstaking than that it be given annually. It is suggested that the examination be given to each pupil at least every third year. The usual pattern is to require an examination in the first grade and then every 3 years through the elementary, secondary school, and college years. Parents should be informed of any disabilities discovered, at the discretion of the examining physician. The records of these examinations can then be forwarded to the counseling office of the school that the student will be attending the next year, thus facilitating program planning.

Some school districts are unable or unwilling to provide physical examinations. In this event, each student should be required to present evidence to the school of an adequate examination from his or her own physician. There is considerable support for requiring an examination from the private physician rather than from the school physician, since the private physician should have a better longitudinal picture of the health or health problems of the student.

Type of examination

The physical examination should consist of the following as a minimum:

1. Information obtained by the school nurse should include the student's health history, vision and hearing tests, a record of height and weight information about the general nutritional status of the student, and a general posture and foot examination.
2. The physician's examination should include the heart (before and after exercise), lungs, blood pressure, abdomen, eye, ear, nose, throat, skin, glands, and posture.
3. The student should be referred to the family physician, to a specialist provided by the school district, or to the city, county, state, or other public agencies for additional examinations by specialists when needed. These special examinations could include psychological examinations, checkups for tuberculosis, or services of other medical specialists such as cardiologists and orthopedists. The service agencies concerned with crippled children and children who have cerebral palsy, neuromuscular disorders, asthma, heart disorders, diabetes, mental retardation, and the like may be consulted as needed.

Medical and physical examination records

A comprehensive record card or file should be begun during the initial examination, and it should follow the student throughout the school years. Many school districts will not forward medical records to a new school district. Since the health record is of such vital importance, provisions should be made to make inexpensive photostatic copies of the record to forward to the new school with the academic records. The card should contain a record of all previous physical examinations, illnesses, immunizations, tests, injuries, referrals (and the findings of them), growth, and defects (and their correction); the health history; and information relative to the assignment of students to special classes and activities in physical education (Fig. 18-4).

It is essential that the physical education department receive from the health office a written recommendation that provides the following informa-

Activity recommendations

Indicate body areas for which physical activities should be minimized, eliminated, or maximized.

	Maximized	Minimized	Eliminated	Both	Left	Right	Comments, including any medical contraindications to physical activities
Neck							
Shoulder girdle							
Arms							
Elbows							
Hands and wrists							
Abdomen							
Back							
Pelvic girdle							
Legs							
Knees							
Feet and ankles							
Toes							
Fingers							
Other (specify)							

Remedial

☐ Condition is such that defects or deviations can be improved or prevented from becoming worse through use of carefully selected exercise and/or activities. The following are remedial exercises and/or activities recommended for this student: (Please be specific.)

_____

_____

_____

_____

_____

_____

_____

_____

Signed _____ M.D.

Address _____

_____ Zip _____

Telephone No. (   ) _____

Date _____ 19_____

Fig. 18-3. Physical education medical referral form approved and endorsed by the Committee on the Medical Aspects of Sports of the American Medical Association, 1975.

SECTION F — CORRECTIVE TEACHER'S NOTES

Date		Signature

SECTION G — DOCTOR'S RECOMMENDATIONS

Date		Signature

SECTION H — PROGRAM EVALUATION

SECTION J — DISPENSATION OF CASE

	First Semester	Sig.	Second Semester	Sig.	Third Semester	Sig.
Case closed (date)						
Pupil to regular P.E.						
Recommended for further exercise						

LOS ANGELES CITY SCHOOL DISTRICTS
Auxiliary Services Division — Health Education and Health Services Branch
CORRECTIVE PHYSICAL EDUCATION HISTORY FOLDER

INFORMATION AND DIRECTIONS FOR USE OF THIS FOLDER

1. **WHAT IS THE PURPOSE OF THIS INSTRUMENT?** This folder has been prepared for the corrective physical education teacher to use during three semesters as a history record of pupil progress in corrective physical education.

2. **WHO IS TO FILL IT OUT?** This folder is to be filled out by the corrective physical education teacher in whose class the pupil is enrolled.

3. **WHEN IS THE FOLDER TO BE FILLED OUT?** The folder is to be filled out when the pupil first enters the class and each semester period during the time the pupil is enrolled in corrective physical education. Use additional folders when necessary.

4. **TO WHOM IS THE FOLDER TO BE SENT?** The folder is to be sent to the Corrective Physical Education Section of the Health Education and Health Services Branch.

5. **WHEN IS THIS FOLDER DUE?** Upon request. However, if the pupil transfers, the folder should be sent immediately to the Corrective Physical Education Section of the Health Education and Health Services Branch, with pupil's new address or school.

6. **DIRECTIONS FOR SECTION A.** Record date in appropriate column. Record body type as L (lithe), M (medium), S (stout). Record muscle tone as good or poor. Record items 4 to 9 inclusive according to degree using a 1 to 4 scale with 1 (little) and 4 (much). Record feet as N (normal), P (pronated), S (supinated), F (flat). Record leg alignment as N (normal), B (bowed), K (knock-knee). Record prominent abdomen as "yes" or "no." Record chest as N (normal), F (flat), P (pigeon). Record items 14 and 15 as "yes" or "no." Record items 16 through 20 as "yes" or "no"; if "yes," indicate whether left or right.

7. **DIRECTIONS FOR SECTION B.** Place in the appropriate space the photographs taken at the beginning of the first semester and at the end of the second and third semesters.

8. **DIRECTIONS FOR SECTION C.** Using a cloth or steel tape, record measurements in inches to the nearest quarter, and weight (including over or under) to the nearest pound.

9. **DIRECTIONS FOR SECTION D.** Describe all exercises planned by the corrective teacher for the pupil and list these according to the following code numbers, putting the appropriate number in the column for numbers:

   1. Specific individual exercises
   2. Relaxation exercises
   3. Coordination exercises
   4. Head and neck exercises
   5. General trunk exercises
   6. Lateral trunk exercises
   7. Foot and leg alignment exercises

10. **DIRECTIONS FOR SECTION E.** The information for this section should be obtained from the pupil's health record card after conferring with the health coordinator and school nurse if a secondary school, or with the school nurse and principal if an elementary school.

11. **DIRECTIONS FOR SECTION F.** This space is for the corrective teacher to use in recording pupil progress and significant information from home or other sources relative to the child's general health problems, including his feelings regarding his defects.

12. **DIRECTIONS FOR SECTION G.** Information for this section should be obtained also from the pupil's health record card or from the school doctor or private physician.

13. **DIRECTIONS FOR SECTION H.** This space is to be used by the corrective teacher to evaluate the corrective program of the pupil. Record significant developments that have been accomplished for the pupil within the corrective class.

14. **DIRECTIONS FOR SECTION J.** This space is for the corrective teacher to use to record the dispensation of the case, that is, when the pupil leaves the class, when the pupil is returned to regular physical education, or in case the pupil is recommended for more than the three semesters of corrective physical education.

CORRECTIVE TEACHER'S SIGNATURE	DATE
1.	
2.	
3.	

Fig. 18-4. Sample cumulative folder.

tion: student's full name, year in school, date of examination, classification for physical education activity, the Individual Education Program, and the signature of the examining physician or of the nurse who transposes the information from the permanent medical record.

This card is filed in the physical education department office. It is then the responsibility of each instructor to check that all students have had a physical examination and that they are enrolled in the types of activity that meet their physical education needs.

CLASSIFICATION FOR PHYSICAL EDUCATION

The handicapped student should be placed in the physical education class that is most normalizing (least restrictive). This placement, as has been noted, is a cooperative arrangement made by the parents, child, and school personnel. A suggested system used in some schools and colleges combines simplicity with accuracy and thus facilitates the transfer of important information from the physician to the faculty (Fig. 18-2).

When the physician, the nurse, and the members of the physical education department are familiar with the information presented in the plan just described, rather detailed information can be forwarded by the examining physician to the physical education department by means of the code described. Busy physicians can therefore furnish more complete information to the physical education department and, specifically, to the adapted physical education instructor than would be possible if they had to write out complete descriptions of the students' conditions and make complete recommendations for their activity programs.

The adapted physical education teacher is often expected to be present during the physical examinations when they are conducted at the school. Although this is a time-consuming procedure, it provides an excellent opportunity for the examining physician and the teacher of adapted physical education to communicate. The doctor can ask specific questions regarding the curriculum and can then approve exercises and activities more adequately. The physical education teacher can seek detailed information from the physician about the nature of the various disabilities and contraindicated activi-

ties. Understanding and free communication between the examining physician and the teacher are essential if the special needs of the child are to be adequately met.

Use of a classification code

In addition to indicating which students should be assigned to adapted physical education classes, the classification code has several other functions (Fig. 18-2). Students who are classified "A" are permitted to enroll in any physical education activity. This often clears them for all intramural and extramural sports. Boys and girls who participate in interscholastic athletic programs are usually given an additional yearly examination to clear them for competition in one or more of the sports activities.

A "B" classification indicates that the student has a disability that limits participation in one or two specific activities. Using the "B" classification to indicate that a student can participate in all physical education activities except one or two reduces the problem of assigning the student to the proper physical education class to one of clerically checking on enrollment in physical education. An example would be "Class B, no swimming." The counseling and physical education departments should be informed to eliminate swimming from the student's schedule.

A very limited number of students have in the past been restricted from all participation in physical education by the examining physician. The number of students in this group should diminish as the quality of the adapted physical education program improves. A good adapted physical education program should provide some type of activity for any student who is well enough to attend regular classes in the school. Students in need of such specialized programs are classified "C" by the doctor and are assigned to an adapted physical education class. Their exercise and activity assignments are then planned by a physical education teacher with special training.

Program adaptations in regular physical education

Students with minor disabilities or posture problems that are functional in nature may receive valuable assistance with their problems if the regular physical education instructor is notified of these conditions and a recommendation is made for a *preventive* program of exercises and activities. Students who need a special sport skill or activity may receive it in the regular class. As an example, a student may need special kicking drills in the swimming pool on a kickboard to strengthen a knee. With a little special help and planning, the regular instructor can make a substantial contribution to the specific educational needs of students who have certain physical deviations and who are mainstreamed in a regular physical education class.

Transfer of students

One of the important features of a quality program of adapted physical education is to provide for the easy transfer of students to a less restrictive physical education class. Although some students are assigned to an adapted class permanently and some for a year or a semester, there are many students in the school who need to be in the class only for a short period of time to recover from an injury or illness or to complete a program of rehabilitation that will prepare them for their return to a regular physical education section. Often, athletes injured during or between seasons can hasten their recovery with a special program of exercises and activities in an adapted class. In addition to the advantage of meeting the needs of all the students in the school more adequately, the provision of a system of easy transfer of students to and from the adapted class does much to erase the stigma sometimes attached to a class for students who have disabilities. When any student in the school may be assigned to this program for rehabilitation—the highly gifted as well as the disabled—there should be no stigma attached to such a transfer.

IDENTIFICATION OF STUDENTS
Identification through activities

All handicapped children should be preevaluated in specific areas of physical education need. For most of these children, specific programming will be under way; however, there may be children who are not legally handicapped that need special physical education programs. These children need to be identified so that special assistance can be provided. There are a number of ways for classroom teachers in the school—and specifically the teachers of regular physical education classes—to help identify students in need of special assistance.

Observation of the students in the classroom or on the athletic field will often disclose physical deviations overlooked by the physician and, often, those of which the students are unaware. Persons with posture deviations, the slow learners in physical education activities, the students with poor coordination or balance, and those with limited strength and endurance may be in need of specially designed programs of exercise and activity to bring them up to levels where they can keep up with their peers in a regular physical education class.

Teachers, counselors, and the school nurse should also watch for the student who has a change of status because of illness or injury. The student should be transferred to an appropriate setting if necessary until the condition is corrected or the fitness level is raised sufficiently for the student to return to a regular class.

Identification through physical education testing

There are a number of different tests that can be administered by the physical educator to aid in the identification of students with some form of physical disability. These tests, combined with the judgment of a qualified instructor, help screen the students who have special needs.

For the selection of the test method, factors such as the following should be considered: the specialized training of the instructors, the number of qualified teachers in the physical education department, the space available, the number of students to be tested, when the examinations are to be given, the amount of time available, and the availability of specialized testing and recording equipment.

Individual examinations by one instructor and by several instructors (station-to-station)

There are two types of individual examinations that are commonly used in schools and colleges. In one type, one instructor examines each student individually, covering all of the tests in the battery. In the other method, several stations are set up with different trained personnel at each station, each responsible for administering one or more tests.

Individual examination by one instructor is usually very thorough and used to evaluate carefully the individual problems of the student. It would involve the procedures described in more detail in other sections of this text. The instructor usually allows 6 to 10 minutes for each student's examination.

Individual examination by several instructors (station-to-station) can be very thorough or can be used to identify the most pronounced cases. These will be reexamined later with more care by the adapted physical education specialist. As many as six to eight stations are set up, either in a large room such as the gymnasium or in a series of small rooms, if they are available. Each tester must be skillful in the administration of one or more tests and the students move from one area to another to receive the complete examination. A typical station-to-station examination plan is shown in Fig. 18-5, A. Students come to the gymnasium properly dressed for the examination. They fill out the appropriate sections of their appraisal sheet, remove shoes and socks, and proceed to station one for anthropometric measurements and evaluation of nutritional status. Age, height, weight, body width, depth, fat measurements, and girth measurements may be taken. The student then proceeds to station two for an examination with the posture screen or plumb line. Station three is a moving (functional) body mechanics examination. The student walks, performs exercises, climbs steps, sits down in a chair, and the like while the instructor evaluates these movement patterns. The student next proceeds to station four, the foot examination. Here evaluation can be made with the podiascope, pedograph, plumb line, foot tracer, and other devices needed. Stations five to eight may be used for physical fitess, range of motion, relaxation, or perceptual-motor tests, as described in the appropriate chapters of the text. The adapted physical education specialist then reviews the total examination results and prepares the final summary evaluation, which will later be used to determine which students are in need of special attention, counseling and placement in the least restrictive environment.

Group examinations

Lowman and Young[9] have suggested procedures for conducting group examinations. A modification of these examinations is presented in Fig. 18-5, B.

The Individual Education Program requires that instructional decisions be made from a data base. Therefore, it is important that expedient procedures be employed to collect such data. There are several ways to collect the data, such as the following: (1) the instructor tests each student, (2) the instructor trains other persons to collect the data, (3) all students are trained to test another person and the testing is done in pairs, (4) all persons are trained to test themselves and record the scores. The type of testing technique chosen depends primarily on the maturity of the students, the complexity of the task, and the difficulty of administering the test. An example of administering a postural evaluation for which the instructor trains others to help is provided.

The entire class is examined by having the students line up in regular (or a predetermined) squad formation. The students are then positioned so that the examiners will have room to pass along each squad and assess each student. The students' names will have been entered previously on a group examination form (Fig. 18-5, C) in the same order as they are arranged in squads. A recorder fills out the form as each student is observed. (This is usually conducted as a gross type of screening to identify students who need special programs to improve fitness, body mechanics, coordination, and the like. These students can be examined more carefully at a later date.) Each student is then checked, using the same procedure, from the side and posterior views. The postural problems most easily identified from each view are so indicated on the group examination form illustrated. The "key" to the abbreviations on the form is found on the back (Fig. 18-5, C). Fitness and coordination can be similarly recorded.

A number of different posture evaluations have been developed using photographic techniques. Still photographs (with or without a plumb line or posture screen), motion pictures, and silhouetteographs provide permanent records to show to a student and to be used for later comparison (Figs. 9-35 and 20-24, E). When certain body landmarks are located on these pictures, various semiobjective measurements can be made to assess static posture.

Many other types of tests can be used to aid in identifying students who require special assistance.

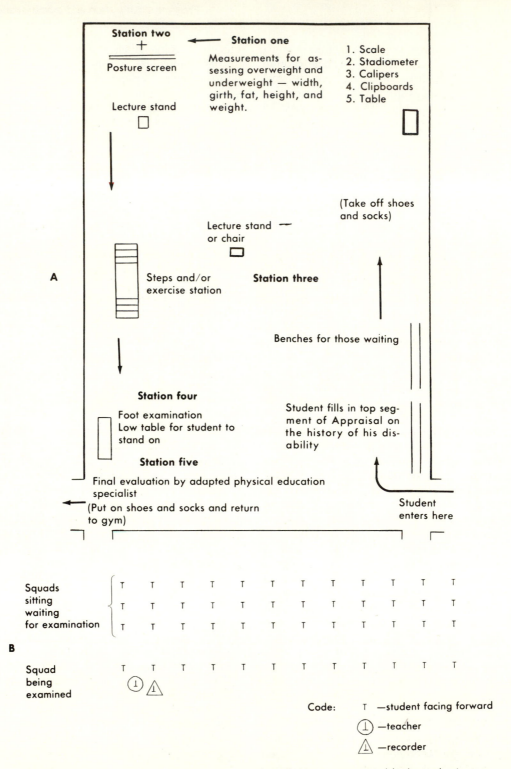

Fig. 18-5. A, Individual method (station-to-station) of conducting a posture and body mechanics examination. **B,** Group method of conducting a posture and body mechanics examination.

ADAPTED PHYSICAL EDUCATION
GROUP POSTURE EXAMINATION CHECK SHEET

NOTE: Fold up bottom of page
for explanation of symbols

SAMPLE FORM

		BODY		FEET			KNEES		PELVIS		ABD.	CHEST		SHOULDERS			SPINE			HEAD		
Check for dev. from Ant., Pos., or Side view		A	S	A&P	A	A	P	A	S	S	A&H	S	S	S	S	S	S	P	A	P	S	S	S	S	A&P
		BB	L	T	L	M	Pro	TT	Hy	Bt	T	FT	BT	Pt	P	F	F	ScW	T	Sc	Lo	Ky	B	F	T
Name of Student																									
Able, Judy																									
Baker, Suzi																									

C

Examine total class from anterior, side and posterior views. Record your eval. of all conditions for each view as you check each student, i.e. check all students from front view and record the major deviations in appropriate columns, then side, then posterior views. (1°=slight, 2°=moderate, 3°=severe)

BODY		FEET		PELVIS		ABDOMEN		SHOULDERS		SPINE	
BB	Body build	L	Long arch	T	Tilt	Pt	Ptosis	F	Forward	Sc	Scoliosis
l	Lithe	M	Meta. arch	FT	Forward tilt			ScW	Winged scap.	Lo	Lordosis
m	Medium	Pro	Pronation	BT	Backward tilt			T	Tilt	Ky	Kyphosis
h	Heavy										
L	Body lean	HEAD		KNEES		CHEST					
T	Body tilt	B	Back	TT	Tibial torsion	P	Pigeon				
		F	Forward	Hy	Hyper-extended	F	Flat				
		T	Tilt (side)	B	Bent						

Fig. 18-5, cont'd. C, Form used to record findings of the group type examination. (The information on the bottom half of the illustration is on the back of the form and is used to indicate the meaning of the code letters on the front of the form.)

These tests are described in other parts of this text or in most standard texts on physical education tests and measurements. Some of the types of tests and evaluations that should be included in the procedures previously described are the following:

1. Range of motion (goniometry, tracings) (Chapter 20)
2. Perceptual-motor tests (Chapters 3 and 20)
3. Relaxation (Jacobson, Rathbone, Benson) (Chapter 6)
4. Physical fitness (American Association for Health, Physical Education, and Recreation; Canadian Association for Health, Physical Education, and Recreation; Clarke; President's Council on Physical Fitness) (Chapters 7 and 12)
5. Health or personal history of student (health, sleep, rest, relaxation, recreation, etc.) (Fig. 5-2)

THE ADAPTED PHYSICAL EDUCATOR AS COUNSELOR

In general, the function of a counselor is to provide a counselee the opportunity to increase self-understanding.[5] Although counseling and guidance in the school or clinical setting are normally carried out by specially trained personnel, there are many instances in which the adapted physical educator must assume this role. Some of the more common of these counseling situations can be categorized under five distinct headings, namely, (1) modulating energy output, (2) reasonable goal setting, (3) daily living practices, (4) family adjustment, and (5) social adjustment.

Modulating energy output

Persons who have problems of low vitality or who must limit energy expenditure must learn to carefully monitor their activity. Examples of conditions that demand careful monitoring are those affecting respiratory and cardiovascular systems. The adapted physical educator plays an integral part in helping these individuals stay within exercise and activity tolerances. Students who tend to rationalize their problems must be guided and assisted in fully understanding the nature of their problems and in accepting the limitations that they impose.

Reasonable goal setting

Instructional goals are set in the Individual Education Program planning conference by the parents, school personnel, and the student (when possible). Very often, persons who plan the goals either underestimate or overestimate the student's ability to learn. Therefore, goals may be set either too low or too high. Goals that are too low "protect" the individual, whereas goals that are too high indicate wishful thinking. This unrealistic attitude may be carried over to everyday living and to the selection of career or occupational goals.

Daily living practices

Handicapped persons often need to develop habits that will enrich their daily lives. The adapted physical educator is often in a position to counsel the student on important aspects of hygienic living, means of coping with and/or avoiding emotional stresses, ways to make life a little easier, and, most importantly, the selection of rewarding leisure-time activities.[3]

Family adjustment

Conducting the Individual Education Program often includes teacher involvement with the student's family. It is of the utmost importance that the adapted physical educator know the students' families and be available to them as a source of information and advice. The lines of communication must always be open between family and teacher.

An interview should take place between the family and teacher at the earliest possible time after the student is admitted to the program. It is highly desirable that the student and both parents be present when the interview takes place. The initial interview gives the teaher an opportunity to describe the program and at the same time discover the expectations of the parents. Moreover, it provides an opportunity for the teacher to determine home enviromental factors that may enhance or deter the adapted physical education program.

Following the initial interview, periodic contacts with the family should be made as a means of providing feedback as to the child's progress. Such contacts give a continuous opportunity for exchanging ideas, clarifying procedures, and counseling as various problems arise. In essence, there should be a spirit of cooperation between the family and teacher for the betterment of the child.

Of major importance to the guidance of both the family and their handicapped child is the right of parents to know what is being done for their child and why. Too often, professionals keep parents in the dark about what services are being rendered to the young client. This attitude is unfortunate and usually stems from the fact that professionals think parents will not fully understand the procedures being employed. Careful communication with parents is provided through Individual Education Program conferences as a part of P.L. 94-142.

To further enhance the counseling and guidance process of parents, several procedures might be tried. The first might be the planning of parent observation periods during the program, after which the teacher should be readily available to answer questions. A second possibility could be the use of parents as aides, assisting children other than their own. A third possibility requiring controlled conditions could be that the parents extend activity in the home.

Social adjustment

One of the most important—and sometimes most difficult—areas to deal with is the social adjustment of the handicapped person. Adapted physical education experiences provide major opportunities for helping the handicapped develop effective social skills.[13]

It is obvious that social acceptance or rejection cannot be entirely controlled by the handicapped person. For example, the public may be repulsed by the prospect of an epileptic having an unsightly seizure, or the drooling individual with cerebral palsy may not be considered aesthetically desirable. The blind person's dependency and the deaf person's communicative problems may often make rewarding relationships difficult. The slowness of the mentally limited child and the uncommon speech quality of the individual with cleft palate may be factors that disallow typical social adjustment.

The adapted physical educator's role in the social growth of the handicapped student is many faceted. One of the major factors is for the teacher to help the disabled individual in understanding his or her own feelings and the reactions of others.

The handicapped student must be guided to make the most of his or her social assets, for example, improving appearance, manners, posture, and personal hygiene. The handicapped individual, although desiring to withdraw from a potentially painful social situation, should be encouraged to take part in group activities whenever possible. Also, it is particularly important that the handicapped student learn many specific game and exercise skills as well as the joy of winning and the ability to lose gracefully.

Adapted physical education offers excellent opportunities for assisting the handicapped student in self-understanding and in acquiring a more rewarding life-style.

ADAPTED PHYSICAL EDUCATION RECORDS

Since most of the work of the adapted physical education teacher is related to the measured instruction progress on the Individual Education Program, it is essential that accurate, complete, confidential records be maintained. These records should be filed in an orderly manner so that they can be located quickly. All records should be dated, for example, letters sent and received, examination information received or examination performed, photographs taken, and student or parent conferences held. Some of the types of records that should be retained are listed below:

1. Medical examination card
2. Physical education progress record card
3. Posture and body mechanics examinations
4. Letters to and from medical personnel
5. Photographic records

STUDENT MOTIVATION

Adapted physical education programs are most successful when they have the support of administrators, physicians, teachers, parents, and students and when the teachers are well qualified, dedicated, and able to highly motivate their students. We have observed programs in adjacent districts and schools having basically the same resources available, with the exception of the qualifications of the adapted physical education teacher: one program proved to be excellent; the other, extremely poor. A good teacher is the single most important factor in providing for a quality program.

The superior teacher is able to motivate students in many ways. Some of the motivation techniques and devices that work especially well in adapted physical education are the following:

1. Keeping students well informed about class rules, regulations, and policies, including grading procedures
2. Maintaining teacher enthusiasm and interest in students
3. Using charts and graphs to record student progress (posture examination cards, weight charts; Fig. 5-44)
4. Utilizing photography, that is, photogaphs of students with posture or disability problems to show them their present problems and to indicate any improvement made (Figs. 20-24, *E*, and 20-26, *B*)
5. Using exercise cards to show day-by-day improvements (Fig. 5-47)
6. Employing aesthetic considerations for girls (nice figure, good posture, proper weight, etc.) and appropriate anthropometric measurements
7. Exercising to music
8. Using good equipment for exercises and testing (Chapters 9 and 20)
9. Maintaining interesting, informative bulletin boards[2]
10. Maintaining contact with the students in games and sports activities
11. Employing interesting adapted sports and games

Each teacher must select the type of motivational techniques that prove successful in the particular situation.[2,9]

Since organization and administration cut across the total adapted physical education program, topics relating to these areas are included in other chapters in this text. Parts of Chapters 3 to 5, 7 to 9, 15, 16, and 19 include detailed information about organizing students for adapted physical education, assignment of exercise routines, and organizational procedures for teaching exercise and adapted sports programs.

REFERENCES

1. Clarke, H. H., and Clarke, D. H.: Developmental and adapted physical education, Englewood Cliffs, N.J., 1963, Prentice-Hall, Inc.
2. Crowe, W. C.: The use of audio-visual materials in devel-

opmental (corrective) physical education, Unpublished master's thesis, University of California, Los Angeles, Los Angeles, 1950.

3. Daniels, A. S., and Davies, E. A.: Adapted physical education, ed. 3, New York, 1975, Harper & Row, Publishers.
4. Guidelines for professional preparation programs for personnel involved in physical education and recreation for the handicapped, Washington, D.C., 1973, American Association for Health, Physical Education, and Recreation and Bureau of Education for the Handicapped, U.S. Department of Health, Education, and Welfare.
5. Hamilton, K. W.: Counseling the handicapped in the rehabilitation process New York, 1950, The Ronald Press Co.
6. Karpinos, B. D.: Fitness of American youth for military service, Milbank Memorial Fund Q. **38:**213, 1960.
7. Karpinos, B. D.: Health of children of school age, Washington, D.C., 1964, U.S. Department of Health, Education, and Welfare.
8. Kelly, E. D.: Adapted and corrective physical education, New York, 1965, The Ronald Press Co.
9. Lowman, C. L., and Young, C. H.: Postural fitness significance and variations, Philadelphia, 1960, Lea & Febiger.
10. Mathews, D. K., Kruse, R., and Shaw, V.: The science of physical education for handicapped children, New York, 1962, Harper & Row, Publishers.
11. Schiffer, C. G., and Hunt, E. O.: Illness among children, Washington, D.C., 1963, U.S. Department of Health, Education, and Welfare.
12. Vodola, T. M.: Individualized physical education program for the handicapped child, Englewood Cliffs, N.J., 1973, Prentice-Hall, Inc.

RECOMMENDED READINGS

Dexter, G.: Instruction of physically handicapped pupils, remedial physical education, Sacramento, Calif., 1973, California State Department of Education.

Drowatsky, J. N.: Physical education for the mentally retarded, Philadelphia, 1971, Lea & Febiger.

Fait, H. F.: Special physical education, ed. 4, Philadelphia, 1978, W. B. Saunders Co.

Geddes, D.: Physical activities for individuals with handicapping conditions, ed. 2, St. Louis, 1978, The C. V. Mosby Co.

Guide for programs in recreation and phyical education for the mentally retarded, Washington, D.C., 1968, American Association for Health, Physical Education, and Recreation and the National Education Association.

Guidelines for adapted physical education, Harrisburg, Pa., 1966, Department of Public Instruction, Commonwealth of Pennsylvania.

Moore, C. A.: The handicapped can succeed, Phys. Educ. **24:**63-164, 1967.

Mosston, M.: Teaching physical education, Columbus, Ohio, 1966, Charles E. Merrill Publishing Co.

Physical activity programs and practices for the exceptional individual, Third National Conference, Long Beach, Calif., 1974, The Alliance.

Physical activity programs and practices for the exceptional individual, Fourth National Conference, Los Angeles, 1975, The Alliance.

Roice, G. R., and Stoner, W.: Administrative aspects of starting a remedial physical education program, Unpublished data, Los Angeles, 1975.

Slader, C. V.: A workable adaptive program, J. Health Phys. Educ. Rec. **39:**71-72, 1968.

Stein, J.: Sense and nonsense about mainstreaming, J. Health Phys. Educ. Rec. **47:**43, 1976.

Techniques and methods for handicapped youth, First National Conference, Los Angeles, 1973, The Office of the Los Angeles County Superintendent of Schools, Division of Special Education.

19

Class organization

Adapted physical education classes can be organized for instruction in several different ways. Conditions vary widely throughout the United States in relation to such factors as the number of days physical education is offered each week, the time allowed for the activity phase of the program, whether the adapted physical education program is integrated with the regular physical education program, the availability of specially trained teachers, and special facilities and equipment. The special abilities and the preferences of the supervisor and teachers may also influence the type of program offered. In any event, it is important to choose the type of class organization that will enable students to progress to the best of their abilities in physical education activities.

THE SPECIAL EXERCISE AND ACTIVITY PHASE OF THE PROGRAM

Many students in adapted physical education need special exercises to help them correct or pre-vent disabilities or to improve their physical fitness or their perceptual-motor abilities. Exercise and activity programs can be conducted by using a combination of the following methods of instruction.

Informal (individual) class organization

Adapted classes can be organized for instruction so that each student has an individual exercise and/or activity program. This method is implicit in the Individual Education Program of P.L. 94-142. Through the use of self-instructional and evaluative standard teaching sequences, children in the early elementary school years can participate in individual exercise programs. The major advantage of this method is that students have programs specifically planned to meet their needs and interests. The exercises, the number of repetitions and the amount of resistance used, the rest periods, and the special equipment needed are all assigned to enable students to meet their predetermined objectives. Students can be strongly motivated to work toward correction or improvement of their disabilities in this type of class. Some teachers may find that control of a group of 20 to 25 students who are all working on individual programs is more difficult than class control of students who are all doing the same program simultaneously. However, the advantages of having each student engage in an individual program of activities would seem to outweigh such problems. Preparation of individual programs is time-consuming, but certain shortcuts can be used to enable the teacher to prepare these individual programs in a minimum amount of time. A complete plan for the choice and assignment of individual exercise programs is presented in Chapter 5.

Formal class organization

A class organized formally for exercises and other selected activities is one in which all students perform the same activity at the same time, usually under the direction of the teacher or a student leader. However, each student performs his or her present level of educational performance on the specific instructional task. This type of program lends itself well to the instruction of younger children in elementary school or to the instruction of boys and girls who cannot accept the resonsibility of an individual program. The advantages of this type of organization are that it gives teachers good control of the class and allows them to observe the performance of all the students more adequately than if they were watching 20 students, each doing something different. A disadvantage of this system is the lack of opportunity to give individually assigned activities to students with special needs. The use of special types of equipment is also more difficult, since each student must have his or her own piece of apparatus in the formal plan.

Group organization

A third method of class teaching involves the organization of an adapted physical education class into homogeneous groups based on similarities in the type of exercise and activity program needed. Students in need of anteroposterior posture correction might be grouped together to perform the same exercises (at their own ability levels), another group might work on foot exercises, and another group might do special adapted activities and exercises for perceptual-motor growth. These groups of students may remain the same throughout the class period or they may change to allow for more flexibility in the programs. Dependable students can lead and motivate those with less interest and drive. The teacher can also take advantage of assigning some individual types of programs and still have adequate supervision because of the several homogeneous groups that perform their programs together.

Combined method

Many teachers prefer to use a combination of the preceding types of class organization to meet the individual needs of the students, to provide for some small group activity, and to include formal exercise and activity sessions during which the teacher more directly controls the amount of work done.

This combination plan might be organized as follows:

5 minutes: Formal warm-up consists of all students doing the same exercises under the leadership and direction of the teacher or a student leader.

5 minutes: Students are divided into homogeneous groups according to their needs and perform three actvities or exercises with the members of their group under direction of a student leader.

10 minutes: Each student performs five exercises or activities specifically assigned to him or her, doing the number of repetitions assigned and recording progress on the exercise card. (Activities using special equipment can be assigned here, since students are able to take turns in the use of special pieces of apparatus.)

5-10 minutes: Games, relays, and contests are organized and led by the teacher, finishing with formal dismissal of the class, if desired.

Additional plans for the organization of the class and of exercise and activity routines are presented in Chapters 3 to 5, 7, 14, 15, and 16.

Activities for daily living and instructional aides

Whether teachers use the individual or the group method of class organization, additional help is always needed, especially as more severely handicapped persons are included in school programs. P.L. 94-142 provides for physical education programs for all; thus, there is a need for a change in emphasis in program content and in class organization. A recent trend in working with handicapped persons is the increased use of aides. Because of the severe disabilities of some handicapped children, more direct help and supervision is necessary to meet the activities for daily living and the instructionally related needs of the handicapped. Both paid help and volunteer help are needed to provide this important function. Standards have been developed for the certification of paid aides, and many junior colleges have training programs for these important members of the instructional staff. Parents, high school and college students in training to become teachers, and members of the PTA and other service groups often serve as volunteers in schools and hospitals. These aides and volunteers allow for an enriched, individualized program of instruction to be given, based on goals and objectives selected for each student. Transfers to and from a wheelchair and getting in and out of bed are examples of activities that might be included or for which special exercise programs would be developed.

THE ADAPTED SPORTS PHASE OF THE PROGRAM

The sports phase of an adapted physical education class can be organized in several different ways, depending on the general plan for adapted physical education in the school, how it is coordinated with the regular physical education program, the availability of regular and special facilities and equipment, and the background and skill of the teacher in charge.

Often, the special class in adapted physical education has, as a part of its yearly program, a certain amount of time scheduled for adapted sports and games. This can be organized in one of the three following ways:

1. A part of each period is devoted to team sport or lifetime sport games.
2. From 1 to 3 days of each week are set aside for these activities.
3. A period of 1, 2, or more consecutive weeks is blocked out for an activity. There can be as many of these blocks of time for sports activities during the semester as are deemed desirable.

Some teachers have found that the first method, in which up to 15 minutes of each class period are devoted to games and sports (usually after the exercise portion of the class is finished), serves as a good motivation device, keeping interest at a high level in the exercise and sports parts of the program. Time, of course, is a limiting factor in this type of organization, tending to rule out sports and games that require extensive preparations, equipment checkout, instruction, or travel to a specialized location for the activity. This method is often used in elementary school classes and, to some extent, in junior high classes.

Where 1 to 3 days a week are set aside for the adapted sports program, activities that require more time, organization, and instruction can be included. Almost any game or sport can be modified

so that handicapped students can participate. Junior and senior high school classes are often organized in this fashion. This type of schedule enables the teacher to keep interest high in the exercise and sports programs throughout the year. It also gives the student an opportunity to work on a special exercise program continuously throughout the semester or year without having to stop the exercise routine for an extended period of time to participate in various sports and games.

Some teachers prefer to organize the adapted sports portion of the class into blocks of time for instruction and activity. This type of program might consist of 4 weeks of swimming, 4 weeks of a team sport, 4 weeks of exercise, and 4 weeks of an individual sport. Thus, student and instructor attention and interest can be focused on one activity at a time. If the regular physical education classes are scheduled on the block system, it is usually easier to obtain facilities and equipment for the adapted physical education classes if they, too, are scheduled for a single activity for a block of time.

However, inasmuch as each parent has the prerogative to participate in the planning of the child's program, great flexibility must be built into the program. Thus, a considerable portion of the physical education program must be individualized so that each child may engage in the specific activities that have been written into the Individual Education Program with the approval of the parents.

Handicapped students in regular classes

Some Individual Education Programs require that students in adapted physical education join a regular physical education class for their work in sports and games. This is in keeping with the concept of mainstreaming. By joining this regular group for various types of activities during the year, handicapped children can learn culturally relevant social behaviors that hopefully will generalize to a normal society in the postschool years. A free interchange between handicapped and nonhandicapped children can do much to eliminate any feelings of stigmatization on the part of the student who is placed in a special class. Physical education teachers who instruct handicapped children in the regular class need skills for the conduct of individualized instruction and for the development of attitudes of the nonhandicapped that are conducive to acceptance of individual differences.

The adapted sports program is more fully discussed in Chapter 8.

Coeducational classes

Some schools have attempted to offer adapted physical education classes to their students on a coeducational basis with varying degrees of success. These programs might be most successful at the elementary school and college levels. At the secondary school level students are especially peer conscious and are sometimes apprehensive about coeducational physical education. Even in the regular classes, it would take a strong teacher with excellent backing from the other teachers and the administration to break down some of the traditional feelings associated with a coeducational program.

If feasible, there are several advantages to be found in the conduct of a coeducational adapted physical education proram; they include the following:

1. The best teacher, male or female, can be used to administer and teach in the program.
2. In small schools, this would increase the flexibility in student scheduling.
3. The arbitrary division of the class because of the sex of the individual student is discouraged.
4. The majority of teachers are trained in corrective or adapted physical education in coeducation classes and thus they are prepared to direct such programs.

The major problems associated with the coeducational class occur in the examination and the exercise phases of the program. Having a male teacher and a female teacher present during the initial posture and other examinations having the students wear appropriate apparel during both the examination and the exercise phases of the program-should minimize these two problems. The traditional pattern of having completely separate classes for boys and for girls in both regular and adapted physical education is gradually being replaced by more coeducational classes. Well-conceived organization and administration of coeducational programs do much to promote quality physical education for the handicapped.

GRADING (MARKING) IN ADAPTED PHYSICAL EDUCATION

A grade in any subject should promote educational goals and should reflect educational aims and objectives. For programs to be most effective, established objectives must indicate the desired goals of instruction so that they may become the criteria on which grades are based. If they are valid criteria, successful measurement will result in valid evaluation. The grade, if one desires to translate behavioral peformance, could reflect how well these criteria have been met.

The complexity of grading physical education classes is magnified when the attempt is made to evaluate the performance of students in an adapted class. The one common denominator among all the students would seem to be the mastery of individual performance objectives. If students are graded on the basis of how well they meet their objectives, a posture student, a cardiac student, an obese student, and a postoperative student can all be properly evaluated for their grades in the class.

The following criteria might be applied to students to determine how well they have met objectives in the adapted physical education class:

1. *Performance:* Standard of performance in reference to individual limitations, such as vigorous work on specific activities and posture exercises for obese students, control of the amount and intensity of work for cardiac and postoperative students, etc.
2. *Persistence:* Accomplishment of individual performance objectives, determined in the Individual Education Program conference.

Suggestions for recording and computing the grade are as follows:

1. Since the grade may involve some subjective judgments on the part of the instructor, the student should be observed and graded many times throughout the semester (weekly, if possible).
2. Either a letter grade or a numerical rating (recorded on the exercise card and in the roll book) can be given to the student; in this way, the student and the instructor are always aware of the student's progress toward stated behavior objectives.
3. These letter or numerical grades can be averaged and then should be considered, along

with other factors that may influence the final grade (knowledge examinations and health factors, if they are considered), to determine the final mark for the semester.

4. Objective measurements should be used to test skill and knowledge.

CURRICULUM PLANNING

Federal and state legislation, administrative codes, and rules and regulations from boards of education provide direction and guidelines for curricular planning at the county and district levels. Counties and large cities also furnish curricular direction and materials to local school districts. The curriculum for programs for the handicapped may be drawn from several resources. To meet state and federal legislative mandates, extensive curricular materials to meet the individual needs of handicapped persons must be developed. Through the use of these instructional materials, pupil progress toward measurable objectives implies teacher accountabilty for the learning of the children.

PLANNING FOR TEACHING AND LEARNING

Teaching and learning are facilitated by careful preplanning, whether this takes the form of a skillfully designed curriculum, a plan for a unit of study within the curricular offerings, or a well organized daily lesson plan.* Unit plans are discussed briefly in this chapter.

Unit plans

Unit plans usually consist of a systematic program of action for organizing and integrating the learning experiences of pupils around some central theme. Adapted physical education classes might have unit plans in physical fitness or in the more traditional areas of swimming, archery, or bowling. In addition, units can be planned to meet the needs of persons with a particular disability.

The organizational plan for the education of handicapped persons in special education programs appears in Fig. 19-1. This provides a guide for the teacher for selection of the behaviors from which handicapped children may benefit. After it has been determined that a child needs to develop a particu-

---

*See references 3, 4, 6, and 7.

lar behavior, a standard teaching sequence should be developed for that behavior. A procedure for constructing a standard teaching sequence follows.

1. *Select the behavior:* 11.1.35 Walks unsupported.
2. *Identify a measure to objectify the behavior:* Number of steps over a specific distance. A decrease in the number of steps represents a longer and narrower walking pattern, which is more normalized.
3. *Identify hierarchies to assist in construction of tasks with varying degrees of difficulty:* (a) Width of the path, (b) length of the stride, and (c) visual attention off the task while walking.
4. *Make a competency statement:* Can walk a path 15 inches wide and 10 feet long in four steps, eyes looking straight ahead.
5. *Construct the standard teaching sequence utilizing the hierarchies of the behavior:* Shift the hierarchical conditions of the objective.

	Number of steps	Width of path	Visual attention
1.	10	20″	On the feet
2.	9	20″	On the feet
3.	8	20″	On the feet
4.	7	20″	On the feet
5.	6	20″	On the feet
6.	9	18″	On the feet
7.	8	18″	On the feet
8.	7	18″	On the feet
9.	6	18″	On the feet
10.	8	16″	On the feet
11.	7	16″	On the feet
12.	6	16″	On the feet
13.	10	18″	Up
14.	9	18″	Up
15.	8	18″	Up
16.	7	18″	Up
17.	9	16″	Up
18.	8	16″	Up
19.	7	16″	Up
20.	6	16″	Up
21.	9	15″	Up
22.	8	15″	Up
23.	7	15″	Up
24.	6	15″	Up
25.	5	15″	Up
26.	4	15″	Up

The standard teaching sequence for teaching a child to walk unsupported involves shifting the conditions of the length of the stride, which re-

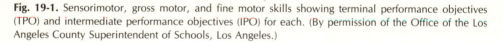

C10. SENSORIMOTOR DEVELOPMENT	C11. GROSS MOTOR DEVELOPMENT	C12. FINE MOTOR DEVELOPMENT
TPO C 10.1 Sensorimotor development (stage I)	TPO C 11.1 Gross motor skills (stage I)	TPO C 12.1 Fine motor skills (stage I)
IPO C 10.1.1 Is aware of auditory stimuli	IPO C 11.1.1 Moves arms and legs randomly	IPO C 12.1.1 Clinches hand on contact
10.1.2 Is aware of tactile stimuli	11.1.2 Turns head to side	12.1.2 Reaches for object
10.1.3 Is aware of visual stimuli	11.1.3 Lifts and holds head	12.1.3 Grasps and holds
10.1.4 Visually tracks	11.1.4 Holds head up	12.1.4 Moves mouth to object (rooting reflex)
10.1.5 Is aware of body parts	11.1.5 Rights self	12.1.5 Sweeps object to body
10.1.6 Is aware of kinesthetic stimuli	11.1.6 Raises chest	12.1.6 Reaches with control
10.1.7 Demonstrates space relationships	11.1.7 Rolls—side to supine	12.1.7 Transfers and releases one object
10.1.8 Demonstrates space perception	11.1.8 Sits on floor (pillow support)	12.1.8 Transfers object from hand to hand
10.1.9 Demonstrates space-time relationships	11.1.9 Demonstrates protective extension (arms)	12.1.9 Pulls peg from pegboard
	11.1.10 Rolls—prone to supine	12.1.10 Picks up object (pincer grip)
	11.1.11 Raises trunk	12.1.11 Unwraps object
	11.1.12 Crawls (on stomach)	12.1.12 Puts three or more cubes in container
	11.1.13 Rolls—supine to prone	12.1.13 Turns pages of book
	11.1.14 Sits on floor (hands support)	12.1.14 Removes object from container
	11.1.15 Sits on floor (unsupported)	12.1.15 Rolls ball
	11.1.16 Maintains hands and knees position	12.1.16 Stacks objects
	11.1.17 Scoots on floor (sitting)	12.1.17 Hurls object
	11.1.18 Stands (supported)	
	11.1.19 Rotates trunk laterally	
	11.1.20 Moves from sitting to prone	
	11.1.21 Moves from back-lying to side-sitting position	
	11.1.22 Moves from prone to sitting	
	11.1.23 Recovers balance while sitting (forward/backward)	
	11.1.24 Recovers balance while sitting (laterally)	
	11.1.25 Creeps (hands and knees)	
	11.1.26 Maintains kneeling position (supported)	
	11.1.27 Maintains kneeling position (unsupported)	
	11.1.28 Moves from back-lying to side-sitting position	
	11.1.29 Maintains side-sitting position	
	11.1.30 Lifts foot while standing (supported)	
	11.1.31 Moves from kneeling to standing position	
	11.1.32 Walks (supported)	
	11.1.33 Walks when led	
	11.1.34 Stands (unsupported)	
	11.1.35 Walks (unsupported)	
	11.1.36 Stoops and recovers	
	11.1.37 Pulls wheeled toy	

Fig. 19-1. Sensorimotor, gross motor, and fine motor skills showing terminal performance objectives (TPO) and intermediate performance objectives (IPO) for each. (By permission of the Office of the Los Angeles County Superintendent of Schools, Los Angeles.)

quires greater balance and motor control; the position of the visual mechanism, which requires greater motor control when the attention is off of the task; and the width of the path within which the student must walk, a measure of motor control of the walking behavior.

The standard teaching sequence cited on pp. 451 to 452 will not accommodate all persons. If the learners cannot enter the standard teaching sequence on the first step, easier tasks must be constructed to accommodate the student's present level of educational performance. On the other hand, if the learner can master the highest level activity on

the standard teaching sequence, activities can be developed that are not within the student's present level of performance. Rarely does a standard teaching sequence accommodate all learners.

Developing the standard teaching sequence

There are different strategies for developing standard teaching sequences. The procedure that was employed to develop the standard teaching sequence for the behavior of walking unsupported was as follows:

1. Reduce the number of steps that it would take to walk 10 feet. This will require the per-

STANDARD TEACHING SEQUENCE

The system requires only that the teacher note the child's progress using the following symbols: X = the steps (activities) in the standard teaching sequence that can be mastered by the student, in this case step Nos. 1, 2, 3, and 4; / = short-term instruction objective, in this case No. 5; * = goal, in this case No. 18.

11.1.35 Walks unsupported (step No.): X̶ X̶ X̶ X̶ 5̶ 6 7 8 9 10 11 12 13 14 15 16 17 18* 19 20 21 22 23 24 25 26

Two-footed standing broad jump

Type of program: Shifting criterion
Conditions
1. Both feet remain behind restraining line before takeoff.
2. Takeoff from two feet.
3. Land on two feet.
4. Measure from the restraining line to the tip of the toe of the least advanced foot.

Measurement: Distance in inches.

Two-footed standing broad jump (inches)	60	62	64	6̶6̶	6̶8̶	7̶0̶	72	74	76	78	80	82*	84
Date mastered				9/7	9/21	10/5							

The scoring procedure of the ongoing development of the person would be explained as follows. The program that the child is participating in is the two-footed standing broad jump. The child began the program at an initial performance level of 66 inches on September 7, and increased performance by 4 inches between September 7 and October 5. Thus the present level of educational performance is 70 inches (note the last number with an X over it). The child will attempt to jump a distance of 72 inches until he or she masters that distance. The child will continue to progress toward the goal, which is 82 inches (note the asterisk). It is a mistake in the applications of learning principles to ask the child to jump the 82 inches when it is known that the goal far exceeds the present level of educational performance. Unreasonable instructional demands from the learner by the teacher violate the principle of learning in small steps, which guarantees success for the child.

The same procedure could be used when teaching a child to throw a ball for accuracy. In the following example, a shifting condition program is used. For instance, two hierarchies that are known in throwing for accuracy are the size of the target and the distance between the thrower and the target. Thus, a standard teaching sequence might be similar to the following sequence of potential objectives: demonstrate the ability to throw a 4-inch ball a distance of _____ feet and hit a target that is _____ feet square five out of five times.

Throwing for accuracy

Type of program: Shifting condition
Conditions
1. Remain behind the restraining line at all times
2. Complete an overhand throw (ball released above the shoulder).
3. If the ball hits any part of the target it is a successful throw.

The above information would be contained in a curriculum book. However, the specific standard teaching sequence would be placed on a bulletin board at the performance area in the gymnasium. This would enable the performer to read his or her own instructional objective. The measurement of the performer's placement in the standard teaching sequence would be indicated on the prescription sheet.

Continued.

STANDARD TEACHING SEQUENCE—cont'd

Criterion for mastery: Three successful hits out of three.

DISTANCE OF THROW	SIZE OF TARGET	DISTANCE OF THROW	SIZE OF TARGET
1. 6'	3' square	10. 18'	2' square
2. 9'	3' square	11. 21'	2' square
3. 12'	3' square	12. 24'	2' square
4. 15'	3' square	13. 27'	2' square
5. 18'	3' square	14. 30'	2' square
6. 21'	3' square	15. 21'	1' square
7. 24'	3' square	16. 24'	1' square
8. 27'	3' square	17. 27'	1' square
9. 30'	3' square	18. 30'	1' square

The steps of the standard teaching sequence can be reduced and tasks can be added that are more or less complex as the situation requires.

Throwing for accuracy (step No.)	1̸	2̸	3̸	4̸	5̸	6̸	7	8	9	10	11	12	13	14*	15	16	17	18
Date mastered																		

---

former to lengthen the stride and narrow the base. However, the central focus is on the length of the stride.

2. The width of the base was reduced from 20 to 18 inches. The focus of development changed to the control of the walking pattern as measured by the width of the pathway.
3. At the thirteenth step in the sequence the attention was diverted from the feet, which required the internalization of the walking pattern.

Standard teaching sequences that are intuitive are relatively easy to develop. However, scientifically valid standard teaching sequences require considerable resources and time to develop. Validation of standard teaching sequence can also be accomplished by observing children attempting to progress through the sequence. If children are not challenged by certain tasks in the sequence, the step size may be too small; on the other hand, if the children have difficulty in progressing, the step size may be too great.

Plotting the student's progress

The standard teaching sequence provides information regarding what the child has learned, what the child's present limits of ability are for the specific task, which short-term instructional objectives will be attempted, and which instructional behavior will be taught next. A suggested recording system to plot the child's development as written on the Individual Education Program is shown above.

The values of planning for units of instruction include the following[2,7]:

1. Making learning more meaningful by avoiding the fragmentation inherent in the daily lesson plans
2. Increasing the retention of learning as a result of the unitary nature of a unit plan
3. Providing flexibility to serve individual differences
4. Helping students develop a stronger feeling of accomplishment as each unit is completed
5. Helping both teacher and learner organize their thinking toward specific goals and objectives
6. Permitting more satisfactory means for evaluating or appraising the progress toward objectives

A unit plan is usually composed of several basic elements that allow teachers to better organize guidelines for learning and consists of the following divisions:

1. *Title:* This identifies the area of study.

CALIFORNIA STATE UNIVERSITY, LONG BEACH

DAILY LESSON PLAN

Student Teacher_____ Date of Lesson_____ Grade_____

Master Teacher_____ Activity_____ Period_____

Primary Behavioral Objective:

Secondary Objectives:

Equipment and Supplies:

Field or Floor Markings:

TEACHER PROCEDURES AND TIME ALLOTMENT	STUDENT PROCEDURES AND CLASS ORGANIZATION	TEACHING CUES
INTRODUCTION:		
EXPLANATION:		
DEMONSTRATION:		
CLASS PARTICIPATION:		
EVALUATION OR CRITERION REFERENCE TEST:		
CONCLUSION AND TRANSITION TO NEXT LESSON:		

Fig. 19-2. Daily lesson plan form.

Continued.

CONSTRUCTIVE STUDENT TEACHER'S SELF-EVALUATION	MASTER TEACHER'S SUGGESTIONS Concerning Lesson Plan and Lesson:
1. Realization of Personal and Professional Objectives	
2. Weakest Part of Lesson	
3. Strongest Part of Lesson	

Fig. 19-2, cont'd. Daily lesson plan form.

2. *Introduction:* This provides an overall view of the content and emphasizes the potential values to participants.

3. *Goals and objectives:* Objectives should be meaningful for the teacher and the student. They should be clearly stated in terms of student behavior; they should provide an outline of the goals to be achieved; and they should indicate the student's performance level.[1,5,6] Objectives are usually developed in several major skill/task categories.

4. *Development of the unit:* This involves procedures for achieving goals by organization of content, methods, and materials related to the unit. Factors to be included in planning are equipment and supplies, grouping for instruction, available space and facilities, teacher resources (including student leaders), standard teaching sequences (weekly and daily plans), and teaching aids such as audio visual materials.[2,4,6]

5. *Culmination of the unit:* This includes plans for a logical and fitting culmination of the activities that have been engaged in by pupils. It can take the form of skill or knowledge tests, demonstration, playoffs, meets, or individual or group evaluations.

6. *Evaluation:* This should involve the appraisal of the student's progress toward objectives in skill, knowledge, and appreciation as indicated in the Individual Education Program. Objectivity should be sought in all forms of evaluation and the process should involve the student, the teacher, and the parents.

Daily lesson plans

The daily lesson plan is taken from the unit plan so that appropriate elements of implementation are followed and all of the essential topics and plans are included in the time scheduled for a given unit. Unit plans should not be rigidly followed, however. As student and/or class needs are discovered or more time is found to be necessary for a student in a particular area, the curriculum should be modified to meet such special conditions.

A daily lesson plan, in a similar way, should help teachers and students plan ahead for desired learning experiences. A typical lesson plan should include the following information:

1. Name (title of unit)
2. Subunit
3. Activities of the day
4. School level or grade
5. Date
6. Major objective(s) for the teacher
7. Procedures
8. Facilities and equipment necessary
9. Evaluation after completion of lesson (Fig. 19-2)

Some adaptations in planning may be necessary when working with severely handicapped persons. The suggested topics can be modified and the order changed if this will facilitate learning.

REFERENCES

1. Bloom, B. S., editor: Taxonomy of educational objectives, the classificatin of educational goals, handbook I: the cognitive domain, New York, 1956, David McKay Co., Inc.
2. Cowell, C. C., and Schwehn, H. M.: Modern principles and methods in high school physical education, Boston, 1958, Allyn & Bacon, Inc
3. Creamer, J. J., and Gilmore, J. T.: Design for competency based education in special education, New York, 1974, Teacher Education Division of Special Education and Rehabilitation, School of Education, Syracuse University.
4. Kemp, J. E.: Instructional design, Belmont, Calif., 1971, Fearon Publishers.
5. Mager, R. F.: Preparing instructional objectives, Palo Alto, Calif., 1962, Pearson Press.
6. Popham, W. J.: Objectives and instruction, AERA monograph series on curriculum evaluation, No. 3, instructional objective, Chicago, 1969, Rand McNally & Co.
7. Project Curriculum Objectives for Physical Education: Curriculum objectives for physical education, Chipley, Fla., 1974. Panhandle Area Educational Cooperative.

RECOMMENDED READINGS

Anderson, M. H., Elliot, M. E., and LaBerge, J.: Play with a purpose, New York, 1966, Harper & Row, Publishers.

Carr, D. B., et al.: Sequenced instructional programs in physical education for the handicapped, P.L. 88-164, Title III, December 1970, Los Angeles City Schools Special Education Branch, Physical Education Project.

Crowe, W. C., Arnheim, D. D., and Auxter, D.: Laboratory manual in adapted physical education and recreation, St. Louis, 1977, The C. V. Mosby Co.

Daniels, A. S., and Davies, E. A.: Adapted physical education, ed. 3, New York, 1975, Harper & Row, Publishers.

Dauer, V. P.: Essential movement experiences for preschool and primary children, Minneapolis, 1972, Burgess Publishing Co.

Davis, E. C., and Wallis, E.: Toward better teaching in physical education, Englewood Cliffs, N.J., 1961, Prentice-Hall, Inc.

Dexter, G.: Instruction of physically handicapped pupils, remedial physical education, Sacramento, Calif., 1973, California State Department of Education.

Drowatzky, J. N.: Physical education for the mentally retarded, Philadelphia, 1971, Lea & Febiger.

Educational Research Council of America: Physical education program guide, Columbus, Ohio, 1969, Charles E. Merrill Publishing Co.

Fait, H. F.: Special physical education: adapted, corrective, developmental, ed. 3, Philadelphia, 1975, W. B. Saunders Co.

Geddes, D.: Physical activities for individuals with handicapping conditions, ed. 2, St. Louis, 1978, The C. V. Mosby Company.

Guidelines for adapted physical education, Harrisburg, Pa., 1966, Department of Public Instruction, Commonwealth of Pennsylvania.

Kirchner, G.: Physical education for elementary school children, Dubuque, Iowa, 1970, William C. Brown Co., Publishers.

Nixon, J. E., and Jewett, A. E.: Physical education curriculum, New York, 1971, The Ronald Press Co.

Physical activities for the mentally retarded (ideas for instruction), Washington, D.C., 1968, American Association or Health, Physical Education, and Recreation.

20

Facilities and equipment

Proper facilities and equipment are as important for classes in adapted physical education as they are for classes in regular physical education. They help the teacher of adapted physical education make the proper adjustment in the student's program of developmental exercises, perceptual-motor activities, modified sports, or rest and relaxation. The lack of such equipment, however, should never be an excuse for the failure to provide an adapted physical education program or for offering a poor program of exercises and activities for the handicapped student. A good teacher of adapted physical education can provide a quality program with minimum facilities and equipment if some imagination is used and the instructor is willing to improvise. However, good facilities and equipment make the teacher's job easier, make the program more meaningful, and provide motivation for the handicapped student.

The facility and equipment needs for adapted physical education programs may vary somewhat according to the type of student served. Such factors as whether the class is coeducational, age and maturity levels of class members, and whether the students dress for activity all have an influence on facility and equipment needs. This chapter includes information about the kinds of facilities and equipment that should be provided for adapted physical education classes at the elementary, junior and senior high school, and college levels.

FACILITIES FOR ELEMENTARY SCHOOLS

Facilities for adapted physical education at the elementary school level vary extensively from district to district and from state to state. They may consist of nothing more than using the regular classroom for physical education or, under more desirable conditions, they may include such other areas as the cafeteria, the auditorium, grass or blacktop areas, or, in a few instances, a gymnasium or a swimming pool.

As the importance of early intervention becomes increasingly apparent, many school districts are beginning to hire adapted physical educators for the elementary school level; however, in some areas of the country the adapted physical education program is woefully lacking for the students enrolled in these schools. Elementary school classroom teachers may, under the best of conditions, have had only one or two courses designed to prepare them for all types of physical education instruction, including adapted physical education. It can readily be seen that an adapted program conducted under these conditions is severely restricted.

P.L. 94-142 mandates instructional programs for all children who qualify. Thus, a qualified teacher on the current faculty or a visiting teacher or supervisor must be provided or a contract with an adjacent school or school district must be made for such a special program. Some school districts have attempted to meet the needs of handicapped children at the elementary school level by providing special centers, located strategically in the district, where the students can be taken for this important part of their educational experience. Students from a number of schools in the district are transported to the center where a specialist in adapted physical education, with a properly equipped facility, is able to offer them expert instruction with the assistance of specialists from the school district and other qualified personnel. Parents should be encouraged to attend these sessions so that the students will be able to engage in a special program of activities at home, in addition to the work done at the center. Some additional supervised work on these special exercises learned at the center may also be a part of the regular physical education program of the students' home school. The Los Angeles and Anaheim, California, schools have used visiting teachers and adapted physical education centers to meet the special needs of the children in their district. Hazleton, Pennsylvania, has provided a mobile unit especially designed for adapted physical education. It travels with two special teachers from school to school. Many rural school districts form special education cooperatives where specially trained teams, including adapted physical educators, are available for consultation. When requested, appropriate members of the team visit outlying schools to discuss specific children's problems, evaluate performance levels, and suggest appropriate intervention programs. This team then designs Individual Education Programs and serves as resource personnel to the teachers in schools throughout the area being serviced. In Kansas, several cooperatives have been formed that provide services to areas ranging in size from one to six counties.

Another possible arrangement that can be used to provide better facilities and equipment for elementary school children is to schedule children for a class at a nearby junior or senior high school where the adapted physical education room and equipment may be available. Using this arrangement, classroom teachers of several elementary schools can bring their children to the nearby secondary school for an exercise and/or activity program conducted by a district specialist. Some modifications may be necessary in providing equipment for such a program, but the room and much of the equipment can be adapted for this type of class.

The minimum equipment needed for adapted physical education in an elementary school program includes six playground balls of various sizes, hoops, one low balance beam, a large mat, one small trampoline or rebound inner tube, three scooters, climbing apparatus, one plumb line or window pole (for assessing postural alignment), and towels. A towel can be substituted for an exercise mat and can be used by a student to perform a large number of special exercises for posture, fitness, and rehabilitation. Testing materials and sports and game equipment can be the same as that used for the regular classes. Individual exercise mats would be preferred to the towels because they are more comfortable, can be kept clean, and allow the students to use the towels for exercise programs while they are in the recumbent position on the mats. However, with some ingenuity, the teacher can provide an excellent adapted physical education program for students at the elementary school with minimum equipment.

Special exercises can be performed in the classroom, if sufficient space is provided, or on a blacktop or grass area outdoors. More extensive equipment for an elementary school program is desirable and may include many of the items that are described in greater detail in later portions of this chapter in connection wth the secondary school and college level programs. Sports and game equipment for adapted physical education students at the elementary school level usually can be borrowed from the regular program and a wide variety of excellent specialized equipment for use with persons of all ages and most types of disabilities have been developed by numerous equipment manufacturers. Any adaptations to modify the activities in terms of size of the equipment, size of the court, and length of the playing time can be worked out by the classroom teacher with the help of a district specialist. For added information about the adapted sports program see Chapter 8. Information on special equipment for perceptual-motor activities is presented in a later part of this chapter.

FACILITIES FOR SECONDARY SCHOOLS AND COLLEGES

Facilities and equipment for adapted physical education in secondary schools and colleges are usually far more extensive than those found in the typical elementary school.

Special exercise room

At least one special room for adapted physical education should be provided for each school at the junior high school, senior high school, and college levels. If the school is large or if the number of students to be accommodated is greater than the number that can be handled in one room, traditionally separate facilities for girls and boys have been provided. Adapted classes should be coeducational, with boys and girls being scheduled into the most convenient class hour.

The size of the adapted physical education room and related facilities adjacent to it are dependent on the philosophy of adapted physical education in each school and in each school district. The adapted physical education room is usually designed to handle a limited number of students. Since students in this program may have individualized programs, whether they are exercise or sports activities, fewer students can be handled satisfactorily than in the regular physical education class. However, it must be remembered that this room must accommodate specialized equipment that occupies a considerable amount of floor, wall, and ceiling space. A clear area must also be provided for exercises and activities that do not involve the use of special equipment. The room therefore must be of sufficient size to meet these special needs comfortably. The minimum size of an adapted physical education room for a junior or

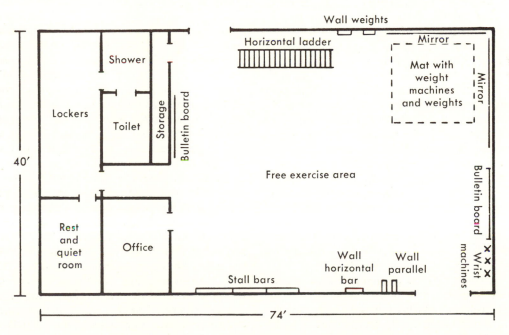

Fig. 20-1. A self-contained adapted physical education room.

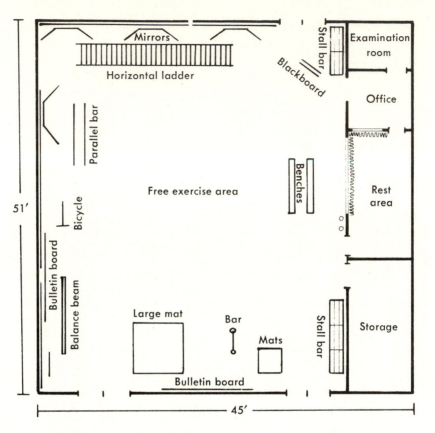

Fig. 20-2. A secondary school girls' adapted physical education room.

senior high school would be 40 feet by 60 feet if the room is limited to the use of adapted physical education classes.[23] If the room is used as a multipurpose facility accommodating regular physical education classes for such specialized kinds of activities as gymnastics or wrestling, additional space is necessary. This multipurpose arrangement has limitations, however, since much of the adapted room equipment should be permanently installed on the floor, ceiling, and walls. An often-recommended 15-foot ceiling height is not sufficient if this room is also used for gymnastics or ball games, in which case the minimum height should be 20 to 25 feet.

A regular spring construction hardwood floor is preferred for this room, although parquet flooring has been used successfully in some facilities. The walls, at least to door height, should be of material

that will withstand hard use. The material used should be resistant to scarring and marking and should provide for the mountings of specialized equipment. The ceiling may be of acoustical tile if ball games are not played in the room. High windows are suggested for two sides of the room to allow for ample light and fresh air and to provide space for equipment on all four walls. Proper lighting and ventilation are important for a special exercise room. Doorways leading to this room from the locker area, hallways, and fields should be extra wide, with ramps leading to them. This arrangement will allow for the easy movement of equipment and for the passing of students who are in wheelchairs or on crutches. Bulletin boards and blackboards should be mounted on the walls (Figs. 20-1 and 20-2).

Considerable planning is required prior to the

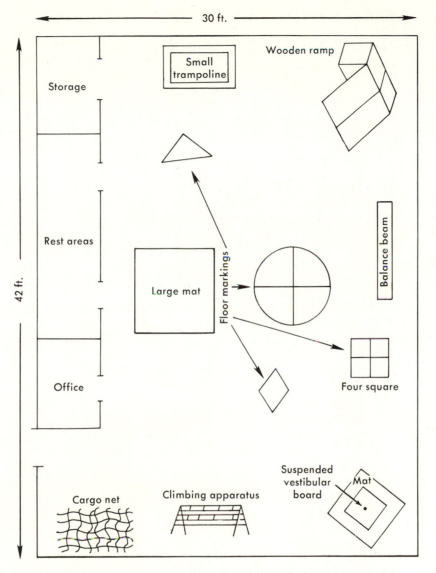

Fig. 20-3. An elementary school adapted physical education room.

time that the equipment is located in the adapted physical education room. It is important that efficient use be made of the space available so that students who are using specialized types of apparatus and equipment are able to use it effectively and so that hazards are not created while students use any special equipment such as barbells, the horizontal ladder, pulleys, and jump ropes (Figs.

20-3 and 20-4). Suitable equipment for such a facility is discussed in a later section of this chapter.

Instructor's office and student rest area

The instructor's office and a room suitable for a rest area and for quiet games should be located immediately adjacent to the adapted room. Observation windows on two sides of the office will al-

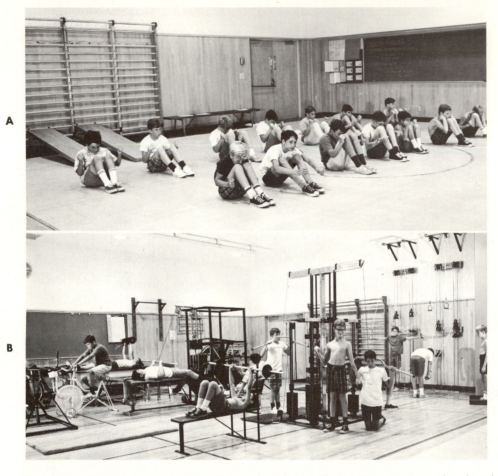

Fig. 20-4. A, Use of the open space area in an adapted physical education room to conduct formal group exercises. **B,** An elementary school class uses a college facility. Each student performs an individual exercise on a piece of equipment.

low the teacher to work at a desk and still supervise both the adapted room and the rest area. Blinds on these windows provide privacy when needed. It is desirable that lavatories be located adjacent to these facilities.

Adapted sports area

An adapted sports area may be located immediately adjacent to the adapted physical education room. A doorway connects these facilities. This area should consist of blacktop and grass for multipurpose use and space for specialized games. Activities that can be conducted on the blacktop in-

clude volleyball, paddle tennis, goal hi, badminton, and deck tennis. A smooth concrete area provides space for shuffleboard, quoits, table tennis, and other adapted activities. A grass or dirt area provides activity space for horseshoes and croquet. The horseshoe-pitching area must be carefully laid out to ensure student safety.

Other adapted sports activities can often be conducted between or adjacent to the regular physical education classes that are using a facility. They can also be conducted when an activity area such as archery, tennis, or swimming is not being scheduled by other classes. Students in the adapted pro-

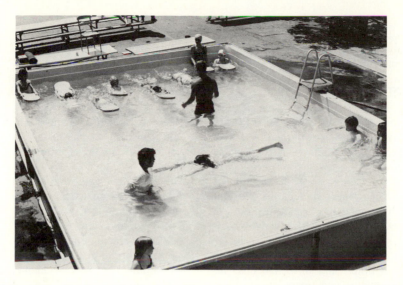

Fig. 20-5. Portable swimming pool. (Courtesy of Lyonel Avance, Los Angeles City Unified School District, Special Education Division.)

gram should have many opportunities to participate in activities that are similar to those engaged in by students in the regular physical education program so that they can be mainstreamed into regular classes at the earliest possible time. Instructors of regular physical education classes can accomplish this by making minor adaptations in the games, sports, and activities that are being conducted in the regular physical education curriculum.

There is a recent trend toward the use of community and private facilities by students in adapted physical education. Nearby recreation centers, private pools, bowling alleys, special exercise facilities, and badminton, racquetball, golf, and archery facilities are often made available and, in some instances, expert instruction is provided for handicapped persons by the personnel at the facility.

In many colleges, swimming for students in the adapted classes is conducted during times when others are not using the pool. Sometimes it is possible to conduct an adapted physical education class in swimming while a small regular class is in session. Since swimming is such an important activity for handicapped persons, every effort must be made to provide pool experiences for as many of the students as possible. A small, warm, therapeutic pool would be an ideal facility for adapted

physical education students, but in most schools both hydrotherapy activities and special swimming classes for handicapped students must be conducted in the regular pool. Some schools have successfully used portable pools (Fig. 20-5) that have been set up on a blacktop or grass area and then moved from school to school every 2 or 3 weeks so that all of the handicapped students in a district can participate in a swimming unit. This works especially well at the elementary school level, for which a swimming pool is seldom included in the physical education facilities. One new practice that can be used in either a school or therapy unit for any age level is the portable pool built on a trailer. This type of pool can be drained and easily transported to a different facility for use without the expense of building a pool or the problems of labor and time required to take down, move, and set up a portable pool at each new locality.

Chapters 5 and 8 present a more complete discussion of aquatic exercises and activities.

SPECIAL EQUIPMENT

The equipment needs of each of the special facilities just described are somewhat unique, depending on such factors as the number of students using each facility; whether the area is used for boys or girls or is coeducational; whether it is for elementary school, junior or senior high school, college, or community use; and whether minimal or ideal equipment is to be furnished.

Minimum equipment

The minimum equipment needed in an adapted room in a secondary school or college level facility includes the following: sufficient individual 1-inch thick plastic-covered body mats to accommodate the peak class load, plus five or six more; 2-inch thick mats of sufficient size to cover the floor under hazardous types of equipment such as the horizontal ladder or the horizontal bar, a platform or firm rubber mats to cover the floor where weight-training activities will take place, towels for use in the exercise program, a plumb line or posture screen for posture examinations, and miscellaneous, inexpensive pieces of testing equipment such as measuring tapes and skin pencils. Ropes for skipping and school benches can usually be obtained from the maintenance department of the school. Since resistance exercises are desired in most programs, homemade weights can be constructed by the instructor or by the students. Thus, with a minimum of expenditure, sufficient equipment can be obtained to start a good adapted program. Special equipment for perceptual-motor training can be purchased or borrowed from regular classes or it can be improvised until funds are available. Equipment for most adapted sports can be borrowed from the regular physical education program.

Standard equipment

Standard equipment for a remedial or adapted room includes the minimum equipment already described plus the following items:

1. A posture screen with a built-in conformator on its side (or a separate conformator)
2. A podiascope
3. Manufactured adjustable barbells and dumbbells and racks for their storage or resistive equipment constructed at the school
4. Stall bars
5. Pulley or chest weights (triplex preferred)
6. Iron boots or special knee exercise apparatus
7. A horizontal ladder
8. An incline board

9. A balance beam
10. Three-way mirrors
11. Special benches
12. Plinths
13. Stall bar stools
14. A wall parallel bar
15. A wall horizontal bar
16. A trampoline or rebound inner tube
17. Special, shaped mats

In addition, the following testing equipment should be included:

1. Breadth, depth, and skin fold calipers
2. A physician's scale
3. A stadiometer
4. A goniometer
5. Joint-tracing equipment
6. Sensorimotor testing equipment

Equipment for special adapted sports should include that used for the following activities:

1. Shuffleboard
2. Horseshoes
3. Table tennis
4. Paddle tennis
5. Badminton
6. Goal hi
7. Medicine ball
8. Rope skipping

Elaborate equipment

More elaborate equipment includes the following:

1. A multistation heavy resistance machine on which students can exercise a number of different areas of the body (this provides six to eight stations)
2. A rowing machine
3. A stationary bicycle
4. Special wrist and forearm exercise machines
5. Shoulder wheels
6. Sound equipment for rhythmical training
7. Dynamometers
8. Tensiometers
9. Isokinetic exercise or testing equipment

In addition, other specialized exercise and testing equipment, plus additional equipment for the adapted sports and games area, may be desired. Elaborate specialized equipment can be purchased for perceptual-motor activities if this constitutes a substantial part of the program.

Equipment for the other specialized rooms described previously includes, in the instructor's office, desks and work tables, filing equipment, and sufficient space for the instructor to do small-group counseling. The rest and quiet game area should have bunks or cots to accommodate 2% of the boys and from 2% to 5% of the girls at the peak period of enrollment. Tables and chairs must be provided for quiet game activities. Mattresses, pillows, sheets, and pillowcases must be provided for this facility. A storeroom must be provided in which the quiet game equipment, adapted sports equipment, and testing equipment can be stored.

Equipment for perceptual-motor activities

Special equipment for perceptual-motor activities should enhance the offerings of the adapted physical education program. Much of the equipment can be made by the teacher, the maintenance or industrial arts department at the school, or, in some cases, by the students themselves.

Inexpensive equipment

1. Pieces of rope and string of various diameters, composition, and length can be used for many types of activities and for testing purposes, including such activities as rope skipping, making shapes and forms, identifying size and texture, jumping over or climbing under, and tying knots (Fig. 20-6, *A*).
2. Cardboard boxes of various sizes and shapes can be used as targets, to sit in, to climb through, to walk in, to catch with, and even as a place to store other pieces of equipment.
3. Masking tape has innumerable uses, including to lay out test areas on the floor or walls, to mark boundaries of courts and play areas, to make symbols to identify (numbers, letters, triangles, squares, etc.), to mark special equipment, to mark a right arm or leg (to help a person identify right from left), and to tape things together.
4. Chalk of different colors may be used to do much of the marking of items included in the previous lists to identify color, to draw on the blackboard (Fig. 20-6, *B*) or on paper (for all types of symbol and color identification), and for "draw-a-man" tests.
5. Plastic bottles or milk cartons can be filled with sand or other materials to serve as weights; different sizes, shapes, and colors can be used for identification; they can be used for games (to run around, to knock over, to catch and throw, to float or sink in the

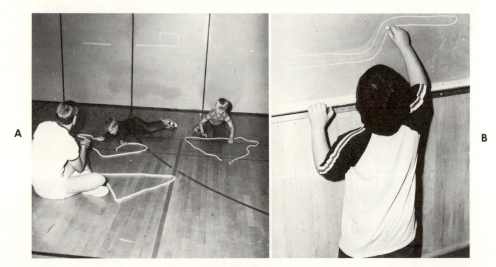

Fig. 20-6. Inexpensive equipment for perceptual-motor activities. **A,** Rope or string. **B,** Chalk. (Courtesy of California State University, Audio Visual Center, Long Beach, Calif.)

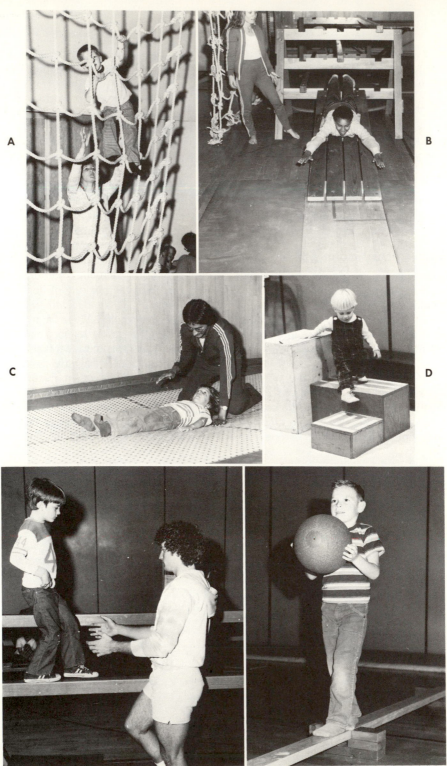

Fig. 20-7. More elaborate equipment for perceptual-motor activities. **A,** Cargo net. **B,** Scooter on incline. **C,** Trampoline. **D,** Wooden boxes. **E,** Stegel. **F,** Balance beam. (Courtesy of California State University, Audio Visual Center, Long Beach, Calif.)

swimming pool) (Fig. 5-49), to hang from strings, to be swung, to be hit, to be avoided, or to be blown.

Low-cost equipment

Since these items can be used fo activities similar to those discussed in the previous section, the low-cost equipment will merely be listed here, as follows, unless there is some special feature to be discussed:

1. Hula hoops
2. Traffic cones
3. Beads and strings
4. Blocks
5. Balance boards for skill development and testing
6. Yardsticks for testing
7. Balloons
8. Beanbags
9. Plastic and Styrofoam balls
10. Stands to hold crossbars, strings, etc.
11. Wooden boxes to stand on or jump from

More elaborate and/or expensive equipment

Equipment on which to bounce may include any of the following:

1. Trampoline (Fig. 20-7, *C*)
2. Mini-trampoline
3. Truck tires or inner tubes (or smaller sizes if desired) with canvas laced across the opening on one side to serve as a trampoline
4. Spring-O-Line bounce boards
5. Spring boards, jumping boards, and inner tubes

Protective and padded equipment may include the following:

1. Mats of various sizes, thicknesses, and consistencies for individual use and to protect under and around the equipment
2. Bolsters to sit on, jump from, or roll on
3. Bataccas to wrestle with, to hit with, and to hit
4. Large padded boxing gloves and head guards
5. Boxers' heavy bag to hit, tackle, etc.
6. King-of-the-mountain pad
7. Jousting clubs
8. Specially shaped mats (inclined, round, square, cylindrical, and cone-shaped)
9. Large rubber balls with plastic covers

Special game equipment may include almost every item of equipment used in the *regular* physical education program, as almost all can be adapted for some use with selected students in the perceptual-motor program. Included would be the following:

1. All types of balls (large, small, light, and heavy; of different textures and air pressures; and special balls like the Whiffle ball, the Fleece ball, the Nerf ball, and knitted balls)
2. Things with which to strike the balls, such as bats, rackets, paddles, and clubs
3. Nets of various sizes
4. Bases and goals
5. Standards to hold up nets, goals, and games (tetherball, basketball, volleyball, and goal hi)

Specialized types of equipment

Some more specialized types of equipment include children's games, especially those requiring manipulation and allowing for identity of color, shape, texture, number, and letter concepts. These may include the following:

1. Balance beams of various widths and heights (Figs. 20-7, *F* , and 20-8, *C* and *D*)
2. A Stegel for balancing and climbing activities (Fig. 20-7, *E*)
3. Stall bars (Fig. 20-11)
4. Incline boards (Fig. 20-7, *B*)
5. A horizontal ladder (Fig. 20-12)
6. Wall parallel and horizontal bars
7. Climbing ropes
8. Ladders
9. A cargo net (Fig. 20-7, *A*)
10. Pulley weights (Fig. 20-11)
11. Rocker boards
12. Scooter boards (Fig. 20-7, *B*)
13. Wheel toys
14. Stilts
15. Bongo boards
16. T stools
17. Wands
18. Three-way mirrors (Fig. 20-10)
19. Pitchbacks
20. Parachutes
21. Endurance equipment such as a treadmill and a bicycle ergometer

Rhythms can provide an opportunity to meet motor development needs, but their use also involves creativity linked to a better self-concept and a broadened self-image (Fig. 20-19). Rhythm equipment might include the following:

1. Lummi sticks
2. Poi-poi balls
3. A metronome
4. A recorder with tapes or records
5. Tambourines
6. Percussion instruments
7. Songbooks or song sheets

Aquatic equipment and activities are discussed in Chapters 5 and 8 (see Figs. 5-48 through 5-51 and 20-5).

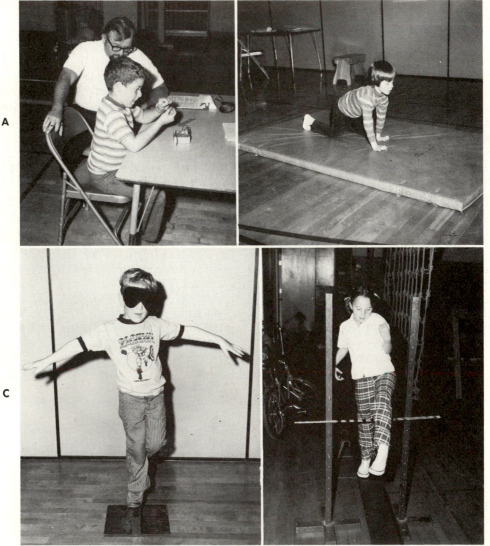

Fig. 20-8. Activities using perceptual-motor testing equipment. **A,** Bead stringing. **B,** Creeping. **C,** Static balance. **D,** Dynamic balance. (Courtesy of California State University, Audio Visual Center, Long Beach, Calif.)

Outdoor play equipment such as slides, swings, teeter-totters, rings, sandboxes, tires, and jungle gyms provides opportunity for a variety of perceptual-motor activities in the fresh air and sunshine.

Tests and testing equipment include markings on mats or the floor, stopwatches, yardsticks and metric tapes or sticks, targets, traffic cones, mats, ropes, hoops, beads, tapping board test equipment, and blocks can be used for *general testing* (Fig. 20-8, *A* to *C*). Some standard tests and test kits that might be used include the following:

1. Roach and Kephart[19]: Purdue Perceptual-Motor Survey
2. Oseretsky[18]: Lincoln Motor Development Scale
3. Stott[21]: Stott Motor Impairment Test
4. Arnheim and Sinclair[2]: Individual Motor Behavior Survey; Diagnostic Motor Ability Test
5. Orpet[17]: Frostig Movement Skills Test
6. Goodenough[12]: Draw-a-Man Test
7. Frostig[11]: Visual Perception Test
8. Fiorentino[10]: Fiorentino Reflex Tests
9. Ayres[3-6]: The Ayres Space Test; Figure-Ground Visual Perception Test; Kinesthesia and Tactual Perception Tests; Motor Accuracy Tests
10. American Association for Health, Physical Education, and Recreation[23]: Physical fitness tests
11. Bruininks[6a]: Bruininks-Oseretsky Test of Motor Proficiency

Proper use of the room and its equipment

Orientation during the first week of school should include information on the rules and regulations that relate to the use of the adapted physical education room and its equipment. These rules include the following:

1. The room should be used only under proper supervision.
2. It is necessary to be instructed in the use of any specialized equipment before using it.
3. Exercises and activities should be performed only when they have been assigned or when they have been approved for use by the instructor; careful instruction in the execution of each exercise must precede its use.
4. It is necessary to be instructed in the proper use and care of barbells, dumbells, and other resistance equipment prior to the time a progressive resistance program is begun. Students should increase the number of repetitions and the amount of resistance used only when they are capable of executing an exercise properly with the previous amount of weight and the assigned number of repetitions.
5. All equipment must be returned to its proper place immediately after use.
6. Information about any faulty equipment must be reported immediately to an instructor.
7. Hazardous types of equipment (weights, horizontal ladders, Stegel, trampoline, ropes, cargo ladder, etc.) must be tested by the instructor before student use and spotters should always be present to prevent accidents and injuries.
8. Students must stop their exercise or activity programs and report to an instructor immediately if they experience undue pain, dyspnea, or general systemic discomfort.
9. Breath holding is discouraged during lifting activities and abdominal exercises, since this may cause an increase in intra-abdominal pressure and thus possible strain. This also causes the Valsalva effect that constricts the carotid artery.

Construction of equipment

Much of the equipment used in an adapted physical education program can be constructed by the instructor or by the maintenance or industrial arts department in a school. Homemade equipment will often suffice for a number of years until an adequate budget can be obtained to buy the more expensive manufactured equipment. Some items that can be constructed are the following: a three-way mirror, which can be mounted on the wall or placed on a rack or on wheels and moved around the room, with the wings on the sides of the mirror being held in place with piano hinges; and posture screens,[9] a podiascope, heel cord stretch boards, foot supinator boards, homemade barbells and dumbbells, pulleys for specialized types of exercises, balance beams, exercise benches, calipers, stadiometers, goniometers, conformators, racks for weights, joint- and foot-tracing devices, bicycle exercisers, and many items for the adapted sports and perceptual-motor programs. *

Description of equipment and uses for it

This section includes illustrations of a number of different pieces of apparatus that can be used in the corrective room, together with a short description and hints about proper use.

Body mats

Body mats are very useful in an adapted program. They are relatively small and light (usually 3 feet wide, 6 feet long, and 1 inch thick). They are plastic covered and therefore easy to clean and some can be folded in the middle and stacked in a small space. They provide safety and comfort for the student while exercising on the floor of the room. If they are always folded or stacked with the clean sides together, a clean surface is available for each student to use. If they are kept off the floor when not in actual use so that they are not walked on and are not used as crash pads underneath weight lifting and similar types of equipment, they will prove quite durable.

Towels

A good, sturdy towel has many uses in the adapted program. Where equipment is limited the towel can be used instead of the exercise mat or if mats are old and soiled, it can be used as a cover for the mat while the student exercises on it. Many exercises can be performed using a towel. Almost every part of the body can be stretched or resistance can be applied by employing the towel in various ways (Figs. 5-16, 5-17, 5-36, and 10-2). The towel can be folded three times lengthwise, then rolled into a tight cylinder and placed directly between the shoulder blades while the individual is resting on the back and can be used thus to stretch the anterior muscles of the chest and shoulder girdle. A folded towel can also be used instead of a headboard and rolled or folded towels can be used for support in certain relaxation exercises (Fig. 20-9 and Chapter 6).

Three-way mirror

Some type of mirror is useful for adapted classes at all grade levels. A mirror with two side wings is

*See references 3, 9, 14 to 17, and 23.

preferable, since it allows the student to see three views of the body and thus to understand posture deviation problems better and to see when the body is in proper alignment (Fig. 20-10). It also allows the student to watch movements during exercise and therefore to be more accurate in the execution of the exercise program. The instructor can use the mirror to point out to students the kinds of deviations in body mechanics observed while using the plumb line, the posture screen, and various other types of measuring devices. Students can check their body positions in relation to a gravity line if a plumb line is hung so that it drops straight in front of a section of the mirror. Mirrors can be mounted permanently on the wall in one section of the room or a three-way or one-way mirror can be mounted on wheels or on slides so that it can be moved to various areas of the adapted physical education room, thus increasing the flexibility of its use. Besides the upright mirror, overhead mirrors have been found beneficial to students performing in the reclined position.

Resistance equipment

Each year, there are many new types of resistance equipment developed for use in adapted physical education and allied fields. Many of these devices are useful for equipping an adapted physi-

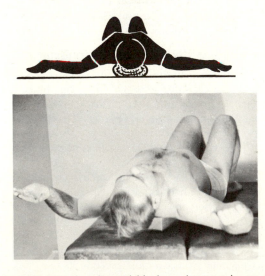

Fig. 20-9. Towel and wood block used to stretch anterior shoulder muscles.

cal education room. In addition to the barbells, dumbbells, iron boots, and pulley weights that have been standard equipment for many years, there are a number of other kinds of special resistance equipment that have been developed, consisting of springs, rubber tubing, and many other types of tension-producing or resistance-producing materials. Special exercise equipment has been designed for specific body parts. Recently, a number of very large and complex exercise machines have been developed for class use. These exercise machines provide 4 to 10 different exercise stations, each of which allow students to exercise a certain part of the body and all of which allow them to apply the principle of progressive resistance in the exercise program. The Universal Gym, the Nautilus, and several new types of isokinetic exercise equipment are examples of this type of machine. The instructor actually has a wide choice of resistance-producing devices, ranging from noncommercial equipment made of bags filled with sand and barbells and dumbbells made from tin cans, cement, and pipe to rather highly sophisticated types of manufactured resistance equipment, some of which actually creates a specific resistance related to the amount of force exerted by the subject. The types of resistance equipment selected by the instructor will depend on preference and on budget limitations.

Stall bars

At least one set (three sections) of stall bars should be included in the equipment of the adapted room. The stall bar is a rather flexible piece of apparatus that allows students to perform many types of stretching and developmental exercises. One set of stall bars provides space for three students to exercise at one time and also can be used as a ladder for incline boards where space is at a premium. When wall space is severely limited, a set of pulley

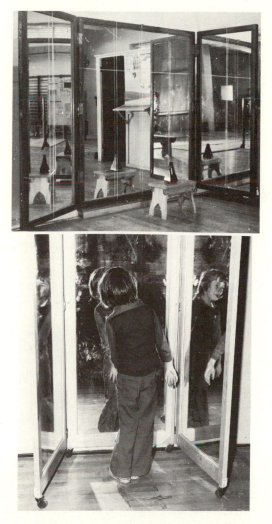

Fig. 20-10. Three-way mirror. Note use of vertical and horizontal lines to aid student with alignment problems. (Lower illustration courtesy of California State University, Audio Visual Center, Long Beach, Calif.)

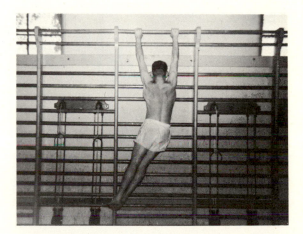

Fig. 20-11. Stall bars and wall weights. Installation of wall weights can be made behind stall bars if space is limited. Note asymmetrical scoliosis exercise.

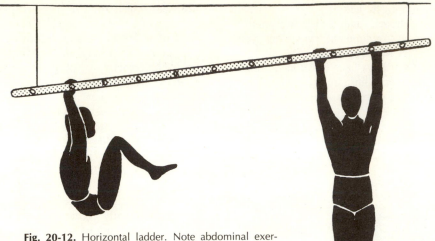

Fig. 20-12. Horizontal ladder. Note abdominal exercise and asymmetrical hanging for scoliosis or low shoulder.

weights can be placed behind one section of the stall bars by the removal of one bar and thus two pieces of apparatus can be placed in the space ordinarily occupied by one (Fig. 20-11). A set of exercises for the stall bars is included in Appendix II.

Horizontal ladder

The horizontal ladder should be placed so that one end is higher than the other. This provides more or less resistance for students as they climb from one end to the other and also allows for certain kinds of asymmetrical hanging exercises to be done by students who have deviations in shoulder height and problems with lateral curvatures of the spine. The horizontal ladder has many uses, ranging from general conditioning exercises for the arms, shoulder girdle, and trunk to very specific stretching and developmental activities for posture and rehabilitation of other disabilities (Fig. 20-12). (See also exercise No. 21, Chapter 5.)

Pulley weights

Pulley weights have been a standard piece of apparatus in the adapted room for many years. There are several types, ranging from those with handles that are placed at the foot level, the chest level, or overhead to various combinations of these positions. The triplex pulley weight, which is a combination of the three just mentioned, provides for a good deal of flexibility in the assignment of exercises and takes a relatively small amount of space in the adapted room. It is also possible to purchase head straps, foot straps, and hand straps so that specific exercises can be provided for special areas of the body that cannot be exercised with the standard pulley weight machine and so that students with loss or paralysis of various can be accommodated (Figs. 20-11 and 20-13). A set of exercises for the pulley weights is included in Appendix III.

Balance beam

The balance beam serves several purposes in the adapted room. It helps students improve their balance and coordination; it helps strengthen and develop the feet and legs; and, when the balance beam is constructed so that it acts as a supinator board, it can also help in the correction of certain foot, ankle, and knee deviations (Figs. 20-7, *E* and *F*, and 20-14).

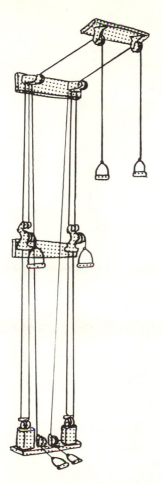

Fig. 20-13. Triplex pulley weight.

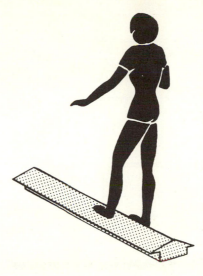

Fig. 20-14. Supinator balance beam.

Hand and wrist machines; shoulder and wrestling wheels

There are a number of wall-mounted commercial machines designed to help students develop the musculature in the hands, wrists, forearms, and upper arms. Most of these machines operate on a friction principle, with the amount of resistance adjustable. Musculature of the shoulder girdle, shoulder, elbow, wrist, and hand can be developed or stretched with properly assigned exercises on these pieces of apparatus (Fig. 20-15 and Chapter 5).

When budget limitations pose a problem, homemade equipment can often be substituted. For example, a hand, wrist, and forearm exerciser can be constructed by attaching a 2- to 4-foot length of clothesline with a weight on one end to a 10-inch long dowel. This simply constructed piece of equipment can be used to perform a whole set of progressive resistance exercises to develop the hand, forearm, and wrist.

Massage plinths

A massage plinth is a very useful piece of apparatus in the adapted room. It can be used by the students for special corrective exercises and by the instructor for taking special measurements. It is possible to adjust the length of the legs of the plinth and therefore the total slant of the top and to adjust portions of the top surface of the plinth to various angles. This affords a large number of possible exercise and test positions.

Benches

Benches similar to regular playground benches can be very useful in the adapted room. They provide sitting stations for execution of foot and ankle exercises and because of their long, narrow construction, they are particularly useful for exercises requiring the subject to assume the prone and supine positions (Fig. 20-16).

Rowing machine

The rowing machine is an excellent piece of apparatus for general conditioning exercises. Specific

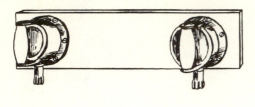

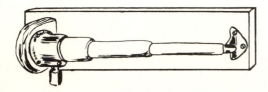

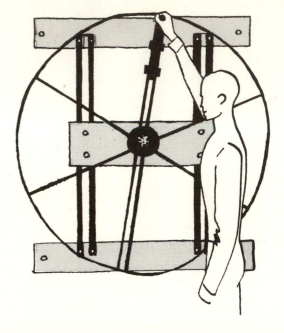

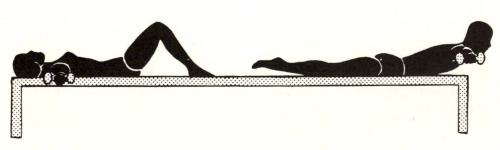

Fig. 20-15. Various types of hand, wrist, forearm, and shoulder exercise devices.

Fig. 20-16. Narrow bench.

exercises can also be designed for various posture and disability problems. Many rowing machines are adjustable so that exercise programs can be graded from easy to difficult.

Ropes

Rope skipping is an excellent activity for many students in the adapted physical education class (Chapter 8 and Fig. 5-43). Since many exercise programs involve, primarily, flexibility and strength development, an endurance activity is often needed. Ropes can be purchased that have handles made of special materials that facilitate turning the rope easily and rapidly. Jump ropes can be made by the instructor from clothesline rope purchased at a local hardware store. Rope $1/4$ inch or $3/8$ inch in diameter makes a jump rope that is quite satisfactory for the adapted class. In addition to being used for varied jumping routines, long and

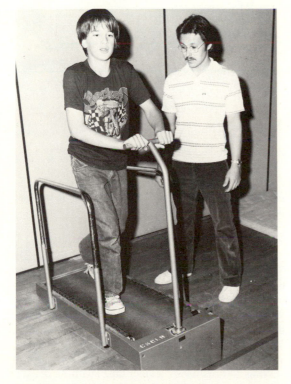

Fig. 20-17. Portable treadmill is used for development of cardiovascular fitness. (Courtesy of California State University, Audio Visual Center, Long Beach, Calif.)

short ropes can also be used for many types of perceptual-motor tests and activities including construction of geometric shapes and letters.

Heel cord stretch apparatus

A number of devices can be used to stretch the heel cord, a desirable activity for certain deviations of the foot and ankle. The heel cord can be stretched while standing on one of the lower rungs of the stall bar. It can be stretched while the student is standing with the forepart of the foot on a block $1^{1}/2$ or 2 inches thick, lowering the heel down over the edge of the block (Fig. 10-10). Various pieces of apparatus can be constructed to provide a straight stretch in dorsiflexion of the ankle or a stretch of the heel cord can be combined with a stretch of the foot everters by employing a supinator board tilted up at one end to provide for a stretch of the heel cord as well. (The supinator board can be leaned up against one of the lower rungs of the stall bar.) (Fig. 20-14.)

Bicycle ergometer and treadmill

The bicycle ergometer and the treadmill are especially useful in improving cardiovascular endurance under controlled conditions. Endurance programs can be carefully graded with these pieces of apparatus. Small portable treadmills are available if cost is a problem (Fig. 20-17). A bicycle ergometer can be modified from any bicycle by persons in the industrial arts or maintenance department.

Bulletin boards and blackboards

Ample bulletin board and blackboard space is needed in the well-planned adapted physical education room. This space can be used for posting announcements, pictures, posters, bulletins, exercise cards, instructional information, and all types of motivational material to interest students in the program. To make the best use of these areas, they should be attractive, material should be interesting and current, and students should be encouraged to contribute materials (Fig. 20-18).

Rhythmic equipment

Many handicapped persons can profit from a variety of rhythmic activities. Some of these include music from tapes or records, which can be used for exercise programs, relaxation, rhythmic training,

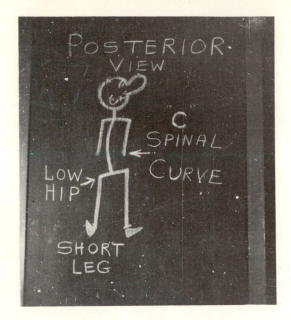

Fig. 20-18. Use of a blackboard as an instructional device.

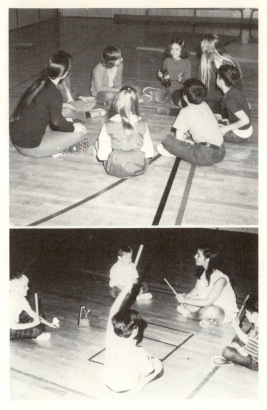

Fig. 20-19. Rhythmic activities. **A,** Using a tambourine. **B,** Using a metronome and sticks. (Courtesy of California State University, Audio Visual Center, Long Beach, Calif.)

and dance activities; percussion instruments; lummi sticks; a metronome; or various musical instruments to help establish a rhythm or beat. If special equipment is not available, rhythmic programs can be lead by a teacher or student, using such techniques as clapping, snapping fingers, marching, walking, running, and exercising to rhythmic patterns. The learners capture these beats and rhythms with the eyes and ears, through feeling the beat, or by various combinations of these senses (Fig. 20-19).

ANTHROPOMETRIC TESTS AND TESTING EQUIPMENT

Tests and measurements are important parts of adapted physical education. Consequently, there are a large number of testing devices available to show students their deviations and to compare tests made at the beginning of the semester with those made at other times during the year. They can be used to identify how much deviation is present in connection with certain kinds of disabilities and therefore to motivate the student in an activity program. A few of the devices having special value

for the adapted program are described in this section.

Stadiometer

The stadiometer is used to measure the height. Stadiometers attached to the physician's scale are not always satisfactory, since it is difficult to obtain accurate measurements with these devices. A very satisfactory stadiometer can be constructed by the instructor or by the maintenance or industrial arts department in the school, or one can be improvised on the wall or the door of the room by installing a yardstick or a steel tape (with its distance from the floor measured accurately). Then, by using either a square piece of wood or a right triangle, the student's height can be measured quickly

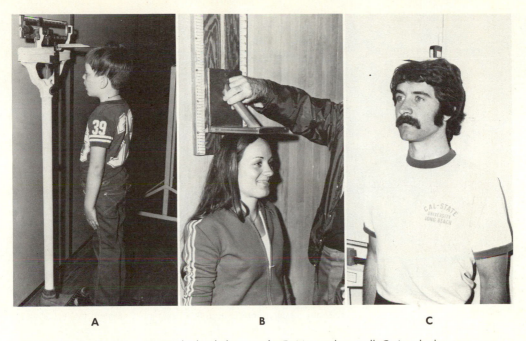

Fig. 20-20. Stadiometers. **A,** Attached to balance scale. **B,** Mounted on wall. **C,** Attached to tape measure. (Courtesy of California State University, Audio Visual Center, Long Beach, Calif.)

by sliding the angle firmly down on to the top of the student's head and reading the correct height from the measuring device mounted on the wall. This method is quick, accurate, and easy and the equipment is inexpensive to construct (Fig. 20-20).

Instructions for use

The technique for measuring height must be standardized so that successive measurements will be as meaningful as possible. The following procedures are suggested for the use of a stadiometer:

1. The student is instructed to stand tall with the heels placed against the wall and with the inner ankle bones touching, if he or she can do so without discomfort. (Shoes must be removed.)
2. The student's head should be pressed back against the wall and the chin should be tucked.
3. The examiner should then slide the right triangle firmly down onto the student's head.

The reading for the correct height of the individual is made to the nearest centimeter or $1/4$ inch.

Successive measurements should be taken at about the same time each day.

Measuring tapes

The adapted physical education teacher can use a metal or plastic measuring tape to perform a number of different tests. Girth measurements can be taken to identify a change in body proportions, particularly those of weight distribution and muscle size. The tape can also be used to measure height, as previously described, and to measure the length of various segments of the body, that is, leg length, the height of various parts of the pelvis from the floor, and the like.

Girth measurements

Description. Girth (circumference) measurements can be taken of many body parts. Tapes with a spring scale attachment at one end can be purchased so that the amount of tension applied during measurement can be standardized. Measurements can be taken of the body and the limbs.

Uses and limitations. Girth measurements,

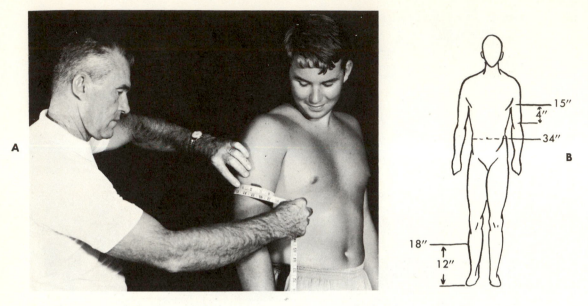

Fig. 20-21. Girth measurements. **A,** Instructor measuring arm girth of student. **B,** System for recording girth measurements by key body landmarks as reference points.

taken as a part of the adapted physical education program, are only as good as the teacher's accuracy. For this reason, it is important that all techniques be standardized and that systems of recording be developed that are simple and that can be compared with the measurements made on successive tests. The tests will be most useful if the following procedures are closely followed each time measurements are made:

1. The identical area must be measured each time.
2. Measurement is taken under the same conditions, for example, with the arm completely extended and relaxed, with the arm flexed and the muscles at work, or with the chest fully inflated or the air completely expired.
3. The tape is pulled snug, but not tight enough to indent the skin. There are no twists in the tape and it passes in a straight line around the body or body part.
4. The student is measured at the same time in relation to the workout program so that only permanent changes in the individual's girth are noted. (The student should not be measured before a vigorous workout at one time

and after a vigorous workout at another time.)
5. The distance from an exact reference point to the part measured and the exact girth measurements are carefully recorded (Fig. 20-21).

These tests are used to measure increases or decreases in body size for students engaged in programs of weight gain or loss and where the size of body parts is being increased or decreased through special exercise or activity programs.

Calipers

Various types of calipers can be used for anthropometric measurements in the adapted program. Three types are in general use: the width caliper, the skin fold caliper, and the depth caliper. The width caliper is used to measure the width of various segments of the body such as the shoulder (biacromial), chest, and the hip (bi-iliac). These widths are sometimes used in determining the breadth of the skeleton in relation to the nutritional status of the student. The depth caliper is most frequently used to measure the anteroposterior depth of the chest. The skin fold caliper is used to mea-

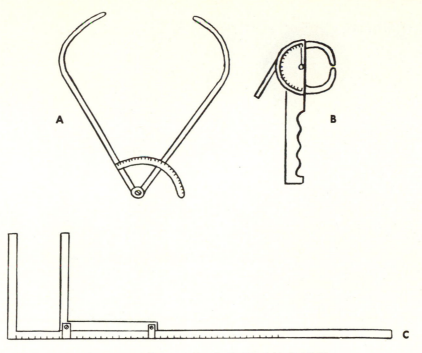

Fig. 20-22. Calipers. **A,** Depth. **B,** Skin fold. **C,** Width.

sure the amount of subcutaneous fat as part of an evaluation of the nutritional status of the student (Fig. 20-22). Techniques for the use of these calipers are discussed in Chapter 7.

Joint angle measurements

Joint angle measurements are made to determine whether the individual has a normal range of motion in the joints and to measure the amount of improvement in joint flexibility following various types of illnesses and injuries.

Three types of devices are commonly used to measure the maximum amount of movement possible in a joint. They include a goniometer, a tracer, and the Leighton flexometer.

Goniometer

Instructions for use. The goniometer most frequently used in the adapted physical education program is a 180- or 360-degree protractor with two extended arms. One of these arms is stationary and the other is movable around the center of the protractor. The measurements are made by placing one of the arms parallel to one part or limb of the

joint to be measured, the axis of the protractor directly over the center of the joint, and the other arm of the goniometer parallel to the other limb of the joint to be measured. The individual moves one body segment as far in one direction as possible and a reading is made on the goniometer. The individual then moves the body segment in the opposite direction to the full range of motion and a second reading is made. Thus, the examiner knows the number of degrees of motion in one direction (flexion) and the number of degrees of motion in the other direction (extension). The number of degrees of motion that exist between the two measurements indicates the range of motion possible for that particular joint.[9]

Uses and limitations. The goniometer is only as accurate as the examiner's skill. Techniques must be standardized so that the protractor is placed on the body parts to be measured in the same way each time. This necessitates the referencing of rather exact landmarks so that the readings obtained will be as accurate as possible. Many of the commercial goniometers have very short arms and therefore are quite difficult to use when measuring

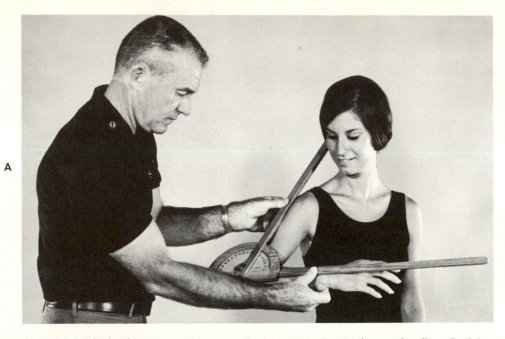

A

Fig. 20-23. Methods of joint measurement. **A,** Goniometer. **B,** Tracing the arm for elbow flexibility. **C,** Elbow tracing. **D,** Flexometer. (**B** and **C** courtesy of California State University, Audio Visual Center, Long Beach, Calif.)

body parts that are more than 12 to 15 inches in length. It is therefore preferable to use a goniometer with arms that are sufficiently long to reach the total length of the arm or leg (Fig. 20-23, *A*). It is possible to construct a goniometer similar to the manufactured types and, in this case, sufficiently long arms can be built into the device. Standardized techniques for goniometry are found in many kinesiology, physical therapy, and physical medicine textbooks.

Tracer

Instructions for use. The tracing device shown in Fig. 20-23, *B,* can be used to measure the flexibility of many of the joints of the human body. This is done by tracing the parts above and below the joint on a large piece of paper spread out on a table or the floor to accommodate the appropriate body part.

To make such a tracing for the upper extremity, the individual is placed in front of a table or a shoulder-high flat surface. A large paper is laid out on the table and the arm is rested on this paper.

The instructor then has the individual extend the elbow as far as possible and, using the device, traces both sides of the upper arm to provide a point of reference for future measurements. Then a tracing is made of either the inside or the outside surface of the lower arm. The student is instructed to flex the elbow as far as possible, keeping the upper arm in the same position. The same surface of the lower arm as was measured previously is then traced in this new position for comparison.

This test gives a reading of the flexibility of the joint in extension and in flexion; the number of degrees of difference between the two positions gives the range of motion for that joint at that particular time. The tracing should be labeled properly, indicating the method of testing, the surface traced, the student's name, and the date of the examination. By using pencils of different colors in the same tracing device, successive examinations can be made on the same paper and comparisons can be made between the amount of flexibility that the individual had on successive dates after the injury (Fig. 20-23, *B* and *C*).

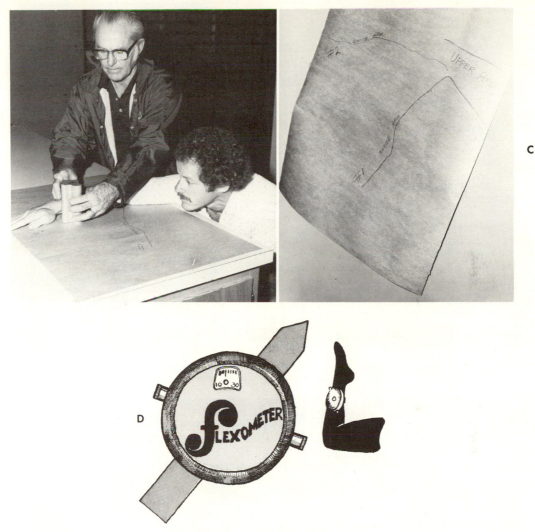

Fig. 20-23, cont'd. For legend see opposite page.

Uses and limitations. The tracer can best be used on the ankle, knee, wrist, and elbow joints, although it can be used, with certain modifications, to measure movement of the hip and shoulder, including rotation at these joints.

Leighton flexometer

Clarke[7] described another device that can be used to measure the range of motion in several joints of the body: the flexometer, developed by Leighton (Fig. 20-23, *D*).

POSTURE AND BODY MECHANICS TEST EQUIPMENT
Posture screen

The posture screen can be used by the instructor to help objectify posture examinations of students in the standing position. The screen helps the instructor make a more accurate evaluation of the degree of deviation present in a student and assists in making a more meaningful follow-up examination. More information is presented on the use of the posture screen in Chapter 9. The screen should

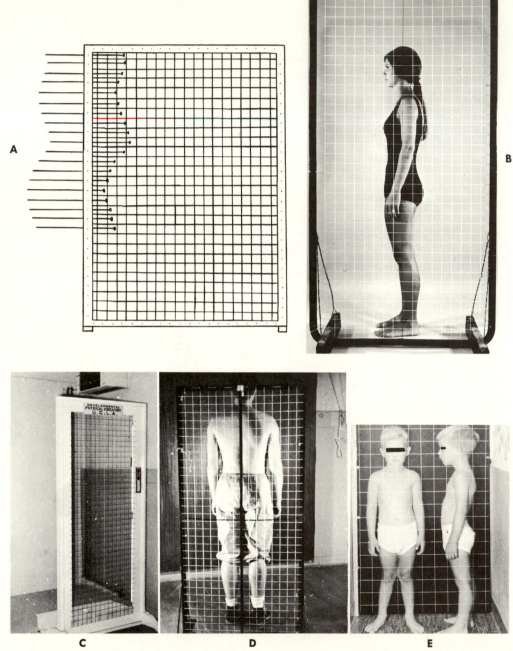

Fig. 20-24. Types of posture screens. **A,** With built-in conformator. **B,** Built from a metal bed frame. **C,** Wood frame with built-in fluorescent lights and platform. **D,** Metal frame that can be folded. **E,** Posture screening through a photographic technique used by Milo Brooks, M.D. It consists of a posture screen painted on the wall. The subject stands in the two positions indicated; a double-exposure photograph is taken, thereby superimposing the screen over the subject.

have an adjustable base so that it can be level, proper tension in the strings so that there is no sagging, and a center vertical line or gravity line of a different color so that it is easily identified. The screen should be light enough to be moved easily around the room and may even be so constructed that it can be folded and carried in a car by a visiting teacher. The posture screen may have a conformator built into one side that will permit the same apparatus to be used for measuring the anteroposterior posture deviations with some objectivity (Fig. 20-24, *A*) and will allow the instructor then to record the results of the conformator examination either on a life-size piece of paper or in graph form on the posture examination sheet. The horizontal and vertical strings form a 2-inch grid on most screens, although some instructors prefer a 4-inch or even a 6-inch grid.*

Plumb line

A plumb line can be purchased from a hardware store, or the instructor can construct one easily by tieing any weight such as a lead fishing sinker to the end of a piece of string. A plumb line is a very useful piece of equipment in the adapted program. It can be used as a gravity line against which both anteroposterior and lateral posture examinations can be taken; it can be used to check the alignment of the leg from the anterior, posterior, and lateral views; and it can be used to check the alignment of the spinal column, all in connection with various posture and body mechanics examinations. It also can be used to align such pieces of equipment as the posture screen and the conformator before they are used to examine students (Fig. 20-25). Chapter 9 describes the use of the plumb line.

Conformator

The conformator is used to identify the amount of anteroposterior curvature in the spinal column. A conformator consists of a number of freely sliding pegs placed in a perpendicular upright frame. The pegs, when placed against the spinal column, conform to the curvature of the skin covering the

---

*Exact specifications of such a posture screen are discussed in Crowe, W. C., Arnheim, D. D., and Auxter, D.: Laboratory manual in adapted physical education and recreation, St. Louis, 1977, The C. V. Mosby Co.

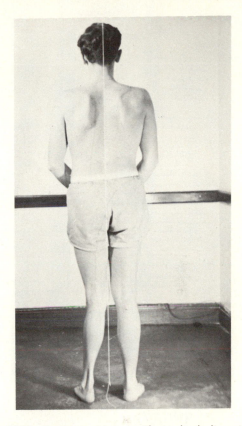

Fig. 20-25. Posture screening with a plumb line. Note knock-knee, atrophy of leg, and winged scapula.

spinal processes of the spine. If all the sliding pegs are exactly the same length and are sliding freely and if the upright is perpendicular to the floor, a fairly accurate measurement can be taken of the anteroposterior curves. Information can be recorded for future reference in several different ways. A photograph can be taken of the student with the conformator adjusted to the back. The photograph in Fig. 20-26 shows the curvatures of the spine of the student as the examiner would see them from the lateral view and also shows the *actual* curvature of the spine as identified by the conformator. (This eliminates the problem of estimating where the spinal column actually is when the ribs or protruding muscles obstruct the actual curves from the view of the examiner.) Some conformators have a piece of wood hinged to the upright so that it swings around and lies flat against the pegs of the

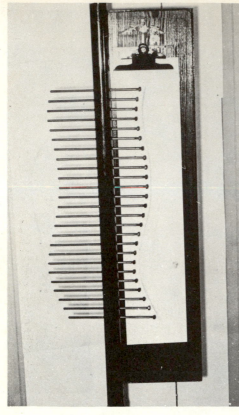

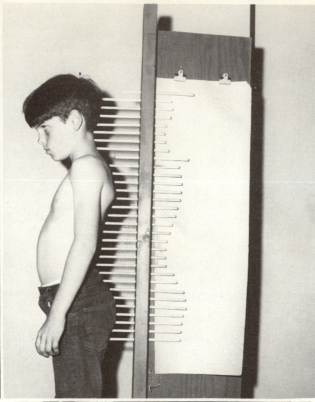

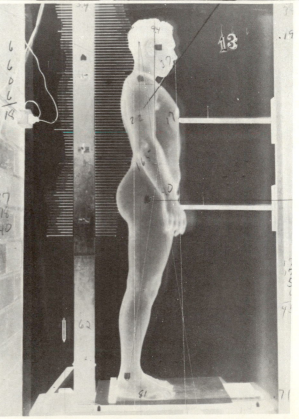

Fig. 20-26. Conformators. **A,** Conformator with attachment to record life-size spinal tracings. **B,** Photography used to record results of a conformator examination. **C,** Silhouetteograph used to record results of a conformator examination. (**B** courtesy of California State University, Audio Visual Center, Long Beach, Calif.)

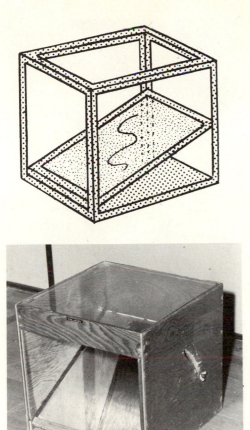

procedure allows the instructor to make successive examinations on this or a different paper and to place them side by side for comparison of the change in curves in each segment of the spine (Fig. 20-26, *A* to *C*).

Podiascope

The podiascope is used to observe the sole of the foot during weight-bearing conditions. This device allows the instructor to objectively determine the mechanics of the foot when the individual has the full weight superimposed on the glass top. To use the podiascope, the student stands on the glass top for approximately 1 minute so that the weight-bearing surfaces of the foot will become readily apparent. The instructor takes a position in front of the podiascope, looking into the slanting mirror to observe the bottom of the foot under weight-bearing conditions. The instructor looks for the areas of greatest stress on the bottom of the foot. A towel draped around the over the student's feet helps to reduce the glare and improve the view. Good lighting in necessary to use this equipment effectively. Photographs of the bottom of the foot can be take through the podiascope (Figs. 9-28 and 20-27).

Foot and ankle tracings

Lowman, Colestock, and Cooper[14] described a technique of making a tracing around the foot to identify the amount of pronation that exists in the foot and ankle. They suggested that it is necessary, in order to standardize techniques in this test, to provide some kind of device that will enable the instructor to hold the marking instument in a perpendicular position in order that lateral deviations of the foot and ankle are reflected in the tracing of the foot. This can be accomplished by fastening some type of marking instrument to an object that will hold it in a constant position or by utilizing a tracing device similar to the one shown in Fig. 20-28. Chapter 9 presents instructions on the use of the tracing device (Fig. 9-30).

Pedograph

An inked impression of the print of the sole of the foot under weight-bearing conditions is known as a pedograph print. The device used to make this print consists of a piece of rubber sheeting that is inked on the underside and is mounted on a frame

Fig. 20-27. The podiascope. (Lower illustration courtesy of California State University, Audio Visual Center, Long Beach, Calif.)

conformator. After the student's spinal curve has been measured, a long piece of paper is mounted on this piece of wood and it is swung around against the pegs to allow the instructor to record graphically the position of the pegs. Using a skin pencil or ball-point pen, a permanent life-size record of the spinal curve is then traced. So that future tests can be performed and comparisons made, at least one landmark should be identified on this record sheet. Usually, this is the seventh cervical vertebra and the nearest rod to the seventh cervical vertebra is pulled out to show this position. This

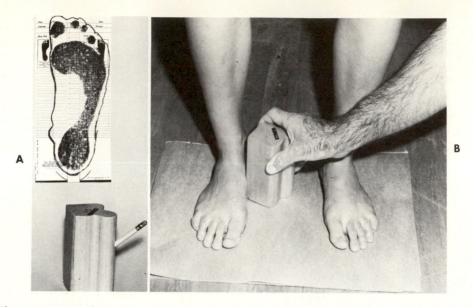

Fig. 20-28. Foot and joint tracer. **A,** Tracing made of foot and ankle and the tracer used. **B,** Making a foot and ankle tracing. (See also Fig. 9-30.) (**B** courtesy of California State University, Audio Visual Center, Long Beach, Calif.)

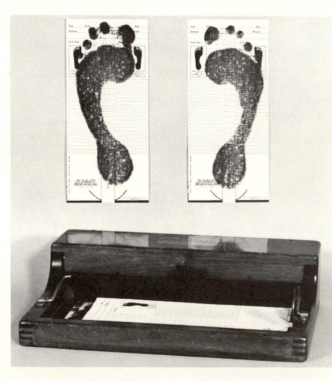

Fig. 20-29. Pedograph machine and pedograph footprints. The pedograph machine and the special paper shown are distributed by the William Scholl Co., Chicago.

so that when the student steps on it, an imprint of the foot will be transferred to a piece of paper placed beneath the sheeting. This provides a permanent print of the sole of the foot and supplies information similar to that obtained during an examination of the foot with the podiascope. Information observed during the podiascope examination can be transferred to this sheet to be used for future reference and for comparison with examinations made at a later time. After the ink has dried, the student can step on the pedograph print and a foot tracing can be made to record pronation and other malalignments of the foot and ankle. Thus, three types of information can be recorded on this print and it can be used as a permanent record for future use and comparison (Fig. 20-29).

REFERENCES

1. Apgar, V.: A proposal for a new method of evaluation of the newborn infant, Curr. Res. Anesth. **32:**260, 1953.
2. Arnheim, D. D., and Sinclair, W. A.: The clumsy child: a program of motor therapy, ed. 2, St. Louis, 1979, The C. V. Mosby Co.
3. Ayres, A. J.: Manual: Ayres Space Test, Los Angeles, 1962, Western Psychological Services.
4. Ayres, A. J.: Manual: Southern California Figure-Ground Visual Perception Test, Los Angeles, 1966, Western Psychological Services.
5. Ayres, A. J.: Manual: Southern California Kinesthesia and Tactile Perception Tests, Los Angeles, 1966, Western Psychological Services.
6. Ayres, A. J.: Manual: Southern California Motor Accuracy Test, Los Angeles, 1964, Western Psychological Services.
6a. Bruininks-Oseretsky Test of Motor Proficiency, Circle Pines, Minn., 1978, American Guidance Service.
7. Clarke, H. H.: Application of measurement to health and physical education, Englewood Cliffs, N.J., 1967, Prentice-Hall, Inc.
8. Crowe, W. C.: The use of audio-visual materials in developmental (corrective) physical education, Unpublished master's thesis, University of California at Los Angeles, Los Angeles, 1950.
9. Crowe, W. C., Arnheim, D. A., and Auxter, D.: Laboratory manual in adapted physical education and recreation, St. Louis, 1977, The C. V. Mosby Co.
10. Fiorentino, M. R.: Reflex testing methods for evaluating C.N.S. development, Springfield, Ill., 1963, Charles C Thomas, Publisher.
11. Frostig. M., et al.: Marianne Frostig Developmental Test of Visual Perception, Palo Alto, Calif., 1964, Consulting Psychologists Press.
12. Goodenough, R. L., and Harris, D. B.: Goodenough-Harris Drawing Test, New York, 1963, Harcourt Brace Jovanovich, Inc.
13. Lowman, C. L.: Technique of underwater gymnastics, Los Angeles, 1937, American Publications, Inc.
14. Lowman, C. L., Colestock, C., and Cooper, H.: Corrective physical education for groups, New York, 1928, A. S. Barnes & Co., Inc.
15. Mathews, D. K.: Measurement in physical education, Philadelphia, 1968, W. B. Saunders Co.
16. Mueller, G. W., and Christaldi, J.: A practical program of remedial physical education, Philadelphia, 1966, Lea & Febiger.
17. Orpet, R. E.: Frostig movement skills tests battery, Los Angeles, 1972, Marianne Frostig Center of Educational Therapy.
18. Oseretsky, N. A.: Metric scale for studying the motor capacity of children. In Lassner, R.: Annotated bibliography of the Oseretsky Test of Motor Proficiency, J. Consult. Clin. Psychol. **12:**37-47, 1948.
19. Roach, E. G., and Kephart, N. C.: The Purdue Perceptual-Motor Survey, Columbus, Ohio, 1966, Charles E. Merrill Publishing Co.
20. Stone, E. B., and Deyton, J. W.: Corrective therapy for the handicapped child, Englewood Cliffs, N.J., 1951, Prentice-Hall, Inc.
21. Stott, D. H.: A general test of motor impairment for children, Dev. Med. Child Neurol. **8:**523-531, 1966.
22. Swisher, I.: Facilities and equipment in adapted physical education, Unpublished data, Santa Monica, Calif., 1952.
23. Youth fitness test manual, rev., Washington, D.C., 1961, The American Association for Health, Physical Education, and Recreation.

RECOMMENDED READINGS

Adams, R. C., Daniel, A., and Rullman, L.: Games, sports and exercises for the physically handicapped, Philadelphia, 1972, Lea & Febiger.
Anderson, M. H., Elliot, M. E., and LaVerge, J.: Play with a purpose, New York, 1966, Harper & Row, Publishers.
Arnheim, D. D., and Pestolesi, R. A.: Developing motor behavior in children—a balanced approach to elementary physical education, St. Louis, 1973, The C. V. Mosby Co.
Cotler, S., and Degraff, A.: Architectural accessibility for disabled of college campuses, New York, 1976, State University of New York.
Cowart, J., and Dressel, M.: Sport adaptions for a student without fingers, J. Phys. Educ. Rec. **47:**46, 1976.
Dauer, V. P.: Dynamic physical education for elementary school children, Minneapolis, 1972, Burgess Publishing Co.
Dexter, G.: Instruction of physically handicapped pupils, remedial physical education, Sacramento, Calif., 1973, California State Department of Education.
Frederick, A. B.: 212 Ideas for making low-cost physical education equipment, Englewood Cliffs, N.J., 1963, Prentice-Hall, Inc.
Huber, J. H., and Vercollone, J.: Using aquatic mats with exceptional children, J. Phys. Educ. Rec. **47:**44, 1976.
Jorris, T. R.: The relationship between abdominal muscle shortening and anterior-posterior pelvis tilt, Unpublished doctoral dissertation, University of California at Los Angeles, Los Angeles, 1960.
Kiphard, E. J., and Leger, A.: Basic psycho-motor education, Hamm, Germany, 1975.

Leighton, J. R.: A simple objective and reliable measure of flexibility, Res. Q. **13:**205, 1942.

Lowman, C. L., and Young, C. H.: Postural fitness significance and variances, Philadelphia, 1960, Lea & Febiger.

Mathews, D. K.: Measurement in physical education, ed. 3, Philadelphia, 1968, W. B. Saunders Co.

Planning areas and facilities for health, physical education and recreation, Chicago, 1970, The Athletic Institute.

Rarick, L. G., Montoye, H. J., and Seefeldt, V.: An introduc-tion to measurement in physical education, vol. 2, Indianap-olis, 1970, Phi Epsilon Kappa Fraternity.

Sloan, W.: The Lincoln-Oseretsky motor development scale, Gen. Psychol. Monogr. **51:**183-252, 1955.

Souter, E. B.: Skinfold measurements of fat in college men, Master's thesis, California State University, Long Beach, Calif., 1968.

Werner, P., and Rini, L.: Perceptual-motor development equip-ment, New York, 1976, John Wiley & Sons, Inc.

Glossary

abduction Moving away from the midline of the body.

accountability Acquisition of short-term instructional objectives of pupils over a specified time frame.

acute Condition having a quick onset and a short duration.

Adam's position Position to determine the extent to which a scoliosis is structural. The subject bends over from the waist with arms relaxed in a hanging position.

adaptive behavior Refers to the effectiveness of adapting to the natural and social demands of one's environment.

adduction Moving toward the midline of the body.

aggression Offensive action or procedure.

agonist Muscle that is directly engaged in action.

allergy Hypersensitive reaction to certain foreign substances that are harmless in similar amounts to nonsensitive individuals.

anemia Condition of the blood in which there is a deficiency of hemoglobin.

angina pectoris Sense of suffocating contraction within the chest, usually associated with organic change in the heart.

ankle and foot pronation Abnormal turning of the ankle downward and medially (eversion and abduction).

ankle and foot supination Refers to the foot turned inward (inversion and adduction).

ankylosis Abnormal immobility of a joint (fusion).

antagonist Muscle that opposes the action of another muscle.

antigravity muscles Muscles that serve to keep the body in an upright posture.

anxiety Uneasiness that is difficult to describe.

aphasia Impairment in use of words as symbols of ideas.

arteriosclerosis Hardening, thickening, and loss of elasticity of the walls of blood vessels.

arthritis Inflammation of a joint.

arthrodesis Fixation of a joint by surgery.

asthma Labored breathing association with a sense of constriction in the chest.

astigmatism Refractive error caused by an irregularity in the curvature of the cornea of the lens; vision may become blurred.

ataxia Clinical type of cerebral palsy that is characterized by a disturbance of equilibrium.

athetoid Clinical type of cerebral palsy that is characterized by uncoordinated movements of the voluntary muscles, often accompanied by impaired muscle control of the hand and impaired speech and swallowing.

atonia Clinical type of cerebral palsy that is characterized by a lack of muscle tone.

atrophy Wasting away of muscular tissue.

aura Warning preceding a seizure.

autonomic seizure Seizure that consists of periods of flushing, sweating, fast heartbeat, gagging, and heightened blood pressure and during which unconsciousness is absent.

Babinski reflex Reflex elicited by stroking the plantar aspect of the foot, resulting in a dorsal extension of the great toe and spreading of other toes.

barrel chest Abnormally rounded chest.

behavior modification Changing of behavioral characteristics through application of learning principles.

behavior training Anxiety reduction of problem situations for particular individuals.

behavioral objectives Objectives that contain an action, conditions, and criteria and that have not been mastered by the learner.

bilateral Pertaining to two sides.

blind Lacking the sense of sight.

"blue baby" Lack of oxygen transportation to the brain, which may occur during birth.

BMR Basal metabolism rate: expenditure of energy of the body in a resting state.

body image System of ideas and feelings that a person has about his or her structure.

borderline retarded Mentally retarded persons who are usually capable of competing with most children in activities other than academic ones.

breech extraction Delivery at birth in which the infant presents himself or herself feet first.

bronchial asthma Condition that affects the respiratory system and usually results from allergic states in which there is an obstruction of the bronchial tubes or lungs or a combination of both.

Bruininks-Oseretsky Test of Motor Proficiency A battery of tests that assesses motor proficiency of children between the ages 4 and 14 years.

cardiovascular disease Inclusive term that describes all diseases of the heart and blood vessels throughout the body.

central deafness Condition in which the receiving mechanism of hearing functions properly, but an abnormality in the central nervous system prevents one from hearing.

cephalocaudal Used to describe development of the individual that proceeds from the head to the feet.

cerebral palsy Conditions in which damage is inflicted to the brain and is accompanied by motor involvement.

chondromalacia Softening of cartilage.

chronic Condition having a gradual onset and a long duration.

circumduction Moving a part in a manner that describes a cone.

competencies Predetermined standards of behavior.

component building Pairing of a positive and a neutral event, then fading the positive in such a manner that there is transfer from the positive to the neutral to make the neutral positive.

condition shifting program Program in which several conditions of behavioral objectives are altered to produce activities that are sequenced from lesser to greater difficulty.

conditions Stipulation of the precise behaviors that are to be displayed when performing an instructional objective; task specifications of the instructional objective.

conductive hearing loss Condition in which the intensity of sound is reduced before reaching the inner ear, where the auditory nerve begins.

congenital Present at birth.

congenital heart disease Condition of the heart at birth.

content referenced test Represents a point on a hierarchical continuum of behaviors.

contracture (muscle) Abnormal contraction of a muscle.

coronary heart disease Condition in which the coronary arteries become sclerotic or hardened and narrowed.

corrective therapy System of therapy utilizing physical activities for the rehabilitation of a disability.

coxa plana Also known as Legg-Calvé-Perthes disease; avascular, necrotic flattening of the head of the femur.

coxa valga Increase in the angle of the neck of the head of the femur to more than 120 degrees.

coxa vara Decrease in the angle of the neck of the head of the femur to less than 120 degrees.

criterion Standard on which judgments may be made for task mastery.

cross education Transfer of a skill from one contralateral body part to another.

cultural-familial mental retardation Mental retardation attributed to child-rearing practices in subcultures, placing children in a disadvantageous position in taking culturally biased intelligence tests.

curriculum Predetermined course of instructional events.

deaf Nonfunctional hearing for the ordinary purposes of life.

decubitus ulcer Bedsore caused by a prolonged pressure.

development To build, to proceed from lower to higher, progression; process of growing to maturity.

developmental period For practical purposes, from birth to approximately age 16 years.

diabetes Chronic metabolic disorder that involves the inability of the cells to use glucose properly.

diagnostic-prescriptive integrity Refers to a direct relationship between the assessment and the programming to remediate the assessed disabilities.

diaphysis The shaft of a long bone.

directionality Perception of direction in space.

disability Physical or mental incapacity.

dislocation Abnormal displacement of a bone in relation to its position in a joint.

displacement Disguising of a particular goal by substituting another in its place.

distal Refers to a point away from an origin, as opposed to proximal.

dorsal Refers to back, back of hand, back of thoracic region, or top of foot.

domain referenced test Represents a cluster of related behaviors.

dorsal Refers to back, back of hand, back of thoracic region, or top of foot.

dorsiflexion Refers to the act of bending the ankle upward (flexion).

dysmenorrhea Painful menstruation.

dysplasia Disharmony between different regions of the body; abnormal development.

dyspnea Difficult breathing.

ecchymosis Black and blue area caused by a hemorrhagic condition of the skin.

ECG Refers to the electrocardiograph test, a record of heart muscle action potential.

edema Extended swelling of organs or parts of organs.

educable mentally retarded Persons who are generally able to succeed in early school-related tasks (IQ 50 to 84).

electromyogram Recording of the action potential of skeletal muscles.

elevation Moving of a part upward.

encephalitis Acute and inflammatory condition of the brain, often characterized by some manifestation of cerebral dysfunction.

epilepsy Disturbance in electrochemical activity of the brain that causes seizures and convulsions.

epiphysis Ossification center at the end of each developing long bone.

equal educational opportunity Compensatory education provided to handicapped children that enables opportunity for attainment of equal benefits or educational goals as compared with the nonhandicapped.

equally effective education Education that is not identical but that provides opportunity to achieve equal benefit or goals through the Individual Education Program in the least restrictive environment.

esophoria A tendency for an eye to deviate laterally toward the nose.

esotropia Refers to a condition wherein an eye deviates laterally toward the nose.

etiology Study of the origin of disease (term often misused for "cause").

eversion Lifting the outer border of the foot upward.

exercise intensity Amount of work load in relationship to the functional capacity of the individual.

exophoria A tendency for an eye to deviate laterally away from the nose.

exotropia Refers to a condition wherein an eye deviates laterally away from the nose.

extension Movement of a part that increases a joint angle.

external evaluation Refers to a situation in which a person independent of the project evaluates the extent to which predetermined behaviors are acquired by pupils and the processes employed for achieving objectives.

extrinsic Pertaining to being outside a part.

fading Sequentially reducing the amount of prompting when a performer is attempting a task.

fibrosis Abnormal amount of fibrous tissue.

flexion Movement of a part that decreases a joint angle.

functional capacity Current level of ability to perform activity.

fundamental motor patterns Motor patterns that are generic to the movement of normal individuals.

fundamental motor skills Motor skills that are generic to several specific sport skills such as catching, striking, kicking, and throwing.

gait Walking pattern.

GAS Refers to the general adaptation syndrome.

general intellectual functioning Assessment of performance on an IQ test.

genu recurvatum Hyperextension at the knee joint.

genu valgum Knock-knee.

genu varum Bowleg.

geriatrics Study of diseases of old age.

gerontology Science of old age.

goal A measurable, observable behavior achieved through attainment of several short-term instructional objectives.

grand mal seizure Seizure that involves severe convulsions accompanied by stiffening, twisting, alternating contractions and relaxations, and unconsciousness.

growth Development of or increased size of a living organism.

hallux valgus (pl. *halluces*) Displacement of the great toe toward the other toes as occurring with a bunion.

handicap Any hindrance or difficulty imposed by a physical, mental, or emotional problem.

hard-of-hearing Conditions of hearing impairment or persons who have have hearing impairments but who can function with or without a hearing aid.

heart murmurs Sounds that can be detected by a stethoscope that are caused by blood flowing past the valves of the heart.

Helbing's sign Medial curving of the Achilles tendon occurring in a pronated foot and ankle.

hemarthrosis Blood in a joint cavity.

hemiplegia Neurological affliction of one half of the body or the limbs on one side of the body.

hernia Protrusion through an abnormal opening.

hierarchy Arrangement of activities in which one task is prerequisite to a higher, more complex task.

hyperopia Farsightedness; inability to see objects close; the light rays focus behind the retina and cause an unclear image of objects closer than 20 feet from the eye.

hyperphoria A tendency for an eye to deviate in an upward direction.

hypertropia Refers to a condition wherein an eye deviates upward.

hypertensive heart Commonly known as high blood pressure, which places a prolonged stress on the heart and major arteries.

hypophoria A tendency for an eye to deviate in a downward direction.

hypotropia Refers to a condition wherein an eye deviates downward.

idiopathic Refers to disease of unknown cause.

Individual Education Program Specially designed instruction to meet the unique needs of a person for self-sufficient living.

inflammation Reaction of the tissue to trauma, heat and cold, chemicals, electricty, or microorganisms.

instruction Organized principles with established technical procedure involving action and practice.

interference method Application of operant conditioning in an educational setting.

intrinsic Pertaining to being within a part.

inversion Turning upward of the medial border of the foot.

ischemia Local anemia caused by an obstruction of blood vessels to a part.

isometric muscle contraction Muscle contraction without any appreciable change in its length.

isotonic muscle contraction Muscle contraction whereby origin and insertion move toward one another.

Jacksonian seizure Seizure characterized by local movements of some part of the body spreading to other parts of the body.

kinesthesis Perception of body in space, including rate and extent of movement.

kypholordosis Exaggerated thoracic and lumbar spinal curves (round swayback).

kyphosis Exaggerated thoracic spinal curve (humpback).

laterality Internal awareness of right and left.

learning ability Refers to the facility with which knowledge is acquired as a function of experience.

least restrictive environment Educational environment that least restricts a person's personal liberty to freely associate with nonhandicapped individuals and enables access and utilization of generic services.

local edema Excess of tissue fluid in an area.

lordosis Exaggerated lumbar vertabral curve (swayback).

luxation Complete dislocation of articular surfaces at a joint.

mainstream placement of handicapped children in regular class with an Individual Education Program.

main task Of less difficulty than a skill and prerequisite to skills.

manualism Means by which the deaf communicate by use of hand signals (signing).

maturation Refers to the rate of sequential development of self-help skills of infancy, development of locomotor skills, and interaction with peers, which would occur irrespective of instructional intervention.

menarche Onset of menstruation.

meningitis Acute contagious disease characterized by inflammation of the meninges of the spinal cord.

menstrual cycle Complex process that involves the endocrine glands, uterus, and ovaries and is manifested by the passing of blood from the uterus on an average cycle of 28 days.

mental retardation Subaverage intellectual functioning that originates during the developmental period and is associated with impairment in adaptive behavior.

met Work metabolic rate divided by resting metabolic rate of a subject.

metaphysis Epiphyseal plate; that portion of the developing long bone that lies between the shaft and the epiphysis.

metatarsalgia Also known as Morton's toe; severe pain or cramp in metatarsus in the region of the fourth toe.

mononucleosis Disease of low virulence that affects the lymphocytes.

monoplegia Neurological affliction of one extremity of the body.

morbidity Number of disease cases in a calendar year per 100,000 population.

Moro reflex Startle reflex elicited by jarring or removing the supporting surface.

mortality Death rate.

motor fitness Characteristics of movement that are essential to the efficient coordination of the body.

motor skill Reasonably complex motor performance.

muscle setting Statically tensing a muscle without moving a part.

muscular dystrophy Chronic, progressive, degenerative, noncontagious disease of the muscular system, characterized by weakness and atrophy of muscles.

myocardial infarcts Limited function of the heart.

myopia Nearsightedness; inability to see objects far away; the rays of light focus in front of the retina when viewing objects 20 feet or more from the person.

neuromotor disorders Conditions in which damage is inflicted to the brain and is accompanied by motor involvement.

nystagmus A continuous horizontal or vertical movement of the eye.

obesity Pathological overweight in which a person is 20% or more above the normal weight (compare *overweight*).

objective Acceptance of events without distortion or prejudice; action toward which effort is directed for a purpose; to achieve goals that can be evaluated without prejudice.

ontogeny Historical development of an organism.

ophthalmologist Licensed physician who specializes in the treatment of eye disease and optical defects.

optician Technician who grinds lenses and makes up glasses.

optometrist Person who provides examination of the eye for defects and faults of refraction and the prescription of correctional lenses and exercises.

oralism Method of teaching the deaf by means of lip reading.

organic brain injury Condition in which damage to the central nervous system exists.

orientation Obtaining the response and reinforcing the response.

orthopedics Branch of surgery primarily concerned with treatment of disorders of the musculoskeletal system.

orthoptic Refers to extraocular muscles that move the eyeball.

orthoptist Person who provides eye exercises and orthoptic training as prescribed by medical personnel.

orthotics Construction of self-help devices to aid the patient in rehabilitation (braces, etc.).

Oseretsky motor development scale A battery of tests that assesses the level of motor development of a child.

Osgood-Schlatter disease Epiphysitis of the tibial tubercle.

osteoarthritis Chronic and degenerative disease of joints.

osteochondritis Inflammation of cartilage and bone.

osteoporosis Increased porosity of bone by the absorption of calcareous material.

overweight Any deviation of 10% or more above the ideal weight for a person (compare *obese*).

paralysis Permanent or temporary suspenion of a motor function because of the loss of integrity of a motor nerve.

paraplegia Neurological affliction of both legs.

paresis Local paralysis.

pathology Study of disease (term often misused for diseased or "pathological conditions").

pattern analysis Study of sequential arrangement of movement behaviors to achieve a purpose.

pelvic tilt Increase or decrease of pelvic inclination.

perceptive deafness Inability to hear caused by a defect of the inner ear or of the auditory nerve in transmitting the impulse to the brain.

pes Refers to the foot.

pes cavus Exaggerated height of the longitudinal arch of the foot (hollow arch).

pes planus Extreme flatness of the longitudinal arch of the foot.

petit mal seizure Nonconvulsive seizure in which consciousness is lost for a few seconds.

phagocytosis Process of ingestion of injurious cells or particles by a phagocyte (white blood cell).

phenylketonuria (PKU) Physiological disturbance caused by an imbalance in the amino acids and resulting in mental limitations.

phylogeny Development of a race or group of animals.

physiatrist Physician in physical medicine.

physical education Refers to development of physical and motor fitness, fundamental motor patterns and skills, and lifetime and team sports and skills.

physical fitness Refers to physical properties of muscular activity such as strength, flexibility, endurance, and cardiovascular endurance.

physical medicine Phase of medicine that utilizes the various therapies to bring about a healing response.

pigeon chest Abnormal prominence of the sternum.

plantar flexion Moving the foot toward its plantar surface at the ankle joint (extension).

pneumonia Disease affecting respiration that is caused by the infection of the air spaces of the lungs.

prescription Specification of action based on diagnosis prior to program implementation.

present level of educational performance The limits of capability in attainment of an unmet goal of the Individual Education Program; the base from which there is postulation of the short-term instructional objectives.

process Steps that lead to objectives in a particular manner; a progressive series of operations to be followed in a definite order that directs action toward achievement of objectives.

profoundly retarded Mentally retarded persons who require complete custodial care.

prognosis Prediction of the course of a disease.

program Sequential order of behavioral objectives that go from lesser to greater difficulty.

programmed instruction Prearranged behavioral objectives in which technical procedures are applied to cope with individual learning differences.

progressive muscular dystrophy Progressive wasting and atrophy of muscles.

projection Disguising a conflict by excluding one's motives; blaming someone else.

prompting Sensory or physical aid to engage the participant in successful activity.

prone position Lying in a face-down position.

prosthesis artificial limb or appliance.

protraction Forward movement of a part, for example, shoulder girdle.

proximal Refers to a point nearest to the origin of an organ or body part, as opposed to distal.

proximodistal used to describe development of the individual that proceeds from the midline of the body outward.

psychogenic deafness Condition in which receptive organs are not impaired, but for emotional reasons, the person does not respond to sound.

psychomotor seizure Seizure in which one may lose contact with reality and manifest bizarre psychogenic behavior.

ptosis Weakness and prolapse of an organ, for example prominent abdomen.

quadriplegia Neurological affliction of all four extremities.

rationalization Resolution of a conflict by hiding a real motive and substituting another reasonable one.

reaction formation Disguised feeling in which a person acts opposite to the response toward which he or she may be motivated.

recreation therapy System of therapy utilizing recreation as a means to rehabilitation.

regular class Public school class in which typical children are educated.

regurgitation Imperfect closure of valves to the heart, which permits backflow of blood.

rehabilitation Restoration of a disabled person to greater efficiency and health.

reinforcer Any consequence that follows an action and strengthens that act.

relaxation Lessening of anxiety and muscle tension.

repression Submerging distressing thoughts into the unconscious mind.

retraction Backward movement of a part, for example, shoulder girdle.

rheumatic heart disease Condition caused by rheumatic fever, which damages the heart, its valves, and blood vessels by scar tissue.

rigidity Clinical classification of cerebral palsy characterized by rigid functional uncoordination of reciprocal muscle groups.

risk Used to describe persons who have a majority of factors pointing toward the potential development of coronary heart disease.

round shoulders Postural condition whereby the scapulae are abducted and the shoulders are forward.

salicylates Salt of salicylic acid used to reduce pain and temperature.

scoliosis Lateral and rotation deviation of the vertebral column.

self-concept How persons view themselves.

self-evaluation Accurate interpretation of the consequences of instructional performance without the aid of outside information.

self-instruction To engage in procedures to achieve one's objectives without personal and direct input from the instructor.

senility A physical and mental infirmity that sometimes accompanies old age.

severely retarded Mentally retarded persons who can be trained to care for some of their bodily needs and to develop language but who have great difficulty in social and occupational areas.

shaping Phase of conditioning in which a person becomes accustomed to routine of environment and tasks required for performance.

short-term instructional objectives A specific observable, and measurable behavior that functions as an intermediate step to extend present levels of educational performance toward the goals of the Individual Education Program.

skill Utilization of abilities to perform complex tasks competently as a result of reinforced practice.

social adjustment Degree to which the individual is able to function independently in the community, achieve gainful employment, and conform to other personal and social responsibilities and standards set by the community.

somatotype Certain body type (endomorphy, mesomorphy, or ectomorphy).

spasm Involuntary muscle contraction.

spastic Clinical type of cerebral palsy characterized by muscle contractures and jerky, uncertain movements of the muscles.

special class Class designed to give special educational help to mentally retarded, emotionally disturbed, deaf, or blind students or children with other handicaps.

spina bifida Congenital separation or lack of union of the vertebral arches.

standard teaching sequence A sequence of hierarchical potential short-term instructional objectives that enable the determination of a pupil's present level of educational performance, of short term instructional objectives, and of learning gains made over a certain time period.

stenosis Incomplete opening of a valve that restricts blood from flowing.

strabismus Crossed eyes resulting from inability of the eye muscles to coordinate.

stress Condition that causes the inability of an organism to maintain its constant internal environment.

sublimation Substitution of one activity for another, more accessible activity.

subluxation Incomplete dislocation of articular surface of a joint.

submaximal intensity Below the functional level of maximum performance.

subtask Subdivision of a task; several subtasks compose the main task.

supination Rotation of the palm of the hand upward or adduction and inversion of the foot.

supine position Lying on the back and facing upward.

system Interdependent items that relate to a whole operation and function as a unit.

talipes (pl. **talipedes**) Generic term for a foot deformity.

talipes equinovalgus Combination of talipes equinus and talipes valgus; person walks on the border of the big toes (plantar flexion and pronation).

talipes equinovarus Walking on the toes and the outside and anterior sections of the foot (plantar flexion and supination)

talipes equinus Walking on the toes or the anterior portion of the foot.

talipes valgus Walking on the inside of the foot (pronated).

talipes varus Walking on the outside of the foot (supinated).

target level Desired performance level of an individual while participating in activity.

task analysis Identification of prerequisite behaviors of tasks to be targets of instruction.

tenotomy Surgical operation on the tendons.

tension State of being strained.

terminal objective Synthesis of all subobjectives that enable mastery of the main or general objective.

tetralogy of Fallot ''Blue babies''; abnormalities of the opening of the septum between ventricles or positioning of the aorta to the right in such a manner that it lies over the defect of the septum of the left ventricle.

therapeutic modality Device designed to bring about a therapeutic response, for example, heat, cold, light, electrostimulation.

therapy Treatment of a disease or disability.

tibial torsion Refers to the medial twisting of the lower leg on its long axis.

torticollis Also known as wryneck; contraction of neck muscles resulting in drawing the head to one side.

trainable mentally retarded Persons who are characterized by the general inability to succeed in problem-solving tasks and who do not have discernible, usable academic skills. They are frequently impaired in both maturation and social adjustment.

tranquilizer Drug that quiets emotionally disturbed patients.

trauma Injury or wound.

tremor Clinical type of cerebral palsy evidenced by a rhythmic movement caused by alternating contractions between flexor and extensor muscles.

Trendelenburg sign Dropping of the pelvis on the un-supported side because of weakness or paralysis of hip abductor muscles.

unique need A behavior that is a target of instruction in the form of goals of the Individual Education Program; deficiencies are determined by a comparison of behaviors required for self-sufficiency in the community and present levels of performance.

valgus (valgum) Angling of a part in the direction away from the midline of the body (bent outward).

varus (varum) Angling of a part in the direction of the midline of the body (bent inward).

vestibular sense Response for balance; located in the nonauditory section of the inner ear.

whiplash injury Deep-tissue neck injury resulting from the head being forcefully snapped forward and backward.

winged scapula Vertebral border of the scapula wings outward because of weakness of the serratus anterior or the middle and lower trapezius muscles.

Wolff's law of bone growth Bone alters its internal structure and external form according to the manner in which it is used.

A reciprocal (partner system) exercise series

A system using the principles of isotonic and isometric muscle contraction has been found to be a valuable adjunct to the adapted exercise program. The benefits are as follows: (1) no equipment is needed, (2) maximum workout takes place in minimum time, (3) all students work at their own levels, and (4) it is highly motivating for participants.

OPERATIONAL TECHNIQUES FOR RESISTANCE

Operational techniques for resistance are as follows:

1. When resistance is applied to a part, it should first be allowed to go through a full range of movement.
2. Isometric resistance should be applied to selected points along the full range of movement.
3. Isometric contractions should be held at least 6 seconds.
4. Three bouts of resistance should be given for each individual exercise.
5. Resistance should be discontinued when fatigue ensues.
6. Participants should express their straining with noise and loud verbal encouragement.

RESISTANCE EXERCISES

1. Neck extension and flexion (Fig. I-1)
    a. Purpose: To strengthen the flexors and extensors of the neck
    b. Starting position: The subject takes a four-point position. The operator stands in front of the subject, with hands placed on the back of the subject's head to resist extension and grasping chin for flexion.
    c. Movement: The subject moves up and down against the resistance of the operator. CAUTION!! Start very slowly, as the neck develops spasms easily.
2. Neck side flexion (Fig. I-2)
    a. Purpose: To strengthen lateral flexors of the neck
    b. Starting position: The subject takes a four-point position. The operator stands in front of the subject, with one leg placed against side of the subject's face.
    c. Movement: The subject pushes the face against the knee of the operator, attempting to move the side of the head toward the shoulder. As the subject applies force, the operator gives way to resistance slowly.
3. Hip extension and flexion (Fig. I-3)
    a. Purpose: To strengthen the hip flexors and extensors
    b. Starting position: The subject takes a four-point position. The operator kneels to rear of the subject, grasping one foot.
    c. Movement: As the operator resists, the subject pulls the knee to the chest and then pushes the thigh backward to full extension.

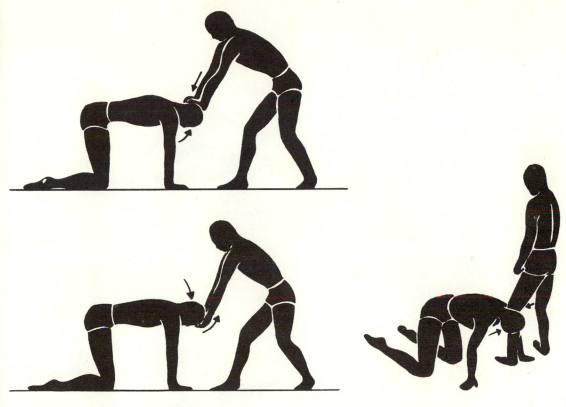

Fig. I-1

Fig. I-2

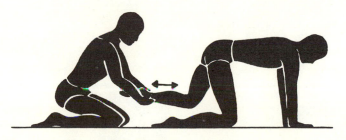

Fig. I-3

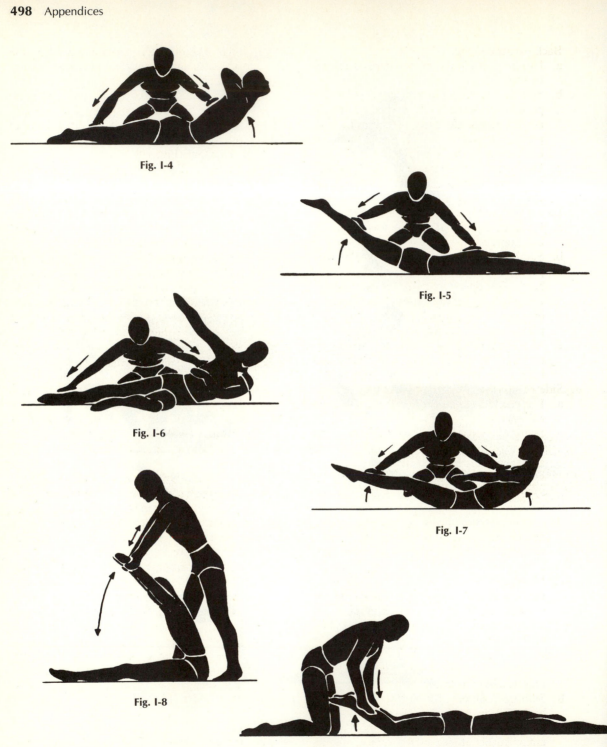

Fig. I-4

Fig. I-5

Fig. I-6

Fig. I-7

Fig. I-8

Fig. I-9

4. Back extension (Fig. I-4)
   a. Purpose: To strengthen the upper back extensors
   b. Starting position: The subject takes a prone position, with the hands clasped behind the head. The operator faces the subject's side, placing one hand on the ankles and one hand between the scapulae.
   c. Movement: The subject attempts to arch the upper back against the resitance of the operator's upper hand.

5. Low back and hip extension (Fig. I-5)
   a. Purpose: To strengthen the low back and hip extensors
   b. Starting position: The subject takes a prone position with the arms extended over the head. The operator kneels at one side of the subject, with the lower hand pressing on the subject's ankles and the upper hand placed between the scapulae.
   c. Movement: The subject holds the upper trunk against the mat and arches the lower back against the operator's resistance.

6. Side sit-up (Fig. I-6)
   a. Purpose: To strengthen the lateral abdominal muscles
   b. Starting position: The subject takes a side-lying position. The lower arm is placed across chest, whereas the upper arm is stretched outward along the body line. The lower leg is bent 90 degrees for support, whereas the upper leg is kept straight. The operator kneels facing the subject's waist and places one hand on the subject's ankle or upper leg and the other hand on the side of the trunk.
   c. Movement: While the operator stabilizes the lower body by pressing down on the subject's ankle, the subject executes a side sit-up against the resistance of the operator's upper hand.

7. Jackknife (Fig. I-7)
   a. Purpose: To strengthen the abdominal muscles and hip flexors
   b. Starting position: The subject lies on the back, lifting the legs and trunk off floor, thereby balancing on the buttocks. The operator kneels at side of the subject, facing

hips. The operator places one hand on the subject's ankles and the other on the subjects chest.
   c. Movement: The subject attempts to maintain the jackknife position. The operator forces the subject's legs and trunk back to the floor.

8. Woodchopper (Fig. I-8)
   a. Purpose: To strengthen the abdominal muscles
   b. Starting position: The subject takes a long sitting position, with the hands clasped and the arms extended over the head. The operator stands behind the subject, bracing the knees against the subject's back, and grasps the subject's clasped hands.
   c. Movement: Against the operator's resistance, the subject pulls both arms down across the body to the floor in a chopping motion. The movement alternates first to the left side and then to the right side of the subject.

9. Leg curl (Fig. I-9)
   a. Purpose: To strengthen the hamstring muscle group
   b. Starting position: The subject takes a prone position, with arms extended over the head. The operator kneels at the foot of subject.
   c. Movement: As the subject curls the leg toward the buttocks, the operator resists by holding down against the subject's ankles.

10. Knee extension (Fig. I-10)
    a. Purpose: To strengthen the quadriceps muscle group
    b. Starting position: Subject takes a prone position, with arms extended over the head. The operator sits on the subject's buttocks, facing footward. With the subject's leg in a flexed position, the operator grasps the subject's ankle.
    c. Movement: The subject extends the leg by kicking downward against the operator's resistance.

11. Front arm raise (Fig. I-11)
    a. Purpose: To strengthen the shoulder flexors
    b. Starting position: The subject stands with

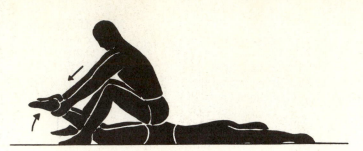

Fig. I-10

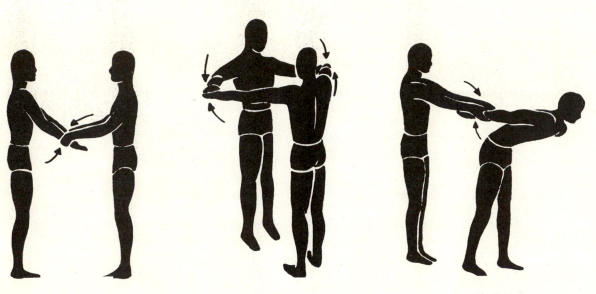

Fig. I-11   **Fig. I-12**   **Fig. I-13**

the arms at the sides. The operator stands facing the subject and grasps the subject's wrists.

c. Movement: The subject attempts to pull the arms straight down to the thighs while the operator resists the movement.

12. Side arm raise (Fig. I-12)

    a. Purpose: To strengthen the shoulder abductors

    b. Starting position: The subject stands with the arms at the sides. The operator stands facing the subject and grasps the subject's wrists.

    c. Movement: The subject abducts the arms

to 90 degrees while the operator applies resistance.

13. Back arm push (Fig. I-13)

    a. Purpose: To strengthen the shoulder extensors

    b. Starting position: The subject stands with the arms at the sides. The operator stands behind the subject and grasps the subject's wrists.

    c. Movement: The subject forces the arms backward through a 50 degree range while the operator resists the movement.

14. Front arm pull down (Fig. I-14)

    a. Purpose: To strengthen the shoulder extensors and chest

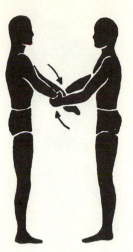

Fig. I-14

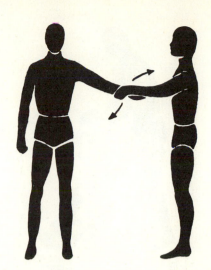

Fig. I-15

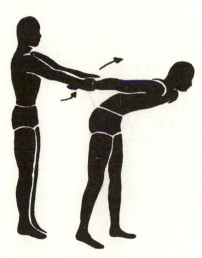

Fig. I-16

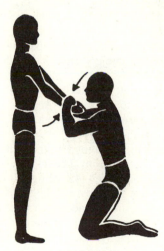

Fig. I-17

b. Starting position: The subject stands with the arms raised 90 degrees to the front. The operator stands facing the subject and grasps the subject's wrists.

c. Movement: The subject attempts to pull the arms straight down to the thighs while the operator resists the movement.

15. Side arm pull down (Fig. I-15)

a. Purpose: To strengthen the shoulder adductors

b. Starting position: The subject stands with the arms raised to 90 degrees at the sides. The operator stands facing the subject and grasps the subject's wrists. NOTE! If the subject is too strong, one arm may have to be exercised at a time as illustrated.

c. Movement: The subject pulls the arms downward to the sides while the operator resists the movement.

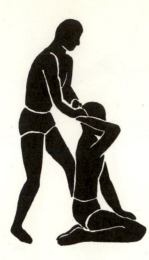

Fig. I-18

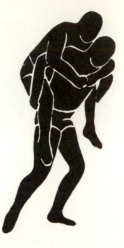

Fig. I-19

16. Arm back pull (Fig. I-16)
    a. Purpose: To strengthen the shoulder flexors and adductors
    b. Starting position: The operator stands behind the subject and grasps the subject's wrists.
    c. Movement: As the subject pulls the arms forward to the sides of the body, the operator resists the movement.
17. Arm curl (Fig. I-17)
    a. Purpose: To strengthen the arm flexors
    b. Starting position: The subject stands with the arms raised 45 degrees to the front, with one hand over the other. Kneeling in front of the subject, the operator places both forearms over the subject's hands.
    c. Movement: The subject curls both arms upward while the operator pulls downward.

18. Arm extension (Fig. I-18)
    a. Purpose: To strengthen the arm extensors
    b. Starting position: The subject kneels with the arm to be exercised raised over the head and bent backward at the elbow. The operator stands behind subject and grasps the wrist of the arm to be exercised.
    c. Movement: The subject straightens the arm over the head as the operator resists the movement.
19. Piggyback exercise for the leg (Fig. I-19)
    a. Purpose: To strengthen the calves and knee, hip, and spine extensors
    b. Starting position: The operator rides the subject in a piggyback fashion.
    c. Movement: With the resistance from the operator's added weight, the subject can do toe raises, half squats, straddle hops, or short runs.

Appendix

II

Stall bar exercises

The stall bar is a traditional piece of equipment in the adapted gymnasium. Figs. II-1 to II-10 provide the reader with a select number of stall bar

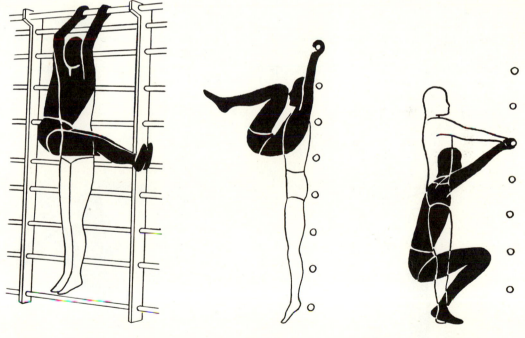

Fig. II-1

Fig. II-2

Fig. II-3

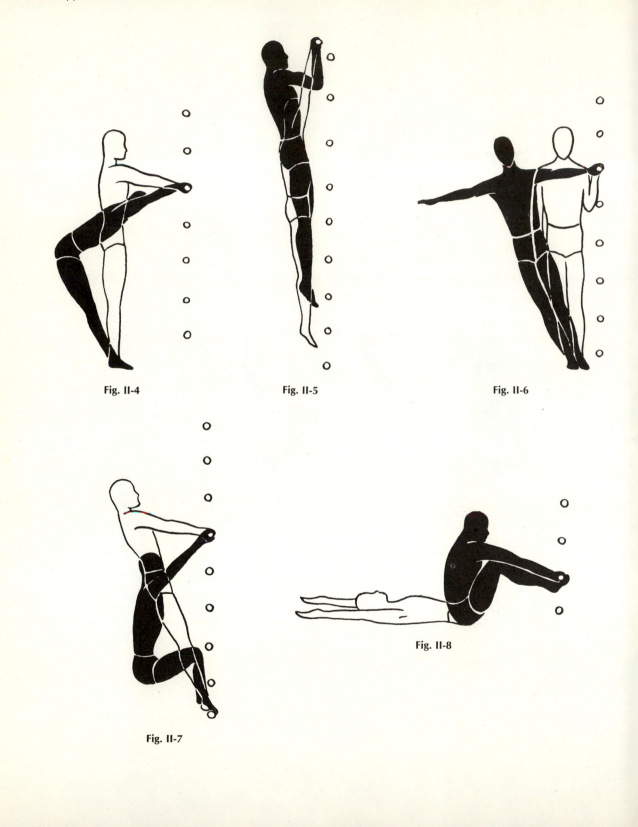

Fig. II-4

Fig. II-5

Fig. II-6

Fig. II-7

Fig. II-8

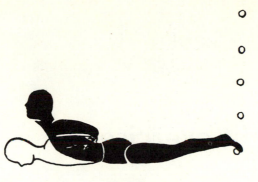

Fig. II-9

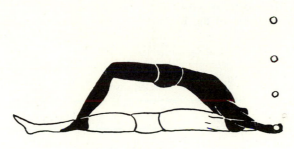

Fig. II-10

Appendix
III

Pulley weight exercises

Pulley weights allow for a variety of progressive resistance exercises. Figs. III-1 to III-10 illustrate suggested routines for various parts of the body. (See also Chapter 5.)

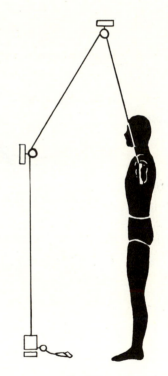

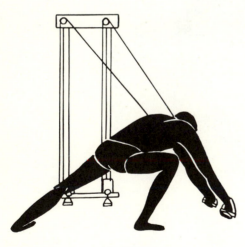

Fig. III-1

Fig. III-2

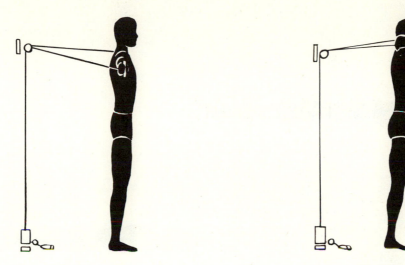

Fig. III-3

Fig. III-4

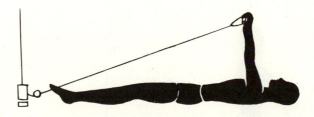

Fig. III-5

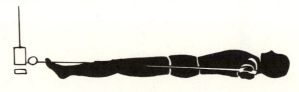

Fig. III-6

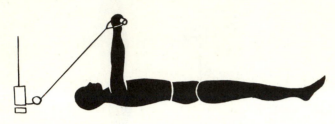

Fig. III-7

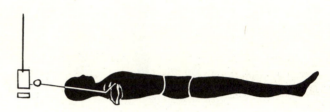

Fig. III-8

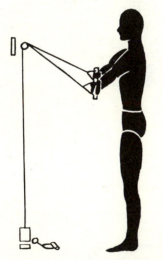

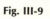

Fig. III-9

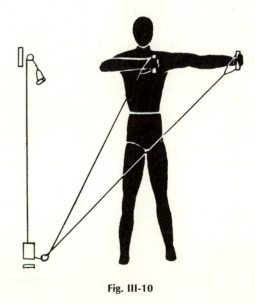

Fig. III-10

Appendix

IV

Crutch and cane walking

It is desirable that the adapted physical educator understand the intricacies of crutch and cane management. Many students, on entering the adapted program, will incorrectly use the crutch or cane. Improper use of these aids can greatly deter the balance and maneuverability of these students. Individuals who require the use of the crutch or cane are many and varied, ranging from amputees or paraplegics to persons who are temporarily incapacitated with some traumatic condition such as a sprained ankle. Whatever the reason for using the crutch or cane, it is imperative that basic principles be practiced by the users.

There are many types of crutches today. The most common, however, are made of hardwood and constructed with a top crosspiece that fits under the armpit and a handgrip that supports the weight of the body. The wood crutch can be made nonadjustable, fitted to the particular requirements of the individual, or, more commonly, as an adjustable type with an extension rod at its support tip and an adjustable handgrip. Metal or leather axillary devices can be added to any crutch in order to better stabilize the arm or wrist. A great number of modifications can be made to provide better support and greater freedom of movement. Recently, the aluminum crutch has come to the fore because of its lightness and adaptability to individual requirements. Aluminum crutches frequently include an arm piece, adjustable handgrips, and a telescopic rod tip; a variation of this type comes with a forearm cup made of spring steel rather than an axillary piece. Like the crutch, the canes used for medical purposes are often made of hardwood or aluminum.

The fitting of the crutch depends on the individual requirements. However, the most prevalent type of fitting is one in which the measurement is taken from 1 inch below the axillary fold to the bottom of the shoe heel. At all times, accessory rubber arm pieces and tips must be taken into account in the measurement. The hand grip is fixed at a point whereby the elbow is flexed in about a 30-degree angle, the wrist is dorsiflexed fully, and the hand is gripped into a fist. The cane, on the other hand, is measured from the top of the greater trochanter to the floor. In this position, the elbow is flexed about 30 to 40 degrees, according to the patient's requirements.

Crutch and cane ambulation are motor skills that require a great deal of physical fitness, along with body control and balance. As in any other motor skill, some individuals have a greater potential than others. It has been suggested that individuals using crutches or canes to any extent should learn as many different gaits as possible in order to be able to adapt to a variety of situations. In the hospital setting, the patient who needs to learn to walk on crutches will go through a progression of developmental activities, all designed to develop strength, balance, and control. Each learned skill is designed to progress to a higher level until ambulation is attained. The progression, in many instances, moves from bed exercises to mat exercises and then continues to standing exercises that provide balance and confidence.

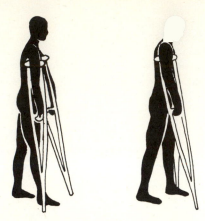

Fig. IV-1. Two-point gait.

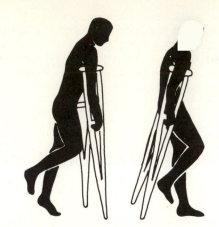

Fig. IV-2. Three-point gait.

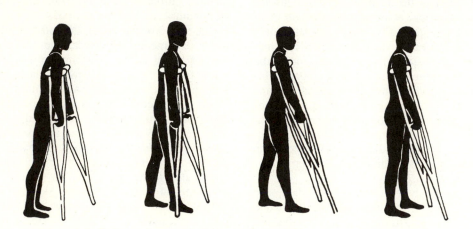

Fig. IV-3. Four-point gait.

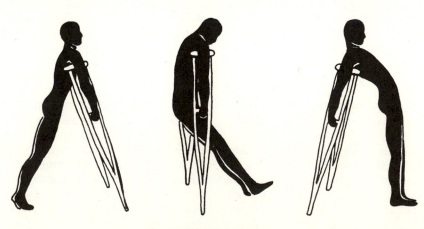

Fig. IV-4. Swing-through gait.

Crutch walking includes two basic types of gait, namely, the point gaits and the swing-through gait. The point gaits are divided into three types: the two point, the three point, and the four point. The two-point gait uses the crutch by moving either the crutch and foot on the same side together or the crutch and the foot on the opposite side (Fig. IV-1). The three-point gait is used by crutch walkers who have the use of one leg that can fully support the weight. While balancing on the nonaffected leg, the individual moves the crutches forward together. The nonaffected leg then is brought through ahead of the planted crutches (Fig. IV-2). In the four-point gait, the right crutch is moved forward, then the left foot; then the left crutch is advanced, followed by the right foot (Fig. IV-3). The swing-through gait, on the other hand, requires greater strength and balance. In the swing-through gait, both crutches are placed ahead of the patient's feet and then the body is swung through to a point ahead of the crutches (Fig. IV-4). The crutches are then recovered and returned to a position ahead of the patient's feet.

In temporary disabilities of the lower limbs, the three-point gait is often used. The patient can either swing to the crutches or swing through, depending on the nature of the disability. From crutch ambulation, patients may progress to two canes and then to single-cane walking when they are able to engage in limited weight bearing. The most stable technique for the single cane is when it is held in the hand opposite the affected side. However, this rule can be varied according to the nature of the patient's disability.

Once the basis of a gait has been learned, the patient may strive to overcome a variety of obstacles such as hill or ramp walking and ascending or descending curbs and stairs. The principles and methods of these skills can be found in a number of articles and books on the subject.

Index

A

Abdominal pumping exercise, 409
Abdominal strengthening, 282, 283
Accountability, 384
Achilles tendon test, 247
Action concept, 89-90
Active games, 202-203
Activities
  for daily living and instructional aides, 446
  identification through, 438
  selected, for speech development, 367
Adam's test, 260
Adaptations
  of program in regular physical education, 437-438
  types of, for learner, 195-196
Adapted games, 200-208
Adapted physical education; *see* Physical education, adapted
Adapted physical education appraisal, 254-255
Adapted physical education records, 443
Adapted physical education rooms, 459, 460, 461
Adapted physical educator as counselor, 441-443
Adapted rooms, games for, 204-205
Adapted sports, selected, 210-215
Adapted sports and games for use in pool, 211-213
Adapted sports area, 462-463
Adapted sports phase of program, 447-448
Adapting activities for blind children, 355-358
Adaptive behavior, deficits in, 371
Administration, 421-488
Administrator's relationship with teacher and student, 430-431
Advisory committee of program, 427-428
Aids, 198, 199
Alignment
  body, tests and measurements for, 242-262
  foot and leg, 230
  leg, 237
    tests for, 248-249
Allergies, 321-324
Alternative programs for disruptive children, 404
Amputations, 291-294
  of lower extremities, 292
  of upper extremities, 292-293
Analysis of task; *see* Task analysis
Anatomy
  of elbow, 288
  of forearm and wrist, 289
  of knee, 272
  of shoulder, 284
Ankle
  bones and ligaments of, 267
  postural deviations of, 225-231
  tests for, 246-247
  tracings of, 246-247, 485, 486

Ankle—cont'd
  trauma to, 266-271
Anterior posture examinations, 237-242
Anterior view with posture screen, 253, 256-257
Anteroposterior deviations of pelvic girdle, 249
Anthropometric tests and testing equipment, 476-481
Antigravity muscles for erect posture, 251
Aphasia, 364-368
Applied behavioral technology in education of emotionally disturbed children, 400-403
Appraisal, adapted physical education 254-255
Aquatic games and activities, 206-207, 208
Arch(es) of foot, 226-227
  longitudinal, test of height of, 246
Archery, 210
Arousal, problems in, in minimal neuromotor disorders, 339
Arthritis, 294-296
Arthropod-borne encephalitis, 415-416
Articulations of shoulder, 285
Assessment, cardiovascular, 318
Assignment of students, 434-437
Asthma, 321-324
Ataxia, 332-333
Athetosis, 332
Atonia, 333
Audiometer, electric, 361
Auditory perception and memory training, 368
Auditory training, 363
Auditory-perceptual disturbance, 338
Aura, 341
Autism, 416-418
Autistic children
  gross motor ability of, 417
  limitations of, 417
  play of, 417-418
Autonomic seizures, 341

B

Back
  flat lower, 233
  flat upper, 234
  lower, stretching, 282-283
Badminton, 208
Balance beam, 472
Balance disturbances, 338
Baseball for blind, 356
Basic skills, development of, by mentally retarded persons, 379-380
Basketball
  for blind, 356
  deep-water, 212
  shallow-water, 211